Stell and Maran's
Head and Neck Surgery

Fourth Edition

John C. Watkinson MSc, MS, FRCS(Ed), FRCS(Glas), FRCS(Otol), DLO
*Honorary Senior Lecturer and Consultant Otolaryngologist/Head and Neck and
Thyroid Surgeon, University Hospital Birmingham NHS Trust, UK*

Mark N. Gaze MD, FRCP, FRCR(Ed), FRCR
*Consultant Oncologist, University College London Hospitals,
Great Ormond Street Hospital for Children and
the Royal National Throat, Nose and Ear Hospital, London, UK*

Janet A. Wilson MD, FRCS(Ed), FRCS
Professor in Otolaryngology/Head and Neck Surgery, University of Newcastle, UK

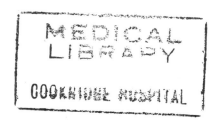
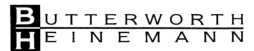
BUTTERWORTH
HEINEMANN

OXFORD · AUCKLAND · BOSTON · JOHANNESBURG · MELBOURNE · NEW DELHI

Butterworth-Heinemann
Linacre House, Jordan Hill, Oxford OX2 8DP
225 Wildwood Avenue, Woburn, MA 01801-2041
A division of Reed Educational and Professional Publishing Ltd

℞ A member of the Reed Elsevier plc group

First published 1972
Second edition 1978
Third edition 1993
Reprinted 1994
Fourth edition 2000

British Library Cataloguing in Publication Data
A catalogue record for this book is available from the British Library

Library of Congress Cataloguing in Publication Data
A catalogue record for this book is available from the Library of Congress

ISBN 0 7506 3366 2

Produced and typeset by Gray Publishing, Tunbridge Wells, Kent
Printed and bound in India

Contents

Dedications

JCW: I wish to thank Sarah Harrison (Research Nurse) and
Sue Boardman (ENT Secretary) for all their help and patience.
To my parents and grandparents for their wisdom and understanding,
and lastly to Esmé, Helen and William as without their love and support none
of this would have been worthwhile

JAW: For my mother, Margaret Penuel MacGregor Robertson,
with love and enduring gratitude, for the brilliance of her academic
example and for her selfless encouragement to all her family

MNG: In loving memory of my mother and father and to Janet and Donald

---

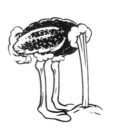

The
'Get A-Head'
Charity Appeal
for Head & Neck Diseases
Including Cancer

A proportion of the royalties from the sales of this book will be donated to the 'Get A-Head' charity
which is for patients who have head and neck diseases, but especially those with cancer.

Foreword to the fourth edition

We became interested in head and neck surgery almost 40 years ago; it was then a fairly new discipline and at that time as many patients were harmed by the treatment of these dreadful cancers as were helped. Not only was this the situation in the UK but also in the developing world, where surgeons still have to practise the generality of surgery, rather than indulge in the comforts of subspecialization. We felt that a one-volume book addressing the entire field would be useful and so it has proved.

One of the attractions of this book was its simple, straightforward approach from first principles, which was a particular help then because of the haphazard state of training in the UK. The approach proved successful as head and neck surgery also became part of the syllabus of training of three surgical specialties.

But by the 1980s a lot of people had been trained to treat a cancer that had the prevalence of cancer of the pancreas. The concept of 'dabbling' thus emerged and it was for this reason that we did not feel it appropriate to continue with the concept. By the 1990s this fault line was being recognized and discussions concerning subspecialization were underway. The third edition was welcomed and was successful.

The discussions between the specialties have now been concluded and the problems of training, recruitment and standards have now been agreed. While all trainees in the three specialties will be exposed to head and neck surgery, only a few will go on to full subspecialty training. This book is thus for the former group since the future specialists will move on to specialist texts in different areas.

Since cancer training centres will be based around radiotherapy institutes, it is appropriate that one of the main authors and editors is now a radiotherapist. We are most grateful for the thought and work that Mark Gaze has put into the project and it is now a much more balanced and helpful book as a result.

John Watkinson and Janet Wilson are two of the new generation of otolaryngologist/head and neck surgeons whose surgical and diplomatic skills cross specialty boundaries.

The most important people in all of these equations are the patients. There are few cancers that cause such a distressing and unfortunate interruption to life than those that arise in the head and neck, and so everything that can be done to improve their care must be welcomed. This book contributes greatly to that, and we are privileged that our names continue to be associated with what we started a very long time ago.

A.G.D. Maran
P.M. Stell

Preface

We are proud to have been responsible for the fourth edition of *Stell and Maran's Head and Neck Surgery*. Between the second and third editions there was a 15-year gap. The present edition appears, however, only 7 years after the third edition. We were keen to reissue this valuable core volume at an earlier date because of a number of key aims:

- to incorporate a flavour of the developments in molecular biology
- to improve and consolidate the quality of the illustrations
- to update the reconstructive chapter in keeping with recent developments
- to augment the endocrinological surgery sections, in which John Watkinson has a particular interest
- to enhance the focus on functional assessments and rehabilitation.

The present edition therefore represents a considerable departure from the last in its chapter structure and content.

The scope of head and neck cancer management now ranges from laboratory science to palliative medicine expertise via major reconstructive surgery, clinical oncology and rehabilitation. Some might therefore question the wisdom of continuing to produce a concise volume attempting to address this range of skills. While the hyperspecialist will graduate inevitably to larger texts, we believe that the pioneering concept of a 'key issues' single volume text for those engaged in the practice of head and neck cancer is as valid today as when it was first conceived a quarter of a century ago by Professors Philip Stell and Arnold Maran.

The book aims to be a key resource for trainees and professions allied to medicine as well as a handy refresher source for established practitioners in otolaryngology, maxillofacial surgery, plastic surgery or clinical oncology whose work includes head and neck practice. Decision-making in head and neck cancer continues to evolve. The UK Effective Head and Neck Cancer Management Guidelines may be found on the website of the British Association of Otolaryngologists (www.orl-baohns.org).

The key principles of assessment and the specifics of tumour resection and irradiation are all covered in an up to date way in this volume. The latest edition maintains the standards of a learning resource that was for all of us our first introduction to the principles underlying the successful approach to the patient with benign and malignant disease of the head and neck.

We gratefully acknowledge the following colleagues for their important contributions:

- Chapter 1 – The nature of head and neck cancer: Mr Michael Kuo PhD, FRCS, SpR, specialist registrar in otolaryngology, University Hospital Birmingham NHS Trust.
- Chapter 3 – Radiology: Dr Julie Olliff MRCP, FRCR, Consultant Radiologist, University Hospital Birmingham NHS Trust.
- Chapter 24 – Conservation surgery: Mr Ian Sheppard FRCS, Consultant ENT Surgeon, Bury Royal Infirmary.

John C. Watkinson
Mark N. Gaze
Janet A. Wilson

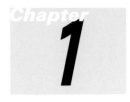

1

The nature of head and neck cancer

'There is a tremendous literature on cancer, but what we know for sure about it can be printed on a calling card'
August Bier 1861–1949

Introduction

Cancers of the head and neck are the sixth most common cancers world-wide, with an increasing incidence in developing countries. Although there are a variety of histological types, squamous cell carcinomas predominate among cancers of the upper aerodigestive tract and, unless otherwise stated, the comments in this chapter refer to squamous cell carcinomas of the head and neck (HNSCC). Rapid developments in molecular biology have made it increasingly clear that the understanding of both the molecular and cellular biological events underlying tumour evolution is central to the work of a clinical and surgical oncologist. This chapter addresses these developments and specifically their clinical relevance.

Aetiology

The larynx and hypopharynx are by far the most common sites of HNSCC in the Western world. There is wide geographical variation in incidence, with the highest in France, Spain and Italy. World-wide, areas of high incidence include Poland, Thailand and Ohio in the USA. The usual sex ratio of laryngeal carcinoma is around 10:1 male:female but there is an abnormally high incidence in Scottish women. Laryngeal tumours are twice as common in heavily industrialized areas and their incidence has shown a slow but steady increase over the last few decades.

Aetiological factors in HNSCC

- Carcinogens
- Viruses
- Iron deficiency
- Familial risks
- Molecular epidemiology

Cigarette smoking and alcohol consumption are the two strongest aetiological factors for the development of HNSCC both independently and synergistically. Smoking filtered cigarettes seems to be associated with a slightly lower risk than smoking unfiltered ones. The dose-dependent relationship between smoking and incidence of HNSCC has been demonstrated in large autopsy and epidemiological studies, with the relative risk over non-smokers ranging from 2.4 for smokers of ≤7 cigarettes a day to 16.4 for smokers of ≥25 per day. Cessation of smoking leads to a gradual reduction in risk by 70% after 10 years. The burning of tar gives off a variety of substances, including methylcholanthrine and benzanthracene which are broken down by aryl-hydrocarbon hydroxylase into carcinogenic epoxides which bind to DNA.

Two studies of *p53* tumour suppressor gene mutations in head and neck cancers have elegantly demonstrated the molecular genetic consequences of cigarette smoking. *p53* mutations were detected in 42% (54/129) of consecutive HNSCC in one study. However, when the analysis accounted for social habits, *p53* mutations were detected in the tumours of 58% of patients who smoked and consumed alcohol, 33% of those who smoked but did not drink alcohol and only 17% of those who neither smoked cigarettes nor drank alcohol ($p = 0.001$). Furthermore, mutation analysis showed that *p53* mutations in the non-smoking teetotal patients occurred exclusively at CpG-rich sites (short stretches of DNA containing a high frequency of cytosine–guanine dinucleotides), which are common sites for endogenous mutations. Conversely, another study examining head and neck cancer cell lines showed that the *p53* mutations detected were principally guanine to thymine transversions, a point mutation which can be effected by the interaction of DNA with benzopyrene. Further molecular evidence of the aetiological role of cigarette smoking is demonstrated by markedly raised blood levels in smokers of interleukin-4 (IL-4) receptor, which is frequently overexpressed in HNSCC cells.

The role of alcohol in the development of cancers of the upper aerodigestive tract appears to be a little more complex. Until the discovery of resveratrol in grapes and wine and the subsequent demonstration of its cancer chemopreventive activity, the many epidemiological studies examining the role of alcohol in carcinogenesis failed to address the association between the type of alcoholic drink and upper aerodigestive tract cancers. The most recently published study which analysed the association between different alcoholic drinks and cancer of the upper aerodigestive tract was a Danish population based study of 28 180. Over a follow-up period of 13.5 years, compared with non-drinkers, subjects who drank 7–21 units of beer or spirits but no wine had a relative risk of 3.0 of developing oropharyngeal or oesophageal cancer. However, subjects who drank a similar amount but who also drank wine as >30% of their total alcohol intake had a relative risk of 0.5. The relative risks for subjects who consumed >21 units of alcohol excluding and including wine were 5.2 and 1.7, respectively. It would seem, therefore, that while there remains a strong association between beer and spirit consumption and upper aerodigestive tract cancer, wine drinkers may be at a lower risk of developing these cancers than drinkers who have a similar intake of beer and spirits.

Clearly central to the differences in susceptibility to xenobiotics between individuals is the ability of an individual to detoxify such agents. The glutathione S-transferases ($GstP$) are a superfamily of enzymes responsible for the detoxification of a wide range of xenobiotics, thereby mitigating against their cellular toxic effects. Given the strength of the causal relationship between chemical carcinogens and the development of HNSCC, it is perhaps not surprising that the glutathione S-transferases may play a pivotal role in HNSCC tumorigenesis. It has recently been shown that mice with a 'knockout' deletion of the pi-class glutathione S-transferases have a four-fold increase in the development of skin papillomas after exposure to the polycyclic aromatic hydrocarbon 7,12-dimethylbenzanthracene and the tumour-promoting agent 12-O-tetradecanoylphorbol-13-acetate. In humans, increased expression of $GstP$ has been reported in many tumours including oral cancers. An important member of this family of enzymes, $GstP1$, is polymorphic in humans with allelic variants showing differences in their catalytic activities towards a range of carcinogens. It has been suggested that carriage of one of the less active allelic variants might result in an increased cancer susceptibility in an individual. Indeed, it has been shown that individuals with oropharyngeal and laryngeal cancers were associated with a significantly lower frequency of the $GstP1 AA$ polymorphism than controls, suggesting that polymorphism at $GstP1$ may mediate susceptibility to these cancers.

Apart from the glutathione S-transferases, other genes mediate individual relative resistance to mutagens, including cytochrome p450. Therefore, an *in vitro* assay of mutagen sensitivity may be more informative and

recently, it has been shown in a case–control study by measuring chromatid breaks in lymphocytes induced by benzo[*a*]pyrene diol epoxide (BPDE) and bleomycin that subjects with sensitivity to both agents were at a 19.2-fold increased risk of upper aerodigestive tract cancer compared with those who were not sensitive to either agent. Furthermore, it was shown that patients with lung cancer sensitive to BPDE exhibited a significantly higher rate of allelic loss at the putative tumour suppressor region 3p21.3, suggesting that as a specific molecular target for BPDE damage.

The observation of synchronous and metachronous tumours in the upper aerodigestive tract has given rise to the concept of 'field cancerization', a term coined originally to account for the presence of multicentric oral cancers. Various molecular studies have addressed the issue of field cancerization to establish whether that is the mechanism underlying the development of multiple primary tumours, or whether multiple tumours share a clonal origin, but which has subsequently migrated within the mucosa and developed distinct later genetic alterations such as is the case in multiple bladder cancers. The detection of $p53$ mutations and the overexpression of growth factors in histologically normal mucosa distant from the primary tumour tend to support the field cancerization theory. However, analysis of tumours in female patients taking advantage of the phenomenon of X (chromosome) inactivation supports a clonal origin of multiple tumours.

Principal carcinogens for HNSCC

- Smoking
- Alcohol

Site-specific carcinogens

- Nickel and chromate dust: nose, larynx, lung and paranasal sinuses
- Hardwood dust: adenocarcinomas of the paranasal sinuses
- Nitrosamines in a salted fish diet <10 years of age: nasopharyngeal carcinoma

---

Site specific carcinogens have been identified for some head and neck cancers. Nickel and chromate dust are principal inorganic chemicals which can cause lesions in the nose, larynx, lung and paranasal sinuses. Clusters of cases in the hardwood industry led to the identification of hardwood dust as an aetiological factor in the development of adenocarcinomas of the paranasal sinuses. Similar epidemiological evidence implicated the nitrosamines in a salted fish diet below the age of ten in the later development of nasopharyngeal carcinoma.

The association of Paterson-Brown–Kelly syndrome (iron deficiency, glossitis, koilonychia and an upper oesophageal web) with postcricoid carcinoma may account for the relatively high incidence of both conditions in the UK and Scandinavia. This may also account for the fact that the postcricoid region is the only subsite of the hypopharynx where the incidence of carcinoma in women exceeds that in men and where the age of incidence is relatively young. The reported risk of post-cricoid carcinoma in patients with an oesophageal web is 4–16%. The decrease in the prevalence of Paterson-Brown–Kelly syndrome in Sweden as a result of dietary changes and education has been mirrored by a similar fall in the incidence of postcricoid carcinoma. Because the symptoms are often mild and slowly progressive, the diagnosis of Paterson-Brown–Kelly syndrome is often missed, but once made, the condition can be reversed with iron replacement and vitamin B therapy.

Two viruses have principally been implicated in the pathogenesis of some head and neck cancers; the human papilloma viruses (HPV) and Epstein–Barr virus (EBV). The E6 and E7 regions of high-risk HPV types (6, 18 and 33) have been shown to inactivate the tumour suppressor gene products *p53* and *pRb*, potentiating neoplastic change and cell immortalization. Using polymerase chain reaction (PCR)-based analysis, HPV DNA has been detected in 15–62% of HNSCC. Although the EBV genome has been detected in other head and neck cancers, EBV is specifically associated with the development of nasopharyngeal carcinoma in this region. Its genome is consistently found in nasopharyngeal tumour cells. Raised serum immunoglobin A (IgA) against the viral capsid antigen has been shown to precede clinical symptoms in nasopharyngeal cancer and the evidence suggests that patients in high-risk regions with an elevated serum anti-EBV IgA level should have an endoscopic examination of the nasopharynx and blind biopsies to include the pharyngeal recesses. Anti-EBV IgA levels have also been shown to be related to tumour burden, but its use as a tumour marker to monitor treatment has not been established.

Family history

Three large case-controlled studies in Canada, The Netherlands and Brazil have demonstrated relative risks, using multivariate analysis, of 3.5–3.79 for HNSCC associated with a family history of HNSCC rising to 7.89 in first-degree relatives of patients with multiple HNSCC. This is supported by similar observations in oesophageal cancer in Turkey and the Far East. These findings suggest that familial factors may be important in determining susceptibility to HNSCC but their exact nature is unclear. The high incidence of nasopharyngeal cancer in south-east China, coupled with its greatly increased incidence in first-degree relatives of patients with nasopharyngeal cancer, has led to linkage analysis pointing to a susceptibility gene near the human leucocyte antigen (HLA) cluster on chromosome 6p. *In vitro* studies have demonstrated increased mutagen sensitivity in HNSCC patients with a family history of HNSCC and further increases in those with two or more affected first-degree relatives or patients with multiple HNSCC.

Molecular biology features

- Proto-oncogenes and tumour suppressor genes
- Apoptosis
- Cytogenetics: chromosomal abnormalities; allelic loss
- Growth factors
- Telomeres, telomerase and cell senescence
- Molecular progression model of head and neck carcinogenesis
- Molecular aspects of invasion and metastasis
- Immune surveillance

Molecular genetics of head and neck cancer

Regulation of the cell cycle is under the control of over 40 genes which include proto-oncogenes and tumour suppressor genes. Under normal conditions, the co-ordinated expression of these genes leads to an equilibrium between growth-promoting and growth-restraining signal transduction, and natural cell loss, such that cell turnover is appropriate to the tissue and the physiological circumstance. An imbalance in these factors, caused by proto-oncogene activation and tumour suppressor gene inactivation, will lead to an unbalanced mitogenic signal and consequent aberrant cell proliferation. This concept of genetic alteration leading to a neoplastic phenotype and subsequent clonal expansion is the basis of the 'clonal evolution model of tumour cell populations'.

Recently, there has been an increasing wave of interest in the significance of apoptosis in the development of cancer and its treatment. Apoptosis, often described as 'programmed cell death', is a distinct mode of cell loss responsible for deletion of cells in normal tissues which is fundamentally different from degenerative cell death or necrosis. Examples of apoptosis within a normal physiological context include the maintenance of the balance of continually proliferating cell populations, the deletion of effete cells such as ageing neutrophils, mediation of involutional processes such as the reversion of the lactating breast to its resting state after weaning and modulation of cell-mediated immunity by cell selection. Apoptosis also occurs in virtually all untreated malignancies and occurs as a 'homeostatic' mechanism by deleting cells which may pose a threat to the host. The induction of apoptosis in untreated tumours is complex and may involve a number of factors including tumour necrosis factor-α and expression of the oncogenes c-*myc* and c-*fos* in certain circumstances. In malignant tumours, the mode of action of the proto-oncogene *bcl-2* has been shown to be a novel one by inhibiting apoptosis rather than stimulating cell proliferation. Ionizing radiation induces apoptosis in normal tissues and tumours to a variable extent and is related to an increase in the level of wild-type p53 protein in the cells.

A number of co-ordinated genetic alterations affecting cell turnover is therefore required to initiate tumour formation and progression. The challenge to the molecular geneticist has been the identification of these genetic alterations and their correlation to known events in the histological progression of tumours from normal mucosa, through dysplastic changes to invasive tumour.

Cytogenetic abnormalities in head and neck cancer

Cytogenetics is the study of chromosomal abnormalities and rearrangements. Cytogenetic analysis has been the mainstay of genetic analysis in reticuloendothelial malignancies, being responsible for the identification of consistent translocations in different leukaemias. Its use in solid tumours has been hampered by the difficulties in establishing short-term primary cultures from head and neck cancers for chromosomal analysis and the erratically acquired chromosomal changes in long-term cell lines which may have occurred *in vitro*, influenced by culture conditions. However, some studies have identified chromosomal areas consistently showing frequent breakpoints suggesting the location of putative tumour suppressor genes (including 3p21, 5p14, 8p11, 17p21 and 18q21) and gain or amplification implying the presence of putative proto-oncogenes at other sites (including 3q, 5p, 8q and 11q13). The advent of molecular cytogenetics has obviated the need for primary short-term cultures and refined the location of chromosomal aberrations. Fluorescence *in situ* hybridization (FISH) allows the analysis of the copy number of a known specific DNA sequence within intact nuclei, whereas comparative genomic hybridization (CGH) permits the rapid screening of the entire genome by comparatively hybridizing matched tumour and normal DNA from a patient on to normal metaphase spreads, thereby detecting areas of deletion or amplification.

Tumour suppressor genes

A statistical analysis of the occurrence of retinoblastoma in children led Knudson to propose, in 1971, that in inherited cancers, two genetic events were required to inactivate the gene responsible for development of the cancer. This became known as Knudson's 'two-hit' hypothesis and together with other work on retinoblastoma, established the paradigm for all future investigations of tumour suppressor genes. While this is the classical model of tumour suppressor gene inactivation in inherited cancers, the two-hit principle also applies to sporadic cancers with the two 'hits' being a variable permutation of gene mutation, chromosomal deletion or hypermethylation of the 5′ gene promoter (in the case of *p16* and many other tumour suppressor genes). The most common permutation is a point mutation in one allele followed by chromosomal deletion in the other (also

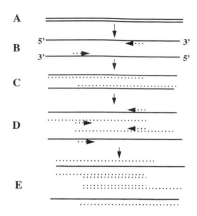

Figure 1.1 Polymerase chain reaction (PCR). PCR amplies specific DNA sequences exponentially. The reaction comprises a variable number of cycles, each of which comprises three steps. (A) The target DNA is double-stranded. (B) The **first** step in PCR involves the denaturing of the double-stranded DNA into single strands by heating to 94°C. This is followed by the **second** step, where specific oligonucleotide primers anneal to the denatured DNA at 55–65°C. (C) The **third** step is the extension of new strands by polymerase at 72°C. (D) The cycle is repeated. (E) With each cycle, the copy number of the target region is doubled. A 28-cycle reaction would generate over 67 million copies.

known as allelic loss). It can be inferred from this fact that areas of frequent allelic loss in tumours may represent the location of putative tumour suppressor genes.

The commonly employed method of molecular detection of allelic losses exploits the presence of highly polymorphic DNA sequences called microsatellites which are abundantly distributed throughout the human genome using the PCR (Fig. 1.1). These microsatellites contain small dinucleotide or trinucleotide repeat units, the number of which may differ between the two alleles in a particular person.

Microsatellite markers are now available which map to these sequences. When DNA sequences containing these microsatellite markers are amplified by PCR in a person heterozygous for that particular microsatellite, the PCR will yield two products of different lengths which will be detected on an electrophoretic gel. Where amplification of tumour DNA from such a subject yields only one product, the tumour is said to show loss of heterozygosity (LOH), implying allelic loss. Persons who are homozygous for a particular marker are said to be non-informative for that marker (Fig. 1.2). Allelotypes generated in this fashion have identified several areas of frequent allelic deletion from which some of the responsible tumour suppressor genes have been cloned or identified. The most common areas of loss are at chromosome 9p21, several discrete regions on 3p, 17p21 and 13q14, and several discrete regions on 8p.

Chromosome region 9p21 loss is the most common chromosomal aberration detected not only in head and neck cancer but in the majority of human cancers, occur-

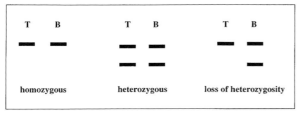

T = tumour DNA

B = blood/leucocyte DNA

━━ = 'band' representing PCR product on electrophoretic gel

Figure 1.2 Schematic representation of microsatellite analysis of matching blood and tumour DNA.

ring in over 70% of head and neck cancers. Positional cloning strategies led to the identification and characterization of *p16* (MTS1 or CDKN2) as a candidate tumour suppressor gene in this area. Unusually, inactivation of this gene by point mutations is an uncommon event. Homozygous deletion and hypermethylation of the 5′ promoter are the predominant modes of gene inactivation. Further support for the key role of *p16* as a tumour suppressor gene is given by the nature of its function as a potent cyclin/cyclin-dependent kinase (CDK) inhibitor involved in the G1–S checkpoint of the cell cycle as well as the demonstration that transfection of full-length cDNA of *p16* and *p16β* into head and neck cancer cell-lines results in marked growth inhibition with cell-cycle arrest in G1. An important aspect of 9p21 deletion is that it is one of the earliest genetic events in the pathogenesis of all the cancers in which it is implicated, specifically non-small-cell lung cancer, bladder cancer and head and neck cancer. The implication of this is that detection of 9p21 deletion or *p16* inactivation may have considerable potential in the definition of early and high-risk pre-malignant lesions.

Several discrete regions of deletion have been identified on chromosome 3p, although only one candidate tumour suppressor gene has been cloned but this has not yet been fully characterized. About 60% of HNSCC show 3p deletion, with the specific regions being 3p14, 3p21.3, 3p22 and 3p25. 3p14.2 is a site of chromosomal fragility across which the *FHIT* gene have been cloned. Mutations and aberrant transcripts of the *FHIT* gene have been reported in up to 65% of head and neck cancers by several groups. However, the function of this gene, and in particular its potential to act as a tumour suppressor gene, remains unclear. There is recent unpublished data to suggest that micro-cell-mediated transfer of a normal chromosome 3 into a HNSCC cell line showing 3p deletion and telomerase activity abolishes the telomerase activity, implying the presence of a putative telomerase repressor gene on chromosome 3p.

Loss of heterozygosity at chromosome 17p has been shown in over half of HNSCC and often correlates with *p53* inactivation. While *p53* mutations are detected in early preinvasive lesions of the head and neck, their incidence increases with tumour progression. Although *p53*

is perhaps the most extensively studied of known tumour suppressor genes, far from reaching a simple function for the p53 protein, research appears to uncover ever more facets to a gene which has a crucial and complex role in tumour suppression whose function is intimately related to that of other tumour suppressor genes, proto-oncogenes and growth factors. What is known, however, is that wild-type p53 protein has a critical role in inducing G1-arrest until repair has been effected; or if that is not possible, in directing the cell into an apoptotic pathway through transcriptional activation of such genes as *p21*/WAF1, *mdm2* and *bax*. Certain mutations of the *p53* gene result in p53 protein which is transcriptionally inactive and therefore unable to execute this function, leading to propagation of acquired genetic alterations and outgrowth of malignant clones.

Allelic loss at 13q14 also occurs in over half of HNSCC. The area of deletion includes the retinoblastoma gene (*RB1*) and is immediately adjacent to the hereditary breast cancer gene *BRCA2*. Immunohistochemical analysis of the RB1 protein product and mutation analysis of *BRCA2* in head and neck tumours showing loss of heterozygosity at 13q14 have discounted both of these known tumour suppressor genes as putative tumour suppressor genes inactivated in this area and imply the presence of another tumour suppressor gene in this region. The exclusion of *BRCA2* is of particular interest as there is evidence that *BRCA2* families show an excess of laryngeal cancer.

Proto-oncogenes

While proto-oncogenes have a more dominant role than tumour suppressor genes in the development of reticulo-endothelial malignancies, the reverse appears to be the case in solid tumours. Consistent amplification of 11q13 implicated *PRAD1* (*CCND1* or cyclin D1) as an important oncogene involved in HNSCC pathogenesis. Further work has shown that amplification of *PRAD1* is associated with increased expression of the gene. On a clinical level, *PRAD1* overexpression correlates with tumour progression and is strongly associated with a reduced disease-free interval and overall survival in patients with operable head and neck cancer.

The role of the *ras* family of oncogenes in HNSCC pathogenesis is unclear. While a high incidence of *ras* mutations has been reported in HNSCC in India, several studies have failed to demonstrate this in the Western world. This finding suggests that there may be a specific mutagenic effect of chewing tobacco or betel nuts upon the *ras* oncogenes.

Growth factors

Polypeptide growth factors and their receptors mediate signals which stimulate cell division and growth in normal cells under physiological conditions. Overexpression of these growth factors and their receptors may promote pathologically excessive cell growth and, as such, they could be considered as protein products of proto-oncogenes, especially when oncogenic retroviruses carry genes (v-onc) showing strong homology to corresponding human genes (c-onc). An example of this is the homology between viral *v-erbB* and human epidermal growth factor receptor (EGF-R). Qualitative analysis of various growth factors in HNSCC at the DNA, mRNA and protein level has consistently demonstrated grossly elevated levels of epidermal growth factor (EGF), EGF-R and transforming growth factor-α (TGF-α) in head and neck cancers as well as surrounding histologically normal mucosa.

Overexpression of other growth factors and their receptors, such as platelet-derived growth factor (PDGF), fibroblast growth factors (FGF-1, FGF-2) and fibroblast growth factor receptor (FGF-R), has been demonstrated in head and neck cancers. The growth factor-like molecule *HER-2/neu* (previously known as c-erbB-2) has shown great promise in prognostic determination in breast cancer and the amplification analysis of the *HER-2/neu* gene is becoming part of the staging process in breast cancer. While *HER-2/neu* amplification has been seen in some HNSCC, it has failed to show any association with clinical parameters. The growth factors and their receptors have been disappointing as potential markers of subclinical tumour recurrence, prognostic determinants or serum monitors of treatment. However, the growth factor receptors expressed on tumour cell surfaces are being intensively investigated with optimistic early results as tumour-specific targets for immunotherapy.

Telomeres, telomerase and cell senescence

Telomeres are specialized structures containing unique, simple repetitive sequences which cap the end of chromosomes. The length of the telomere is maintained in germ-line cells by the enzyme telomerase which is absent in normal somatic cells. This observation led to the theory that progressive shortening of telomeres with each cell division leads to cell senescence and ageing of the organism. Several mechanisms for this have been proposed. A critical shortening of the telomere may leave a nontelomere free DNA end which signals cell-cycle arrest. Telomere loss could also extend to the deletion or inactivation of genes located subtelomerically, again leading to cell-cycle arrest. Two important consequences of critical telomere shortening in cells which survive the cell crisis are genomic rearrangements and chromosomal loss which may in turn lead to malignant transformation. This is particularly relevant to rapidly dividing and regenerating tissues such as skin and mucosa. Paradoxically, while some of these survivors will subsequently go into cell-cycle arrest owing to critical telomere length shortening, a proportion will then express telomerase activity. Such activity is capable of cell immortalization by maintaining telomere length indefinitely. Telomerase

activity has been demonstrated in 80% of oral cancers and around 50% of oral leucoplakia lesions. While detection of telomerase activity in oral rinses from head and neck cancer patients remains limited by technical problems of test sensitivity, the potential for antitelomerase drugs as a novel treatment remains promising.

Molecular progression model of head and neck squamous cell carcinogenesis

The identification of the temporal relationships of genetic alterations in tumorigenesis and their relationship to the histological progression of tumours is more than a scientific intellectual exercise. An understanding of the genetic processes underlying tumour initiation and progression has important therapeutic implications such as the detection of known early genetic alterations in primary screening and early detection of tumour recurrence. The pioneering genetic progression model for colorectal tumourigenesis was proposed by Fearon and Vogelstein in 1990. Specific genetic alterations were assigned to each step of the well-established adenoma–carcinoma sequence in colorectal tumorigenesis. A similar model has been more difficult to establish in HNSCC but a number of models has been suggested by different groups from analysing published allelotype data; from microsatellite analysis of adjacent areas of histologically normal tissue, dysplasia, carcinoma *in situ* and invasive carcinoma; and from microsatellite analysis of 'matched' normal, dysplastic and carcinomatous tissue from individual patients biopsied at different times. These are largely in agreement with one another and a proposed molecular progression model is given in Fig. 1.3.

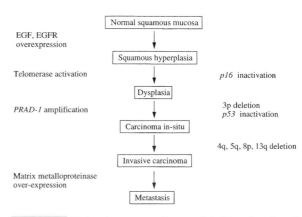

Figure 1.3 Molecular progression model of head and neck carcinogenesis.

Tumour immunology

Although the first cases of 'immunotherapy for cancer' were reported by Coley in the nineteenth century when he published the results of his treatment of advanced malignancy with repeated injections of erysipelas-derived serum, the nature of the immune response to cancer and its potential exploitation for therapy was only recognized in the 1980s. The concept of tumour immunosurveillance, whereby the immune system constantly detect and kill malignant cells before they can form a tumour, is strongly supported by the demonstration of activated immune effector cells [tumour-infiltrating lymphocytes (TIL)] within tumours and the hugely increased incidence of malignant disease in immunosuppressed patients. The successful development of a tumour depends on neoplastic cells escaping either recognition or destruction by the immune system. Such escape in HNSCC may arise from the functional down-regulation of TIL by tumour-secreted factors such as prostaglandin E_2 (PGE_2) and TGF-β.

Activation of cytotoxic T-cells (CTL) requires two signals. The first is provided by the binding of the T-cell receptor to the major histocompatibility complex (MHC) class I molecule present on the tumour cell. The down-regulation of this molecule in some malignant cells is another way in which some tumours can escape immunosurveillance. The second signal is provided by the binding of a costimulatory molecule to its ligand on the T-cell. An example of this is the B7.1 molecule which is expressed on the surface of professional antigen-presenting cells (e.g. macrophages and dendritic cells) and which binds to the CD28 ligand on T-cells. In the absence of this binding, the T-cell may become anergic or undergo apoptosis. As these molecules are not present on malignant cells, one form of immunotherapy successfully tried in animal models exploits this system by introducing the co-stimulatory molecule cDNA into tumour cells using a viral vector which results in its surface expression. Furthermore, promise has been shown by combining this approach with the use of cytokines.

The identification of tumour-specific antigens has both diagnostic and therapeutic implications. The monoclonal antibodies E48 and U36 bind to peptides expressed on HNSCC, stratified squamous epithelium and transitional epithelium. Technetium-99m (^{99m}Tc)-labelled E48 IgG has been used for clinical imaging of head and neck cancer while both E48 and U36, coupled with iodine-131 and rhenium-186, respectively, have successfully been used for immunotargeting HNSCC in nude mice.

The clinical trials of immunotherapy showing the greatest promise in head and neck cancer have arisen from the observation that HNSCC cells secrete immunoregulatory cytokines (e.g. the interleukins IL-2, IL-4 and IL-6) which effect growth inhibition both directly and indirectly. Local treatment with IL-2 given by intratumoural injection in one trial of patients with recurrent HNSCC has been shown to give total or partial responses in around 30% of patients. This may be related to an increase in T-cells and lymphokine activated killer (LAK) cells within the tumours. Systemic treatment with cytokines such as IL-2, IL-12 and interferons has been limited by treatment-associated toxicity. IL-2 has also been used to expand TIL *in vitro* followed by the reintroduction of autologous IL-2-activated TIL. Although such cellular adoptive immunotherapy showed early promise in animal models which has yet to be translated into full clinical trials, immunotherapy looks set to assume its place as the third non-surgical treatment modality for cancer.

Cancer invasion and metastasis

As tumours acquire the capacity for invasion and metastatic spread, the therapeutic window of opportunity rapidly closes and there has been much recent investigation into the molecular and cellular basis of cancer invasion. Invasion is the active translocation of neoplastic cells across tissue boundaries and through host cellular and extracellular matrix barriers. It is a dynamic and active rather than a passive process resulting from a combination of angiogenesis and co-ordinated alternation between matrix proteolysis and cellular adhesion involving a complex interaction of proteolytic enzymes, motility factors and cell–cell adhesion molecules which propels the tumour front forwards.

Folkmann proposed in the 1970s that tumour growth was dependent upon the recruitment of new blood vessels. Such tumour-induced angiogenesis occurs in parallel with the transition to tumour invasiveness and may indeed be permissive for the progression of carcinoma *in situ* to invasive carcinoma.

Endothelial cell proliferation

- Prostaglandin E_2 (PGE2)
- Transforming growth factor-β (TGF-β)
- Fibroblast growth factor (FGF)
- Vascular endothelial growth factor (VEGF)

Endothelial cell proliferation is stimulated by a number of tumour produced growth factors such as prostaglandin E2 (PGE-2), transforming growth factor-beta (TGF-β), fibroblast growth factor (FGF) and perhaps most importantly, vascular endothelial growth factor (VEGF). The degree of vascularization may have implications on pathology and treatment; a high degree of vascularization may provide better access to the circulation for metastatic spread and yet it provides a less hypoxic environment for tumour cells, theoretically rendering them more sensitive to ionizing radiation. Angiogenesis has been demonstrated immunohistochemically in a number of tumours, including HNSCC, with antibodies to vascular antigens such as factor VIII-related endothelial antigen. Published data correlating the degree of tumoural microvessel development and clinical parameters in HNSCC is inconsistent, but there is good evidence that high microvessel density may predict a favourable response to radiotherapy, particularly in nasopharyngeal carcinomas.

Perhaps the most promising novel therapy suggested recently attacks this Achilles' heel of cancer, the fact that a new blood supply is crucial to its continued existence. Endostatin is an endogenous protein which is a potent inhibitor of endothelial cell proliferation, a process which underpins angiogenesis. Convincing animal data has shown that endostatin treatment of mice with implanted tumours overcomes almost all of the problems which have dogged other non-surgical adjuvant therapies, principally the development of resistance to treatment and the inability to repeat treatment with tumour recurrence. Furthermore, all of the implanted tumours disappeared competely without recurrence after two to six cycles of treatment. Clearly, it is a large step from tumours implanted in nude mice to endogenous tumours in humans; however, large clinical trials of endostatin have already begun in many cancers.

The extracellular matrix which surrounds normal tissues and tumour cells supports and regulates those tissues and cells. Disruption of this matrix is a prerequisite for local tumour invasion and subsequent penetration of blood vessels and lymphatics gives rise to tumour dissemination and metastasis. Degradation of the extracellular matrix involves several families of enzymes, of which the most extensively investigated are the matrix metalloproteinases (MMP) and their tissue inhibitors (TIMP), both of which are produced by tumour cells and an imbalance of which leads to proteolysis. Among MMP, the type IV collagenases (gelatinases) have most convincingly been demonstrated to be associated with a metastatic phenotype. Clinical trials of matrix metalloproteinase inhibitors in the treatment of a variety of human cancers are already underway and show early promise as adjuvant therapy in advanced tumours.

Clinical applications: present and future

Aside from increasing our understanding of tumour behaviour, the assembly of knowledge of critical genetic events in head and neck carcinogenesis is directed at its application in prediction of tumour behaviour and development of novel therapeutic options. The potential for molecular assessment of surgical resection margins and detection of occult lymph-node metastases has been demonstrated in a paper from the Johns Hopkins University. Tumours harbouring a *p53* mutation were identified and the mutation was characterized by sequencing. A probe unique for each specific *p53* mutation was synthesized and used to probe histologically uninvolved surgical margins and locoregional lymph nodes in 25 tumour resections. The phage clone technique employed was very labour intensive but sufficiently sensitive to detect one cell with the specific *p53* mutation within 10 000 normal cells. With a median follow-up of 15 months, 38% of patients with specific *p53* mutations

detected at the surgical margins exhibited site-specific recurrence compared with no recurrences at *p53* mutation-negative margins. Lymph-node analysis showed specific *p53* mutations in 21% of lymph nodes which led to upstaging of the tumours. The same group has also shown the utility of gene mutation detection in saliva for head and neck cancers, in sputum for lung cancer and in faeces for colorectal cancer; however, these tests have yet to reach a sufficiently high sensitivity for routine use in screening and detection of subclinical recurrence.

Possible future therapeutic strategies

- Virus-directed enzyme prodrug therapy (VDEPT)
- Tissue inhibitors of matrix metalloproteinases (TIMP)
- Antiangiogenesis agents

Genetic determination of phenotype and prognosis in head and neck cancer will be important and as more genes become identified, greater precision in such determination will be achieved. Several cytogenetic breakpoints have been shown to be associated with radioresistance *in vitro* and certain apoptotic markers show promise as indicators of resistance to chemotherapy. As these become better defined, treatment strategies may be tailored to the tumour genotype. The development of less labour-intensive methods and 'gene-chips' for simultaneous mutation analysis of up to hundreds of genes will make genotyping of both tumours and margins an integral part of tumour staging and treatment monitoring in the future.

Finally, perhaps the holy grail for the molecular oncologist is perceived to be gene therapy. Even before the successful cloning of known tumour suppressor genes, a crude form of gene replacement therapy by the introduction of whole chromosomes suspected of harbouring putative tumour suppressor genes had been shown to suppress tumorigenicity *in vitro*. The introduction of wild-type *p53* and *p16* into human head and neck cancer cells either by transfection *in vitro* or via a recombinant adenovirus *in vivo* in nude mice has consistently shown growth suppression in both situations. Several trials of virally mediated *p53* gene replacement therapy in head and neck cancer are already under way but the results have not yet been published.

Cancer treatment involving genetic modulation is not restricted to the replacement of inactivated tumour suppressor genes. Virus-directed enzyme prodrug therapy (VDEPT) for head and neck cancer has been extensively investigated in experimental animal work. An example of this is the introduction of the herpes simplex virus thymidine kinase gene into tumour cells, resulting in expression of thymidine kinase in those cells and its conversion of gancyclovir into a phosphorylated compound which halts DNA synthesis. This type of treatment can be combined with IL-2 immunotherapy which exhibits synergistic effects in animal models.

In summary, therefore, recent advances in molecular biological research in cancer have improved our understanding of the genetic and cellular events underlying the development of cancers of the head and neck. Some of these events correlate well with clinical parameters while others remain poorly characterized. The identification of new genes and further characterization of the oncogenic process hold promise for radical improvements to established methods of tumour evaluation and treatment as well as exciting new developments in novel therapeutic strategies.

Acknowledgement

The important contribution to this chapter of Mr Michael Kuo PhD, FRCS, specialist registrar in otolaryngology, University Hospital Birmingham NHS Trust, is gratefully acknowledged.

Further reading

Ah-See K. W., Cooke T. G., Pickford I. R., Soutar D. and Balmain A. (1994) An allelotype of squamous carcinoma of the head and neck using microsatellite markers, *Cancer Res* 54(7): 1617–21.

Boehm, T., Folkman, J., Browder, T. and O'Reilly, M.S., Anti-angiogenic therapy of experimental cancer does not induce acquired drug resistance [see comments]. *Nature*, 1997 390, 404–7

Boyle J. O., Mao L., Brennan J. A., Koch W. M, Eisele D. W., Saunders J. R. and Sidransky D. (1994) Gene mutations in saliva as molecular markers for head and neck squamous cell carcinomas, *Am J Surg* 168: 429–32.

Brennan J. A., Mao L., Hruban R. H., Boyle J. O., Eby Y., Koch W. *et al.*, (1995) Molecular assessment of histopathological staging in squamous cell carcinoma of the head and neck, *N Engl J Med* 332: 429–35.

Clayman G. L., El-Naggar A. K., Roth J. A., Zhang W. W., Goepfert H., Taylor D. L. and Liu T.-J. (1995) *In vivo* molecular therapy with *p53* adenovirus for microscopic residual head and neck squamous carcinoma, *Cancer Res* 55: 1–6.

El-Naggar A. K., Hurr K., Batsakis J. G., Luna M. A., Goepfert H. and Huff V. (1995) Sequential loss of heterozygosity at microsatellite motifs in preinvasive and invasive head and neck squamous carcinoma, *Cancer Res* 55(12): 2656–9.

Gronbak M., Becker U., Johansen D. H. T., Jensen G. and Tia S. (1998) Population based cohort study of the association between alcohol intake and cancer of the upper digestive tract. *BMJ*, 317: 844–8

Latchman D. S. (1997) *Basic Molecular and Cell Biology*, 3rd edn, BMJ Publishing Group, London.

Lemoine N., Neoptolemos J. P. and Cooke T. (1994) *Cancer – A Molecular Approach*, Blackwell Scientific Publications, Oxford.

Mao L., El-Naggar A. K., Fan Y. H., Lee J. S., Lippman S. M., Kayser S. *et al.* (1996) Telomerase activity in head and neck squamous cell carcinoma and adjacent tissues, *Cancer Res* 56(24): 5600–4.

Sidransky D. (1995) Molecular genetics of head and neck cancer, *Curr Opin Oncol* 7: 229–33.

Strachan T. and Read A. P. (1999) *Human Molecular Genetics*, Bios Scientific Publishers, Oxford.

Waridel F., Estreicher A., Bron L., Flaman J.-M., Fontolliet C., Monnier P. *et al.* (1997) Field cancerisation and polyclonal *p53* mutation in the upper aerodigestive tract, *Oncogene* 14: 163–9.

2 Assessment

'Get it right first time'

Clinical examination

Those patients with head and neck cancer who are both incurable and untreatable and some of those who are treatable and might be curable are sometimes best left well alone. Deciding which patients with this disease should be treated, however, is often more difficult than in many other fields of surgery because there are seldom any objective signs to show that the patient is beyond treatment. When the patient is first seen, the tumour is often confined to the head and neck with no clinical evidence of distant metastases; furthermore, although a head and neck tumour may be incurable, there are very few that are unresectable and virtually every structure in the head and neck to which a tumour may be fixed can be removed in continuity and repaired in some way, shape or form.

This means that the vast majority of patients with head and neck cancer are potentially treatable but not all are curable. Some of them should not be treated, usually because a combination of advanced stage and poor general condition makes the mutilating effects of surgery not worthwhile. In general, the first decision to be made in a patient with a confirmed head and neck cancer is whether or not to treat the patient before deciding what form of management strategy is appropriate. If a patient is unfit for surgery because of advancing age or poor general health, then consideration will have to be given to whether or not palliative treatment is appropriate by radiotherapy and/or chemotherapy, or whether purely supportive measures will suffice with no active anticancer treatment at all. Hence, a final decision on treatment often hinges on a full assessment of the patient including physiological age and general condition. It is advisable to obtain as many opinions as possible and not to rush in with a treatment plan, remembering that 'young men kill their patients – old men watch them die'. The best option for all concerned is to 'get it right first time'!

There are four possible end-points to the initial assessment exercise:

- the patient is potentially curable
- the patient has a potentially curable primary tumour but is likely to succumb to another illness within a few months
- the patient is incurable of the tumour but ought to be treated actively with palliation
- the patient is incurable and should be treated symptomatically.

Much of the following discussion in this chapter shows how these clinical end-points may be reached.

History

Taking the history from a patient with a head and neck tumour is no different from taking the history of a patient with any other medical or surgical condition. There are however, three points that are of particular importance when it comes to making the ultimate decision with regard to treatment planning. These are the age of the patient, their social circumstances and tumour biology.

Head and neck tumours often occur in people over the age of 45 years. If someone has a cancer under this age, then they may do less well than somebody aged over 45 years. Something bizarre may have altered their immune status to have caused this tumour to develop. Most head and neck tumours are epithelial carcinomas and reflect years of abuse of the epithelium by cigarettes and tobacco, often combined with alcohol. Therefore, when a young person develops such a tumour, it often carries a sinister significance. Elderly people often have impaired functional organ reserve or frank comorbidity, and are often less able to be successfully rehabilitated with regard to speech and swallowing than are younger patients after major surgery.

The next important issue to consider is that of social circumstance. Most head and neck operations violate normal anatomy and physiology and usually the psyche of the patient. Every patient who has a head and neck operation requires not only physical support but psychosocial support afterwards. If they live alone and are unable to read and write (as sometimes occurs, even today) or are alcoholics, then these factors should play a part in deciding whether or not the patient has surgery or radiotherapy as primary treatment.

Finally, it is important to assess tumour biology. This has been discussed in Chapter 1, but it is important to realize that certain biological factors may be important when considering other prognostic indicators such as tumour (T) and node (N) stage. Poorly differentiated tumours often have a worse prognosis than well-differentiated tumours and tumours in the young may do worse than those in the old. In addition, tumours that develop in immunocompromised individuals seldom do well by any modality.

The late John Conley (the famous New York surgeon) used to have a useful teaching aphorism, namely: 'Listen to what the tumour tells you – sometimes it says "I am going to kill you". In other words "the cancer is trying to tell you something doctor"!'

A tumour that is growing very quickly may not be amenable to treatment by any modality and can act as a 'clinical biological indicator' so that any treatment may indeed be worse than the end-point of the disease itself. The situation where the operation was a success and the patient a failure is not a desirable end result.

The patient's general condition should always be classified using one of the methods of measuring performance status such as the Eastern Co-operative Oncology Group (ECOG) scheme or the Karnofsky status (Table 2.1).

Finally, if one is assessing a patient who has had treatment elsewhere, it is important to remember not to assume anything that has gone on before and to start again both in the history taking and in the clinical examination in order not to get caught out. In patient assessment,

a useful aphorism to remember is 'good judgement is usually the result of experience but experience has usually resulted from previous bad judgement'.

Examination

Examination of the primary site

When examining a patient with a head and neck tumour, one should always think in terms of 'T' staging. When assessing the local lesion for treatment, its borders can be delineated exactly both by inspection and by palpation and a permanent record of these findings made on a preprinted set of illustrations (see Appendix 2.1). This is done both in the clinic and in the operating room.

Every region should be documented from different angles. It is important to have a copy of the current TNM (tumour, node, metastasis) staging system (UICC, 1997) both in clinic and in the operating room to facilitate quick and accurate staging. It is also important to assess the patient's dentition and where there is any cause for concern, particularly if the patient is to undergo radiotherapy, the advice of a restorative dentist should be sought.

Examination of the neck

Involved lymph nodes rarely produce symptoms until they are quite large. Therefore, the surgeon must depend mainly on physical examination to detect clinically enlarged nodes. It takes between 2 and 5 min to conduct a careful examination of each side of the neck. It is important to repeat the examination at every opportunity and to compare findings amongst several examiners. Detailed drawings using prepared diagrams (Appendix 2.1) complement the written report and are essential. As soon as possible, each clinician develops his or her own technique which he or she can then perform in the same systematic manner each time the examination is conducted.

The triangles of the neck and the lymph nodes that they contain (Fig. 2.1) are examined in turn. Having inspected the neck from the front, the clinician stands behind the patient and flexes his or her head slightly. Clothing should be removed until the points of the shoulders can be seen. The index fingers are placed on both mastoid processes and the clinician works down the trapezius muscle until the fingers meet at the clavicle. There are nodes under the trapezius muscle and, because of this, fingers should be inserted under the anterior border of the muscle with the thumb pressing down on the top with the shoulder blades forward. When the clavicle is reached, the posterior triangle (level V) is palpated. Here the nodes lie between the skin and muscles of the floor of the triangle and therefore can be rolled between these two surfaces. Tension is taken off the sternomastoid muscle by passive, gentle lateral movement of the head to the examined side. The fingers are placed in front of, and medial to, the sternomastoid with the thumb behind it, thus forming a 'C' around the muscle. The examination progresses down

Table 2.1 Eastern Co-operative Oncology Group (ECOG) scale

Grade	Description
0	Fully active, able to carry on all predisease activities without restriction (Karnofsky 90–100)
1	Restricted in physically strenuous activity but ambulatory and able to carry out work of a light or sedentary nature, e.g. for example, light housework, office work (Karnofsky 70–80)
2	Ambulatory and capable of self-care but unable to carry out any work activities. Up and about more than 50% of waking hours (Karnofsky 50–60)
3	Capable of only limited self-care, confined to bed or chair 50% or more of waking hours (Karnofsky 30–40)
4	Completely disabled. Cannot carry out any self-care. Totally confined to bed or chair (Karnofsky 10–20)

(a)

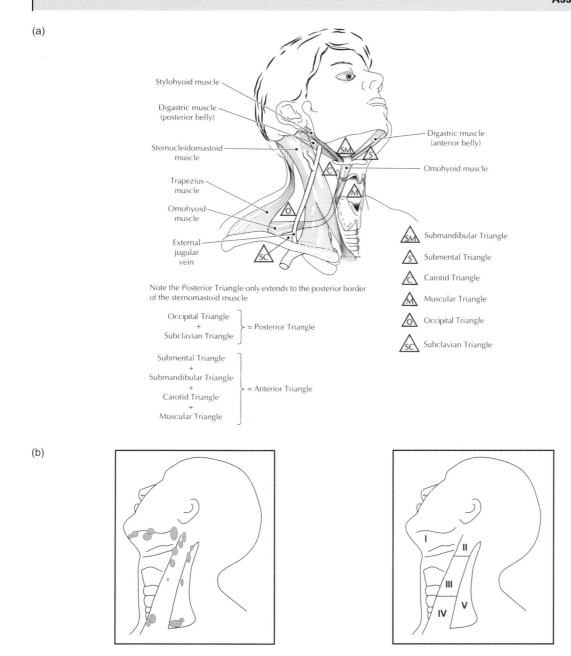

Note the Posterior Triangle only extends to the posterior border of the sternomastoid muscle

Occipital Triangle
+
Subclavian Triangle
} = Posterior Triangle

Submental Triangle
+
Submandibular Triangle
+
Carotid Triangle
+
Muscular Triangle
} = Anterior Triangle

(b)

Figure 2.1 (a) The triangles of the neck and (b) lymph-node levels.

the muscle carefully because 80% of the nodes lie under the muscle within the jugular chain (levels II–IV) of the deep cervical lymph nodes. The smallest node which can be easily palpated in the jugular chain is probably 1 cm. The jugulodigastric node is the largest normal node in the neck and can be palpated in many normal people. Most clinically positive nodes occur in the upper jugular chain (levels II and III) but the most superior jugular nodes (level II), including the junctional nodes, are difficult to palpate, particularly in men, and positive lymph nodes in the lower jugular area (level IV) may be difficult to feel since they are often small, deep and mobile.

Attention should be paid to the suprasternal notch and the space within it (the space of Burns), as clinically positive cricothyroid and pretracheal nodes may be discovered. The trachea is palpated and at this point the size of the thyroid gland is assessed. Then, working upwards, the mobility of the larynx and pharynx on the prevertebral fascia is assessed and, in particular, a note made of any pain on palpation of the trachea which may indicate direct invasion of this structure by direct extension from a postcricoid carcinoma.

The submandibular gland and nodes along with the submental nodes (level I) should now be examined.

These are all easier to feel and nodes down to 0.5 cm can usually be palpated. At the posterior border of the submandibular gland, the examination continues upwards over the face to assess the preauricular nodes.

A number of normal structures can be confused with a lymph node in the neck. The lateral tips of the transverse processes of both C_1 and C_2 can simulate lymph nodes, as can the parotid tail, superior horn of the thyroid cartilage and the carotid bulb. Irradiated and obstructed submandibular glands may also simulate lymph-node enlargement.

The reliability of the neck examination depends on the experience and ability of the examiner, the gross anatomy of the individual neck and whether or not there has been previous treatment such as surgery and/or radiotherapy. A fat, thick or a muscular neck can make evaluation difficult, as can a recent incisional biopsy or tracheostomy.

It is important to remember that there is a well-recognized error in tumour palpation in general, with considerable intraobserver and interobserver variation when estimating tumour size. These pitfalls of tumour measurement are particularly common in head and neck cancer. There is considerable error in palpating the neck, with significant variation between experienced observers.

Failure to detect disease in the neck may directly affect prognosis. The incidence of false-positive nodes is important for two reasons. First, a false-positive node may result in unnecessarily aggressive treatment, and secondly, a patient with unilateral primary but bilateral palpable nodes may be condemned to inadequate treatment on the basis that he or she has incurable disease.

General examination

The patient's general health should be assessed with the usual investigations. All patients undergoing major surgery should have a full blood count, urea and electrolytes, liver function tests along with a chest X-ray, electrocardiogram (ECG) and thyroid function tests. Occult hypothyroidism is not uncommon in the elderly nor in those patients having revision treatment when previous surgery or radiotherapy to the thyroid gland can affect its function. Patients should be assessed for deep vein thrombosis (DVT) prophylaxis (see Chapter 6). Specialist head and neck imaging is discussed subsequently (Chapter 3) but in those patients at risk of a second primary within the chest, a computed tomographic (CT) scan of the chest should be considered as an alternative to a chest X-ray.

A decision as to whether the patient is fit for surgery and a general anaesthetic should be made following discussion with the anaesthetist who shares the final responsibilities for the patient's health during any such procedure. The anaesthetist may well decide to order further investigations that may be deemed appropriate over and above those discussed previously such as chest X-ray, ECG and thyroid function tests. The patient's nutritional status should be assessed with a dietician and preopera-tive feeding may be required. This may be done orally, intravenously, via a nasogastric tube, feeding gastrostomy or jejunostomy or, more commonly nowadays, a percutaneous gastrostomy (PEG). The type of feed and route of administration should be a joint decision with the dietician and where postoperative feeding problems may be encountered, i.e. in oral, oropharyngeal and laryngeal surgery, it is commonplace for head and neck surgeons to request preoperative PEGs.

Staging of cancer

Cancer is a heterogeneous disease, or rather group of diseases, and the natural history and response to treatment can be both wide and varied. There are obvious advantages in subdividing cases of cancer into groups in which the behaviour may be similar and this process is called staging.

A staging system for head and neck squamous cell carcinoma (HNSCC) is important for both clinical and therapeutic research and as an acceptable and reproducible method of staging all sites within the region. It is mandatory to allow any meaningful comparison to be made between different centres, both nationally and internationally. The goals of any cancer staging system are therefore, by definition, far reaching and multiple in nature. The system should act as a dictionary, allowing individual physicians and surgeons to compare and exchange information using language and vocabulary that they can all understand. The staging data obtained (and suitably recorded as at least a minimum data set; see Appendix 2.2) should reflect prognosis and provide guidelines for treatment selection, allow an analysis of isolated clinical factors such as pretreatment findings, age, complications and survival, and should be easy both to comprehend and to update. It is worth looking at a few of these points in more detail.

First and foremost, staging acts as a guide to the appropriate treatment. The question, 'how should a patient with carcinoma of the larynx be treated' cannot be answered without reference to staging. A patient with a small tumour confined to the true vocal cord which remains mobile can be successfully treated either by surgery or by irradiation with voice preservation, but a patient with an advanced transglottic carcinoma, causing airway obstruction and invading the thyroid cartilage with nodal metastases, usually requires laryngectomy and neck dissection.

Secondly, the stage of a tumour acts as a guide to prognosis. Multivariate analysis of one large recent study showed stage, anatomical site and age in that order to be the most significant predictors of survival. Accurate prognosis is important, not only to satisfy a patient who wants to know the likelihood of successful treatment but also to ensure the equivalence of groups in clinical trials. For example, suppose a new form of treatment is being compared with standard practice in the treatment of oropharyngeal carcinoma. If there arises by chance a preponderance of more advanced cases in the conventional treatment arm, the survival rate in the experimental arm may be greater, even if in reality there is no difference between the treatments, stage by stage. Prerandomization stratification by stage will prevent this source of error.

Staging also permits more reliable comparison of results between centres by allowing an estimate of case mix. For example, if hospital A publishes better survival figures for laryngeal cancer, it may be assumed that it is a better hospital offering better treatment than other hospitals. Yet, different hospitals serve different populations and consequently the pattern of cancer cases they see may be different. The observed discrepancy may therefore result from the fact that hospital B serves a large population of socially disadvantaged patients who present late with advanced disease. If survival figures are published separately for each stage, it may be found that there is no difference between hospital A and hospital B or even that truly better results from hospital B have been masked by the large proportion of poor prognostic cases treated there.

Finally, staging allows a more reliable examination of reasons behind time trends. For example, the incidence of both malignant melanoma and testicular cancer is increasing in Scotland, yet the proportion of patients dying from these diseases is diminishing. It might be assumed that the improved survival from melanoma has been caused by the development of effective systemic therapy, as is the case for testicular tumours. In fact, examination of the distribution of stages at presentation shows that more cases of melanoma are now being diagnosed early as a result of a public education campaign but the prognosis of advanced cases has not changed.

Benefits of staging

- Planning therapy
- Aid to prognosis
- Comparison of results
- Epidemiology

Most of the reasons for staging do not immediately appear to benefit the individual patient and so it might be tempting for the busy surgeon to make no attempt at the staging process beyond a brief assessment for the purposes of choosing either treatment A or B, or worse still for him or her to assign hurriedly a wholly inaccurate stage. Yet, if the biology of cancer is to be more fully understood and if treatments are to be improved, it is imperative that staging should be carried out fully and accurately on every patient

So, how do we stage cancer? The basic requirement is to define in each patient all of the factors relevant to the natural history and outcome of the relevant disease, thereby enabling a patient with cancer to be grouped with other similar cases. The first subdivision of cancer is, of course, by primary site since no sensible physician would con-

template applying generalizations about lung cancer to skin cancer. However, this grouping is still inadequate and mention of histological type is necessary to distinguish basal cell carcinoma of the skin from malignant melanoma, and small cell from squamous carcinoma of the lung.

Even amongst tumours of one histological type arising at one primary site, there are still variations in prognosis. The most important factor determining these variations is usually the size and extent of the primary tumour, and whether or not lymphatic or bloodborne metastases are present. Together these constitute the stage of the tumour. While assessment of the tumour, nodes and metastases is usually sufficient for the staging purposes, other factors which are sometimes taken into account include the histological differentiation or grade of the tumour, along with the patient's age and sex, for example, in cases of soft-tissue sarcoma and differentiated thyroid carcinoma. For tumours such as lymphoma, which do not follow an orderly progression from primary tumour to nodal involvement and then distant metastases, special staging systems have been devised.

Even for epidermoid cancer, there are a variety of different staging classifications. Although these have similar aims and use similar data, the systems differ in important regards and therefore lead to groupings which may not be directly comparable and may thus preclude meaningful exchange of data not only between centres but also between countries.

Fortunately, over the years, the two principal staging classifications for head and neck cancer, those of the American Joint Committee on Cancer (AJCC) and the Union Internationale Contre le Cancer (UICC), have undergone a convergent evolution and are now identical for all intents and purposes.

Details can be found in the current UICC handbook (UICC, 1997). For each primary site in the head and neck, the factors taken into account in the stage classification are described in the appropriate chapter of the UICC handbook, to which every head and neck surgeon should have access. The following general definitions apply to all sites.

The TNM system for describing the anatomical extent of head and neck cancer is based on the assessment of three components, namely T, the extent of the primary tumour, N, the presence or absence and extent of regional lymph-node metastases and M, the presence or absence of distant metastases. All cases are identified by T, N and M categories, which must be accurately determined and recorded before treatment is commenced. The system is confined to carcinoma for all sites and malignancy must be confirmed by histological examination.

The extent of primary tumour is indicated by the suffixes 1, 2, 3 or 4, representing progressively more advanced disease. Increase in size is usually the sole criterion for categories 1, 2, and 3, while 4 often indicates direct extension (spread by continuity and contiguity) from outside the primary site, or invasion of underlying bone or cartilage. Other criteria are applied in special circumstances, such as fixation of the vocal cord in laryngeal carcinoma and the degree of extrapharyngeal extension in nasopharyngeal carcinoma. T_0 is used when there is no evidence of a primary tumour, T_{1s} used when the primary is non-invasive or carcinoma *in situ* and T_x when for some reason the extent of the primary tumour cannot be assessed.

Two classifications have been described for each head and neck site. There is a clinical classification (pretreatment clinical classification, designated cTNM) and a pathological classification (postsurgical histopathological classification, designated pTNM). For cTNM, traditional staging demands that certain prerequisite patient assessment be performed and its use reflects the level of certainty according to the particular diagnostic method used.

The UICC classification suggests that for each site the specific methods of investigation available for TNM classifications should be listed. These include mandatory methods such as clinical examination and biopsy which should always be employed to establish the extent of the tumour, and additional methods such as conventional radiography, along with other special investigations. The pTNM classification is based on evidence acquired before treatment, supplemented or modified by additional information acquired either surgically or pathologically. Further information regarding the primary lesion may be recorded under the headings 'G' for histopathological grading, 'L' for lymphatic invasion and 'V' for venous invasion. The presence or absence of residual tumour after treatment may be described by the symbol 'R'.

Within the TNM classification, the oral cavity, pharynx, larynx, maxillary sinus, salivary and thyroid glands are all listed as primary sites, the pharynx being subdivided by convention into the nasopharynx, oropharynx and hypopharynx. The cervical oesophagus is listed as a subsite.

Multiple tumours should be classified independently and in the case of multiple synchronous tumours in one organ, the tumour with the highest T category should be classified and the multiplicity or number of tumours indicated in parentheses.

Each site is described under a TNM heading (mandatory) and a cTNM and pTNM classification (optional). After being assigned various TNM categories, patients are grouped into a number of clinical stages (Table 2.2).

Three categories are used to describe progressive involvement of the regional lymph nodes. These apply to all head and neck sites except for the thyroid gland, the nasopharynx and the cervical oesophagus which have different classifications and are discussed in Chapters 20 (nasopharynx) and 23 (thyroid).

Under the current joint classification, the clinical findings regarding regional cervical lymphadenopathy are defined for each site independent of the primary tumour. N_0 indicates no palpable adenopathy whilst the designation of N_1 indicates metastasis in a single ipsilateral lymph node, 3 cm or less in its greatest dimension. The N_2 category is subdivided into three sections. N_{2a} indicates metastasis in a single ipsilateral lymph node, more than 3 cm but not more than 6 cm in greatest dimension. N_{2b} indicates metastasis in multiple ipsilat-

eral lymph nodes, none more than 6 cm in greatest dimension. N_{2C} indicates metastasis in bilateral or contralateral lymph nodes, none more than 6 cm in greatest dimension. N_3 disease is any lymphatic spread more than 6 cm in size in greatest dimension.

As in the case of T staging, the suffix 0 means no evidence of regional lymph-node involvement and the suffix X means that the node cannot be assessed.

Lymph nodes are described as ipsilateral, bilateral, contralateral or midline; they may be single or multiple and are measured by size, exact number and anatomical location (Fig. 2.1). Midline nodes are considered ipsilateral. During clinical examination, the actual size of the nodal mass should be measured and allowance made for the intervening soft tissues. It is well recognized that most masses over 3 cm in diameter are not single nodes but represent confluent nodes or tumour in the soft-tissue compartments of the neck. The current UICC classification recommends that, although the level of involvement of cervical lymph nodes is not incorporated into the current N classification, it should be recorded whenever possible. The logic behind this is that the level of involvement may directly affect treatment and prognosis and further changes in the staging system to incorporate this are therefore likely. However, the current UICC booklet only recommends the use of four levels when most head and neck surgeons now use five (Fig. 2.1).

The presence or absence of distant metastases is indicated by M_1 or M_0, respectively. If the presence of metastases cannot be assessed, the X suffix is used. M_1 can be subdivided further to include the anatomical area involved such as pulmonary (PUL), hepatic (HEP) or brain (BRA). With the five principal options for the T stage, four for the N stage and two for the M stage, there are at least 40 possible TNM options for each site and

Table 2.2 Current stage grouping for head and neck carcinoma

Stage	T	N	M
0	T_{is}	N_0	M_0
I	T_1	N_0	M_0
II	T_2	$N0_0$	M_0
III	T_3	N_0	M_0
	T_1	N_1	M_0
	T_2	N_1	M_0
	T_3	N_1	M_0
IVA*	T_4	N_0	M_0
	T_4	N_1	M_0
	Any T	N_2	M_0
IVB*	Any T	N_3	M_0
IVC*	Any T	Any N	M_1

UICC (1997).
*New inclusion.

more if the various subcategories are included. This is clearly too many for easy use. Even in the largest reported patient series, there will be some combinations with too few patients for meaningful comparison. Therefore, the different TNM categories are aggregated into stage groupings, designated by Roman numerals. In general terms, stage 0 disease is carcinoma *in situ*, stage I disease comprises a node-negative operable primary, stage II is an operable primary with operable nodes, stage III is disease considered inoperable by virtue of either an advanced primary tumour or advanced nodal disease and in stage IV disease, distant metastases are present (Table 2.2).

Despite the obvious value of staging, both in the management of individual patients, and for the grouping of patients in trials and reports of treatment, it does have its limitations. The most insidious of these is that attempts to increase the accuracy of staging lead to greater complexity, and hence paradoxically to more errors and an increased likelihood of non-compliance by the person responsible for staging. Advances in methods of collecting and recording data will hopefully reduce these errors.

Although the TNM system is the best that is currently available, problems exist with it that the surgeon should be aware.

Limitations of T staging

- Crude system
- Tumour size not related to prognosis
- Hard to assess clinical extent
- Debatable anatomical boundaries
- Inconsistencies
- Omissions

The TNM system provides head and neck surgeons with a common means of communication that is clinically orientated and based on pretreatment diagnostic studies. No one system is perfect and the criticisms that were aimed at the old classifications focused on the numerous subcategories that contained so few cases per category that statistical conclusions could not be drawn. In addition, there was lack of agreement on anatomical boundaries, the staging of cervical lymphadenopathy and the fact that host tumour responses and histopathological findings were not taken into account.

On reviewing the current handbook, changes have been made to classifications representing the nasopharynx, hypopharynx, supraglottic larynx, salivary glands and overall stage grouping. Emphasis is still placed on tumour size, although it is well recognized that this alone is of little prognostic significance in many head and neck carcinomas.

In addition, head and neck surgeons are aware of the difficulties in assessing the extent of primary disease in the oral cavity, pharynx, larynx or paranasal sinuses. For tumours of the oral cavity and oropharynx, the progressive assignment of levels T_1–T_4 is based on

the assumption that the size of the tumour can be readily measured. The increasing severity with T_4 is reserved for tumours of any size with evidence of deep invasion into muscle, bone or other adjacent structures. There can be little difficulty in establishing the difference between T_1 and T_4 disease but treatment planning and prognostic significance become less clear when the tumour measures between 1.5 and 3 cm. Bony invasion of the mandible demonstrated radiographically is classified as T_4 disease. The question arises, 'what constitutes bony erosion?'. The 2 cm lesion in the anterior floor of the mouth that involves the alveolar ridge and is adherent to the periosteum will not necessarily demonstrate bony erosion on radiographic evaluation. However, most surgeons agree that the underlying bone should be included in the surgical resection and therefore T_2 and T_4 disease may require essentially the same treatment. A similar problem is encountered in determining the depth of invasion of lesions into the soft tissue of the floor of the mouth. Superficial invasion of the sublingual area as opposed to invasion of the mylohyoid muscle can be subtle.

In contrast, the tumours of the larynx and hypopharynx are classified according to the number of anatomical surfaces involved, although a size measurement is now also included for the latter. However, in the past there has been considerable disagreement over the definition of the anatomical boundaries of these lesions and in particular of the larynx and hypopharynx. Such confusion still continues, although the current classification (UICC, 1997) now defines the lateral limits of the posterior pharyngeal wall (the apex of one pyriform sinus to another). In addition, the T_3 extent of a laryngeal lesion does not have the same grave consequences of a T_3 hypopharyngeal tumour with fixation of the hemilarynx. What then of a T_3 supraglottic tumour with fixation of the supraglottic larynx? Surely fixation of the latter suggests invasion of the soft tissues of the neck and should therefore qualify as T_4 disease.

Further prognostic staging of primary disease relates to the confusion surrounding the fact that bony involvement of the medial or inferior walls of the maxillary sinus receive only a T_2 classification but when oral carcinoma involves the antrum (erosion of the inferior wall of the sinus), the classification is T_4. Apparently, this disparity is based on the discrepancy in behaviour of the two separate bone involvements.

For salivary gland cancer, the presence of a facial paralysis now means automatic mandatory stage IV classification. Within the larynx, $T_4 N_0$ supraglottic cancer remains stage IV disease (albeit now-stage IVA), which now recognizes the favourable prognosis of this specific disease subset.

There is no mention of the cervical trachea as a subsite within the current lung staging system and this is surely an omission since it was included in previous UICC and AJCC manuals. The reason for its exclusion is that there is currently too little information on outcome to construct a realistic staging system (L. Sobin, personal communication). In addition, there is no mention in either system of a TNM classification for carcinoma of the external auditory meatus or middle ear, although one has been proposed in the past (see Chapter 21).

Limitations of N staging

- No mention of levels
- No immunological status
- No mention of extracapsular spread
- Bilateral involvement implies better prognosis than large nodes greater than 6 cm

The current staging system for cervical lymph nodes can also be criticized on the basis that it is not sophisticated enough to provide a description of the level of nodal involvement, which is a recognized prognostic indicator. Similarly, the immunological and pathological status of lymph nodes is not included, despite the fact that both the immunology of lymph nodes and the presence of extracapsular nodal invasion are important prognostic indicators. In addition, inclusion of bilateral or contralateral disease as N_2 is confusing since it implies a better prognosis than N_3 disease. The word fixation has, at least, been removed from previous nodal classifications since it was open to wide and varied subjective interpretation. However, it is worth noting that the present classification of N_3 disease includes nodes which are greater than 6 cm in size which are usually fixed. At present, the UICC defines four levels and their inclusion into TNM staging is not mandatory. However, the AJCC makes no mention of the lymph-node level, but recommends that the position of any lymph-node involvement should be recorded pictorially. The Memorial Sloan-Kettering Cancer Centre has used five levels of distribution for some years, these are included in standard American textbooks and it is likely that these five levels will be incorporated into a future classification to standardize cervical lymph-node level nomenclature (Fig. 2.1). A prospective study is surely needed to show whether the level of the node is more prognostic than its size and, if so, whether the difference is statistically significant.

All of the above inconsistencies make the head and neck a complicated region in which to apply a single concept of classification. However, the end result embraces the orderly description of disease with increasing size and extent and one which lends itself to incorporation into a staging system so that comparisons of treatment results might be meaningful. The current system, while fallible, is founded on sound principles and represents the combined work and experience of many physicians and surgeons who have spent years treating head and neck cancer. Any shortcomings or criticism of the system must reflect the complexity of the disease rather than any actual deficiencies within the staging classification, although it is interesting to note that of the five UK representatives on the current UICC Committee, not one is a head and neck surgeon.

Recognizing that current staging systems do not discriminate perfectly between good and poor prognostic categories, investigators have often created their own staging systems to report their own results. When reading the literature it is important to know which system is being used. It is perhaps in the case of nasopharyngeal carcinoma (NPC) that the greatest number of staging systems were, until recently, in operation. One recent study, for example, reported superior prognostic prediction by NPC using not only disease extent but also parameters such as the presence of cranial nerve involvement and the duration and number of other associated symptoms. Unless results are reported using an internationally recognized staging classification, it is virtually impossible to compare different series meaningfully and this is reflected in the recent changes in the TNM classification for nasopharyngeal carcinoma.

As mentioned previously, the anatomical site classification is for the most part satisfactory, showing a significant difference in survival between laryngeal and pharyngeal tumours, but the dual listing of the aryepiglottic fold in both categories presents problems with the occurrence of large tumours involving both sites. It would therefore appear to be better to classify these large tumours as being pharyngeal in origin as many are marginal lesions coming from the pharynx into the larynx rather than vice versa.

Finally, in recent years the advent of sophisticated imaging technology has made assessment much more accurate. Cases are often demonstrated to be more extensive than is clinically apparent, and are accordingly put into higher stages. Table 2.3 shows the results of treatment for a form of cancer, as staged by an older,

Table 2.3 Comparison of results of treatment for cancer using an old and a new staging system

Stage	Old staging systems			New staging systems		
	No. of patients	% Cured	No. cured	No. of patients	% Cured	No. cured
I	30	80	24	25	84	21
II	30	50	15	25	60	15
III	30	20	6	25	28	7
IV	10	10	1	25	12	3
All	100	46	46	100	46	46

less accurate clinical method and using modern sophisticated imaging techniques.

The cure rate for each stage of the disease is higher in those staged with the more modern technique, yet the overall cure rate for the entire cohort of patients, at 46%, is identical whichever staging system is used. This illustrates the phenomenon of stage migration, where apparently superior results are produced by the upstaging of patients. This is called stage creep and is sometimes referred to as the 'Will Rogers' phenomenon'. Will Rogers was an American wit from Oklahoma who stated that every time an Oklahoma man moves to California, the average IQ of both states improves.

While it would be inadvisable to contemplate major surgery before excluding the presence of distant metastases, in practice very few patients with squamous cell carcinoma have disease outside the head and neck at presentation. The converse situation, of a secondary lesion in the head and neck, should be considered when adenocarcinoma occurs in the cervical lymph nodes or salivary glands, and a primary lesion in the breast, bowel or chest should then be excluded.

Radiology

Important advances in radiological techniques over the last 15 years have established CT and magnetic resonance imaging (MRI) as the mainstay investigations in the preoperative work-up of patients with head and neck cancer. The types of investigation and their appropriate role in the evaluation at different sites are dealt with in Chapter 3. As a general rule, at present, not every patient with head and neck cancer will require a preoperative CT or MRI scan but the following guidelines may be helpful in the assessment of head and neck tumours as to whether or not to obtain a scan of the primary site, the neck or both of these areas.

Primary site

In the assessment of the primary tumour, an anatomical scan may be helpful to:

- assess the size of the primary lesion
- assess the neck at the same time
- stage the disease accurately
- assess the chest and abdomen when searching for an occult primary, a second primary or the presence of distant metastases
- confirm the diagnosis, e.g. glomus tumours
- aid assessment for conservation surgery
- stage and assess inaccessible tumours such as those in the maxillary sinus and the parapharyngeal space
- aid baseline and postoperative assessment in tumours that have a high risk of recurrence or recur slowly, i.e. adenoid cystic carcinoma.

The neck

Neck imaging (CT or MRI) should not be performed routinely but may be useful:

- if the neck is being scanned as part of the evaluation of the primary tumour
- if there is a high chance of occult disease (>20%) as an alternative to elective treatment
- in an N_{2a}, N_{2b} or N_3 neck, when the presence of deep fixation or contralateral neck disease may alter therapy from surgery to no surgical treatment at all
- in the short, stocky neck where clinical examination is difficult
- for restaging following previous surgery and irradiation.

Endoscopy

The patient with a head and neck tumour undergoes endoscopy for three reasons:

- To define the tumour accurately for staging and treatment planning
- To exclude a second synchronous primary tumour (or to try to find an occult primary)
- To obtain a biopsy.

It has been suggested that out-patient videolaryngoscopic examination can, in some hands, be adequate and this may be true in certain instances, particularly for small tumours if they have been biopsied elsewhere, but most otolaryngologists will require rigid endoscopy under a general anaesthesia to allow appropriate assessment and the necessary biopsies to be taken.

The surgeon tries to define the limits of the tumour in all directions and relate them to anatomical landmarks. It is often necessary to use adjunctive techniques such as the paediatric endoscope and angle telescopes to look at extension into the ventricle of the larynx and the subglottis. Next, a biopsy is taken from the viable part of the tumour, i.e. not from its centre, which may be necrotic, and not from its edge, which may only show dysplasia. A large piece is taken with cutting forceps that do not crush the tissue and placed directly into formalin: it should not be poked with needles or put in on a swab as these manoeuvres may distort the tissue. A biopsy of a tumour in the mouth is best taken with a knife; if lymphoma is suspected, the conventional method was to send half the specimen fresh and half in formalin. New immunological staining techniques now mean that fresh specimens are no longer required, but this will depend on local laboratory facilities. Finally, a drawing is made of the operative findings.

Synchronous primary

In general, the presence of a synchronous primary tumour is more likely than the presence of distant metastases. The cumulative incidence of second lesions following primary lesions at any head and neck site is up to 15%. Fewer than half will have a detectable synchronous primary lesion, almost half of which will be detected by a thorough ear, nose and throat examination. The pick-up rate of routine endoscopy at the time of primary diagnosis of synchronous primary upper aerodigestive tract carcinoma is thus likely to be in the order of 2–3%. While detection of such a tumour may modify the therapy of the original tumour, there is no substantial evidence about the effect on survival. Certainly, every patient must undergo a chest X-ray as most head and neck cancer patients are also high-risk candidates for lung cancer. In addition, it is now accepted practice in any patient having CT of the head and neck for staging advanced disease prior to definitive surgery to carry on and perform staging chest CT as well, to exclude both distant metastases and a second primary. The liver can also be assessed at the same time or alternatively some authors suggest liver ultrasound in high-risk patients.

The reported incidence of synchronous oesophageal primaries ranges from 0.7 to 1.7%. In some series, radiology is as accurate as endoscopy in detecting these lesions, while others find oesophagoscopy to be superior. There are few, if any, data on the later development of oesophageal neoplasia in patients with negative screening at the time of presentation, perhaps because in that situation there is no way to distinguish a missed synchronous lesion from a metachronous lesion. One small study of laryngopharyngo-oesophagectomy with gastric pull-up had a 17% incidence of oesophageal primaries detected at endoscopy, rising to 25% when the resected specimens were examined pathologically. All were small (and, by inference, potentially curable) lesions, the development of which was associated with a 33% incidence of Barrett's oesophagus. In another study, only four out of 69 patients were asymptomatic and had a normal chest X-ray when their synchronous or metachronous oesophageal or bronchial neoplasms were diagnosed. All four died from a variety of causes soon after therapy and the 5-year survival of 43 similar patients elsewhere (0.7% of those endoscoped) was just 7%. It is perhaps the generally poor status and outcome in patients with multiple primaries, as much as the cost ($1000 in the USA) or potential morbidity, which leads surgeons to question the value of triple endoscopy at presentation.

Fine-needle aspiration cytology

Fine-needle aspiration cytology (FNAC) is now the mainstay initial investigation for the patient who presents with cervical lymphadenopathy. There is an argument that there is no need to carry out the investigation on somebody who has a palpable lymph node in the presence of a biopsy-proven primary squamous cell carcinoma as, when surgical cure is anticipated, a management plan will usually include surgery on cervical lymph nodes. This is because even if the FNAC result were negative, it would

take a brave person to ignore such palpable nodes. However, as the FNAC result is obtained easily and quickly, it is usually performed so as to speed up management decisions.

Incisional biopsy of a lymph node is rarely justified. A squamous carcinoma may be implanted into the tissues, although recent studies have shown that as long as the correct form of management is instigated within 6 weeks of the incisional biopsy, prognosis is not affected. If the tumour is a lymphoma, the specimen will not give nodal architecture information if only a small piece is obtained and in vascular tumours the procedure can even be fatal! The former practice of Tru-cut needle core biopsies has now been superseded by FNAC. In certain instances, such as in the diagnosis of anaplastic carcinoma, adequate information may be obtained from an out-patient Tru-cut needle core biopsy if tissue cannot be obtained under general anaesthesia for various reasons.

FNAC of head and neck lesions increased at the same rate as the development of skills in exfoliative cervical cytology and in FNAC at other sites, particularly the breast. In the head and neck, it is of great value because of the multiplicity of accessible organs and the heterogeneous pathology encountered (Fig. 2.2). An early clue as to the tissue or tumour of origin may thus greatly influence the early management of a patient with head and neck swelling, reducing dramatically both patient

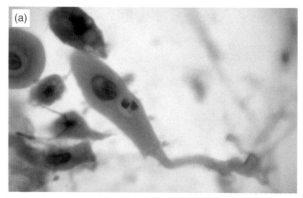

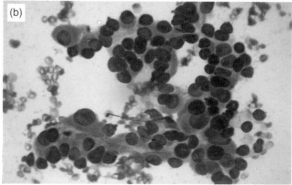

Figure 2.2 Fine-needle aspiration cytology showing (a) squamous cell carcinoma and (b) papillary carcinoma of the thyroid gland.

anxiety and resource consumption. The early detection of, for example, a goitre, lymphoma or adenocarcinoma will lead to a very different clinical approach from the detection of a pleomorphic adenoma or a squamous cell carcinoma. It is this very plethora, however, which makes head and neck FNAC particularly challenging. The involved cytologist needs to be skilled and committed. Under these circumstances the overall accuracy exceeds 92% with few false negatives and, very occasionally, a false-positive report. Although not every open biopsy is conclusive either, FNAC is clearly no substitute for histology, especially in the determination of nodal architecture in lymphoma, the malignant potential of a follicular thyroid tumour or of extracapsular spread in squamous carcinoma, or in the distinction of a pleomorphic from a monomorphic adenoma. Conversely, open biopsy is contraindicated in pleomorphic adenoma or nodal deposits of squamous carcinoma. All series report a small but appreciable false-negative rate (2%) and any suspicious lump should, therefore, be explored or otherwise investigated as appropriate.

FNAC is simple and cheap, as the only specialist input is that of the cytologist. Although ultrasound or CT-guided aspiration may be required in postnasal or parapharyngeal space lesions, most lumps are readily accessible. The financial savings compared with excisional biopsy in the USA are estimated to be between $1000 (out-patient) and $2000 (in-patient). One of the most common reasons for failure is the submission of inadequate material for diagnosis, in which case the best course is often simply to repeat the aspirate.

The necessary equipment should be kept in a small box ready for use and comprises a 20 ml syringe, 21 G needles, microscope slides, slide carriers, fixative spray and skin swabs. Air is expelled from a syringe and a needle attached. The lump is stabilized with the left hand as the needle enters (Fig. 2.3). Suction is applied, and while this is maintained, several radial passes are made within the substance of the swelling. The suction is released and the needle withdrawn through the skin. The tissue core should thus be retained within the needle itself, rather than transferred to the syringe. The needle is disconnected and 10 ml of air aspirated into the syringe. This is then reconnected it to the needle and the specimen expelled on to a slide. The yield may be improved by sending the needle separately in cytospin fluid so that further cells can be obtained, but the laboratory must be aware of the presence of a 'sharp'. A second slide is used to smear the specimen and this process repeated with further slides until the smear is of the right thickness. This can be judged only with experience and feedback from the cytologist. Both fixed and air-dried slides should be sent to the laboratory. The slides should be sprayed at once with alcohol fixative, if Papanicolaou or similar stains are to be used. In addition, they should be air-dried for May–Grünwald–Giemsa to be used. Blood in the specimen will cause a drying artefact but may not render it useless. If fluid is aspirated, this should be sent in a clean universal container so that a cytospin preparation can be obtained.

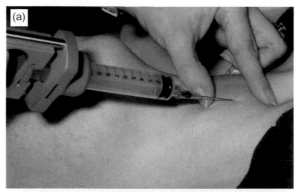

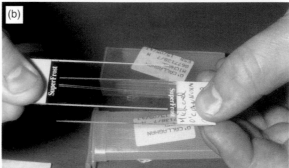

Figure 2.3 Technique for fine-needle aspiration cytology showing (a) aspiration of a solitary thyroid nodule and (b) smearing.

Several clinical and animal experiments have been performed to assess the safety of FNAC. Some report no cell seeding at all, while others have detected spillage of 10^2–10^4 cells but have also shown that the number of cells required to cause a seeded growth in humans is about twice that observed. Transperitoneal implantation of advanced retroperitoneal lesions has been reported in a small number of cases to have been followed by seeding but there are no reports of seeding of head and neck tumours, including parotid tumours. One fatality has, however, been reported, following aspiration of a carotid body tumour! Suspicion of this lesion is variously regarded either as a contra-indication or an indication for the use of a finer (23 G) needle.

Pathology

It is important to have a relationship with the head and neck pathologist, to discuss regularly cases at monthly or more frequent meetings and to record details in the agreed and systematic manner. Specimens should be pinned out and details relating to the primary and nodal disease recorded accordingly. It is important to record the type of growth (histology) along with the pathological TNM stage and overall stage. Pathological tumour size should be recorded along with tumour thickness, which is important in tumours such as the oral cavity and melanoma, and the margins relating to microscopic resection should be commented on. Multifocality of the tumours should also be recorded, along with the presence or absence of perineural, vascular, lymphatic and bone invasion. Differentiated thyroid tumours should be reported as thyroglobulin positive or negative. Cervical lymph nodes should be recorded on a diagram relating to the levels involved and the report should include which nodes were sampled and the number of nodes sampled, along with the number of positive nodes found and their pathological site and whether or not there was extracapsular spread. This report should form part of the minimum data set (Appendix 2.3). The allocation of a pN_0 classification to a neck dissection must satisfy the following criteria. Histological examination of a selective neck dissection specimen will ordinarily include six or more lymph nodes while histological examination of a radical or modified radical neck dissection will ordinarily include 10 or more lymph nodes.

Follow-up policies

Follow-up of patients treated for cancer is performed for several reasons which are of different importance. Some of these are for the direct benefit of individual patients, whereas others are for the benefit of future cohorts of patients. Possible reasons for follow-up are given below.

- To monitor the primary tumour site and nodal areas after completion of initial radical therapy. This has the aim of detecting residual disease or relapse at an early stage when it is still possible to institute potentially curative salvage treatment.
- To ensure that the patient is being successfully rehabilitated with regard, for example, to speech and swallowing after radical treatments which may have interfered with normal head and neck physiology.
- To reassure the patient that the team which treated them still cares about their progress and wants to know if any problems develop. Patients can be educated about which symptoms should lead to clinical review earlier than planned. Advice given about secondary prevention strategies such as smoking cessation can be reinforced and monitored.
- To prevent treatable morbidity such as dental decay and hypothyroidism before it becomes clinically significant by the monitoring and early detection of problems.
- To obtain accurate data about important outcome measures for the purposes of medical audit and clinical governance, these include local and regional control, treatment-related morbidity, second malignant neoplasms, functional impairment and survival.
- To provide training opportunities for trainees in surgery and oncology and the professions allied to medicine.

Reasons for follow-up

- To detect relapse and institute salvage treatment
- For speech and swallowing rehabilitation
- For patient support and education
- For prevention and treatment of late morbidity
- To collect outcome data systematically
- For training

In patients with head and neck squamous carcinoma, the appropriate frequency of routine follow-up varies, depending on several of the factors mentioned above, but principally on the likelihood of relapse and the possibility of salvage treatment.

For example, a patient with T_2N_0 cancer of the anterior tongue treated with brachytherapy alone, without prophylactic neck irradiation or surgery, has a significant likelihood of nodal relapse which may be subsequently cured by neck dissection if detected early, but which might become inoperable if there is a 3-month delay. Similarly a patient with early laryngeal cancer treated by radiotherapy alone requires frequent follow-up so that salvage surgery can be performed without delay in the event of local failure.

In such patients, follow-up should be monthly in the first year after completion of treatment, 2-monthly in the second year, 3-monthly in the third year, then 6-monthly to 5 years (Table 2.4). Subsequently, annual follow-up may be deemed appropriate, but in many cases discharge to the care of the general practitioner is a reasonable alternative.

By contrast, a patient who has undergone composite resection of a T_2N_0 oropharyngeal cancer with postoperative radiotherapy to the primary site and both sides of the neck requires less frequent follow-up to detect relapse, as there is very little chance of effective salvage. Nonetheless, follow-up is still necessary to monitor deglutition, nutrition and dentition.

In this case, an appropriate follow-up schedule might be 6-weekly for the first year, 3-monthly for the second year and then 6-monthly to 5 years, with optional annual follow-up after that.

Table 2.4 Follow-up frequency after treatment for squamous cancer of the head and neck

Time after treatment	Good possibility of successful salvage of local or nodal relapse	Little chance of successful salvage
First year	Monthly	Six-weekly
Second year	Two-monthly	Three-monthly
Third year	Three-monthly	Six-monthly
Fourth year	Six-monthly	Six-monthly
Fifth year	Six-monthly	Six-monthly
After 5 years	Annually or discharge	Annually or discharge

Different follow-up plans may be more appropriate for patients with rare tumours such as lymphoma or sarcoma. In patients who have a thyroid cancer, follow-up is usually lifelong as recurrences can occur many years following initial treatment.

References and further reading

American Joint Committee (1993) *Manual for Staging of Cancer*, 4th edn, J.B. Lippincott, Philadelphia, PA.

BAHNO (1999) National minimum and advisory head and neck cancer data sets, *The British Association of Head and Neck Oncologists*.

Hermanek P. and Sobin L. H., eds (1992) *Union Internationale Contre le Cancer*, 4th edn, 2nd rev., Springer, Berlin.

The Royal College of Pathologist (1998) Minimum data set for head and neck carcinoma histopathology reports.

UICC (1997) International Union against Cancer. *TNM Classification of Malignant Tumours*, 5th edn, Wiley-Liss, New York.

Watkinson J. C. (1991) Some aspects of imaging squamous cell carcinoma using technetium 99m (V) Dimercaptusuccinic acid, MS Thesis, University of London.

Watkinson J. C. (1993) The clinically N₀ neck – investigation and treatment (Editorial), *Clin Otolaryngol* 18, 443–5.

Watkinson J. C., Johnston D., Jones N., Coady M., Laws D., Allen S. and Hibbert J. (1990) The reliability of palpation in the assessment of tumours, *Clin Otolaryngol* 15, 405–9.

Appendix 2.1: Standard diagrams to document the site, size and extension of a head and neck primary tumour and/or cervical metastases

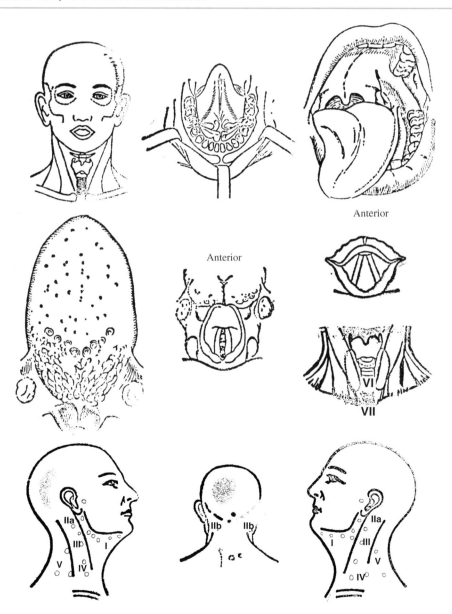

Appendix 2.2: British Association of Head and Neck Oncologists (BAHNO) National Minimum Data Set (1999)

1. Patient registration details

NHS Number: .... Hospital code: .... Hospital number: ....

Surname: .... Forename: .... Name at birth: ....

Date of birth: .... Sex: (*M=male, F=Female, U=Unknown*): ....

Address at time of diagnosis: ....

Current postcode address at diagnosis: ....

■ Marital status at diagnosis: ....
  (*1=single, 2=married, 3=first marriage, 4=re-marriage, 5=divorced, 6=widowed, 7=separated, 8=cohabiting, 9=unknown*)

■ Ethnic origin: ....
  (*0=White, 1=Black Caribbean, 2=Black African, 3=Indian, 4=Pakistani, 5=Bangladeshi, 6=Chinese, 7=Black other (non-mixed origin), 8=Black other mixed, 9=unknown*)

■ History of non-head and neck cancer

  Site: ....
  (*0=none, C50=breast, C34=lung and bronchus, C18=colon, C20=rectum, C16=stomach, C15=oesophagus, C67=bladder, C61=prostate, C62=testis, C71=brain, C81=Hodgkin's lymphoma, C83=non-Hodgkin's, C96=malignant neoplasm lymphoid haemopoeitic & related tissue, 99=unknown*)

■ Year of diagnosis: ....

2. Referral (first presentation only)

Date first symptom: .... Date primary referral: ....

Date first seen by Hospital: ....

■ Tumour Event (New section to be completed for each primary, if recurrence only those items marked with '*'):

  *primary head and neck tumour number
  (*1=first primary, 2=second primary, 3=third primary, 4=fourth primary, 5=unknown primary*): ....

  *Current event (*1=original, 2=recurrence, 9=unknown*): ....

  *Type of recurrence *1=local, 2=regional, 3=distant, 9=unknown*): ....

  *Date of diagnosis or Date of recurrence: ....

■ How diagnosis reached: ....
  (*1=death certificate, 2=clinical, 3=X-ray, 4=scan, 5=exploratory, 6=marker, 7=cytology, 8=haematology, 9=histology, 10=histology of mets, 11=postmortem, 12=other, 98=not applicable, 99=not known*)

■ Treating 'lead' surgeon or oncologist: ....

■ Previous treatment for current head and neck cancer elsewhere? (*Y=Yes, N=No, U=Unknown*): ....

■ Performance status at presentation: ....
  (*0=fully active, 1=restricted in heavy activity, 2=ambulatory and capable of self-care, 3=capable of only limited self-care, 4=completely disabled*)

- (Site of Primary (ICD-10)): ....
- Laterality (side of tumour): ....
  (*1=left, 2=right, 3=bilateral, 4=midline, 8=not applicable, 9=unknown*)
- Final pre-treatment: T: ....   N: ....   M: ....   Stage overall: ....
- Biopsy histology: ....
- Differentiation: ....
  (*1=well-differentiated, 2=moderately diferentiated, 3=poorly differentiated, 4=undfferentiated/anaplastic, 5=unknown*)
- Date clinical management planned: ....
- Treatment offered: ....
  (*C=curative, P=palliative, R=refusal of treatment by patient, U=unknown*)

  *Planned treatment modality: ....
  (*1=primary surgery, 2=primary radiotherapy, 3=planned combination therapy (pre-op RXT and surgery), 3=planned combination therapy (surgery post-op RXT), 5=chemotherapy in trial, 6=chemotherapy non trial, 7=supportive therapy, 8=other, 99=unknown*)

3. Surgery and post surgery pathology details

Date surgery: ....   Date discharge: ....

Consultant surgeon(s) responsible for case: ....

- Main surgical procedure: ....
- Second surgical procedure: ....
  Third procedure: ....   Fourth procedure: ....
  Fifth procedure: ....   Sixth procedure: ....

Date of pathology: ....   Number positive nodes: ....

- Surgical specimen pathology: ....
- Differentiation: ....
  (*1=well-differentiated, 2=moderately differentiated, 3=poorly differentiated, 4=undifferentiated/anaplastic, 9=unknown*)
- TNM pathological surgery: T: .....   N: ....   M: ....   Stage overall: ....
- Tumour thickness (mm): ....
- Margins (microscopic): ....
  (*1=clear/adequate (>5 mm), 2=close/marginal (1 to 5 mm), 3=inadequate (<1 mm), 4=severe dysplasia at margin, 9=unknown*)
- Invasive front: ....
  (*1=cohesive, 2=non-cohesive, 9=unknown*)
- Extracapsular spread of lymph nodes: ....
  (*0=none, 1=extracapsular spread, 9=not stated*)
- Perineural invasion: ....
  (*1=no perineural invasion, 2=yes perineural invasion, 8=not applicable, 9=not known*)
- Vascular/lymphatic invasion: ....
  (*1=no vascular/lymphatic invasion, 2=yes vascular/lymphatic invasion present, 8=not applicable, 9=not known*)
- Bone/cartilage invasion: ....
  (*1=no bone/cartilage invasion, 2=yes bone/cartilage invasion present, 8=not applicable 9=not known*)
- Extrathyroid invasion: ....
  (*1=no extrathyroid invasion, 2=yes extrathyroid invasion, 8=not applicable, 9=not known*)

4. Radiotherapy details

Start date: .... Finish date: ....

■ Consultant oncologist responsible for case: ....

■ Hospital for radiotherapy: ....

■ Site treated: ....
   (*P=primary, N=nodes, C=primary and nodes T-adjuvant/prophylactic, M=metastases, O=other*)

5. Chemotherapy

Start date first cycle: .... Start date last cycle: ....

■ Hospital treatment: ....

■ Oncologist: ....

■ Course (no cycles) given: ....

6. Performance status and quality of life

■ Performance status at one year from date of diagnosis: ....
   (*0=fully active, 1=restricted in heavy activity, 2=ambulatory and capable self-care, 3=capable of only limited self-care, 4=completely disabled*)

7. Current Status

■ Vital status (*A= alive D=dead*): ....

■ Current disease status: ....
   (*1=no evidence of head and neck cancer, 2=head and neck cancer present (inc. mets), 3=non-head and neck cancer present, 4=immediately post treatment, 5=status unknown*)

■ Date last known alive or date of death: ....

■ Current follow-up status: ....
   (*1=under follow-up, 2=lost to follow-up, 3=discharged*)

■ Date gone abroad: ....

Form completed by: .... Date: ....

Appendix 2.3: Head and Neck Carcinoma Histopathology Report (National Minimum Data Set). Royal College of Pathologists, November 1998

Surname:	Forenames: ....
Date of birth:	Sex: ....
Hospital:	Hospital No.: ....
NHS No.:	Date of receipt: ....
Date of reporting:	Report No.: ....
Pathologist:	Surgeon: ....

1. Primary tumour

■ Size: ....

■ Subsites(s): ....

■ Right ☐   Left ☐   Midline ☐

■ Type of resection: ....

■ Maximum diameter (mm): ....

■ **Histological type:**   squamous carcinoma ☐

   Other/subtype: ....

■ **Differentiation:**

	well	☐
	moderate	☐
	poor	☐
Invasive front	cohesive	☐
	non-cohesive	☐

■ Clinical TNM stages: ....

■ T: ....   N: ....   M: ....

■ Previous radiotherapy: Yes ☐ No ☐ Unknown ☐

■ Previous chemotherapy: Yes ☐ No ☐ Unknown ☐

■ Distance from invasive tumour to:

   Muscosal margin (mm): ....

   Deep margin (mm): ....

	Yes	No
Vascular invasion	☐	☐
Nerve invasion	☐	☐
Bone/cartilage invasion	☐	☐
Severe dysplasia present	☐	☐
Severe dysplasia at margin	☐	☐

2. Neck dissection

■ **Right neck dissection:** Yes ☐ No ☐

   Comprehensive ☐   Selective ☐

   Node level present: 1 2 3 4 5 6 other

   Total number of nodes: ....

   Number positive nodes: ....

   Levels with metastasis: 1 2 3 4 5 6 other

   Largest metastasis (mm): ....

   Extracapsular spread: Yes ☐ No ☐

   Levels with ECS: ....

■ **Left neck dissection:** Yes ☐ No ☐

   Comprehensive ☐   Selective ☐

   Node level present: 1 2 3 4 5 6 other

   Total number of nodes: ....

   Number positive nodes: ....

   Levels with metastasis: 1 2 3 4 5 6 other

   Largest metastasis (mm): ....

   Extracapsular spread: Yes ☐ No ☐

   Levels with ECS: ....

3. Comments/additional information

....

....

....

4. Summary of pathological data

■ Tumour site: ....

■ New primary ☐ Recurrence ☐ Not known ☐

■ Tumour type: ....

■ Resection of primary tumour:...............................

   Clear ☐   Close ☐   Involved ☐

■ pTNM stage: pT: ....   pN: ....   pM: ....

■ SNOMED CODES:

   T: ....   M: ....

   T: ....   M: ....

Signature: ....   Date: ....

Radiology

'X-rays are only as good as the doctor who requests
them and the radiologist who reports them'

Introduction

Many of the exciting advances in medicine have
occurred in imaging. In some cases, these advances have
overtaken the available treatment options for many of the
conditions under discussion in this book. Because of this,
a patient should only usually be imaged if it helps with
their management, or there is some other potential gain.

Imaging techniques that utilize ionizing radiation carry
with them a potential increased lifetime risk of developing
another cancer and this should be kept in mind when
selecting which imaging technique to use. If the patient
is young and/or is likely to undergo multiple imaging
examinations during the course of his or her illness and
follow-up, then it may be more appropriate to choose an
imaging modality such as magnetic resonance imaging
(MRI) or ultrasound (US). Knowledge of the normal
anatomy as displayed by cross-sectional imaging
techniques is the key to understanding the imaging of
head and neck cancer. A combination of tumour
localization, history and imaging appearances can sometimes allow a definitive diagnosis to be made. Often, however, imaging is used to aid the clinician in the
subsequent management of the patient. It can be used to
act as a guide for biopsy or fine-needle aspiration cytology
(FNAC) to obtain a histological diagnosis.

Plain films

A chest X-ray is the most common examination request-
ed. It is used to assess the head and neck patient as part
of the pre-anaesthetic assessment but should also be
performed to exclude co-existing bronchogenic carcinoma, the presence of pulmonary metastatic disease or other
co-existent pathology. Some authors recommend that
computed tomographic (CT) scanning of the chest should
be performed as part of the preoperative staging of
patients with head and neck cancer since only approximately 30% of malignant tumours detected on CT are
visible on chest radiographs.

Retrosternal extension of a thyroid goitre may be
apparent as a superior mediastinal mass which may
displace or narrow the trachea. Thoracic inlet views
may be obtained to further assess tracheal narrowing, but
respiratory flow loops have been shown to be more
sensitive than plain films (Gittoes *et al.*, 1996).

Contrast studies

The barium swallow examines the oesophagus. The
pharynx and upper oesophagus are examined using either
videofluoroscopy – or cinefluoroscopy. Contrast examinations are able to assess the act of swallowing by analysing
the following features:

- tongue movement
- soft palate elevation
- epiglottic tilt
- laryngeal closure
- pharyngo-oesophageal segment (cricopharyngeal
  opening) and pharyngeal peristalsis.

The barium swallow can be used to assess oesophageal
motility and double-contrast films can be used to demonstrate morphology. Barium should not be used as a contrast agent when aspiration is present or suspected, or when
anastomoses are being assessed postoperatively since aspiration can be fatal. Malignant pharyngeal and oesophageal
tumours can be diagnosed by their irregular narrowing of
the lumen associated with mucosal destruction, ulceration
and shouldering. The length of the tumour can be measured, which is important for staging hypopharyngeal
tumours and planning operative intervention for possible
free jejunal transfer as well as radiotherapy field planning.
Previous radiotherapy, caustic ingestion and dermatological
disorders can cause smooth oesophageal narrowing.

Ultrasound

Ultrasound (US) does not use ionizing radiation. It is
readily available in most hospitals but is an operator-

dependent technique. The ultrasound beam will not readily penetrate bone, cartilage or gas, making it an inappropriate technique for staging many primary head and neck cancers. The US beam is also attenuated (weakened) as it passes through the tissues, making examination of fat necks and deep structures (e.g. the deep lobe of the parotid gland) more difficult. It is extremely useful in differentiating solid from cystic mass lesions.

An assessment can be made of the margins and texture of neck masses, which may give information about the nature of a palpated neck mass. This appears to be particularly useful in the evaluation of neck nodes.

Doppler US is flow sensitive and can be used to evaluate the neck vessels and relationship of masses to important vascular structures. It may also give information regarding the vascularity of neck masses.

Computed tomography

Computed tomography (CT) uses ionizing radiation. It is now readily available in most hospitals and is the imaging modality most used to stage head and neck malignancy. Spiral CT scanners image while the patient is moved through the gantry obtaining a three-dimensional (3D) volume block of data. These scanners are faster than conventional rotate–translate scanners and a spiral CT scanner will be able to obtain an examination of the neck in under 1 min. Axial images are obtained with the patient supine. On most machines, the gantry of the CT scanner has a maximum tilt of 25°. This enables scan acquisition in a plane perpendicular (or parallel) to the area of interest in many instances. For example, scanning patients with suspected laryngeal cancer is ideally performed with CT sections obtained parallel to the vocal cords. It may be necessary for the patient to extend the neck in either a supine or prone position to obtain direct coronal scanning of the skull base in patients with nasopharyngeal carcinoma, the hard palate and paranasal sinuses. The gantry may also be tilted to avoid artefacts from dental amalgam.

All studies should be performed with the administration of an intravenous contrast agent. This allows identification of rim enhancement in pathological nodes and increases the definition of the primary tumour.

The scans should be performed as quickly as possible to maximize vascular opacification and, if present, tumour enhancement. Spiral CT is the preferred technique, allowing rapid scan acquisition, reducing patient motion artefact and, if appropriate, facilitating multiplanar scan reformats.

CT scans may be displayed on different settings. Soft tissue and bone settings are routinely used in the head and neck. Scans of important bony or cartilaginous structures, for example, the laryngeal cartilages in a patient with suspected laryngeal carcinoma, should also be reconstructed using a bony algorithm which is helpful for demonstrating bone and cartilage invasion. The pulmonary parenchyma should be reviewed at lung window settings if the chest is also being examined.

CT has disadvantages in comparison with MRI. Artefact from dental amalgam can severely degrade the image of the oral cavity. Beam hardening artefact can also occur from bony surfaces. The dose of ionizing radiation must always be taken into consideration when an imaging modality is chosen and in young patients in whom repeated scans are necessary, MRI is to be preferred. The speed of acquisition with CT minimizes motion artefact from swallowing and respiration and CT has a superior spatial resolution.

It has been shown that the addition of CT will improve staging of laryngeal and hypopharyngeal cancer compared with clinical evaluation (CE) which alone was 52% accurate; CT alone was 68% accurate while combined CE–CT evaluation was 84% accurate (Thabet *et al.*, 1996).

Magnetic resonance imaging

MRI does not use ionizing radiation but requires a very homogeneous magnetic field which in most clinical scanners ranges from 0.5 to 1.5 Tesla. It also requires radiofrequency waves.

These conditions impose some limitations on which patients may be examined by this technique. Claustrophobic patients may not be able to tolerate the long bore of the conventional magnet although some open systems are now available. Patients with ferromagnetic surgical clips, embolization coils, etc., may not be suitable and MRI is contraindicated in patients who have cardiac pacemakers.

MRI has superior soft-tissue contrast to CT and allows multiplanar imaging. The nasopharynx is an area where both these qualities are useful. MRI may be able to identify small nasopharyngeal masses not seen on clinical examination and sagittal scanning is a good imaging plane to assess skull base extension. Although MRI images the bone marrow very effectively, it will not (unlike CT) examine cortical bone. CT also has superior spatial resolution and is generally a faster technique, which may be very important in a patient with a compromised airway.

The most common sequences used in head and neck imaging are T_1-weighted spin echo (SE), T_2 weighted SE and short tao inversion recovery (STIR) sequence. The T_1-weighted SE sequence displays anatomy well with fluid-containing structures, e.g. cerebrovascular fluid appearing of low signal intensity, i.e. black, and fat appearing of high signal intensity, i.e. white.

The T_2-weighted sequence displays fluid-containing structures as high signal intensity. The STIR sequence suppresses the high signal intensity from fat and fluid-containing structures are of high signal intensity. This allows easy recognition of fluid. Many tumours have a higher water content than normal tissue and have surrounding peritumoral oedema. This is readily displayed on the STIR sequence.

Intravenous gadolinium contrast agent may be administered to look for pathological enhancement of

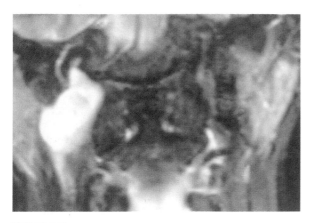

Figure 3.1 Coronal STIR MRI scan revealing abnormally high signal intensity and a recurrent tumour extending up into the foramen lacerum on the right.

involved nodes. It is useful for assessing perineural spread of the primary tumour. Postcontrast scans are obtained using T_1-weighted images. Frequency selective fat suppression should be used on these sequences following intravenous contrast since both fat and gadolinium are of high signal. MRI is better than CT for the assessment of perineural and intracranial tumour spread (Parker and Harnsberger, 1991).

Perineural tumour is seen as perineural thickening and enhancement with widening of the affected foramen (Fig. 3.1). The most commonly affected nerves are the mandibular and maxillary divisions of the trigeminal nerve and the facial nerve.

Nuclear medicine

Nuclear medicine techniques use ionizing radiation. Spatial resolution and anatomical detail are poorer than with other cross-sectional techniques but, whereas US, CT and MRI generally depict morphology, these investigations predominantly demonstrate physiology.

Traditionally, iodine-based radioisotopes have been used in the assessment of thyroid disease. Functioning thyroid nodules will take up iodine-123 (^{123}I) and iodine-131 (^{131}I) can be used to treat iodine-avid differentiated thyroid tumours. Radioisotope bone scanning using the conventional agent technetium-99m (^{99m}Tc) methylene disphonate and ^{99m}Tc dimercaptosuccinic acid (DMSA) for medullary thyroid cancer can both be used to investigate suspected bony metastatic disease. Positive scans using [^{99m}Tc]MDP will also be seen in the presence of infection and radiotherapy-induced osteonecrosis.

Positron emission tomography (PET) is a relatively new imaging technique based predominantly on glucose analogue uptake and metabolism in tumours using fluorine labelled deoxyglucose (^{18}FDG). It may improve the detection of head and neck cancer, especially recurrent disease, but lacks anatomical detail. Coregistration may be performed with CT or MRI to improve this. It may also be

useful in the search for an unknown primary in patients who present with malignant neck nodes. It appears to have a role in the differentiation of postoperative change or radiation fibrosis from recurrent or residual tumour.

Specific sites

The following sites can be imaged:

- larynx
- oral cavity (lip, floor of mouth, tongue, gingiva and hard palate, retromolar trigone)
- pharynx (nasopharynx, oropharynx, hypopharynx)
- neck nodes
- paranasal sinuses
- salivary glands
- parapharyngeal space
- thyroid.

Larynx

The supraglottic larynx extends from the tongue base and valleculae to the laryngeal ventricle. It contains the epiglottis, aryepiglottic folds, false vocal cords, laryngeal ventricle and the arytenoid processes of the arytenoid cartilages. The glottis consists of the true vocal cords and the anterior and posterior commissure. The subglottis extends from the undersurface of the true vocal cords to base of the cricoid cartilage.

Scans of this region should be performed parallel to the plane of the true vocal cords. The slice thickness should not exceed 5 mm and should preferably be less than this.

The key to the imaging of this region is the understanding of the anatomy of the pre-epiglottic and paraglottic fat spaces. These are readily seen on both CT and MRI but are major clinical blind spots.

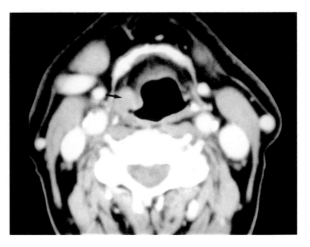

Figure 3.2 Axial contrast-enhanced CT scan. The C-shaped area of normal fat in the pre-epiglottic space can be seen. On the right side, there is abnormal soft tissue from submucosal spread of a tongue base lesion down inferiorly into the right paraglottic fat (arrow).

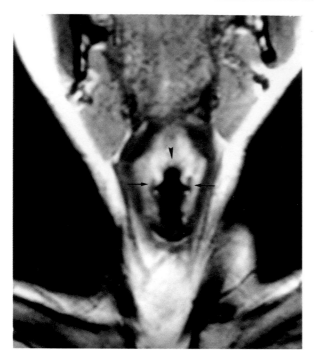

Figure 3.3 Coronal T$_1$-weighted MRI scan in a normal patient demonstrating the paired paraglottic fat spaces (arrows) which are of high signal intensity on this T$_1$-weighted sequence. Superiorly, they merge with the pre-epiglottic fat (arrowhead).

The pre-epiglottic fat space is a C-shaped area of fat lying anterior to the epiglottis (Fig. 3.2). The paraglottic fat spaces are paired fatty areas lateral to the true and false cords. They end at the undersurface of the true cords and merge superiorly with the pre-epiglottic space (Fig. 3.3). These regions are not visible on endoscopy and deep spread of disease may occur here. The addition of CT and/or MRI will improve staging accuracy in assessing submucosal spread into these areas and into the extralaryngeal soft tissues.

Detection of thyroid cartilage involvement is important in the staging of laryngeal cancer. It is more common in glottic than supraglottic cancers. Variable ossification of the cartilage makes the radiological staging difficult. It is much easier if the cartilage is ossified. The normal marrow within the cartilage has a high signal intensity on T$_1$-weighted SE images owing to its fat content. Tumour will have a lower signal intensity. The higher fluid content of tumour gives rise to a high signal within the cartilage on STIR images. If the cartilage is not ossified, cartilage will be seen as a low or intermediate signal on T$_2$-weighted scans, with tumour remaining of high signal. MRI is slightly better than CT, with a reported sensitivity of 89–94%, specificity of 74–88% and negative predictive value of 94–96% (Castelijns *et al.*, 1988; Becker *et al.*, 1995; Zbaren *et al.*, 1996). For practical purposes, however (i.e. availability, speed and spatial resolution), CT continues to be used to evaluate and stage patients with

endoscopically proven laryngeal carcinoma. A recent study (Becker *et al.*, 1997) found that sclerosis of a laryngeal cartilage was the most sensitive criterion for invasion for all laryngeal cartilages (Fig. 3.4) but was not very specific since it can also be seen as a response to reactive inflammation.

The presence of extralaryngeal tumour with cartilage erosion or lysis (Fig. 3.5a, b) was the most specific indicator of invasion in the thyroid cartilage (sensitivity 71% and specificity 83%; negative predictive value 89%). In practice, it may be worthwhile staging with CT and if laryngeal cartilage invasion is uncertain, then a tailored MRI can be performed. Neither CT nor MRI can differentiate between radionecrosis and tumour following radiotherapy (Briggs *et al.*, 1993).

Supraglottic carcinoma

Imaging issues: supraglottic carcinoma

■ Pre-epiglottic space and extension into tongue base
■ Paraglottic space
■ Thyroid cartilage involvement

Tumours involving the epiglottis tend to grow circumferentially with extension into the pre-epiglottic space. More advanced tumours may spread into the tongue base and below into the paraglottic space. Tumours of the aryepiglottic fold tend to grow exophytically with spread into paraglottic space (Fig. 3.6) and the fixed portion of the epiglottis.

Lesions involving the false cords and laryngeal ventricle spread submucosally into the paraglottic space. More

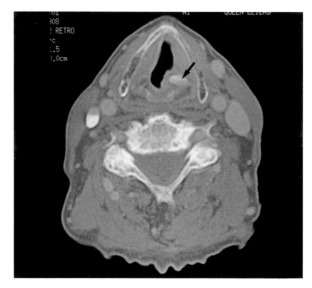

Figure 3.4 Axial contrast-enhanced CT scan through the true cords displayed on bone window settings. The left vocal cord tumour has extended posteriorly. The left arytenoid cartilage is sclerotic (arrow) and added soft tissue is seen on its medial aspect. The right arytenoid cartilage can also be seen but does not appear sclerotic.

advanced lesions may spread inferiorly to involve the true vocal cords and into the subglottis. This may be demonstrated using coronal MRI or reformatted CT.

Glottis

> **Imaging issues: glottic carcinoma**
>
> ◾ Subglottic or supraglottic submucosal extension (paraglottic and pre-epiglottic spaces)
> ◾ Extension outside the larynx
> ◾ Thyroid cartilage destruction

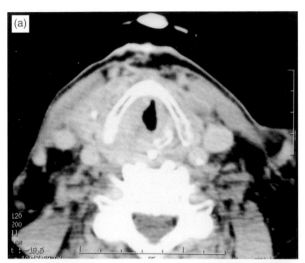

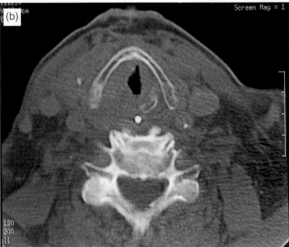

Figure 3.5 (a) Axial contrast-enhanced CT scan through the glottis displayed on soft-tissue settings revealing abnormal soft tissue on the right extending anteriorly to involve the right paraglottic fat space with added soft tissue extending posteriorly to involve the pharynx. Soft tissue is seen extending into the soft tissues of the neck and is seen on the external aspect of the right thyroid cartilage lamina. (b) The same CT section displayed on bone window settings revealing destruction of the posterior aspect of the right thyroid lamina with a mixture of lysis and sclerosis.

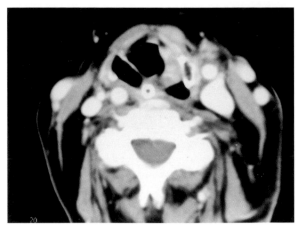

Figure 3.6 Axial contrast-enhanced CT scan demonstrating a supraglottic tumour with involvement of the left aryepiglottic fold. Anteriorly, the abnormal soft tissue has extended towards the epiglottis with extension laterally into the paraglottic fat.

Glottic tumours may spread anteriorly to the involve the anterior commissure (Fig. 3.7) and beyond. The normal anterior commissure should not measure more than 1 mm in thickness. Tumour may then spread into the contralateral vocal cord or submucosally into the pre-epiglottic space, or directly invade the thyroid cartilage. Posterior spread to involve the posterior commissure may be identified with thickening. Sclerosis of the arytenoid or cricoid cartilages may be due to either abutting or invading tumour (Fig. 3.4). Inferior extension in the subglottis should be carefully looked for. If the lesion reaches the upper margin of the cricoid, a vertical hemilaryngectomy cannot be performed.

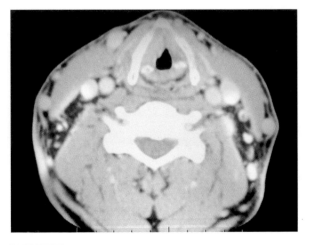

Figure 3.7 Axial contrast-enhanced CT scan demonstrating a tumour involving the right vocal cord with extension into the paraglottic fat. Anteriorly, there is thickening of the commissure indicative of tumour spread across the midline.

Evaluation of the postsurgical larynx may be difficult with imaging. There may be thickening of the mucosa which is seen overlying the arytenoid, as well as other distortions including dilatation of the lateral hypopharyngeal recess (Maroldi *et al.*, 1997).

MR imaging and clinical assessment have been compared with outcome following radiotherapy. Cord mobility, tumour volume and cartilage invasion have been shown to be important prognostic indicators (Castelijns *et al.*, 1996). Three risk groups may be recognized using the findings from pretreatment CT if radiotherapy is being considered.

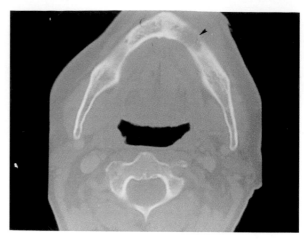

Figure 3.8 Axial CT scan of the mandible displayed on bone window settings showing bone erosion and involvement (arrowhead) from an alveolar ridge tumour.

Risk groups for radiotherapy recurrence

- The **best** prognosis is seen with a small tumour volume of less than 3.5 cm³ with sclerosis involving one or no cartilage
- A **moderate** risk group is one with a small tumour volume and sclerosis of two laryngeal cartilages or a volume greater than 3.5 cm³ with one or no cartilage sclerosis
- The **poor** risk group has a high tumour volume and ipsilateral arytenoid and adjacent cricoid cartilage sclerosis

---

The patients in the moderate and poor risk groups are at higher risk for recurrence following radiotherapy and should be closely observed (Mendenhall *et al.*, 1997). Abnormal signal intensity in the thyroid cartilage combined with a tumour volume of >5 cm³ in the untreated patient also appears to confer a worse prognosis following radiotherapy (Castelijns *et al.*, 1996).

Following radiotherapy, symmetric thickening of the epiglottis, aryepiglottic folds and false cords will occur. The paralaryngeal fat will have an increased attenuation due to oedema, and thickening of the anterior and posterior commissures is also a regular feature (Mukherji *et al.*, 1994).

Identification of recurrence may be difficult clinically as well as with CT or MRI. A mass greater than 10 mm spreading beyond the larynx, thickening of the anterior commissure or erosion of residual cartilage may be seen with recurrent tumour (Maroldi *et al.*, 1997). PET with labelled fluorodeoxyglucose (^{18}FDG) appears to be useful in differentiating postradiotherapy and surgical change from recurrent tumour (Greven *et al.*, 1994; McGuirt *et al.*, 1995; Wong *et al.*, 1997).

Oral cavity

The oral cavity is made up of the lip, upper and lower gingiva, buccal mucosa, hard palate, floor of the mouth and oral portion (anterior two-thirds) of the tongue.

Imaging issues

- Objective size of tumour (T1–T3)
- Invasion of maxillary antrum, pterygoid muscles or tongue base

---

Lip

Imaging has little role to play in early lesions which may not be distinguishable from the normal obicularis oris muscle. The margins of more advanced infiltrative lesions may be defined more readily with imaging.

Bone erosion which usually occurs along the buccal surface of the mandibular or maxillary alveolar ridge is best detected with CT (Fig. 3.8). The presence of bone erosion upstages these lesion to T$_4$ and necessitates bony resection.

Imaging issues: lip carcinoma

- Bone erosion
- Soft-tissue invasion

Floor of mouth

Imaging is used to assess the presence of bone erosion and tumour size, which may clinically be underestimated if there is submucosal extension. It is important to determine the relationship of the tumour to the midline septum and to the contralateral neurovascular bundle since this will alter treatment (Fig. 3.9a–c). Thin-section CT is again the imaging modality of choice if bone involvement is suspected, e.g. fixed lateral floor of mouth tumours, but otherwise MRI may give more information about the tumour, especially if there is artefact from dental amalgam.

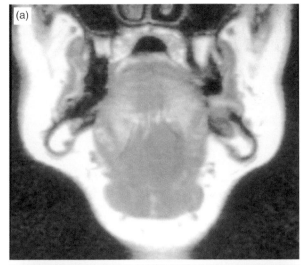

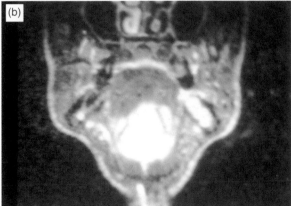

Imaging issues: floor of mouth carcinoma

■ Extent of bone erosion
■ Deep invasion along the mylohyoid and hyoglossus muscles
■ Relationship to ipsilateral lingual neurovascular bundle
■ Extension across the midline and relationship to contralateral neurovascular bundle
■ Tongue base invasion
■ Extension into the soft tissues of the neck

Tongue

The majority of tumours arise from the lateral aspect or undersurface of the tongue (Fig. 3.10). Large ones of the anterior and middle third of the tongue tend to spread to the floor of the mouth and coronal imaging can be useful in the evaluation. Spread to the tongue base may occur from the more posteriorly based tumours. Imaging should assess the size of the lesion and whether it has crossed the midline. Identification of the relationship of the mass to the neurovascular bundle is important since this will alter management.

Gingiva and hard palate

Cross-sectional imaging may understage these lesions which are better assessed by direct visual examination. Low-volume superficial tumours may not be visible on imaging but more advanced lesions with suspected bone involvement should be examined using CT. Direct coronal CT should be performed to stage tumours involving the hard palate.

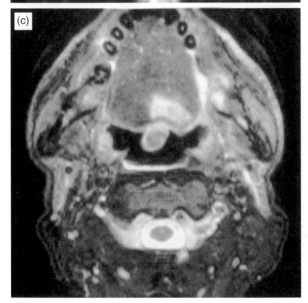

Figure 3.9 (a) Coronal T$_1$-weighted and (b) STIR scans through the floor of mouth revealing a large mass involving the floor of the mouth on both sides of the midline. (c) An area of abnormally high signal from tumour extension is seen on MRI in the same patient in the posterior third of the left tongue extending towards the tongue base.

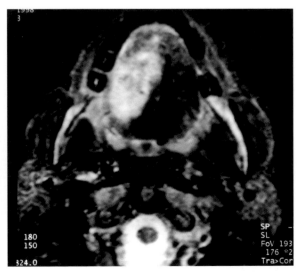

Figure 3.10 Axial STIR MRI sequence displaying a high signal intensity carcinoma involving the lateral aspect of the right side of the tongue. This tumour has extended from the middle third of the tongue to involve the posterior third.

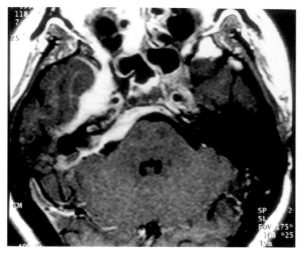

Figure 3.11 Axial contrast-enhanced T₁-weighted MRI scan demonstrating abnormal enhancing tumour in the right pterygopalatine fossa, which extends into the medial aspect of the right temporal fossa and the right cerebellopontine angle. This was due to recurrent adenoid cystic carcinoma.

Adenoid cystic carcinoma commonly shows perineural spread into the pterygopalatine fossa (Fig. 3.11) via the greater and lesser palatine nerves. This extension may be better imaged using MRI with gadolinium enhancement.

Retromolar trigone carcinoma

The retromolar trigone is a small triangular area posterior to the last mandibular molar tooth. Tumours arising in this region may grow anteriorly into the buccal region or posteriorly into the tonsil via the superior constrictor muscle. Superior extension may occur into the skull base and inferiorly into the floor of the mouth. Bone involvement is often not detected clinically and may occur early. This should be assessed with appropriate imaging and, if present, will alter management.

Mandible

It is important to consider the presence or absence of mandibular invasion prior to resecting any oral or oropharyngeal tumour. The presence of mandibular invasion increases with the size of the primary tumour, its proximity to the mandible and whether or not there has been previous surgery or irradiation. Preoperative imaging can be very useful in the detection of mandibular invasion.

An orthopantogram (OPG) is useful to assess the state of dentition and the possible siting of any mandibulotomy incision. It will demonstrate gross mandibular invasion. A positive bone scan ([^{99m}Tc]MDP) may occur in the presence of either benign (peridontal disease, recent extractions, sinusitis, etc.) or malignant involvement. However, a negative bone scan usually means no bony invasion unless there is very aggressive bony destruction or myeloma is present.

CT and MRI can detect subtle bony invasion as well as the extent of significant invasive disease. However, the decision as to whether or not conservation mandibular surgery is feasible is best based on a combination of the radiological findings together with operative assessment.

Imaging issues: the mandible

- State of dentition
- Position of the mental foramen
- Presence or absence of bony invasion
- Extent of bony involvement
- Any inferior alveolar nerve/canal extension

Pharynx

Nasopharynx

Squamous cell carcinoma accounts for 70% of superficial malignant tumours in the nasopharynx. Imaging should aim to provide an assessment of the pattern of spread of the tumour, especially into areas not easily examined clinically, i.e. deep extension as well as spread superiorly to the skull base and beyond. Lateral extension into the deep structures of the nasopharynx can occur via the sinus of Morgagni, a natural fascial defect sited in the superolateral wall of the nasopharynx which allows the passage of the eustachian tube and levator veli palatini muscle. Tumour can then gain access to the masticator, prestyloid, poststyloid and parapharyngeal spaces. This can result in involvement of the third division of the fifth cranial nerve. Retrograde perineural spread to the skull base can then occur. The most common sites of skull base invasion are the petroclinoid fissure and foramen lacerum (Fig. 3.1). This can result in internal carotid artery encasement and extension into the cavernous sinus.

Skull-base invasion

- Cavernous sinus involvement is best assessed using coronal or axial MRI and contrast enhancement may be useful
- Extension of tumour into the clivus is best evaluated on sagittal and axial T₁-weighted SE (Fig. 3.12a) and STIR sequences
- Involvement of the cribriform plate and orbits is evaluated using a coronal imaging plane (Fig. 3.12b), and although MRI is better than CT for the detection of marrow involvement, CT is more sensitive for detection of subtle bone erosion/destruction (Fig. 3.12c)
- MRI has been shown to be better than CT for soft-tissue infiltration and arterial encasement as well as cavernous sinus involvement (Fig. 3.13)

Because of this, CT and MRI can be complementary for skull-base evaluation. Combining radiographic tumour staging reliably predicts surgical findings for skull-base involvement in a number of tumours but MRI

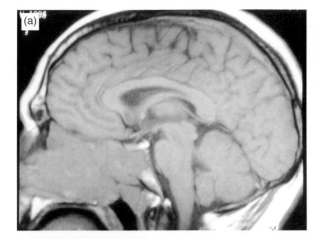

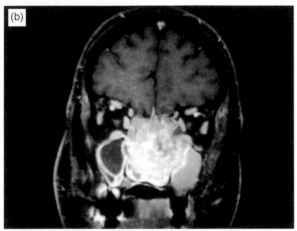

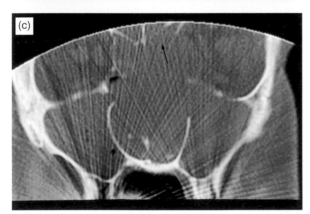

Figure 3.12 (a) Sagittal T_1-weighted MRI sequence revealing a large soft-tissue mass expanding the nasal cavity and extending posteriorly to involve the clivus, with replacement of the normal high signal intensity of marrow fat within the superior aspect of the clivus which exhibits an intermediate signal intensity tumour. This was due to a neuroendocrine tumour. (b) Coronal T_1-weighted fat-saturated MRI scans post-gadolinum showing heterogeneous tumour enhancement. There is involvement of the medial walls of the orbit with extension of abnormal tissue into the orbital fat. (c) Erosion of the cribriform plate (arrow) is better demonstrated by a direct coronal CT scan using bone window settings.

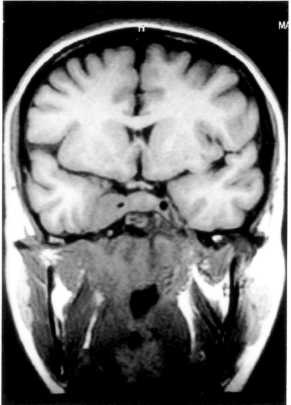

Figure 3.13 Coronal T_1-weighted MRI scan through the pituitary fossa revealing added soft tissue in the right cavernous sinus with encasement of the right internal carotid artery which has a much smaller diameter than the left. This was due to recurrent adenoid cystic carcinoma of the nasopharynx.

alone will usually yield sufficient information (Kraus *et al.*, 1992).

It has been suggested that single photon emission computed tomography (SPECT) may be more sensitive than CT for the detection of skull-base involvement by providing better anatomical localization (Keogan *et al.*, 1994), but the CT technique was not ideal in this study.

Anterior extension into the posterior nasal cavity can be clinically assessed but further extension into the pterygopalatine fossa (Fig. 3.11) is better assessed using axial CT or MRI scanning.

Retrograde spread may occur along the path of the maxillary branch of the fifth cranial nerve to again involve the skull base. Inferior extension with involvement of the lateral pharyngeal walls and tonsils is relatively common. This spread may be submucosal and thus not easily seen on clinical examination.

Pitfalls in imaging the nasopharynx

- Normal asymmetry of the lateral pharyngeal recess
- Variability in normal lymphoid tissue

Oropharynx

> **Imaging issues**
>
> ■ Objective size of primary tumour
> ■ Perineural and deep spread of tumour:
> ■ Soft palate to pterygopalatine fossa (V2) and foramen rotundum
> ■ Palatine tonsil to masticator space (V3) and foramen ovale
> ■ Lingual tonsil to neurovascular bundle of tongue
> ■ Posterior oropharyngeal wall to retropharyngeal space

The oropharynx is made up of the pharyngeal wall between the nasopharynx and pharyngoepiglottic fold, the soft palate, the tonsillar region and the tongue base.

Either CT or MRI may be used to evaluate the tongue base. Information about the ipsilateral and contralateral (if the lesion crosses the midline) neurovascular bundle should be sought. This determines whether a partial glossectomy is a treatment option. Both the anterior extent of the lesion and whether there is any involvement of the floor of mouth should be assessed.

Treatment of tonsillar and soft-palate lesions depends on the size of the tumour and involvement of surrounding structures. MRI has been recommended as the

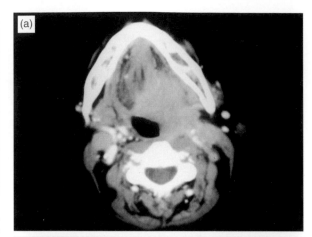

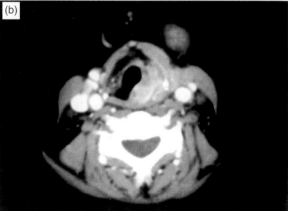

Figure 3.15 (a) Large oropharyngeal tumour extending anteriorly to involve the muscles of the floor of the mouth. It is involving the tongue base and extending out into the soft tissues of the neck with arterial encasement on the left. (b) More inferiorly, the extent of submucosal spread is seen with tumour occupying the left paraglottic fat and extending round into the pre-epiglottic fat space.

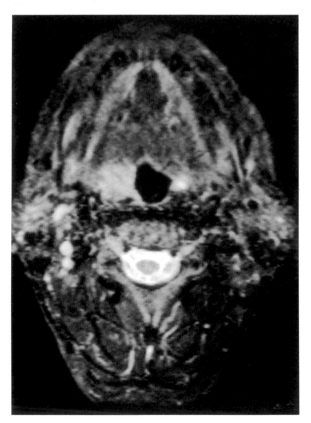

Figure 3.14 Axial STIR MRI scan revealing an abnormally high signal due to a right tonsillar carcinoma.

imaging modality of choice (Fig. 3.14). There should be a detailed evaluation of submucosal extension into the soft tissues of the neck (Fig. 3.15a). In addition, the prestyloid and poststyloid parapharyngeal space as well as the nasopharynx and the tongue base (Fig. 3.16) should be assessed. Encasement of the carotid artery (Fig. 3.15a) will alter management. Bone erosion and invasion of the prevertebral muscles can occur in advanced lesions. Submucosal extension (Figs 3.15b, 3.17a, b) may not be visible clinically (Fig. 3.2) and bulky disease close to or invading the skull base, together with evidence of encasement of the internal carotid artery, may preclude surgery.

Hypopharynx

The hypopharynx extends from the hyoid bone superiorly to the inferior aspect of the cricoid cartilage. The three major subsites of the hypopharynx are the piriform sinus (Fig. 3.18), the postcricoid area (Fig. 3.19) and the

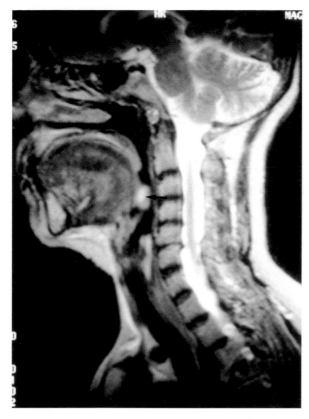

Figure 3.16 Sagittal T$_2$-weighted MRI scan showing a small squamous cell carcinoma limited to the tongue base (arrow).

posterior hypopharyngeal wall. Carcinomas are most common in the piriform sinus (60%) followed by the postcricoid area. These tumours often present late. Piriform sinus carcinomas commonly spread into the soft tissues of the neck and may destroy the posterior margin of the ipsilateral thyroid cartilage (Fig. 3.18).

Assessment of soft-tissue invasion by postcricoid carcinoma (Fig. 3.19) is difficult because of the normal variation seen in the thickness of the prevertebral muscles and inferior constrictor muscle. Posterior wall tumours may invade the retropharyngeal space and extend up into the oropharynx and nasopharynx.

Imaging issues: hypopharyngeal carcinoma

- Invasion of soft tissue, bone or cartilage
- Anterior extension into paraglottic space
- Extension into oesophageal inlet
- Retropharyngeal extension and adenopathy

Neck nodes

The presence of involved neck nodes is the most important prognostic indicator in patients with head and neck cancer and palpation is known to be an inaccurate technique for the assessment of the neck. Elective neck treat-

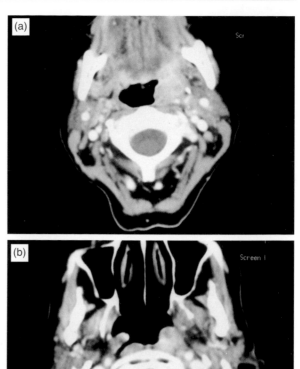

Figure 3.17 (a) Axial contrast-enhanced CT scans demonstrating a left tonsillar mass. (b) The patient presented with left otalgia and scans reveal submucosal extension up into the left side of the nasopharynx.

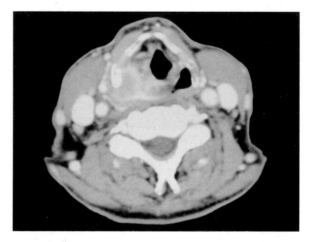

Figure 3.18 Axial contrast-enhanced CT scan demonstrating abnormally enhanced tumour filling the right piriform sinus with extension into the soft tissues of the neck and involvement of the right thyroid cartilage with increased sclerosis of this cartilage. Anterior extension into the paraglottic space is seen on the right.

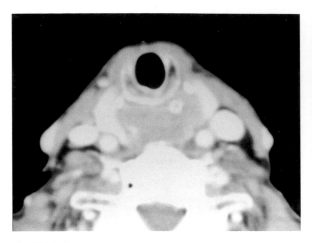

Figure 3.19 Axial contrast-enhanced CT scan revealing a large soft-tissue mass involving the postcricoid oesophagus. A nasogastric tube is noted.

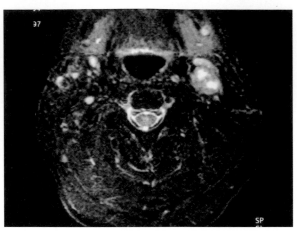

Figure 3.20 Axial MRI STIR sequence showing an enlarged node at level II on the left with separate areas of increased signal intensity due to necrosis within this pathological node.

ment may be performed in patients with a primary head and neck cancer when there is a risk of nodal neck disease which exceeds 20%. Either contrast-enhanced CT or MRI can be used to image neck nodes and will upstage approximately 20% of patients who are thought to have clinically negative necks. Ideally, this should be done while staging the primary tumour or while hunting for an unknown primary. The first- and second-order drainage nodes should be assessed. Often the entire neck to the clavicles is imaged. Some centres use ultrasound to stage nodal disease combining imaging with image-guided FNAC or biopsy (Van den Brekel *et al.*, 1993). The anatomical classification system and patterns of drainage are discussed in Chapter 12 and nodes in each of these groups may be recognized using cross-sectional imaging techniques. All of the lymph nodes in the neck with the exception of intraparotid nodes are surrounded by fat, which allows identification of nodes measuring only a few millimetres.

Between 10 and 20% of clinically occult metastatic nodes may be detected using CT or MRI. Nodes may not be palpable because of a deep location such as the retropharyngeal or high deep cervical chain. The neck becomes more difficult to palpate following previous surgery and/or radiotherapy.

Abnormal nodes are identified on CT and MRI using size criteria or by the presence of pathological enhancement (Som, 1992). If a node greater than 1.5 cm in diameter near the angle of the mandible (or 1 cm in diameter elsewhere in the neck) is taken as being abnormal then the diagnosis will be wrong in 20–28% of cases. Some argue that sensitivity is more important than specificity and recommend the use of a 1 cm maximum nodal diameter anywhere in the neck. It has also been suggested that nodes in the retropharyngeal chain should not measure more than 8 mm in maximum diameter. Metastatic nodes are often spherical in shape, unlike normal nodes which are elliptical, so that a ratio of maximum nodal length to

the maximum axial nodal diameter of less than 2 has been suggested to be abnormal. Whichever criteria are used, the false-positive and false-negative rates are between 10 and 20%.

Central necrosis occurs in lymph nodes which have been invaded by tumour (Fig. 3.20). This is more likely to be seen in larger nodes but remains a specific sign of nodal involvement even if the node is not enlarged using conventional size criteria. It is demonstrated on post-contrast CT and MRI scans as a central area of non-enhancement (Fig. 3.21) and may be mimicked by postinflammatory fatty infiltration (Fig. 3.22) but, in these cases, the fatty node usually remains an oval shape and the fat is not located centrally. The presence of central necrosis is not diagnostic of invasion by squamous cell carcinoma and may be seen in other conditions such as lymphoma and melanoma. It may also be seen in suppurative adenopathy.

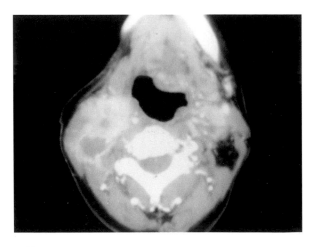

Figure 3.21 Axial contrast-enhanced CT demonstrating bilateral rim enhancing nodes with central areas of necrosis.

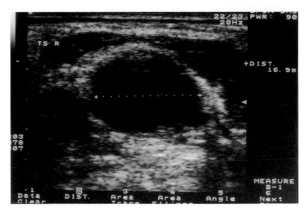

Suspicious nodes on cross-sectional imaging

- Size greater than 1 cm
- Rim enhancement following IV contrast
- Central necrosis
- Spherical shape

A T_1-weighted, fat-suppressed sequence following intravenous gadolinium chelate appears to be the optimum MRI sequence to visualize central necrosis. High signal within neck nodes on a T_2-weighted sequence is common.

Extranodal extension of tumour results in a loss of clarity of the nodal margin with soft tissue extending into the fat surrounding the node (Fig. 3.21). Extranodal spread is seen better on CT than MRI. The presence of macroscopic tumour beyond the nodal capsule correlates with a much greater risk of recurrence. Vascular invasion

Figure 3.24 Transverse ultrasound scan through the right side of the neck revealing an enlarged node with an area of central necrosis causing posterior acoustic enhancement.

also worsens prognosis. If the artery is entirely surrounded by tumour it is likely to be invaded (Fig. 3.23) but this is not completely reliable. Conversely, the vessel is less likely to be involved if tumour just abuts it but microcopic invasion may be present and undetected.

US with US-guided fine needle aspiration may be used in the evaluation of nodal disease in the neck. Enlarged metastatic nodes often exhibit inhomogeneous reflectivity due to necrosis (Fig. 3.24) or tumour, but nodes containing fat may also be inhomogeneous. Small metastatic nodes are less likely to be inhomogeneous.

If a minimal axial diameter of 7 mm (8 mm in the subdigastric area) is used (or a group of three or more nodes with diameters not more than 12 mm smaller in axial diameter) then ultrasound has been shown to have an accuracy of 70% with a sensitivity of 60% and specificity of 77% for metastatic nodal disease.

PET using ^{18}FDG may enable differentiation of normal and reactive nodes from malignant nodes due to abnormal glucose metabolism in malignant tissue. However, the technique is expensive and its spatial resolution is less than that of the other techniques. Its role has yet to be established but at present it seems to be most useful in the treated neck.

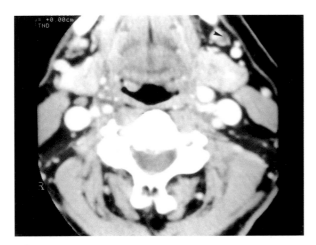

Figure 3.22 CT scan showing a small left-sided level I node which has an eccentrically placed area of low attenuation (arrowhead) due to postinflammatory fatty infiltration, in a patient who does not have head and neck malignancy.

Paranasal sinuses

The maxillary sinus is most commonly involved (80%). Approximately 18% have malignant adenopathy at presentation. These are usually from posterior wall tumours with retropharyngeal node involvement. CT and MRI will demonstrate a sinus mass usually with associated wall destruction, rather than expansion (Fig. 3.25). Axial images are best for the demonstration of posterior extension into the infratemporal fossa and pterygopalatine fossa, while coronal images are best for the spread of tumour superiorly into the orbit and intracranially. Imaging should be performed following intravenous contrast and if CT is used, both axial and coronal scans should be performed with a higher radiation dose than is used for imaging inflammatory paranasal sinus disease.

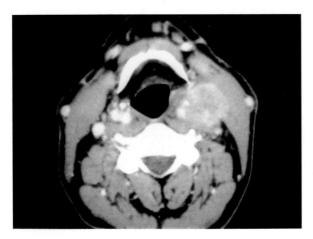

Figure 3.23 Axial contrast-enhanced CT scan demonstrating an enlarged left-sided level II/III node which has encased the left carotid bifurcation. There also appears to be some involvement of the left sternomastoid muscle.

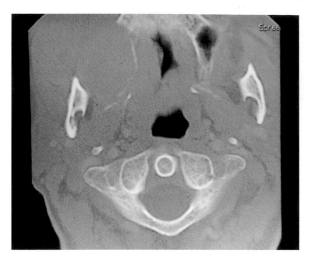

Figure 3.25 Axial CT scan displayed on bone window settings revealing a large soft-tissue mass which is involving and destroying the floor, medial and lateral walls of the right maxillary antrum.

Imaging issues: maxillary sinus carcinoma

- Infrastructure (T_1) versus suprastructure (T_2)
- Invasion of cheek, orbit, anterior ethmoid sinuses, pterygoid muscles (T_3)
- Invasion of cribriform plate, posterior ethmoid sinuses or sphenoid sinus (T_4)

Salivary glands

The pleomorphic adenoma is the most common salivary gland tumour. Most occur in the parotid gland. On CT, it is a well-defined mass with a higher attenuation (appearing denser) than the surrounding parotid parenchyma. It does not enhance significantly following intravenous contrast. Larger tumours may be heterogeneous with areas of lower attenuation due to necrosis, old haemorrhage and cystic change. Most often these tumours are of low signal intensity on T_1-weighted MRI images and of high signal intensity on T_2-weighted images (Fig. 3.26a, b). Again, larger tumours may be heterogeneous on MRI.

Mucoepidermoid carcinoma accounts for approximately one-third of all malignant salivary gland tumours. Almost 50% arise in the parotid gland, with most of the remainder being seen in the minor salivary glands, especially in the palate and buccal mucosa. Low-grade lesions behave almost like benign lesions but the high-grade tumours are aggressive with metastatic spread to subcutaneous tissues, lymph nodes, bone and lung.

The imaging findings depend on the grade of tumour, with low-grade lesions appearing similar to pleomorphic adenomas and high-grade tumours having indistinct margins with low to intermediate signal intensity on both T_1- and T_2-weighted MRI images.

Adenoid cystic carcinoma occurs most commonly in the parotid gland (2–6% of all tumours), the submandibular gland (12% of all tumours) and the palate. Perineural spread is common (Fig. 3.11). Skull-base extension may occur from the parotid gland via the facial or mandibular nerve and is best imaged using contrast-enhanced MRI.

Imaging of a parotid mass may not be necessary if the tumour is well defined, mobile and contained within the superficial lobe. MRI has been shown to be an excellent modality to determine the relationship of a parotid mass to the plane of the facial nerve (Ariyoshi and Shimahara, 1998).

Malignant tumours are more common in the minor salivary glands, e.g. in the palate and upper lip region. Malignant tumours generally have irregular, ill-defined margins (Kaneda *et al.*, 1994), demonstrate invasion and

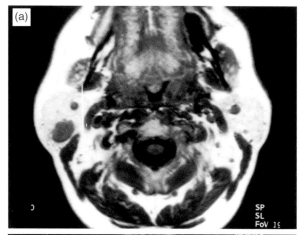

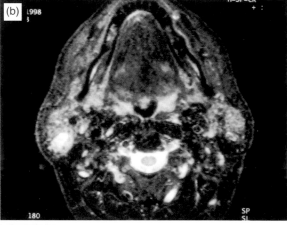

Figure 3.26 (a) Axial T_1-weighted scan through the level of the parotid glands demonstrating an intermediate to low signal intensity mass which is fairly well defined lying in the superficial lobe of the right parotid gland. A line has been drawn from the posterior border of the mandible to the anterolateral margin of the posterior belly of the digastric muscle. This line may be used to determine whether masses arise within the superficial or deep lobe of the parotid. (b) STIR MRI scan on the same patient demonstrating the mass to be of predominantly high signal intensity.

are hypointense on T_2-weighted images, but there are no specific features to indicate malignancy. PET has not been found to be useful in this regard.

Imaging issues: salivary glands

- Location: deep or superficial lobe of parotid
- Perineural spread
- Spread by contiguity into surrounding structures (i.e. mandible)
- Skull-base extension
- Lymph-node involvement

Parapharyngeal space

Imaging is essential in the work-up of a mass apparently pushing into the pharynx. It can be used to determine accurately the site of origin of the mass and thus its likely aetiology.

The key to understanding this area is the anatomy of the parapharyngeal fat space (Fig. 3.27), which is the central space of the deep face. The surrounding spaces include

- the pharyngeal mucosal space
- the masticator space

(a)

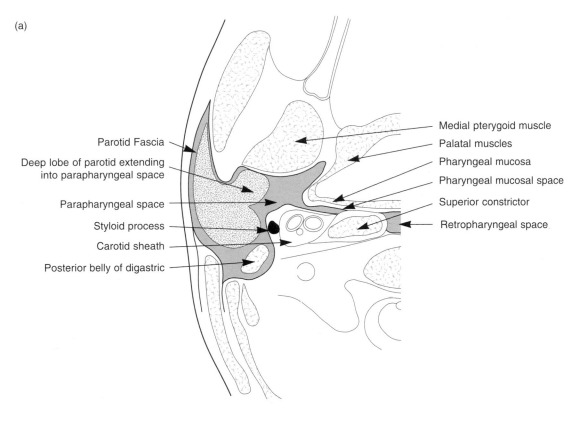

(b)

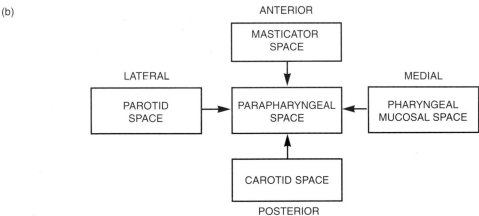

Figure 3.27 Anatomy of the parapharyngeal and surrounding spaces. (a) The intimate relationships of the parapharyngeal space. (b) Note the central strategic location of the parapharyngeal space.

- the parotid space
- the carotid space
- the lateral retropharyngeal spaces.

Few lesions actually arise from the parapharyngeal space because of its limited normal contents. The main content of this space is fat and it is the **displacement pattern** of this fat that allows the localization of mass lesions arising from the structures surrounding the face.

A mass arising from the parotid space will lie **lateral** to the parapharyngeal fat and will displace the fat of the pharyngeal space **medially**. A parotid mass will widen the distance between the angle of the mandible and the styloid process. Masses arising from the deep lobe of the parotid gland have been discussed in the section on salivary gland tumours.

A mass arising from the carotid space will displace the parapharyngeal fat **anteriorly** and will be accompanied by anterolateral displacement of the styloid process. A mass arising from the posterior portion of the carotid space, e.g. vagal schwannoma, neurofibroma or paraganglioma, will be seen **posterior** to the internal carotid artery.

Masses arising within the carotid space have some characteristic imaging features. A pseudomass may be possible owing to ectasia of the common or internal carotid artery or an asymmetric internal jugular vein. This will readily be identified with contrast-enhanced imaging. Inflammatory conditions arising from this space are usually apparent from the clinical history and examination. Vascular lesions such as jugular vein thrombosis or carotid artery aneurysm are also usually diagnosed readily following contrast-enhanced CT.

Paragangliomas are benign tumours arising from neural crest cells. The glomus tympanicum is found on the cochlear promontory, while the glomus jugulare arises from within the jugular foramen. The glomus vagale occurs in the nasopharyngeal and oropharyngeal carotid space and the carotid body tumour at the carotid bifurcation. These tumours show intense enhancement following intravenous

contrast medium (Fig. 3.28). Lesions greater than 2 cm in diameter have characteristic features on MRI, with serpiginous flow voids being seen within the mass. Again, there will be intense enhancement following intravenous gadolinium. A schwannoma will appear as a well-encapsulated soft-tissue density mass displacing the internal carotid artery **anteriorly**. Flow voids are absent on MRI but contrast enhancement is seen, usually of lower intensity than a paraganglioma. If bone involvement is present at the jugular foramen a schwannoma will cause smooth scalloping, whereas a paraganglioma will demonstrate more permeative bony change with erosion of the jugular spine.

A neurofibroma is seen on CT as a well-defined, low-density mass. MRI may not be able to differentiate a neurofibroma from a schwannoma, unless the neurofibroma is of plexiform type. The appearances of squamous cell nodal metastases have already been described.

A primary lesion of the masticator space will invade the parapharyngeal space from **anterior** to **posterior**, displacing the parapharyngeal fat **posteriorly** and **medially**. Benign and malignant tumours from muscle and bone origin make up the bulk of tumours. Inflammatory conditions from the mandible and teeth should also be considered.

Thyroid

There are six main types of primary thyroid malignancy. The most common type is differentiated thyroid cancer, which includes papillary, papillary/follicular mixed (80%) and follicular (10%). These tumours are often radioiodine avid and this group has the best prognosis. Hürthle cell carcinoma is a variant of follicular carcinoma which is not radioiodine avid. The other tumour types include medullary, lymphoma and lastly anaplastic carcinoma, which has the worst prognosis of all. The most common way for thyroid carcinoma to present is as a solitary nodule when the incidence of malignancy is approximately 10%. The diagnosis is usually made by FNAC (which may be image guided) so that formal imaging is not usually required in many cases. An open biopsy is often necessary to distinguish lymphoma from anaplastic carcinoma.

However, in some instances US may be helpful. US can differentiate solid from cystic masses but cannot differentiate benign from malignant. Even the diagnosis of a cystic mass does not preclude the presence of malignancy. Cystic areas occur in up to 40% of malignant masses. The presence of multiple nodules lessens the chance of malignancy but does not exclude it. Ultrasound may be useful to:

- diagnose a multinodular goitre
- assess tumour size
- evaluate the state of the contralateral lobe
- assist in aspiration and FNAC.

Scintigraphy can be of value in:

- assessment of the contralateral lobe
- identification of residual functioning tissue in the thyroid bed
- identification of metastatic disease.

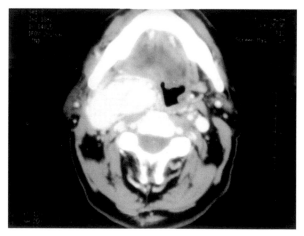

Figure 3.28 Contrast-enhanced CT demonstrating an intensely enhancing mass at the level of the right carotid artery bifurcation consistent with a carotid body tumour.

Cross-sectional imaging is used to stage advanced thyroid cancer (T_2N_1 and above). It can assess the state of the contralateral lobe, direct extension into local visceral structures, major vessels and the presence of any cervical metastases. CT and MRI can also give information regarding extension into the mediastinum (which is not available with either US or scintigraphy), as well as the presence of distant metastatic spread. It is also used to routinely stage lymphoma and to exclude a phaeochromocytoma. If contrast-enhanced CT is used, the iodine load which is given in the form of intravenous contrast may prevent treatment with radioiodine for up to 6 months. MRI should be used if the tumour is iodine avid and early treatment is anticipated with ^{131}I. The use of coregistration using CT or MRI with SPECT ^{99m}Tc(v) DMSA can be particularly useful in distinguishing tumours and scar tissue from recurrent disease in medullary carcinoma of the thyroid gland (Fig. 3.29).

Examples of anatomical images in thyroid carcinoma are shown in Chapter 23.

Imaging issues: thyroid carcinoma

- Extracapsular extension
- Contralateral lobe
- Vascular invasion
- Mediastinal involvement
- Pharyngeal and oesophageal involvement
- Laryngeal and tracheal involvement
- Nodal disease (levels I–VII)
- Distant metastatic spread
- Lymphoma staging
- Exclusion of phaeochromocytoma [multiple endocrine neoplasia (MEN) syndrome]

Papillary carcinoma is the thyroid tumour with the greatest likelihood of nodal spread. The nodes may be small and appear hyperplastic. They are sometimes cystic or haemorrhagic or contain calcification. They may enhance following intravenous contrast. Haematogeneous metastases are much less common (4–7%) and spread is usually to the lungs, bone or central nervous system.

Follicular carcinoma spreads to nodes less often but is more likely to spread haematogeneously. It is more likely to demonstrate vascular invasion than papillary carcinoma and is usually a solid tumour.

Anaplastic carcinoma is a very aggressive tumour with an extremely poor prognosis. It occurs with a background of a multinodular goitre in approximately 40% of patients. Calcification is seen in over 50% of tumours. Vascular and aerodigestive tract invasion is relatively common and nodal or distant disease occurs in up to 80% of patients.

Medullary carcinoma is seen as part of the multiple endocrine neoplasia (MEN) syndromes 2A and 2B (see Chapter 23). The primary tumour and nodal metastases may show calcification. Nodal disease is present in over 50% of cases.

A previous history of Hashimoto's thyroiditis is almost always present in patients with thyroid lymphoma. This more commonly presents as a solitary mass but multiple nodules are present in approximately 20% of patients. Response to chemotherapy and radiotherapy is variable. These tumours do not take up technetium or iodine radioisotopes but may be gallium avid. Vascular invasion and nodal disease may occur.

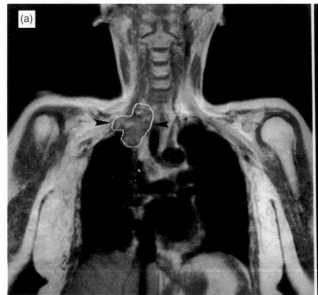 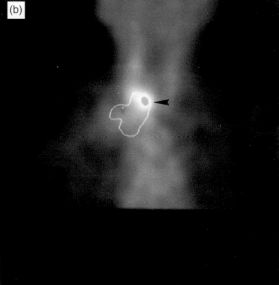

Figure 3.29 (a) Coronal MRI in a patient with medullary carcinoma of the thyroid. Recurrence is suspected clinically and biochemically, and the MRI indicates the presence of a mass in the right superior mediastinum. (b) Coronal SPECT ^{99m}Tc(v) DMSA scan (with image interposition) showing increased activity at the upper aspect of the mass. (Courtesy of Professor M. Maisey.)

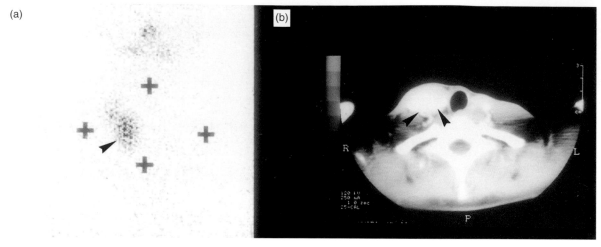

Figure 3.30 (a) Post-radioiodine-131 ablation scan suggesting recurrent disease in the right lower neck. The serum thyroglobulin was elevated. (b) CT scan confirmed an enlarged node at level IV. Treatment was by neck dissection and further radioiodine ablation. The patient remains alive and well 4 years later.

Residual and recurrent disease

The detection of residual and recurrent disease is fraught with difficulty. Clinical examination is impeded by swelling and the presence of scar tissue, while the normal anatomical planes have been distorted, which hampers the interpretation of CT and MRI images. In the future, PET scanning may have a role to play in the assessment of residual and recurrent carcinoma in the head and neck, but the results of current research are awaited.

Recurrent thyroid carcinoma is usually suspected when the serum thyroglobulin is rising despite adequate TSH suppression. Physiological imaging with ^{131}I whole-body diagnostic scanning may suggest the site of any possible head and neck recurrence, which should then be assessed with anatomical imaging using CT or MRI (Fig. 3.30) prior to further surgery.

Acknowledgement

The important contribution to this chapter of Dr Julie Olliff MRCP, FRCR, Consultant Radiologist, University Hospital Birmingham NHS Trust, is gratefully acknowledged.

References and further reading

Ariyoshi Y. and Shimahara M. (1998) Determining whether a parotid tumour is in the superficial or deep lobe using magnetic resonance imaging, *J Oral Maxillofac Surg* **56**: 23–6.

Becker M., Zbaren P., Laeng H., Stoupis C., Porcellini B. and Vock P. (1995) Neoplastic invasion of the laryngeal cartilage: comparison of MR imaging and CT with histopathologic correlation, *Radiology* **194**: 661–9.

Becker M., Zbaren P., Delavelle J., Kurt A.M., Egger C., Rufenacht D.A. and Terrier F. (1997) Neoplastic invasion of the laryngeal cartilage: reassessment of criteria for diagnosis at CT, *Radiology* **203**: 521–32.

Braams J. W., Pruim J., Kole A. C., Nikkels P. G., Vaalburg W., Vermey A. and Roodenburg J. L. (1997) Detection of unknown primary head and neck tumours by positron emission tomography, *Int J Oral Maxillofac Surg* **26**: 112–15.

Briggs R. J., Gallimore A. P., Phelps P. D. and Howard D. J. (1993) Laryngeal imaging by computerized tomography and magnetic resonance following radiation therapy: a need for caution. *J Laryngol Otol* **107**: 565–8.

Castelijns J. A., Gerritsen G. J., Kaiser M. C., Val, K. J., van Zabten, T. E., Golding R. G. *et al.* (1988) Invasion of laryngeal cartilage by cancer: comparison of CT and MR imaging, *Radiology* **167**: 199–206.

Castelijns J. A., van den Breckel M. W., Tobi H., Smit E. M., Golding R. P., van Schaik C. and Snow G.B. (1996) Laryngeal carcinoma after radiation therapy: correlation of abnormal MR imaging signal patterns in laryngeal cartilage with risk of recurrence, *Radiology* **198**: 151–5.

Gittoes N., Miller M. R., Daykin J., Sheppard M. C. and Franklyn J. (1996) Upper airways obstruction in 153 consecutive patients presenting with thyroid enlargement, *BMJ* **312**: 484.

Greven K. M., Williams D. W. III, Keyes J. W. Jr, McGuirt W. F., Harkness B. A., Watson N. E. Jr *et al.* (1994) Distinguishing tumor recurrence from irradiation sequelae with positron emission tomography in patients treated for larynx cancer, *Inte J Radiat Oncol Biol Phys*, **29**: 841–5.

Kaweda T., Minami M., Ozawa K., Akimoto, Y., Okada, M., Yamamoto, H. *et al.* (1994) Imaging tumours of minor salivary glands, *Oral Surg Oral Med Oral Pathol*, **78**: 385–90.

Kraus D. H., Lanzreri C. F., Wanamaker J. R., Little J. R. and Lavertu P. (1992) Complementary use of computed tomography and magnetic resonance imaging in assessing skull base lesions, *Laryngoscope* **102**: 623–9.

Keogan M. T., Antouri N. and Wright E. P. (1994) Evaluation of the skull base by SPECT. A comparison with planar scintigraphy and computed tomography, *Clin Neck Med* **19**: 1055–9.

Lowe G. H. S. and Rubasin S. E. (1993) Contrast evaluation of the pharynx and oesophagus, *Radiol Clin North Am* **31**:1265–91.

Maroldi R., Battaglia G., Nicolai P., Cappiello J., Cabassa P., Farina D. and Chiesa A. (1997) CT appearances of the larynx after conservative and radical surgery for carcinomas, *Eur Radiol* **7**: 418–31.

McGuirt W. F., Williams D. W. III, Keyes J. W. Jr, Greven K. M., Watson N. E. Jr, Geisinger K. R. and Cappellari, J. O. (1995) A comparative diagnostic study of head and neck nodal metastases using positron emission tomography, *Laryngoscope* **105**: 373–5.

McGuirt W. F., Greven K. M., Keyes J. W. Jr, Williams D. W. III, Watson N. E. Jr, Geisinger K. R. and Cappellari J. O. (1995) Positron emission tomography in the evaluation of laryngeal carcinoma, *Ann Otol Rhinol Laryngol* **104**: 274–8.

Mendenhall W. M., Parsons J. T., Mancuso A. A., Pameijer F. J., Stringer S. P. and Cassissi N. J. (1997) Definitive radiotherapy for T3 squamous cell carcinoma of the glottic larynx, *J Clin Oncol* **15**: 2394–404.

Mukherji SK, Mancuso AA. Kotzur IM, Kubilis PS, Tart RP, Lee WR, Freeman D. (1994). Radiologic changes of the irradiated larynx. Part 1. Expected changes. *Radiology* **193**: 141–8.

Mukherji S. K., Pillsbury H. R. and Castillo M. (1997) Imaging squamous cell carcinomas of the upper aerodigestive tract: what the clinicians need to know, *Radiology* **205**: 629–46.

Parker G. D. and Harnsberger H. R. (1991) Clinical–radiological issues in perineural tumour spread of malignant diseases of the extracranial head and neck, *Radiographics* **11**(3): 383–99.

Reiner B., Siegel E., Sawyer R., Brocato R. M., Maroney M. and Hooper F. (1997) The impact of routine CT of the chest on the diagnosis and management of newly diagnosed squamous cell carcinoma of the head and neck, *AJR* **169**(3): 667–1.

Robert Y., Rocourt N., Chevalier D., Duhamel A., Carcasset S. and Lemaitre L. (1996) Helical CT of the larynx; a comparative study with conventional CT scan, *Clin Radiol* **51**: 882–5.

Som P. M., Sacher M., Stollman A. L., Biller H. F. and Lawson W. (1988) Common tumours of the parapharyngeal space: refined imaging diagnosis, *Radiology* **169**: 81–5.

Som P. M. (1992) Detection of metastasis in cervical lymph nodes: CT and MR criteria and differential diagnosis, *Am J Roentgenol* **158**: 961–9.

Thabet H. M., Sessios D. G., Gado M. H., Gnepp D. A., Harvey J. E. and Talaat M. (1996) Comparison of clinical evaluation and computed tomographic diagnostic accuracy for tumours of the larynx and hypopharynx, *Laryngoscope* **106**: 589–94.

Van den Breckel M. W. M., Stel H. V., Castelijns J. A., Nauta J. J., van der Waal I., Valk J. *et al.* (1990) Cervical lymph node metastasis: assessment of radiologic criteria, *Radiology* **177**: 379–84b.

Van den Brekel M. W. M., Castelijns J. A., Stel H. V., Golding R. P., Meyer C. J., Snow C. B. *et al.* (1993) Modern imaging techniques and ultrasound-guided aspiration cytology for the assessment of neck node metastases: a prospective comparative study, *Eur Arch Otorhinolaryngol* **250**: 11–17.

Watkinson J. C. (1997) Principles and use of nuclear medicine, in *Scott-Brown's Otolaryngology*, 6th edn, Vol. 1, *Basic Sciences*, Butterworth-Heinemann, Oxford, Chap. 23, pp. 1–22.

Wong W., Hussain K., Chevretton E., Hawekes D. J., Baddeley H., Maisey M., McGurk M. (1996) Validation and clinical application of computer-combined computed tomography and positron emission tomography with 2-(18)fluoro-2-deoxy-D-glucose head and neck images, *Am J Surg* **172**: 628–32.

Wong W. L., Chevretton E. B., McGurk M., Hussain K., Davis J., Beaney R. *et al.* (1997) A prospective study of PET-FDG imaging for the assessment of head and neck squamous cell carcinoma, *Clin Otolaryngol* **22**: 209–14.

Yousem D. M., Som P. M., Hackney D. B., Schwaibold F. and Hendrix R. A. (1992) Central nodal necrosis and extracapsular neoplastic spread in cervical lymph nodes: MR imaging versus CT, *Radiology* **182**: 753–9.

Zbaren P., Becker M. and Laeng H. (1996) Pretherapeutic staging of laryngeal cancer: clinical findings, computed tomography and magnetic resonance imaging versus histopathology, *Cancer* **77**: 1263–73.

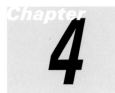

4 Treatment options: the principles of surgery

'Look before you leap'

Preparation

The patient

It is vital to prepare both the patient and their relatives psychologically before major surgical treatment options are undertaken for a potentially fatal disease, particularly when there is the possibility of considerable morbidity and even mortality. Statements made here are the opinions of the authors and are not intended to be in any way dogmatic.

One of the perennial problems of cancer therapy is what to tell the patient about the disease. An abdominal malignancy can often be treated without the patient or relatives being aware of the precise extent of the resection and therefore it is possible to treat the patient without telling him or her exactly what is being done, if this is the preferred option. In head and neck cancer this is not so. Many operations may mutilate the patient to some extent and deprive him or her, temporarily or permanently, of an important function such as speech or swallowing which will be immediately apparent to friends and relatives. Therefore, it is essential that the patient should be given an accurate account of all the facts.

Many patients now use the words 'malignancy' and 'cancer' with greater ease than a few years ago. These words can therefore now be used much more freely by the medical profession. At the first interview, the authors usually confine themselves to telling the patients and relatives that he or she may have cancer, a malignancy or a growth. Further in-depth explanations at this stage are usually pointless because the news has induced a massive mental block in most patients, and their minds concentrate on other factors such as family and possible outcomes; to talk further at this stage is simply a waste of time. Some degree of optimism should, however, be expressed at this first interview but the full explanation of the details of treatment is better left until the patient is seen again, often in the hospital environment for a biopsy or definitive treatment, when they are more receptive.

It is common nowadays to have in the clinic either a Macmillan head and neck nurse or a community liaison head and neck nurse who is trained in information skills, counselling and all aspects of head and neck oncology. They can then take over and perhaps give the patient and their relatives some more information following the initial consultation, so that the consultant's time is freed up to see the next patient.

Informed consent

The doctrine of informed consent has not yet been enshrined in English or Scottish law but may well be soon. It is essential to explain what is involved in the patient's illness, both to the patient and to the relatives or friends (with the patient's agreement). It is better to carry out this part of the interview with the relatives and the patient together at the same time. Talking to the patient and relatives separately can easily lead to suspicion and to misinterpretations in a situation which is already fraught with the opportunity for misunderstanding.

Informed consent consists of the following:

- details of the nature and severity of the cancer
- advice on the alternative treatments available
- recommendation of the optimal treatment plan
- effects of not taking advice
- specific risks of the operation
- risks of surgery in general.

Details of the nature and severity of the cancer

It is essential before going on to discuss treatment options to ensure that the patient has a realistic concept of the histological diagnosis and stage of the disease. For example: 'we have shown that your hoarse voice is due to a cancer in your voice box. The cancer has been detected at an early stage, and we hope to cure you with simple treatment'; alternatively: 'our investigations have shown that the pain in your ear has been caused by a cancer which started in your throat – in the tonsil. Unfortunately, this cancer has spread to glands in your neck. This is a very serious situation which can be difficult to treat successfully. You may need to have both a major operation and follow-up treatment'.

Advice on the alternative treatments available

In the management of head and neck cancer, a number of alternative treatments exist and, depending on whom the patients sees, different treatment options are available. Indeed, it has recently been said that a treatment plan for head and neck cancer depends on which specialist, i.e. surgeon or oncologist, the patient goes to see. For this reason, patients should be assessed in a multidisciplinary clinic prior to the formulation of a treatment plan. It is important to discuss with the patient alternative treatments (i.e. radiotherapy, surgery plus or minus post-operative radiotherapy, palliative treatment with radiotherapy and/or adjuvant chemotherapy or no treatment at all) and indicate the results that can be achieved in that particular own department. High cure rates may be achievable in some institutions, but these results will not be transferable to every practice. This applies both to surgery and to radiotherapy.

Recommendation of the optimal treatment plan

To discuss one type of therapy to the exclusion of another would be entirely wrong but at this point in the discussion the surgeon should indicate to the patient, from their experience, which modality they think is preferable both for the patient and for this particular tumour.

Effects of not taking advice

If the patient opts for surgery when radiotherapy has been suggested or vice versa, then the explanation of the effects has been covered by the previous part of the interview. If, however, the patients opts for no treatment, then no term of life should ever be given to patient and relatives for two reasons. First, one cannot begin to be accurate in estimating somebody's lifespan with an untreated carcinoma, and secondly, anything that is said may be taken as definitive and quoted back to you. Nonetheless, the patient must know that untreated cancer will sooner or later prove fatal.

Specific risks of the operation

Strictly speaking, in English law, according to the Sideway case, all that the patient needs to be told about is serious risks such as paralysis, death and blindness. Most courts, however, would judge that the wise doctor would expect the prudent patient to be told of any complications and effects of surgery that would materially alter his or her quality of life. Nowadays, most surgeons will inform patients of all major and important complications that

occur more often than in 2% of cases, e.g. recurrent laryngeal nerve injury and thyroid surgery, facial nerve injury and parotid surgery. It is not enough just to use these words; one must be prepared to explain the effects of complications such as aphonia, dysarthria, dysphagia and the problems of prosthetic replacement.

While it is often difficult for patients to appreciate the difference, it is important to try to explain the differences between the severity of a complication (trivial, significant, severe or fatal), the likelihood of it occurring (very rarely, seldom, usually or always) and its duration (whether it will be transient or permanent).

Risks of surgery in general

The risks of surgery in general include the problems of the anaesthetic, which should form part of the interview between the anaesthetist and the patient before any surgery is undertaken. However, the surgeon should check that this has been done and it may be prudent to go over any queries that the patient may have following the discussion with the anaesthetist or, if he or she has not mentioned such risks, they should be discussed with the patient. It is the duty of the surgeon to discuss the generic complications of surgery, such as haemorrhage, thromboembolism and wound and chest infections.

Finally, a note should be made in the case records that all of the above have been discussed with the patient. A consent form, which is now available in most British hospitals, is insufficient to take care of what has just been discussed and some surgeons have their own consent forms to include serious specific complications, e.g. thyroid surgery. While it is not yet necessary for statements to be signed and countersigned this may well come to pass in the UK within the next decade and if there is any worry about any specific problems relating to consent of a patient, it is better to obtain the patient's consent in front of a witness than to ask them to countersign the document.

Opinions are divided about whether or not to let a patient see a successful patient who has had a similar operation prior to surgery. The authors feel that it may not always be helpful for a patient who is to undergo a total laryngectomy to talk to one who has undergone the same operation and has been fully rehabilitated. This is because first, even the very best rehabilitation from a laryngectomy is ill considered by the normal population and by no means every laryngectomee is fully rehabilitated. Second, a target may be set which may never be reached by the patient in question. However, as a general rule, if the patient wishes to see and meet somebody who has undergone successful surgery, it should be considered a reasonable request.

Occasionally, a surgeon will be asked to perform head and neck surgery (and very occasionally head and neck cancer surgery) on a Jehovah's witness. There is a special consent form for these patients and they should be given the appropriate advice not only relating to informed consent as discussed above but also about not receiving a blood transfusion.

Once this has been done, the authors think it is reasonable to perform major head and neck surgery to include cancer surgery for those operations that do not normally require significant blood transfusion. This would include the operations up to laryngectomy or neck dissection. The most experienced surgeon in the unit or centre should carry out this surgery and (like all head and neck cancer operations) it should not be performed by the occasional head and neck dabbler. Operations over and above those just described which in experienced hands usually require blood transfusion should not be offered to a Jehovah's Witness without consent for a blood transfusion. In this situation the patient will either opt for an alternative form of treatment or request a second opinion.

The surgeon and team

It is important to remember that the surgeon is in charge and that everybody in theatre is there because the surgeon has decided to operate on the patient in question. Cancer surgery is an art, not a science, and a treatment plan must be formulated which you have discussed with the oncologist and other colleagues in the multidisciplinary team. As the surgeon approaches the operating table, this is not the time to start thinking what to do and whether, for example, a neurosurgeon, cardiac or vascular surgeon will be required. The surgeon should have come up with a plan, and a plan for that plan, and have rehearsed it in his or her mind, so that on the approach to the operating table the surgeon's thoughts are clear and he or she does not hesitate on taking the pen to mark out the incisions. One must 'get it right first time', because it is better to be radical early and conservative late rather than vice versa. Like the athlete preparing for an important race, a night's rest is important to give a clear mind and for those doing microvascular surgery, a steady hand may be enhanced by abstinence from caffeine and alcohol.

The smooth running of an operation is greatly enhanced if the procedure has been discussed beforehand with all the surgical team to include policy issues and individual duties. A good assistant makes head and neck surgery look easy.

The anaesthetist should be warned of any potential problems, including difficult intubation and whether or not the operation involves free tissue transfer. The nursing team should be warned about the major steps of the operation and the order in which they will be performed, e.g. endoscopy followed by major head and neck resection, which may include bone resection. If microvascular surgery is being performed the specific nursing team that is skilled in that technique needs to be informed so that they come on the late shift, since often they will not be required until later on in the operation.

It is important to try to operate as part of a team and nowadays most people have two teams, one playing a major part in the resection and the other in the reconstruction. This means that no one person is operating for long periods without a break, lunchbreaks can be taken

and the operation is usually completed within the normal working day.

Sir Harold Gillies, the father of plastic surgery and himself an ear, nose and throat (ENT) surgeon and Rhodes scholar from New Zealand, had some famous sayings regarding surgery. Although they were applied to reconstructive surgery they can be applied to any operation and are as true today as when they were written over 50 years ago. The important ones are listed in the box below.

> ■ Observation is the basis of surgical diagnosis
> ■ Make a diagnosis before treating the patient
> ■ Make a plan, and a pattern for this plan
> ■ Aftercare is as important as the planning
> ■ Consult other specialists
> ■ Make a record
> ■ Thou shalt not have a routine
> ■ Thou shalt have a style

In summary, 'look before you leap'.

Skin preparation

Some patients require shaving prior to surgery. If this is done the day before surgery it increases the bacterial count on the skin so the patient should receive prophylactic antibiotics. An alternative is to shave the patient immediately before the procedure.

Before the skin is prepared in theatre, the position of the patient should be adjusted exactly, either by the surgeon before scrubbing up or by trained theatre staff under supervision. The patient's neck is extended by placing a small sandbag underneath the shoulders. If the patient is to undergo a neck dissection, the neck is extended and turned to the other side by placing the sandbag mainly under the ipsilateral shoulder. There should be a plastic sheet under the patient's head and shoulders because wet towels allow bacteria from the theatre table to pass through them.

A separate trolley may be used to clean the patient's skin. If desired, the surgeon may wear two pairs of gloves and once cleaning up is completed, the outer pair may be discarded when the skin is clean and the towels are in place.

When carrying out thoracic or abdominal work the whole of the area (head, chest and abdomen) can be prepared, draped, covered in a steridrape and then covered with a green towel until required. This similarly applies to the arm or the leg if free tissue transfer is being undertaken.

By now the patient will be prepared for surgery. For a major operation, a urinary catheter will have been inserted and the patient have on both thrombo-embolic deterent (TED) and flowtron stockings. These can be removed at the end of the procedure prior to taking a skin graft.

When operating on the face when the facial nerve is at risk, it is important to steridrape the face so that full facial movements can be visualized.

Many sterilizing solutions are available for head and neck surgery and surgeons tend to use whatever the current fashion is in their hospital, together with what they have used in the past. It used to be said that the only important point about sterilizing solutions is that the particular preparations should not be coloured so that any changes in skin flap colour can be seen at an early stage but nowadays this does not matter. A good option is to use povidone iodine on the neck and lower face, and reserve Savlon or chlorhexidine for around the eyes.

After the skin has been prepared, the edges of the operative field may be sprayed with nobecutaine so that the towels stick to the skin. An amputation dressing may be placed at the base of the neck between the shoulders on either side to eliminate the dead space and this technique, along with spraying the edges of the operative field, helps to eliminate potential dead spaces and keep infection to a minimum. Towel clips often get during the way in a long operation and tend to slip, so it is wise to sew the towels to the skin with 3/0 silk.

The incision

Principles of incisions

Incisions for operations in the head and neck must conform to the basic requirements of any incision and as such should provide adequate access. Because of this, the incisions made in head and neck surgery are fundamentally different to those in abdominal or thoracic surgery, where access is obtained by a cut that is deepened through the overlying structures, and by retraction of the edges of the incision, so that skin flaps are not raised. In neck surgery, large skin flaps must be developed to provide adequate access; these flaps must sometimes be so large that their blood supply becomes tenuous, particularly in a patient who has been irradiated.

This is best illustrated by the operation of radical neck dissection in which the operative field extends from the clavicle below to the mandible above, from the border of the trapezius laterally to the midline medially; thus the entire skin of the neck must be elevated (see Chapter 13).

There is a well-known surgical aphorism that a wound heals from side to side and not from end to end, implying that a long wound heals as well as a short one. Doubtless this is true of incisions used for abdominal or thoracic surgery in which flaps are not developed, but in neck surgery, where extensive flaps must be elevated, this aphorism is untrue; blind adherence to this principle will lead, on occasion, to avoidable disasters.

Any incision must be capable of extension, during the operation or later, so that any present or future eventuality can be dealt with. It is particularly important when operating on the neck for the first time to bear in mind that another operation may be required at a future date, so that the incision used must be capable of being reopened to deal with the problem, of being extended or even excised as part of further definitive surgery.

An example of this is a laryngectomy in which a neck dissection may later be needed. In this instance, if the laryngectomy is performed through a narrow apron type of flap, it may subsequently be difficult to fashion a satisfactory incision through which to carry out an appropriate neck dissection.

An incision must not damage vital structures in or beneath the skin. The most important structures running in the skin are the cutaneous blood vessels. Cadaver studies have shown that the blood supply of the neck is taken largely from two pedicles, one anterosuperior derived from the carotid artery, and one inferomedial derived from branches of the subclavian artery. There is thus a watershed running in an inferomedial direction in the neck and it is said that incisions which take advantage of this are particularly safe (Fig. 4.1). This is probably not the whole story, because in the live patient, a flap delineated by horizontal incisions is very safe and very rarely undergoes necrosis, which is not true of flaps delineated by vertical incisions.

The most important structures beneath the skin are the branches of the facial nerve, and elevation of the flap in the upper part of the neck must proceed in such a manner as to preserve these. This matter is dealt with in Chapter 13.

An incision must always heal well, producing a scar that is cosmetically acceptable. Remember that a surgeon will be judged by these scars and that proper incisions come together and improper ones tend to gape. To achieve this an incision should, if possible, be placed in the lines of election for scars in the neck or in relaxed skin tension lines. These run in a horizontal direction and usually coincide with the skin creases, which should be used wherever possible for siting a scar (Fig. 4.2). It should be noted that the lines of election for scars do not coincide with Langer's lines, which run vertically on the neck. A further factor which may mitigate against healing is the use of the three-point junction. A well-known surgical principle states that the use of such a junction increases the incidence of wound breakdown and wherever possible such a junction should not be used; when performed it should be sewn up in the conventional manner for such an incision.

In summary:

- wherever possible, an incision in the neck should lie in the horizontal plane
- it should be designed to be extended if complications are encountered
- the flaps raised should be as small as possible to be compatible with the intended operation.

It is important to look before you leap. It was Sir Harold Gillies who said 'Seven times seven turn your knife in your hand err you cut the skin of a fellow man' and Last in the same year (1968) said 'seven times seven make up your mind err you cut across Langer's line'. Such statements make it clear that it is important to have a plan when operating within the head and neck.

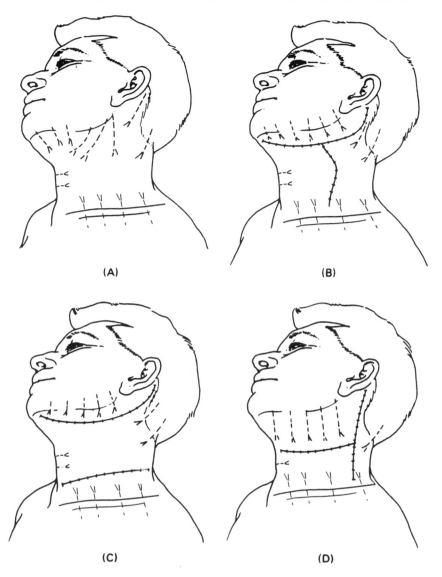

(A)　　　　　　　　　　　　(B)

(C)　　　　　　　　　　　　(D)

Figure 4.1 Blood supply to the skin and neck in relation to various incision lines. Note the watershed in the middle of the neck under normal conditions in (A).

When operating on the face (particularly for skin cancer and scar revision), one should remember two cardinal rules. First, 'one must not obtain incomplete clearance during excision of the tumour' and secondly 'one must not unknowingly create any secondary deformity'. Both of these problems can be prevented by prior thought and proper marking of the incision.

Marking the skin incision

The site of incision is marked with methylene blue using a mapping pen. The marks should be made without traction and counteraction, which distorts the skin, and once the incision is marked, points on either side of the incision line may be made with a needle dipped in methylene blue to facilitate closure (Fig. 4.3). It is

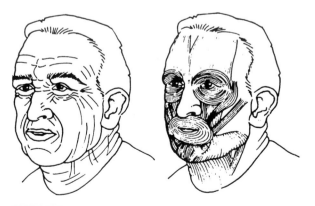

Figure 4.2 Lines of election for scars related to wrinking and the underlying musculature.

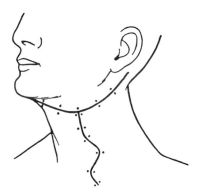

Figure 4.3 Skin incision marked.

important to spend some time, particularly when operating on the face, in marking out the incision; if there is any doubt the line should be erased and the incision redrawn.

At this stage, the site of the incision may be injected using 1:200 000 adrenaline in normal saline. This reduces the bleeding, inflates the underlying soft tissues and identifies the surgical planes more easily, e.g. in parotid surgery. It is also possible to use up to 60 ml of xylocaine 0.25% with 1:80 000 adrenaline along the incision site to help with postoperative pain relief.

The local anaesthetic in the skin prevents the weal and flare reflex when the skin is cut, and the infiltration of the soft tissue markedly reduces bleeding during the operation. With the preparation of the operative site in this way, coupled with careful operative technique and controlled hypotension, the blood loss should be minimal. For example, the blood loss during a radical neck dissection or a total laryngectomy should be less than 200 ml.

In view of the increasing difficulty in obtaining blood, increasing anxiety about diseases transmitted via transfused blood and adverse prognosis relating to patients who receive blood transfusion, the advantages of minimizing blood loss are obvious.

Making the incision

The knife should be held at right angles to the skin, which in some parts of the body can be difficult to achieve. Where the skin is very loose, the pressure of the knife can distort it, causing the resulting cut to be slanted and untidy, which may make subsequent resuturing difficult. In addition, skin edges cut on the bevel may undergo necrosis (Fig. 4.4). The answer is to provide external tension. In most cases, this can be achieved by spreading

the skin with the other hand and using traction and countertraction. Occasionally, it is necessary to create tension in all directions and a useful trick is to ask an assistant to stretch the skin in the line of the cut as well as using a pair of skin hooks.

The cut should be made with sufficient boldness to part the skin with one clean stroke rather than a process of erosion, but not so bold as to damage underlying structures. The knife blade is held at right angles to the skin using the belly of the blade. Where a small cut is required, a small blade such as a number 15 is easiest to use, whereas for larger incisions, larger blades such as a number 10 or number 22 will suffice.

Remember that the knife is an extension of the hand. It is not a rigid structure but should be used like a paintbrush to glide over and through tissues. Head and neck surgery is unique in that it combines the finesse of delicate microsurgery with subtle small movements of the fingers and progresses through various movements at the wrist, elbow and shoulder, occasionally to employ the more vigorous manoeuvres of the orthopaedic surgeon. The combination and timing of subtle and rapid vigorous movements make head and neck surgery unique.

The assistant now retracts the flaps vertically with double skin hooks in the subcutaneous tissues (Fig. 4.5). This demonstrates a clear plane deep to the platysma; sharp dissection in this plane is bloodless. Allis forceps should never be applied to the skin and in the past it has been stated that tooth forceps should not be used to hold the skin. It is the authors' opinion that rather than applying crushing pressure with non-tooth forceps to the skin, it is better to hold the skin for a short period with tooth forceps. The assistant must never fold the flap completely on itself as this may lead to button-holing.

After elevating the flaps, the skin surface must be excluded completely from the wound either by stitching the flaps back to the towels or by retracting them with a Joll's clamp and side towels. If the skin flaps are stitched to the towels, the needle must not be passed through the skin, only through the subcutaneous tissues. If the upper skin flap has been folded over the chin on to the face to hold it out of the way, tension from the sutures to the underlying face should be avoided by placing a swab between the suture and the face.

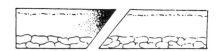

Figure 4.4 Bevelled skin edges.

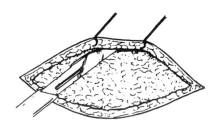

Figure 4.5 Skin edges elevated and retracted.

Dissection

The surgeon should use a limited range of instruments, know each instrument by name and become thoroughly familiar with each one. Some of the basic rules of surgery are 'pick it up, use it and then put it down; do not wave the instrument about; and keep your eye on the ball and your mind focused on the job'.

Another secret regarding head and neck surgery is adequate access. Each individual step of surgery is then easy, but access to allow that manoeuvre to be executed properly can be difficult. Access requires space and once the appropriate incision has been made, the creation of further space demands the ability to think in three dimensions and move important structures out of the way.

Dissection is performed with a sharp blade with an assistant providing traction and countertraction. Scissors are useful in certain circumstances but as a general rule it is advisable not to use them for the technique of dissection as this will cause bleeding that will then have to be stopped. Using a knife, the 'bleeders' can be seen and diathermied before they bleed. This subtle point makes all the difference and the surgery more elegant.

As regards bleeding points, a good rule is to use coagulation diathermy on the specimen only and to tie named vessels left in the patient using vicryl. The surgeon should not leave long-ended ligatures, tie a large mass of tissue or coagulate a large area, since all of these factors lead to possible abscess formation and subsequent postoperative infection.

Incision and excision of bone

There are two main reasons for incising bone in head and neck cancer surgery. The first is to provide access and the second is to excise bone as part of the tumour excision.

A common example of access surgery where bone must be divided to provide access is in mandibulotomy for access to tumours in the oral cavity and oropharynx. Here, the bone will be put back together again and it is important that the cut has been made in the appropriate place with the appropriate equipment to facilitate good surgical realignment.

Preoperative orthopantogram (OPG) will allow the surgeon to plan where best to place the mandibulotomy but it is common practice to perform a paramedian mandibulotomy just anterior to the mental nerve. Reconstruction will be completed using titanium plates, the alignment for the two plates is then marked prior to incision and the screw holes are drilled first. The bone is then incised using a reciprocating saw. There is no need to step the incision since a straight cut will suffice, and on completion of the surgery realignment is easily achieved.

Excision of bone for the treatment of cancer is dictated by the extent of the tumour but in the absence of previous irradiation, **conservation surgery** is possible and using the reciprocating saw or fissure burr excision of part of the mandible is possible. Once the bone is rejoined following access surgery or excision with reconstruction, the area should be covered with vascularized tissue to promote healing. It is important to remember that heavily irradiated bone may become infected postoperatively if it is divided and exposed to saliva.

For complete bony excision of the mandible, it is also possible to use a Gigli saw if access to a reciprocating saw is not possible. Once one starts to use it, there must be no pause because the wire curls up and sticks in the bone if it is not kept taut, and this can result in a broken wire. The handles should be kept as far apart as possible, cutting with the wire almost straight, and being aware of fragments of bone, blood and even part of the saw flying off and hitting the operator in the face.

Tumour excision

After excising the specimen, in continuity, leave the table with the specimen and examine the edges. In oral and pharyngeal cancer the margin around the tumour often appears narrow, probably because mucosa retracts after it has been cut. However, if there is no margin at one edge the surgeon should go back and excise another strip of mucosa at this point. Specimens from the edges nearest the tumour are sent for frozen section to ensure that excision has been complete.

After examining the specimen the theatre sister takes away all of the instruments used in the removal of the tumour, because they are contaminated. The surgeon takes off the gown and gloves, puts on new ones and makes sure that everybody else does the same.

In the past, didactic recommendations were made regarding safe margins. However, pathological studies have refined our knowledge of this area and it is now known that the margin must be dictated by the tumour. Lip cancers require a margin of not more than 1 cm, and the excellent results from supraglottic laryngectomy have shown that only millimetres of clearance are needed near the vocal cords. Conversely, some tumours require a margin of more than 2 cm, the most notorious of these being tumours of the tongue, oropharynx and hypopharynx. Each case should be treated on its merits but one should always strive to perform as wide a removal as possible within the limits of subsequent reconstruction and inevitable cosmetic deformity.

If radiotherapy has been used previously to treat the head and neck cancer, it is important not to be fooled by the subsequent reduction in the size of the tumour. The margin to be excised is the same as if the patient had not had radiotherapy and this is also true of chemotherapy.

Tissues become distorted during excision, so tattoo a line of clearance around the tumour before starting to remove it. If preoperative radiotherapy is to be used, tattoo the selected line of excision before irradiation. This is best done at the time of biopsy under general anaesthetic.

Wound irrigation

Before beginning to close the wound it must be washed out well. Many different solutions are available and as long as they are toxic to cells, it does not matter which one is used. Sterile water, Savlon, hydrogen peroxide and other cytotoxic solutions are all as good as each other but the important part of this process appears to be the mechanical action of the washing rather than the lytic action on the cells. All areas must be washed thoroughly with at least 1 litre of solution. It is the author's preference to use Savlon followed by half-strength hydrogen peroxide. This washout process often restarts bleeding from several small points, which facilitates the opportunity to secure final and absolute haemostasis.

Drains

It is a good surgical regime always to drain the neck. Suction drainage is usually employed. A wick type of drain is as likely to allow bacteria into the wound as it is to let serum out, although occasionally when draining infected wounds, a corrugated wound is required.

Methods

Polythene tubes

These are the simplest and easiest method of establishing suction drainage. Holes are cut in thin polythene tubing and connected to a suction machine or wall suction. However, they tie the patient to the bed and therefore he or she cannot walk about without disconnecting the drain. They are seldom used now unless a suction vacuum cannot be maintained.

Vacuum systems

Various closed suction systems are available but are expensive. These are the simple Redivac drains or the slightly more expensive 'Surgidenc' variety, which are larger and softer. These tubes are already perforated and sterilized and drain into bottles or canisters which are evacuated of air. In accordance with the laws of technology, the best and cheapest of these is no longer made. These systems have the advantage that the patient is mobile and are the most commonly used variety. Care is needed to keep an eye on the indicators at the top of the drain to detect when the vacuum becomes exhausted and the drain stops working.

Fixation of the drainage tube

There is a lot of nonsense written about how to tie in a drain. A drain will not come out if it is sewn in properly. The best way of fixing a Redivac drain is to take a silk suture and place it through the skin, and then halve the suture, remove the needle and tie a knot about 2 cm from the skin. This means that a knot is not tied directly on to the skin, which is painful and can promote infection. The stitch pulled is tied around the drain using a double hitch, i.e. over and over, and the stitch pulled tight so that it just compresses the tube. The knot is completed in the conventional manner and if required the knot may be repeated once more, but there is no need to go round and

round the stitch using the 'Roman garter' method. This is laborious and untidy, and often does not do what it is required, which is to fix the drain.

Sometimes there may be leaks from where the drain exits from the skin. This may be prevented by spraying the site with Nobecutaine and covering it with a swab at the end of the procedure. The other thing to do is to check that a drainage hole is not exposed on the exterior, which will lead to loss of vacuum. The latter is easily corrected by recognizing the problem and pushing the drain further in, if possible, or closing the hole with a stitch.

Sometimes after surgery to the trachea, i.e. laryngectomy, there will be a through-and-through leak with constant devacuuming of the drains. In this situation the drains should be connected to either a Robert's pump or wall suction to facilitate constant suction drainage. The wounds are covered with Nobecutaine and dressings and after 48 h, conventional suction drainage can be reapplied and there are usually no further problems.

Closing the skin

It is important to produce a good scar after any head and neck surgical procedure: the scar is the only visible sign to the patient and relatives for assessing the surgeon's skill. Remember: 'by your scars you will be judged'.

The principles of sewing the skin are accurate apposition, good surgical technique with no tension and the avoidance of dead spaces and haematomas. This may be achieved by using suction drainage, closing the skin in two layers and using the appropriate suture material together with proper meticulous surgical techniques.

Instruments

Healthy tissues should not be pinched, crushed or otherwise abused. There is no doubt that having the right instrument for the right job makes the procedure less of a trial for the surgeon and patient alike. For example, closing a small wound with a fine suture using a pair of heavy forceps and a pair of Kilner needle holders (which have a particularly strong ratchet) irritates the experienced and is likely to make the inexperienced feel unnecessarily clumsy. Fine work requires fine instruments.

The skin should not be grasped with forceps unless it is absolutely necessary. Non-toothed forceps crush the skin and can do more damage than using toothed forceps quickly and efficiently. The wound, where possible, should be grasped by the subcutaneous tissues using a skin hook or, as previously stated, using toothed forceps. A good technique is to use these as a hook and lever. This means using the forceps with the tips open, hooking the subcutaneous tissues with one tip and exerting gentle pressure with this tip to lever the skin backwards, thus facilitating the passage of the needle (Fig. 4.6). This is a habit which is worth acquiring early, as the novice's frustration at trying to place a suture with one hand is directly proportional to the force applied to the forceps held in the other hand, with consequent damage to the skin

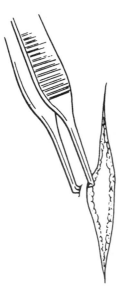

Figure 4.6 One tip of a toothed forceps used as a hook and the other as a lever.

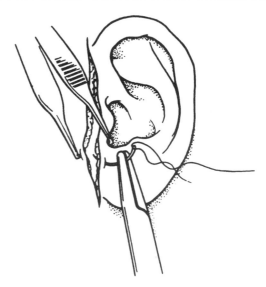

Figure 4.7 Open forceps used for simultaneous counter-pressure and eversion.

edges. Otherwise, a skin hook may be used. This is even harder to learn but once mastered is an excellent technique. The purpose of forceps is to evert the skin whilst the suture is being placed. This can often be achieved by pressing the open forceps down on either side of the wound, which has the effect of pushing the skin edges up (Fig. 4.7), and then passing the needle through both sides with one movement. The same effect can be produced by using fingers instead of forceps.

Sutures

An increasing number of sutures are becoming available and a list of those most frequently used is given in Table 4.1. Absorbable sutures are used when the suture is not expected to be removed, i.e. in subcutaneous closure, suturing mucosa or where removal may be difficult, e.g. behind the ear in a young child. They are absorbed at different rates and this is reflected in their ability to take the tension of a sutured wound. Plain catgut loses its tensile strength most rapidly (after 5 days), although chromic catgut lasts longer. Vicryl lasts for around 4 weeks and polydioxanone (PDS) lasts longest (about 60 days). These sutures are all absorbed by varying degrees of inflammatory response, except for PDS, which is absorbed by hydrolysis, although what practical difference this makes has yet to be determined. From the above, two points emerge:

- if possible, absorbable sutures should not be placed too close to the skin, because of the inflammatory response
- longer lasting absorbable sutures should be used where there is a tight skin closure or where the skin tension is naturally high, to take the weight and tension of the wound.

Table 4.1 Suture materials

	Non-absorbable	Absorbable
Monofilament	Nylon (Ethilion) Prolene Polybutester (Novafil) Stainless steel	PDS II (polydioxanone) Monocryl (polyglecaprone) Catgut (chromic and plain) Softgut
Multifilament	Silk Nurolon (polyamide) Polyester (Ethibond) Linen	Vicryl (polygalactin) which is available both dyed and undyed Dexon (polyglycolic)
Tissue glue/adhesives	Cyanoacrylate	
Clips	Stainless steel Titanium	
Steristrips	1/2, 1/4 and 1/8 inch	

Catgut is easy to work with and ties a good knot but is absorbed quite quickly. Dexon and Vicryl are easy to work with but require very careful multiple knots. PDS is harder to work with but ties an excellent knot, lasts the longest and is particularly useful when sewing in flaps in the pharynx. Non-absorbable materials are used as either skin sutures or permanent subcutaneous sutures. Silk is the easiest of any suture to handle and ties the best knot; best here meaning the most secure knot with the least number of throws. There is some evidence that because it is multifilament and therefore has some capillary action, it is more likely to cause hatch marks (suture marks) than the equivalent monofilament and should not be used routinely on the skin. However, it is of particular use when resuturing wounds following dehiscence, when it works well with the through-and-through one-layer closure stitch. Linen is also easy to handle and may be used to ligate larger vessels but is becoming less available. Nuralon is very similar to silk, but ties a less secure knot.

Monofilaments are in general harder to handle and require more care in tying the knot than Nylon. When removed early, they cause minimal scarring to the skin. Prolene, Ethilon and Novafil are more slippery than Nylon, and are therefore better for subcuticular closure of wounds and tie better knots. Clips are quicker, more expensive, give an excellent end result and are particularly useful in closing following thyroid surgery, surgery for branchial cysts, thyroglossal duct cysts and neck dissections.

Suturing

The wide variety of sutures available has been described above. The decision remains as to which type of suture to use for any given situation, but many surgeons will find that as they develop a busy practice, they will tend to use fewer types of suture. It is good advice to use the finest suture that will hold the wound and to consider carefully how long the sutures will have to remain in place. Subcutaneous sutures are used to close the dead space and take the weight of a wound, while skin sutures should do no more than provide fine edge approximation of a wound that already has a 'kissing fit' from the subcutaneous closure. Wounds heal from side to side and not end to end. Although sutures can be removed (after 5 days), it is the deep sutures which hold the wound and the time taken for a wound to heal properly is the time that it used to take to sail around the world (80 days).

The incidence of hatch marks on the wound is directly related to the length of time for which the sutures are left in, their tightness and the type of suture used. If a suture needs to be left in for any length of time, a subcuticular one should be considered.

Most sutures are not atraumatic, that is to say, the needle is swaged on to the suture. All needles discussed in this chapter, except for the one used for subcuticular sutures, are meant to be used with needle holders, which means that they are curved. They may be round-bodied, taper-cutting or true-cutting. Round-bodied needles have a simple tapering tip and are used where minimal tissue

trauma is obligatory, such as in the bowel, on pharyngeal mucosa or on vessels during microvascular surgery. However, they are extremely difficult to pass through tough tissues such as skin. A cutting needle must be used for suturing skin or subcutaneous tissues. As the name implies, cutting needles have a cutting tip, in a variety of types, which permits them to be passed easily through most tissues. The taper-cutting or reverse-cutting needles are a compromise between cutting and round-bodied needles and combine maximum efficiency of passage through tissue with minimal trauma.

Curved needles should be mounted in the needle holder in their flattened midsection at the tip of the holder for maximum efficiency (Fig. 4.8a). If they are mounted at the swaged section, which is round, there is a tendency for the needle to twist in the needle holder and bend or break off (Fig. 4.8b). Individual preference will indicate which needle holder the surgeon prefers to use but some needle holders have particular advantages. The Nievert needle holder is favoured by some plastic surgeons; it sits comfortably in the hand and allows the tip of the needle holder to be manoeuvred in many directions with minimal hand movements. Another favourite is the Gillies and Foster Gillies needle holder which allows accurate placement of sutures under direct control and the suture to be cut without an assistant.

Subcutaneous sutures may be used to obliterate dead spaces and approximate the wound edges. An absorbable suture should be used on a cutting needle. The platysma is closed with either an interrupted or a continuous suture

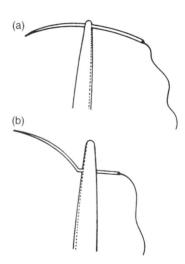

Figure 4.8 (a) Correct and (b) incorrect method of holding a needle.

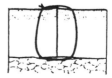

Figure 4.9 Correct position of skin suture.

and the final knot inverted. This layer is the main strength layer of neck closure and should be airtight. Skin sutures are used to provide accurate edge approximation with skin eversion. To achieve eversion, the deep tissue should push the edges upwards when the knot is tied (Fig. 4.9), which is the reason for turning the skin back with forceps or a skin hook as the needle is passed. Eversion of the wound edges is mandatory for primary healing with a good scar: an inverted wound may look fine until the sutures are removed; then, the edges gape and healing is by secondary intention.

There are many different methods by which to close the skin and each has its place in different situations at different times. On the face with no tension, if the deep closure is done properly, sometimes no sutures are required and steristrips will suffice. The simplest way to close a wound is using an interrupted stitch and, for increased strength and tightness, the mattress suture may be used. However, putting in stitch after stitch is laborious and sometimes continuous sutures have their advantages. They are faster and easier to remove for both the patients and the doctor and nurses and there are fewer knots to accumulate blood clots. This makes them easier to clean and reduces the infection rate. However, continuous sutures have to be placed with proper regard to edge eversion and tightness and are unsuitable where the suture might need to be removed prematurely, unless it is a locked suture, for once one side is cut the whole wound is at risk of separating.

Continuous sutures may be over and over. Some surgeons favour the blanket suture, particularly for the curved incision of a major neck procedure. Both types of suture use a non-absorbable material such as Nylon or Ethilon. It has been said that mattress sutures are for mattresses and blanket sutures for blankets, but in the right situation, both techniques have their uses (Fig. 4.10). When performing the blanket suture, the needle is positioned at more than a right angle to the skin edge to obtain a larger bite of the dermis together with the fat and skin. The needle is placed 2 mm in from the skin edge and the sutures placed 5–10 mm apart, depending on the length of the wound, in order to distribute tension evenly. Equal bites should be taken because unequal ones lead to poor skin apposi-

tion. This stitch should evert the skin edge. When sewing up a wound with a continuous stitch, the length of the suture should be four times the length of the wound, the entry points either side of the wound should be 5 mm from the skin edge and each stitch should be 1 cm apart. Wounds that are sewn up properly heal well.

In cases where sutures are to be left in for more than 10 days, and where a good scar is of overriding importance and the wound is relatively short and straight (e.g. surgery for a pharyngeal pouch), a subcuticular suture is useful. This may be either absorbable Dexon or preferably a non-absorbable suture, which should be a monofilament. Prolene and Novafil are easiest to remove. Either a straight or curved needle may be used, depending on personal preference.

Satisfactory and rapid skin closure can now be achieved using staples in a disposable handpiece. A three-point junction must be sewn up first if staples are to be used on the main wound. To prevent necrosis of the corners and bunching of the tip of the flap the three-point junction is closed in a conventional manner. First, the needle is placed 1 cm in from the edge of the reception side of the wound and a subcutaneous bite of the tip taken. Then the needle is brought out again 1 cm from the skin edge on the reception side and the knot tied, making sure that the suture enters and leaves the reception side at the same level as it does in a 'V' flap (Fig. 4.11).

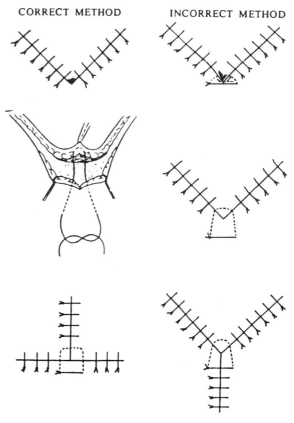

Figure 4.11 Suturing of a three-point junction. Note the incorrect method may lead to tip necrosis of the flap.

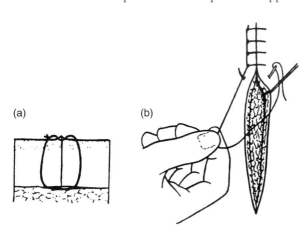

Figure 4.10 (a) Mattress suture and (b) blanket suture.

Postoperative care

Tracheostomy nursing care

A trained nursed should be in attendance at all times for the first 24–48 h following a tracheostomy. The nurse should be acquainted with all of the complications of the operation and the principles of sterile suction and humidification, and should be able to remove and replace the tube if necessary. Often, the inclusion of a rescue stitch will facilitate replacement of the tube. This involves placing a non-absorbable suture (usually silk) through the lower tracheal wall of the cut window in the trachea at the time of the tracheostomy. This is then tied in a loop and taped to the patient's chest. If the tube comes out in the middle of the night, gentle traction on the suture will bring the trachea forwards and open the window, thus identifying the route for reinsertion.

The patient must be informed before the operation that he or she will not be able to speak until the tracheostomy is closed. They may find a 'magic slate' or pad on which to write useful, along with a bell with which to summon assistance.

Fixation of the tracheostomy tube

A tracheostomy tube can be difficult to replace if it is dislodged within the first 48 h. Therefore, it should be taped in and stitched to the skin as well. These stitches can be cut out when the tube is changed for the first time, and then only tapes used for the second tracheostomy tube. The tapes are tied so that they are doubled over with the head in the neutral position; if they are tied in the extended position, they will be too loose when the head is in the neutral position. A reef knot is used and the knot placed so there is one on each side of the neck, which is achieved by placing the tapes through the tracheostomy tube and doubling them over, with the lengths being two-thirds to one-third. A long length and a short length should then be used on each side, the long length being passed through to the other side and tied to the corresponding short length. The tapes should not be tied so tightly that they obstruct the lymphatic drainage, causing oedema of the skin flaps above the ties. It is best not to take the tapes across a pedicle of a skin flap from the chest, and if there is any concern about obstructing the flow in a pedicled or free flap, the tube should simply be stitched in. The use of a rescue stitch has been described already.

Removal of secretions

Excess secretions are inevitable after a newly created tracheostomy because the tube acts as a foreign body and stimulates secretions, and the trachea has never been exposed to cold dry air before. In addition, there may be some oozing of blood from the operation site. Secretions should be removed by suction every 30 min or more often if indicated. After the first 48 h, this period may be lengthened but suction will always be required at least every 4 hours in the immediate postoperative period. The nurse should wear sterile gloves and use the special suction tubes that minimize tracheal and bronchial trauma.

Humidification

The normal channels for warming and humidifying the air have now been bypassed, so artificial humidification is required to prevent the crusting of secretions. Humidification is provided by hot water bath humidifiers or by nebulizers delivering cold droplets. An alternative is heat and humidity exchangers. The humidified air is delivered by a mask or a 'T' tube applied to the tracheostomy tube. A satisfactory alternative to prevent crusting is the instillation of saline into the trachea. If secretions (and therefore crusting) are particularly severe, it is often useful to administer nebulized mucolytics for a few days. This problem is not uncommon since many patients have chronic obstructive airways disease. If crusting in the trachea becomes significant, daily inspection may be necessary with a flexible nasopharyngoscope and significant obstructive crusts and clots can be evacuated from the trachea and upper bronchi.

Changing the tracheostomy tube

The various types, designs and indications for using these tubes are discussed in Chapter 9. Normally for the first 48 h, a cuffed plastic or silastic tracheostomy tube is used since this will cater for the prevention of secretions and blood reaching the trachea and also allow ventilation. It is now mandatory to use a tracheostomy with both an inner and an outer tube. This facilitates cleaning of the inner tube so that tube obstruction is avoided. The first two changes normally take place after 48 h when a slightly smaller tracheostomy tube may be inserted. Thereafter, the tube is changed twice a week in order to avoid wound infection or crusting. After a tracheostomy tube is inserted into the trachea, it must be established with absolute certainty that it is actually in the trachea lumen, as it is easy to place the tube in the anterior mediastinum. When inserting the tube, the patient should be asked to breathe in and breathe out and hold the breath in expiration. This caters for easy tube insertion when the trachea is at its maximum diameter. Once the tube is inserted, the patient is asked to take deep breaths and feel the air coming in and out of the tube. The safest method of changing the tube at 48 h when any difficulty is anticipated is to insert a sterile catheter into the old tube, which is then withdrawn over the catheter. The new tube is then threaded over the catheter into the trachea. There is always a risk of failure of reintubation and this can result in unnecessary and untimely death. A pair of tracheal dilators should always be taped to the head of the bed, and a tracheostomy set, a battery laryngoscope and a bronchoscope should be available on the ward in case of dire emergencies. A doctor should always be present at the first tube change.

Care of the inflatable cuff

When a cuff is inflated to occlude the airway, its pressure can exceed the systolic blood pressure. This means that the area of the tracheal wall with which it is in contact is in danger of ischaemic necrosis. The tracheostomy cuff should be inflated for the first 12 h following surgery and during this time deflated for 5 min every hour. After 12–24 h, it may then be let down as long as there is no excessive bleeding or the patient is not being ventilated. New high-volume, low-pressure cuffs are now standard on most makes of tracheostomy tubes and these minimise the risk of tracheal damage. However, it is still good practice to deflate the cuff as indicated since occasionally, complications such as tracheal stenosis or very rarely ulceration with subsequent vascular haemorrhage from the innominate artery can still occur.

Breathing exercises

Most patients require postoperative breathing exercises from the physiotherapist. It is customary that a dedicated physiotherapist is present on most head and neck wards, who will see the patient preoperatively and then visit them in the postoperative period. If secretions are excessive, more vigorous treatment by intermittent positive-pressure breathing triggered by the patient is used. If this is not available, the patient's lungs can be inflated with an Ambu bag after suction has been performed. This gives greater ventilation and deep-breathing exercises can be performed more often. After sucking out the trachea, the Ambu bag is fitted on to the tracheostomy connection, the cuff of the tracheostomy tube is inflated and the patient ventilated for 3 min. The Ambu bag is then taken off and the cuff deflated. The temporary tracheostomy tube can be removed on the fifth day after surgery as long as the patient is progressing well. The tracheostomy tube may be spigoted off during the day. The following day, the tracheostomy tube may be blocked overnight as well. Therefore, on the next day if all goes well, the patient will have been blocked off for 24 h so that the tracheostomy tube can be withdrawn. The wounds are then dressed and allowed to close by secondary intention. It is important to recognize when spigoting a tube off, that only a small tube or fenestrated tube should be spigoted since if one tries to block off a large tube, particularly one that is cuffed, this may cause total respiratory obstruction in its own right even when the patient's upper airway is patent. So, in summary, it is wise not to remove a tracheostomy tube unless it has been spigoted off for 24 h.

Dressings

Special waterproof squares (melanin) can be used to care for the tracheostomy; they have a slit on their top surface which can be passed around the edge of the tube and may be left open at the top or secured with a safety pin. They require changing regularly because they absorb secretions and blood. They also play the important role of applying pressure between the tracheostomy tube and the wound, which is particularly useful when there is a small air leak from the skin through the trachea into an associated neck wound.

While it is often not a good idea to cover neck wounds, it can be helpful in the first 24 h to apply Nobecutaine or Opsite spray to the wound. It can then be covered with blue gauze dressing and the end of the dressing is wrapped around the drain site before activating the drains. This helps to seal the wound and one should now listen for any air escape which will indicate the location of a leak. This is discussed in the next section.

Drains

A suction drainage tube will have been inserted in the operating theatre. Continuous suction must be maintained since bacteria are as likely to go up a drainage tube as serum is to come down it, unless the vacuum is maintained. Whenever suction is taken off the tube, it should be clamped. It is also important not to allow the patient to wander around the ward with a drainage tube dangling free; the canister or the bottle should always be fixed to the patient's dressing gown and where the tube comes out from the skin, it should be secured with adhesive tape (e.g. Micropore).

In some situations where drainage may be prolonged and the formation of a seroma is not uncommon (e.g. latissimus dorsi donor site), the prolonged use of suction leads to the persistent production of serous fluid. In this situation, one solution is to cut the drain and allow free drainage. Once covered with a dry dressing the drainage will quickly subside.

Leaking drains

All of the advantages of suction drainage are lost if air is allowed to leak into the drainage tube from either an anastomosis, the skin incision or the tracheostomy site. This then means that saliva, air or infected secretions are drawn underneath the skin flaps, almost certainly leading to wound infection and skin breakdown. The leak must be stopped immediately to prevent this. Once a leak is noted, the wound should be examined to ascertain whether the leak comes from the tracheostomy, the skin incision or the internal suture line.

The best method of preventing an air leak from a tracheostomy is to keep the tracheostomy wound separate from the main wound. This is possible if the tracheostomy is temporary and care should be taken to keep the incision small and over to the other side if, for example, a neck dissection is being performed on one side. If the two incisions are joined by accident, then the junction may be closed carefully to provide an airtight seal. A permanent tracheostomy should be fashioned with great care in layers to prevent a leak, as described in Chapter 9.

If air is heard leaking around the tracheostomy, local packing with saline-soaked swabs or 'jelonet rolls' will usually stop it. This is the easiest site of an air leak to diagnose and the site of the leak can easily be localized if the tracheostomy tube is moved around.

If the incision has been stitched properly in two layers, it should not leak. However, if leakage does occur, a useful manoeuvre is to go along the suture line pulling the edges apart slightly. When the site of the leak has been found, there will be a large gush of air into the suction tube. Apply local pressure to the leak after stopping the suction and 5 min later start the suction again; alternatively, insert another stitch under local anaesthetic. If this does not work, the drains should be placed on a Robert's pump or low wall suction for 24 h and then closed suction reapplied.

Air leaks can also occur where the drain exits from the skin if the exit holes have been made with anything other than a special needle introducer, or if a drain has slipped and a perforation lies outside the skin. In this situation, leaks around the tube may be covered with a swab or a pursestring suture inserted to narrow the hole. If a perforation lies outside the skin, it may be quite difficult to push the tube back but it can be done. Alternatively, one could use Nobecutaine or Opsite spray together with adhesive tape to cover the hole. Otherwise, a Robert's pump or low wall suction will have to be applied.

After stitching up the mucosa, the suture line should be watertight; the easiest way to check this is to pour some water into the pharynx. If the closure is watertight, it will also be airtight. If the suture line is leaking, this is particularly bad news, because the air will be mixed with saliva, and the flaps will very soon lift up and then become infected. If this is the leaking site, the diagnosis is usually made by exclusion of leakage from the two previous sites above. In this situation, the suction should be stopped for at least 24 h and a pressure dressing applied. After 24 h the tube may be moved a little and gentle suction restarted; if the original leak was small it will usually have sealed itself.

Type of drainage

Within the first 24–48 h, the drainage from a radical neck dissection usually consists entirely of blood and measures approximately 200 ml/day. After 48–72 h, it becomes serous and after 4 days usually only 25 ml drains in 24 h. A lot may be learnt about the character of the drainage and its smell. Air, saliva or a malodour is often the first sign of an internal fistula; if this has occurred there are two alternatives. If a drain is still *in situ*, it may be left to deal with the drainage so that healing in the rest of the neck may take place and one may convert a general problem into a local problem. A localized fistula will occur which may then be packed and allowed to heal by secondary intention. If the drain has been removed, there will be leakage from an area of the wound, which should be opened to facilitate drainage and subsequent packing.

Alternatively as soon as any evidence of leakage occurs, the fistula under the neck flap may be localized with a finger, a small hole may be made in the skin over it and suction applied directly to the fistula. This converts a long fistulous tract into a small one which may heal spontaneously. The presence of chyle or lymphatic fluid within the drainage tube indicates a chyle or lymphatic leak and this complication is dealt with in Chapters 6 and 13.

Removal of drains

The old dictum of 'remove a drain when it stops draining' is not entirely true. If there are problems with drainage tubes, particularly with intractable failure or blockage, it is better to remove them early rather than risk ascending infection under the flaps. The drainage tubes should not be removed until the drainage is less than 25 ml and when the colour of fluid within the tube changes from bright red blood to serous fluid, indicating that the drain is actually sucking serum from the capillaries. This is due to the high pressure (approx. 750 mmHg) that exists within a vacuum drain. However, as a drain cannot be left *in situ* indefinitely and as it causes some secretion, it can usually be removed by the fourth or fifth day if the daily drainage has been consistent for 48 h. Very occassionally, they have to be left longer.

Intravenous fluids

Following head and neck surgery some patients will have nasogastric tubes *in situ*, some will have a percutaneous gastrostomy (PEG) and some will be fed via an open gastrostomy or jejunostomy. However, most head and neck patients will not require enteral or parental feeding and can be fed within 48 h of the operation. In the first 48 h, the patient must not be given too much water and salt as this could result in pulmonary oedema. Between the end of the operation and the next morning, the prescription of intravenous fluids should be the joint responsibility of the anaesthetist and the on-call surgical team. Fluids, and blood if required, can usually be given via a central intravenous line which has been left in at the end of surgery. This can be removed the next day if the haemoglobin and electrolyte levels are satisfactory, if nasogastric feeds are tolerated and the central line is not needed to give any other solution or antibiotic. Other fluids that might be required are mannitol for patients undergoing a second neck dissection, dextran 40 which may be given in the first 12 h following microvascular surgery, calcium replacement following total thyroidectomy and intravenous hyperalimentation.

It is worth noting that during a long procedure the total fluid loss is often underestimated, resulting in a significant reduction in urinary output in the early hours of the following morning. When examining the patient, it is important to ascertain an accurate assessment of fluid balance because often all that is required is a fluid challenge (plus or minus some frusemide) and normal fluid balance is promptly restored.

Oral feeding

In contrast to most major abdominal operations, after which the gut does not function properly for several days, gastrointestinal function after most forms of major head and neck surgery is normal. Provided bowel sounds have returned, most patients can be fed via the gastrointestinal tract from day one. This is generally desirable since many patients undergoing major head and neck surgery are already malnourished. Many commercial enteral feeding preparations are now available that provide a balanced intake and usually contain about 1 kcal (4.2 kJ)/ml. In the absence of gastrointestinal disease, the more expensive elemental feeds are unnecessary and the prescriptive use of such preparations will usually be controlled by the head and neck dietician.

Such feeds may be administered via a nasogastric tube, a PEG, or an open gastrostomy or jejunostomy. Where enteral feeding is anticipated for a short period following surgery a nasogastric tube will suffice. Where feeding is anticipated for longer periods, or where complications are more likely to occur such as surgery to the oral cavity, oropharynx, hypopharynx and even larynx, it is now common practice in major head and neck centres to perform a preoperative PEG. These can be inserted easily, they are performed under a local anaesthetic with sedation and provide access to the upper gastrointestinal tract without the problems of nasogastric tube insertion. A PEG is particularly helpful if the patient is likely to need postoperative radiotherapy.

In cases where the abdomen is being opened as part of the procedure, such as in jejunal transfer or stomach transposition, postoperative feeding may be procured through an open jejunostomy. In cases where a nasogastric tube is used, it is placed during the operation and feeding can normally be started on the following day. The best way of ensuring an adequate intake is to give the feed continuously throughout the 24 h using gravity feed or a special pump. Intermittent bolus feeding is associated with abdominal discomfort and it is often impossible to maintain an adequate intake this way. On the day after the operation a graduated regime such as that in Table 4.2 is begun. Full-strength feeds providing about 2400 kcal (10 MJ) in 24 h can be achieved on the second day, which is adequate for most adult patients. Before feeding starts, care be taken to ensure that the feeding tube is in the stomach by aspirating the stomach contents or listening over the epigastrium while air is injected. Details of feeding regimens following free jejunal transfer or gastric transposition are given in Chapter 17.

Although narrow-bore feeding tubes are often used for feeding as they are more comfortable, they are initially less than ideal after major head and neck surgery as they are more likely to be displaced if the patient vomits and more likely to become blocked when multiple prescriptions are being pushed down them. Displacement of a feeding tube after major head and neck surgery is undesirable, as it may be impossible to replace it until after the pharyngeal wound has healed and in this situation a PEG is preferable.

In patients who are particularly malnourished, who have had surgery involving the gastrointestinal tract (ileal

Table 4.2	Feeding regimen following head and neck surgery
1st hour	30 ml warm sterile water
2nd hour	60 ml warm water with glucose
3rd hour	30 ml water and 30 ml warm milk with glucose
4th hour	60 ml water and 30 ml warm milk with glucose
5th hour	30 ml water and 60 ml warm milk with glucose
6th hour	60 ml water and 60 ml warm milk with glucose
7th hour	30 ml water and 90 ml warm milk with glucose
8th hour	120 ml warm milk with glucose
9th hour	200 ml milk feed
11th hour	Full feed

loop, etc.), and who do not have (or cannot have) either a nasogastric tube, PEG or feeding jejunostomy, it may be judged desirable to provide intravenous nutrition for several days after the operation until full gastrointestinal function returns. However, if possible, intravenous nutrition should be avoided at all costs owing to the associated problems of sepsis that can occur with infection of the line.

Deep vein thrombosis prophylaxis

Patients should be assessed for the risk of deep vein thrombosis (DVT) prophylaxis as discussed in Chapter 6. Patients are divided into high, moderate and low risk and are treated accordingly. Low-risk patients are mobilized early, those with a moderate risk are mobilized early and graduated compression (TED) stockings used until full mobility is achieved. For high-risk patients (including all head and neck oncology patients), perioperative and postoperative subcutaneous low molecular weight heparin (tinzaparin 3500 units once daily) is given until the patient is mobile, along with the prescription of graduated compression (TED) stockings. The use of perioperative intermittent pneumatic compression is also recommended. Patients who develop a DVT and subsequent pulmonary emboli should be treated in the conventional manner.

Monitoring of flaps

Any flap requires monitoring in the postoperative period. Local flaps in the head and neck require observation, as do distant pedicled flaps which should be observed for 1 week following surgery. Any gross vascular changes in a pedicled flap may well indicate that the stitches are too tight or that the pedicle is under some compression or tension, and revision may be required. Usually, there are very few early indicators that there will be a problem with the flap and then later there is partial or complete loss of the skin paddle with preservation of the underlying muscle. In this situation, it is important to sit tight and initially do nothing. Subsequent débridement may be necessary for superficial necrotic skin which, with survival of the underlying muscle, will normally heal by secondary intention or take a skin graft later on. It is very rare that a pedicled myocutaneous flap requires replacing.

In contrast, free tissue transfers require constant monitoring as they are an 'all or none' phenomenon. Free flaps most often to go wrong in the first 48 h following surgery and they should be monitored vigorously during this period. This is dealt with in Chapters 6 and 7.

Medications

Antibiotics

Prophylactic antibiotic cover in head and neck cancer surgery is indicated in a number of situations. It is not required for clean operations such as superficial parotidectomy and modified radical neck dissection, which usually last for less than 3 h. However, for longer procedures or where shaving has been carried out within the last 24 h before surgery, then a short 48 h course of prophylactic antibiotic therapy is appropriate, with antibiotics such as co-amoxiclav or cefuroxime.

Unless there is a specific indication to do so, preoperative swabs taken from the mouth and throat in the clinic are no longer required. One indication is in a patient who has been in the ward and has had methicillin-resistant *Staphylococcus aureus* (MRSA) which has been successfully treated, who then is readmitted for further surgery. They should have their MRSA status evaluated on admission. Prophylactic anti-MRSA therapy should be considered.

The main indication for the role of prophylactic antibiotics in head and neck surgery is for operations on the mouth, pharynx, larynx and upper oesophagus. In this situation, the mouth and pharynx normally contain Gram-positive cocci and anaerobes. Gram-negative cocci are seldom present but can colonize the mouth within 2–3 days of the passing of a nasogastric tube, which allows the ascent of intestinal organisms. As long as the patient has no nasogastric tube at the time of surgery, any prophylactic antibiotic prescribed need only cover the Gram-positive cocci and anaerobes.

The majority of head and neck surgeons in the UK now use either co-amoxiclav or a combination of cefuroxime and metronidazole for prophylactic cover, although the use of the latter antibiotic is not strictly necessary. Another option is to use erythromycin since this is highly effective and is not frequently used for other purposes. However, it causes significant gastrointestinal upset and is not tolerated well intravenously.

Although the use of these antibiotics is deemed prophylactic, there is a significant risk of postoperative infection following major surgery and antibiotic cover should be continued for 5 days. Once postoperative infection becomes established, despite using the above regimens, swabs should be taken for culture in the usual way and further antibiotics prescribed accordingly.

Chest infections should be prevented as far as possible by attention to dental hygiene, preoperative treatment of any sinusitis and chronic bronchitis, and sterile precautions during tracheostomy care. Established chest infection is treated as described in Chapter 6.

If the patient has a tracheostomy before the operation, a swab should be taken from it a few days before the operation and the appropriate antibiotic cover started immediately.

Thyroid and parathyroid replacement

A total thyroidectomy is carried out either for benign or malignant disease of the thyroid gland or in continuity with a pharyngolaryngectomy for carcinoma of the pharynx, larynx or upper trachea, and usually includes removal of the parathyroid glands. If the parathyroids are not involved with tumour, they may be preserved and even if they are supposedly removed, the patient may remain normocalcaemic in the postoperative period because of ectopic parathyroid tissue. Some of the problems of postoperative head and neck surgical management relate to calcium balance and thyroid hormone replacement.

The half-life of thyroxine is approximately 10 days, so that thyroid replacement need not begin for at least 1 week after operation, after which time the patient is usually swallowing or being fed by the enteral route. Treatment begins with thyroxine 100 μg/day but care should be exercised in the elderly, in whom lower doses (50 μg/day) should be introduced. On discharge from hospital, the dose is increased to 150 μg/day and then, after 3 months, further assessment of thyroid function allows fine tuning to maintain a normal thyroid profile.

Parathyroid replacement is more difficult. The parathyroid glands are very sensitive to handling, temporary and permanent ischaemia as well as trauma, and despite not being removed or even devascularized, some degree of hypocalcaemia in the postoperative period following near-total or total thyroidectomy should be regarded as inevitable. The management of this is discussed in Chapter 6.

Dressings and sutures

Wound dressings

Wound dressings have several adverse effects: they can make the wound warm, macerated and liable to infection, they successfully conceal impending complications, such as haematomas, and they encourage the inquisitive to draw them aside with a dirty finger to inspect the wound. If all of the bleeding points have been secured and the incision properly closed, dressings usually have no other contribution to make to the care of the patient. As mentioned previously, a small amount of gauze dressing laid along the suture line in the immediate postoperative period may help to seal and prevent a small leak but this will not hide the major part of the wound and can be removed after 12–24 h.

It is not a good idea to apply any pressure bandages around the neck. However, an extended head and neck bandage can be of value following parotidectomy, when firm pressure for 24 h following surgery helps to seal the flaps down and prevent troublesome haematomas. A bandage must never be applied around the neck after bilateral neck dissection or a second neck dissection as it would occlude the remaining venous return via the vertebral veins.

If neck flaps have been elevated by saliva tracking out of a fistula, they can be encouraged to reseat themselves by fenestrating the fistula and applying a pressure dressing to the flaps. This has been described previously.

Necrotic areas should be cleaned twice daily and dressed (see Chapter 6). Surgical débridement is performed on the ward; usually no analgesia is needed as dead tissue has no nerve supply.

Sutures

If an adequate subcutaneous layer has been used to close the wound, skin sutures may be removed after 7 days if the wound appears normal. This should be extended to 10 days if patient has received previous radiotherapy. Sterile sutures after laryngectomy are usually left for 10 days to 2 weeks as the mucocutaneous junction is often under great tension and it is difficult to remove sutures when a stoma button or laryngectomy tube is *in situ.*

Monofilament synthetic sutures can be left in place longer than silk, which is braided and has a wick action that causes microabscesses within 72 h. For this reason, silk stitches should be removed as early as possible. Intra-oral sutures are usually made of vicryl and do not need to be removed. Sometimes silk in used and should be removed 7 days later. Before removing the stitches, the wound edge is cleaned of all crusts. The material is cut flush with the skin on the opposite side to the knot and then the knot is pulled over the wound to remove the stitch. The loose ends must never be pulled away from the skin edges as this can cause wound disruption. When a blanket suture is removed, care is taken not to disrupt the wound edges: the free end is cut when it becomes more than about 4 cm long.

Postoperative examination

Patients in the postoperative period following head and neck surgery should be examined twice a day. Examination should include not only the head and neck, but also the chest, abdomen and the calves. Such vigorous follow-up is the best way to detect early complications. Patients who are in intensive care should be cared for jointly with the staff on that unit.

Getting up

As soon as possible after surgery, patients are propped up in bed at 45° in order to avoid lymphatic stasis in the head and neck. A patient who has had a bilateral neck dissection must never lie flat, because of the danger of cerebral oedema. If the common or internal carotid artery has been ligated, for example, after a carotid blow-out, the patient must be nursed flat for 48 h (see Chapter 6). Thereafter, the patient's head may be raised by one pillow per day.

There are very few head and neck procedures that stop the patient getting out of bed on the next day. The patient should be walking freely around the ward within 72 h, carrying any drainage bottle with them. This helps to prevent postoperative chest infection and DVT.

This is in sharp contrast to patients who have an operation such as a thorocotomy or laparotomy, since significant pain in the postoperative period prolongs their morbidity and subsequent confinement to bed.

Follow-up

Any patient who has had a surgical procedure for head and neck cancer is at risk of developing recurrent disease and should be followed up at regular intervals. This has been discussed in Chapter 2.

At each follow up visit, the primary site is examined for recurrence and the neck for enlarged lymph nodes. Any primary recurrence may be treated by further surgery and an enlarged lymph node is often treatable and may even be cured by neck dissection. A lymph-node metastasis is more likely to present within the first 2 years but it is important to note that these nodes may grow rapidly and within 6 weeks may be incurable. After 2–3 years, follow-up every 6 months is satisfactory because recurrence after this time is uncommon and any nodes that develop will almost certainly be slow growing.

The above follow-up principles also apply if radiotherapy has been used as the primary form of treatment.

Further reading

Gillies H. D. and Millard, D. R. (1957) *The Principles and Art of Plastic Surgery*, Butterworth, London.

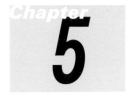

5 Principles of non-surgical treatment

'Difficult as it may be to cure, it is always easy to poison and to kill'
Elisha Bartlett

Treatment options for head and neck cancer

Treatment intent

Before considering the treatment options for an individual with head and neck cancer, the multidisciplinary team must first ascertain all relevant information about not just the tumour but also the patient. The key tumour variables are the histological type and the stage. Those related to the patient include age, general health, occupation and social support. Then a decision can be made by the team, taking into account the viewpoint of the patient and any family or friends, as to the aims of treatment. Is cure a reasonable goal, considering the possibility of success and the cost in terms of toxicity and functional loss? Or is the disease too extensive or the patient too frail for more than symptom control and supportive care? In other words, should the treatment be radical or palliative?

> *Key issues in treatment planning*
> - Tumour stage
> - Patient fitness
> - Social factors
> - Goal: cure versus palliation

Radical and palliative treatment

In radical treatment the aim is to cure the patient, even though the chances of achieving this end may be recognized to be slim. Complex, time-consuming and unpleasant treatments can be justified if cure is a possible outcome. However, when the disease is recognized to be incurable, palliative treatment aimed solely to alleviate symptoms is recommended. This should be simple and quick and should not produce side-effects worse than the symptoms that it aims to treat.

Radical treatment with palliative intent

In head and neck cancer the division between radical and palliative treatment is often less clear-cut. There are many occasions where a radical style of treatment is rightly used in an attempt to achieve local tumour control, despite the fact that the disease is considered to be incurable. This may be justified by the particularly horrible nature of uncontrolled cancer in some head and neck situations. In addition, unlike many forms of advanced malignancy such as lung cancer or bone metastases, where a short course of low-dose radiotherapy, or even a single treatment, may greatly improve symptoms, this is rarely the case for head and neck cancer. Here a full course of radiotherapy – radical radiotherapy with palliative intent – usually needs to be given to achieve adequate palliation, and conventional palliative radiotherapy is rarely used.

Modalities of treatment

Once treatment intent has been decided upon, the attention of the team can turn to how best to achieve that aim. There are three principal therapeutic modalities available for the treatment of cancer: surgery, radiotherapy and chemotherapy. Squamous head and neck cancer is, by and large, a locoregional disease. The majority of patients who die from this cancer do so as a result of uncontrolled disease at the primary site or in cervical lymph nodes. Distant metastases are uncommon. It follows that local treatments which are successful in eradicating the disease from the head and neck are likely to be curative. Both surgery and radiotherapy are local treatments, and either individually or in combination often effect a cure.

The choice between surgery and radiotherapy is not made entirely on medical grounds. Logistic factors, such as the availability of radiotherapy within a reasonable time frame, need to be considered. Waiting lists for radiotherapy commonly exceed good practice guidelines. Because of the inadequate provision of radiotherapy facilities in some areas prompt treatment is impossible, and so surgery may be preferred. Similarly, some patients may choose to have surgery closer to home than travel to a big city where most radiotherapy facilities are located.

Chemotherapy has had tremendous impact in improving the cure rates for some types of cancer such as lymphoma, testicular germ cell tumours and various paediatric malignancies. It has had a more marginal benefit in most of the common solid tumours, and squamous carcinoma of the head and neck is no exception. If chemotherapy is to make a substantial contribution to the management of head and neck cancer, it is more likely to do so by improving the local control probability in conjunction with radiotherapy and surgery than by eradicating distant spread.

Radiotherapy

Rationale for radiotherapy

Radiotherapy, that is, treatment with ionizing radiation, has been recognized as a valuable modality in the management of cancer for a century. Over this period, radiotherapeutic technology has evolved and there have been significant advances in surgery, and disease that some years ago was best treated with one modality may now be better treated with the other or with both. It can be misleading to base judgements of the value of current treatment practices on reports published decades ago about the outcome of patients treated in the preceding quarter-century. The modalities of surgery and radiotherapy should be considered complementary rather than competitive. As mentioned above, radiotherapy, like surgery, is a local treatment, at least as far as head and neck cancer is concerned. Its purpose is to eradicate tumour at the primary site, and in some cases the regional lymph nodes. Its principal advantage is that it can often do so while sparing normal tissue function. For example, radiotherapy is certainly no better, and perhaps slightly worse, at curing advanced laryngeal cancer than surgery, yet it offers the chance of preservation of the natural voice, which is not possible with laryngectomy.

How radiotherapy works

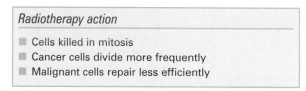

Radiotherapy action

- Cells killed in mitosis
- Cancer cells divide more frequently
- Malignant cells repair less efficiently

Radiation causes damage to DNA in both normal and malignant cells. If cells are unable to repair this damage by the time of their next division, then they die in mitosis. The response of both normal and malignant cells to radiation is qualitatively similar, but in general malignant cells have a lower repair capacity and a shorter cell cycle than normal ones. Thus, the chances of a dose of radiation killing a malignant cell are greater than those of killing a normal cell. It is on these quantitative differences in the response to radiation of normal and malignant cells that radiotherapy depends.

Relationship between cure and complications

The basic principle of radiotherapy is to achieve as high a radiation dose into the tumour and any occult extensions as possible to ensure a cure, while minimizing the dose to surrounding normal tissue, in order to avoid complications as far as possible. In the head and neck the situation is more complex for several reasons. First, squamous cancer is less radiosensitive than some other tumours such as lymphoma and requires a high dose for cure which is at the level of radiation tolerance of much normal tissue and exceeds the tolerance of the more sensitive normal structures. Secondly, radiotherapy in the head and neck requires greater technical precision than at other anatomical sites, because of the close juxtaposition of critically radiosensitive organs such as the eye and brainstem to the tumours requiring treatment. In addition, other structures such as the salivary glands and mucosa, while not as critically susceptible to radiation damage as the brainstem, should nonetheless be spared unnecessary irradiation in order to minimize both acute and long-term sequelae.

For these reasons, the therapeutic ratio, that is the relationship between the dose that is required for cure and the dose which causes unacceptable damage, is low. In general terms, a tumour is more likely to be cured if a higher dose is given. Similarly, complications are more likely if a higher dose is used. This relationship is shown graphically in Fig. 5.1. It is a matter of philosophy and judgement what incidence of serious complications can be justified in the pursuit of cure, although 5% is generally accepted as reasonable. For some potential complications, such as spinal cord damage, the acceptable threshold is set much lower. It can be seen that the likelihood of an uncomplicated cure diminishes beyond a certain critical dose level. Another factor to be noted from this graph is that the central part of both curves is quite steep. This means that a relatively small increment in dose may greatly increase the likelihood of cure or greatly increase the risk of complications. Conversely, a small dose reduction, as may occur if the last one or two treatments

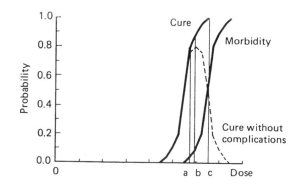

Figure 5.1 Relationship between radiation dose and the probability of tumour cure, severe late normal tissue morbidity and uncomplicated cure, with a particular treatment regimen.

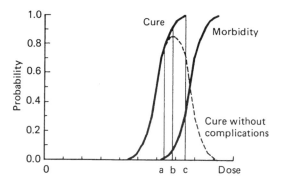

Figure 5.2 Using an alternative treatment schedule the therapeutic ratio is enhanced.

in a fractionated course are omitted because of acute side-effects, may greatly diminish the likelihood of cure. The aim of any modification in treatment technique is to enhance the therapeutic ratio. This enables a higher dose to be given, achieving a greater cure rate for a given complication rate (Fig. 5.2).

Low therapeutic ratio for squamous carcinoma of the head and neck

- Squamous carcinoma is relatively radioresistant
- Adjacent normal tissues are sensitive to radiation
- Vital organs must be spared

Combined modality treatment

Although radiotherapy is often used as the sole modality, it is frequently used in combination with surgery or chemotherapy, and sometimes both. It may be decided at the initial assessment to use radiotherapy in combination with surgery either preoperatively or postoperatively. Alternatively, while surgery may originally have been intended as the sole treatment, radiotherapy is sometimes subsequently indicated in the light of operative findings because of residual disease, or at a later date because of the development of recurrence. Similarly, surgery is sometimes required to salvage recurrent or residual disease following primary radiotherapy.

Uses of radiotherapy with curative intent

- Radiotherapy alone as principal treatment
- Radiotherapy planned in conjunction with surgery
  - preoperative radiotherapy
  - postoperative radiotherapy
- Pathology-guided postoperative radiotherapy
- Salvage radiotherapy for recurrence after surgery

Sometimes in an individual patient radiotherapy is used both as the definitive treatment and as an adjunct to surgery. An example might be someone with a small tonsillar carcinoma and bulky cervical lymph nodes. Radiotherapy

alone has little chance of sterilizing a large lymph node mass, and the greatest probability of tumour control in the neck is with a radical neck dissection with postoperative radiotherapy. In contrast, there is a high likelihood of controlling the small tumour in the oropharynx, and radical radiotherapy may be less morbid than a composite resection.

Preoperative and postoperative radiotherapy

The patterns of failure of surgery and radiotherapy are different. Surgery is good at removing the central bulk of disease, but residual viable tumour, often microscopic, can be left at the resection margins. Radiotherapy is best at eradicating small volumes of disease and is more likely to fail if there is a large bulky tumour. The two modalities can therefore be combined usefully, the advantages of each overcoming the shortcomings of the other. Preoperative radiotherapy was once advocated on the grounds that the tumour will shrink prior to surgery, making the operation easier, and that by sterilizing the majority of viable cells the risk of tumour dissemination at the time of operation was reduced. In most circumstances, however, postoperative irradiation is now considered preferable for several reasons. First, proper pathological staging of the tumour and nodes is now possible and is a better guide to the extent of irradiation required. Secondly, the recent introduction of free as opposed to pedicled flaps in reconstructive surgery has meant that postoperative radiotherapy can commence sooner than was previously the case. In addition, tumour dissemination at the time of operation is now considered more of a theoretical problem than a real one. Finally, following surgery, only microscopic, well-vascularized tumour should be left behind, which should be relatively easy to cure with radiation.

Adjuvant radiotherapy

Adjuvant radiotherapy is given following the definitive treatment which has apparently removed the malignancy, in order to reduce chances of recurrence. In the radiotherapy of head and neck cancer this includes elective postoperative irradiation following complete surgical excision of a tumour and prophylactic irradiation of a clinically negative neck. The irradiation of known residual disease following incomplete surgery is not considered to be adjuvant. Adjuvant radiotherapy entails giving a high-dose fractionated course, similar to that used in radical treatment.

Types of radiation treatment

There are three ways of administering ionizing radiation to a tumour, of which by far and away the most important is external beam radiotherapy or teletherapy. Interstitial radiotherapy and unsealed sources have a small part to play in the treatment of head and neck cancer.

External beam radiotherapy

Photons and particles

External beam radiotherapy is also known as teletherapy. In this form of treatment, a beam of radiation is directed by a machine to the tumour-bearing part of the patient who is some distance away, usually lying on a couch. A variety of different types of radiation are in current use. Others have been tried in the past and have now been superseded. In general terms, ionizing radiation is either particulate or high-energy electromagnetic radiation, called photons, similar to radiowaves or visible light, but with a much shorter wavelength. These photons are either X-rays or gamma rays. The only particulate radiation in common use is the electron beam.

Types of external beam radiotherapy

■ Photons (X-rays or gamma rays)
■ Particles (e.g. electrons)

Energy of photon beams

The X-rays used in therapy are classified by their energy level, which is measured in volts (V). The least energetic have an energy up to about 100 000 V or 100 kV. This type of radiation, called superficial, is poorly penetrating, treating an effective depth of only about 1 cm, and is used exclusively for treating small skin tumours. Until the 1950s, the most penetrating beams generally available came from orthovoltage equipment. They had an energy of about 300 kV and were also called deep X-rays, a name which still lingers on although this type of equipment is virtually obsolete.

Types of photon radiation beam

■ X-ray photons
  – superficial, e.g. 100 kV
  – orthovoltage, e.g. 300 kV
  – megavoltage, e.g. 6 MV
■ Gamma ray photons
  – cobalt, ~2 MV

Advantages of megavoltage radiotherapy

Supervoltage or megavoltage machines such as linear accelerators are now universally available. They operate at 4–20 million volts (MV) and produce much more penetrating beams than was possible in the orthovoltage era. Although increased penetration is the principal advantage of megavoltage irradiation, there are also other benefits.

With orthovoltage beams, the maximum dose was delivered to the skin, with progressively lower doses to underlying tissues. As a consequence, damage to the skin limited the amount that could be given to deep-seated tumours. With 4 MV beams, the skin is relatively spared, with the maximum dose at a depth of 1 cm and a much more gradual fall-off of dose at depth. In addition, the edges of linear accelerator beams are much more precisely defined – in technical terms there is less penumbra (literally the edge of the shadow) – meaning that narrower margins can safely be used around a tumour than was possible with orthovoltage. A final important benefit for megavoltage irradiation is that its absorption in different tissues is quite homogeneous. Orthovoltage beams had a much greater absorption in dense materials such as bone and calcified cartilage, and so complications such as osteoradionecrosis and laryngeal cartilage necrosis, which are now only rarely seen, were a considerable problem.

Radioactive isotopes emitting megavoltage gamma rays

In addition to X-rays, the gamma rays emitted by some radioactive isotopes are of megavoltage quality and can be used for teletherapy. The beam from a radium 'bomb' was the earliest form of high-energy external beam treatment available. Radium was superseded as a source after World War II when artificially radioactive isotopes of caesium and cobalt became available. Cobalt, which produced more penetrating radiation, was preferred in most circumstances. The physical characteristics, especially the penetration and penumbra, of the beams from a linear accelerator are in many respects preferable to those of a cobalt unit. However, the latter is comparatively low-technology equipment which is cheaper and requires less maintenance by skilled staff, and so cobalt units are still used fairly widely throughout the world for economic and logistic reasons.

Particle beam irradiation

Types of particle beam

■ Electrons
■ Neutrons
■ Protons

Some linear accelerators are dedicated to the production of X-ray photon beams, whereas others are dual-purpose and can also be used to produce electron beams. While the bulk of radiotherapy is carried out using photons, there are some circumstances in which **electrons** are preferable. They give a relatively uniform dose up to a certain depth of penetration and then the dose falls off very rapidly. They are, therefore, used to treat superficial parts, where it is desired to spare an underlying structure from excess irradiation. For example, they can be used to boost the dose to a nodal mass overlying the spinal cord, following initial photon treatment to a cord tolerance dose. Orthovoltage treatment also has limited penetration but electrons are superior as the fall-off of dose at depth is more rapid, they show some skin-sparing and they are not preferentially absorbed by bone or cartilage. For this last reason they are also the radiotherapeutic treatment of choice for lesions of the pinna and nose.

Neutron beam therapy is the only other form of particle radiation to have been widely used. Despite radiobiological predictions that neutrons would be advantageous, a large number of clinical trials conducted in various centres throughout the world on many different tumour types, including head and neck cancer, has failed to demonstrate the anticipated benefit. It remains possible that neutrons may have a role in a few circumstances, but most neutron therapy facilities have closed and are not being replaced.

Proton beam therapy has very limited applications and is not widely available. The only current UK facility for proton beam therapy is in Liverpool and is used exclusively for the treatment of ocular melanoma. Higher energy protons are available in some parts of the world and may be beneficial for some tumours such as cordoma of the clivus.

Interstitial radiotherapy

In interstitial radiotherapy, or brachytherapy, sealed sources of radioactive isotopes are either implanted into the tumour or placed in a natural body cavity, for example, the maxillary antrum or nasopharynx (intracavitary therapy). Implants of long half-life materials which require removal after about 1 week are most commonly used. As an alternative, short half-life elements may be permanently implanted. Originally, radium needles were used for removable implants and radon for permanent implants. The former were superseded initially by caesium and later by iridium, and radon has been replaced by gold or iodine. Thick, rigid needles were previously the principal type of implant but over the last few years, more versatile, flexible systems have become more widely used. This form of treatment is obviously more easily used in anatomically accessible parts of the body such as the oral cavity, and a detailed description of the use of iridium implants for oral cavity cancer is given in Chapter 15. The main reason for using interstitial therapy is that it enables a very high radiation dose to be given to a very limited volume. Because of the inverse square law, there is a very rapid fall-off of dose from the surface of the source. Interstitial therapy can be used either on its own to treat small tumours or to give a boost to a residual mass after initial external beam therapy.

Whereas at one time radioactive implants had to be directly inserted by the operator, resulting in radiation exposure for operating theatre staff, afterloading techniques are now widely available. With afterloading, empty applicators are inserted initially. Time can be spent making the geometrical parameters of the implant as ideal as possible without fear of unnecessary radiation exposure. Once the applicators have been correctly positioned, they can be afterloaded with the radioactive material either manually or by a remote afterloading machine.

A newer use of brachytherapy in the field of head and neck cancer is for the retreatment of recurrent neck nodes which have previously been irradiated. During a radical neck dissection there is intraoperative insertion of tubes for subsequent afterloading. The tubes can then be covered with a well-vascularized myocutaneous flap. In this way the tumour bed is reirradiated without overdosing the neck skin which was previously treated to tolerance levels.

Use of unsealed sources

Radioactive isotopes can be used in the form of drugs given orally or intravenously. These drugs are then concentrated by metabolic pathways in malignant tissue, enabling large radiation doses to be given to the tumour, with relative sparing of the normal tissue. There is only one example in the treatment of head and neck malignancy, and that is the treatment of differentiated thyroid carcinoma of follicular cell origin with radioactive iodine. This is discussed fully in Chapter 23.

Volume to be treated

It might reasonably be thought that the volume to be treated by radiotherapy is self-evident. Surely it should be enough to cover the bulk of the tumour as defined by clinical examination and imaging, allowing a reasonable margin for microscopic infiltration. In fact, the volume which should be treated remains a matter of some controversy, and practice varies. Nonetheless, despite the fact that the size of the margin treated around tumours varies, and that in some centres clinically uninvolved nodes are irradiated prophylactically, reported survival rates are remarkably constant. The need for salvage treatment may be greater if elective neck irradiation is withheld in tumours which have a high incidence of occult nodal involvement, but this does not appear to compromise overall survival. It becomes a matter of philosophy whether one chooses, despite the increased morbidity, to overtreat a proportion of patients to ensure that the maximum number of patients are cured first time around, or whether one prefers to minimize initial treatment so as to spare side-effects, recognizing that more patients will require salvage treatment. Another factor to be considered is that when a smaller volume is treated a higher dose may be given. This might enable more tumours to be cured. One way to combine the treatment of a large volume, so as to treat some part prophylactically, with giving the highest possible dose to a small volume, is to use a shrinking field technique. Initially, a large volume is covered and taken to a modest dose deemed to be adequate to treat subclinical disease, then the volume is reduced to cover only the bulk of the disease which is then boosted to a high dose. Alternatively, a boost may be given by interstitial therapy.

Fractionation of radiotherapy

Conventional fractionation

The maximum amount of radiation that can be given as a single dose is limited by normal tissue tolerance and, with the exception of a small skin tumour, is inadequate to cure cancer. If the total dose is divided up into a number of small doses, called fractions, given for example daily, the maximum dose tolerated by normal tissues increases, and cure becomes more likely. For this reason radical radiotherapy is given as a fractionated course over a number of weeks. As the practice of radiotherapy has to a large extent developed empirically, the precise fractionation schedule varies considerably from centre to centre. Despite the variation in total dose, number of fractions per week, total number of fractions and overall time, each institution reports broadly similar results. At one end of the spectrum, a patient might be treated in 16 fractions over 3 weeks; at the other a patient might receive 35 treatments over 7 weeks. A higher total dose, say 65 Gy, will be given for the protracted treatment, compared with perhaps 50 Gy for the shorter regimen. The shorter course treatment is standard in some British centres, but the longer course is regarded as the international conventional fractionation schedule. The short course is regarded as hypofractionation in international circles.

A number of clinical trials have addressed the question of fractionation. One of the largest, organized by the British Institute of Radiology, showed no significant differences in outcome comparing three with five fractions per week, or a short with a long overall treatment time in the management of laryngeal and hypopharyngeal carcinoma. As the acute mucosal reaction is more severe when the overall treatment time is short more protracted fractionation is recommended when a large area of mucosa requires irradiation. As brain tissue is more likely to be damaged if large doses per fraction are used, a protracted schedule is preferred if any of the central nervous system is included within the treated volume. Except in these circumstances there is probably no reason to opt for longer treatment courses.

Conventional and alternative fractionation schedules

- Conventional: 60 Gy in 30 × 2 Gy fractions over 42 days
- Hypofractionation: smaller number of fractions each larger than 2 Gy
- Hyperfractionation: larger number of fractions each smaller than 2 Gy
- Acceleration: shortened overall time
- Split course: gap to allow acute reactions to settle

Experimental fractionation

Hyperfractionation is when the number of fractions is increased beyond conventional levels and the dose per fraction is reduced correspondingly. In order to keep the overall treatment duration the same, treatments need to be given more than once (twice or three times) a day. With multiple treatments per day, the interfraction interval becomes critical to allow for repair of sublethal damage in normal tissues. The minimum safe interfraction interval is usually regarded as 6 h.

Acceleration is when the overall treatment time is reduced. These two modifications are combined in the treatment regimen known as CHART (continuous, hyperfractionated, accelerated radiation therapy). This gives a radical course of treatment in just 12 days, using three fractions per day, 7 days per week. The short overall time is designed to overcome the repopulation of malignant cells which is believed to occur during long courses of treatment and the reduced fraction size is used to prevent increased late tissue damage. CHART has been shown in large multicentre clinical trials to be advantageous in some circumstances, but the magnitude of benefit is not as great as had been hoped for.

Split courses

It has already been mentioned that the acute mucosal reaction may be dose limiting. In an attempt to overcome this problem, some workers have divided the radiotherapy course into two halves, separated by a gap of about 2 weeks, allowing the mucosal reaction to settle. However, this gap gives time for the remaining tumour cells, stimulated by the first phase of treatment, to divide rapidly and repopulate the tumour. Studies have shown that split-course regimens produce inferior results to continuous schedules and this practice is mentioned only to be condemned.

If an unplanned gap in treatment occurs, perhaps because of machine breakdown or intercurrent illness, tumour cell repopulation threatens to diminish the likelihood of cure. In these circumstances there are several strategies for compensation. For example, the total dose may be increased by increasing the size or number of the remaining fractions. Perhaps the best way is to treat to the same planned total dose with the same fraction size in the same overall time treating with multiple fractions per day.

Units of radiation measurement

In physical terms, radiation dose is prescribed using the SI units of absorbed dose, the gray (Gy). This unit of measurement, like the renowned research establishment, the Gray Lab, is named after the pioneering British radiobiologist L. H. Gray. Some people prefer to talk in terms of the centigray (cGy), which is one hundredth of a gray. This unit has replaced the previous unit of radiation absorbed dose, the rad, which is equivalent to 0.01 Gy. However, in biological terms it is not adequate to describe the dose to a tumour in terms of the physical dose alone.

Other factors which must be mentioned are the number of fractions, fraction size, interval between fractions, overall time, volume treated, radiation quality (e.g. photons or neutrons) and beam energy.

Units of radiation measurement

■ Gray = Gy = SI unit
■ Centigray = cGy = 0.01 Gy
■ Rad ≡ cGy

Formulae of equivalence

Over the years, a variety of complex mathematical formulae has been invented by which time, dose and fractionation factors can be rolled into one number to describe a course of treatment. However, the biological factors which affect probability of tumour cure and risk of complications are different. Thus, a time–dose–fractionation formula may say that two different treatment schedules are equivalent. While this may be the case as far as likelihood of tumour cure is concerned, the two regimens may be very different in terms of complications. For this reason, such formulae are best avoided and treatment schedules should be fully described in terms of all of the relevant factors.

Planning and quality control of radiation therapy

Selecting the treatment volume

When it has been decided to treat a patient with radiation, the precise technical details of the treatment must be decided upon before it is commenced. The extent of the tumour will be known from clinical examination and radiological studies. This information, combined with a knowledge of the natural history of that tumour type and its usual patterns of spread, determines the volume that needs to be treated. In the head and neck it is important to confine the treatment to this volume, in order to protect vulnerable structures such as the eye, lacrimal and salivary glands, the brainstem and spinal cord.

Preparation of a shell

For accurate treatment of the target volume with sparing of adjacent structures to be possible, the patient needs to lie still during treatment, in a constant position from day to day. To ensure this, the patient's head is immobilized in a plastic shell. Such shells, sometimes called masks, moulds or casts, are prepared individually for each patient. This process takes about 3 working days and requires skilled technical staff, working in a well-equipped mould room. First, with the patient lying in the intended treatment position, strips of plaster of Paris bandages are applied like a mask to the head and neck. When these have set, the mask, which has an impression exactly the same shape and size as the patient, is removed. This impression is filled with liquid plaster and a cast is formed. A thermoplastic vacuum-forming machine is used to shape a piece of plastic over the cast. The shaped plastic is then trimmed, holes are cut for the eyes and nostrils, and it is fitted to a neck rest and base board. The shell is then checked on the patient, to ensure that it fits snugly and comfortably. It has been shown that the use of a shell, by avoiding the possibility of a 'geographical miss', improves the likelihood of cure when small volume tumours, such as early laryngeal cancer, are being treated.

Simulation

The treatment simulator is a diagnostic X-ray machine with image-intensification facilities. It can rotate around the patient, like the treatment unit with exactly matching geometry. The screen shows a pair of parallel wires perpendicular to another pair. The distance between the wires in each pair can be adjusted to make rectangles of any size, indicating the treatment field. The patient lies in the shell in the treatment position on the simulator couch. Using the image intensifier, a treatment field of appropriate size is chosen. A radiograph is taken as a permanent record of treatment intent, showing the position of the selected field and any areas to be shielded, in relation to the tumour and normal structures. As in most cases more than one field is used to cover the tumour, this process is repeated for the other fields.

Beam shaping

Blocks can be introduced into the beam to produce an irregularly shaped field to shield any vulnerable structures. Either standard blocks can be used, or for irregular shapes customized blocks can be prepared for an individual patient. Modern linear accelerators are now equipped with multileaf collimators which allow automatic beam shaping without the need for blocks to be made and manually positioned for each treatment. The position of the beam and any blocked areas are marked on to the shell to guide radiographers during treatment. The shell is also used to ensure that the beam alignment, as well as beam position, is correct.

Wedges and compensators

The aim of treatment planning is to ensure that the target volume which contains the tumour receives a high and uniform dose, and the surrounding areas, particularly if they are prone to radiation damage, receive a minimal dose. Beyond the depth where the absorbed dose is maximum (about 1 cm for 4 MV photons), the dose received from one beam decreases as it penetrates further into the patient. Two or more beams are thus often used. These are fired from different angles and intersect at the tumour, which therefore receives the highest dose. Because of the oblique incidence of a beam on the surface of the patient, or because two beams from the same side of the patient converge, the dose received by the tumour can vary across its depth. In order to achieve a uniform dose distribution, therefore, metal wedges may be inserted in the head of the treatment unit into the beam to attenuate the dose differentially across its width.

In certain circumstances it may be necessary to use individually prepared devices to achieve dose homogeneity. These are called compensators as they compensate for the variations in dose which would otherwise exist.

Isodose plans

A computer is used to create a map or plan of the radiation dose distribution within the patient. Usually this plan is of one cross-section through the middle of the tumour, although in complicated cases several sections at different levels are required. The plan shows the outline of the patient and the position of the tumour and any adjacent vulnerable structures. The position of treatment fields is indicated and contour lines are drawn joining points which receive the same dose (isodose lines). The isodose plan is checked to ensure that the tumour is contained within the high dose volume and therefore receives an adequate and uniform dose, and that the dose received by any critical structure is within its limits of tolerance.

Planning systems are becoming more sophisticated, and now true three-dimensional (3D) computer programs are available which can determine rapidly the dosimetry of multiple, shaped, non-coplanar beams in relation to the tumour and normal tissues. Precise delineation of the patient contour, the tumour volume and the location of critical structures comes from computed tomographic (CT) images, where necessary supplemented by CT/magnetic resonance imaging (MRI) image fusion. This technology offers the prospect of maintaining cure rates with diminished radiation morbidity in complex anatomical areas such as the head and neck. For some tumours it may be possible to increase local control rates by tumour dose escalation if the dose to critical normal structures can be minimized.

Treatment verification

During the first treatment session, radiographs may be taken using the beam from the treatment unit. These verification or check films are compared with the simulator films to ensure that the treatment field is positioned as planned and that any blocks are correctly located. Many modern linear accelerators are equipped with on-line portal verification equipment so that each field can be checked daily for accuracy before it is administered.

Chemotherapy

Development of chemotherapeutic practice

The first use of cytotoxic chemotherapy for the treatment of malignant disease was in the 1940s. More drugs were developed in the 1950s, and by the 1960s combinations were developed which proved to be curative for some chemosensitive cancers. The euphoria of anticipated success in the 1970s led to the establishment of many academic units of medical oncology and fuelled the belief that it would not be long before improvements in chemotherapy would make radiotherapy and even surgery for cancer treatment obsolete. While there have certainly been advances in chemotherapy practice in the 1980s and 1990s, especially in the field of supportive care, progress towards the cure of common solid tumours in adults remains disappointing. The principal reason why chemotherapy fails to cure cancer is that malignant cells have either intrinsic or acquired drug resistance. Very few completely novel cytotoxic drugs have been developed in the 1990s. Perhaps the greatest advance has been the recognition that chemotherapy may be used to good effect, not alone, but in combination with radiotherapy.

For squamous carcinoma of the head and neck, chemotherapy may be used in combination with surgery and radiotherapy as an adjuvant in radical treatments, or alone as a palliative treatment for advanced or recurrent disease. The drugs most widely used in the treatment of head and neck cancer are listed in Table 5.1. In other malignancies occurring in the head and neck region, chemotherapy has a much more important role. Many patients with lymphoma, for example, or rhabdomyosarcoma may be cured with chemotherapy alone.

Chemotherapy is a specialist area of medical practice, and cytotoxic drugs should only be prescribed by oncologists with the relevant expertise. Chemotherapy should only be administered in settings where there there are the necessary support staff such as cytotoxic pharmacists and clinical nurse specialists, and facilities for monitoring of toxicities and supportive care. It is still, however, important for specialists in other disciplines who refer patients for treatment to know the basics about chemotherapy.

Classes of chemotherapeutic agents

The 30 or so cytotoxic drugs in general use today have various origins and work in different ways. They also have different patterns of side-effects. They can be grouped together into the following five classes.

Alkylating agents

These are reactive compounds which exert cytotoxicity by binding covalently to DNA, often forming cross-links, and effectively interrupting DNA replication. Other functional cellular molecules can also be alkylated in this way. Examples of drugs in this class are cyclophosphamide, ifosfamide, melphalan, chlorambucil and the nitrosoureas, carmustine and lomustine.

Antimetabolites

These are simple chemicals with a structural similarity to normally occurring cellular compounds. They act by interfering with essential cellular metabolism. Methotrexate, for example, is an antifolate compound which acts as a false substrate for the enzyme dihydrofolate reductase, thereby preventing the conversion of dihydrofolate to tetrahydrofolate. Folinic acid bypasses this block and

Table 5.1 Cytotoxic drugs used in head and neck cancer

Drug	Class	Usual route of administration	Major toxicities	Precautions
Methotrexate	Antimetabolite	i.v. bolus	Myelosuppression Mucositis	GFR Monitor blood levels Hydration Action terminated by folinic acid
Vincristine	Plant derivative	i.v. bolus	Neuropathy	Never give intrathecally
5-Fluorouracil	Antimetabolite	i.v. bolus i.v. infusion	Diarrhoea	Action enhanced by folinic acid
Bleomycin	Antibiotic	i.m. injection	Fever, rigors Lung fibrosis	Steroids Lung function
Cisplatin	Miscellaneous	i.v. infusion	Ototoxicity Nephropathy Emesis	Audiogram Hydration GFR
Carboplatin	Miscellaneous	i.v. infusion	Myelosuppression	GFR Platelets
Doxorubicin	Antibiotic	i.v. bolus	Myelosuppression Cardiotoxicity Alopecia	Ejection fraction
Cyclophosphamide Ifosfamide	Alkylating agent	i.v. bolus	Myelosuppression Alopecia Cystitis	Use uroprotective drug mesna with ifosfamide and high-dose cyclophosphamide

i.v.: intravenous; i.m.: intramuscular; GFR: glomerular filtration rate.

it can be administered to terminate the cytotoxic effect of methotrexate. Blood methotrexate levels can be measured and provide a guide as to whether folinic acid is necessary or not. Other antimetabolites include the purine antagonists 6-mercaptopurine and 6-thioguanine, and the pyrimidine antagonists 5-fluorouracil and cytarabine. These drugs act in the DNA synthesis (S) phase of the cell cycle. Folinic acid can be used with 5-fluorouracil to potentiate its efficacy. This is a very different role from its use in conjunction with methotrexate.

Classes of cytotoxic drugs
■ Alkylating agents
■ Antimetabolites
■ Plant derivatives
■ Antitumour antibiotics
■ Miscellaneous

Plant derivatives

Various substances derived from plants are cytotoxic. The vinca alkaloids vincristine and vinblastine come from the Madagascar pink periwinkle and act by binding to the protein tubulin, preventing spindle formation during mitosis and leading to metaphase arrest. The epipodophyllotoxin derivatives etoposide and teniposide are inhibitors of the enzyme topoisomerase II which is involved in DNA processing. The yew tree derivatives paclitaxel and docetaxel inhibit microtubule disassembly.

Antitumour antibiotics

Various naturally occurring drugs have been extracted from bacterial and fungal cultures. They include actinomycin D, bleomycin and the anthracyclines doxorubicin and daunorubicin. They work by intercalating between DNA base pairs, preventing cell division.

Miscellaneous drugs

The platinum derivatives carboplatin and cisplatin form cross-links with DNA. Asparaginase breaks down asparagine, depriving some malignant cells of an essential nutrient. Procarbazine is a monoamine oxidase inhibitor, but is also a cytotoxic prodrug which is metabolically activated to produce an alkylating effect on nucleic acid.

Assessment of new drugs

Because of the limited efficacy and significant toxicity of all presently available cytotoxics, new drugs and analogues of existing chemotherapeutic agents are being developed with the hope of improving efficacy or diminishing toxicity. Following initial assessment of *in vitro* and *in vivo* laboratory models, the place of a particular agent is assessed by passing it through a series of clinical trials called phase I, II and III.

Phase I studies are usually carried out by or in close collaboration with a drug company to assess dosage levels and toxicity. Heavily pretreated patients with recurrent untreatable disease are used. Three patients are treated at one dosage level and the toxicity and response, if any, are assessed. The dose is then increased by increments on further groups of three patients each, until intolerable toxicity is reached. If the drug shows any signs of activity it then passes to a phase II study.

Patients with previously treated end-stage disease are the usual subjects for **phase II** studies. The maximum tolerated dose established in a phase I study is used. The main end-points of interest in a phase II study are toxicity and response. The toxicity in various organs is assessed on a five-point scale laid down by the World Health Organization for each course of treatment. The size of the tumour is measured before treatment (not always an easy or possible task) and after each course of treatment. If the tumour disappears completely this is counted as a complete response. If the product of two perpendicular diameters decreases by more than 50% of the original, this is counted as a partial response. For head and neck cancer median survival in a study of this sort is usually around 6 months.

The disadvantages of this type of trial are, first, that an untreated control arm is virtually never included. Secondly, the value of response of the tumour in terms of palliation of the patients' symptoms is unmeasured. Thirdly, about one-third of all patients eligible for such a study do not receive treatment for a variety of reasons. They are rarely reported, so that the results of the treatment are artificially inflated because only favourable patients are included. Finally, many reports of studies of this type compare the survival of responders with non-responders. Most authors then make the completely illogical and unjustified conclusion that the responders have benefited. Unless treated responders are compared with an untreated group no such conclusions can be drawn. These phase II studies usually contain about 20 patients and can be completed in a year or less.

Clinical trials

- Phase I: to determine toxicity and dose levels
- Phase II: to demonstrate efficacy
- Phase III: randomized comparison with standard treatment

A **phase III** trial has two or more arms and the main end-point is survival of the patient. It usually compares best standard treatment with an experimental treatment. Sometimes, two treatments regarded as standard in different centres are directly compared. This type of trial requires several hundred patients and several years to complete. In this type of trial, toxicity and response are recorded, but the main criterion is survival. Furthermore, all patients, once randomized, are included in the analysis whether they were treated or not. This type of trial therefore provides a much more objective answer. It is important when designing such a trial to estimate the number of patients likely to be required in order to judge whether the trial is feasible; most clinicians have a very optimistic view of the size of the trial. There are various statistical formulae for calculating the trial size. These depend on the likelihood of events, the anticipated difference between the two arms of the trial and the power required to detect a difference.

Errors in clinical trials

- Type I: false negative
- Type II: false positive

Planning the size must take into account the chances of a type I and type II error. A type I error is the chance of rejecting a hypothesis when it should be accepted, usually because the trial contains too few patients to have the required power to detect a difference between the two arms. A type II error is the chance of accepting a result as significant when it should be rejected. The minimal acceptance level for power is 80% and for significance the minimum is 5%. (The probability of the difference being a chance finding is <5%: '$p < 0.05$'.) The calculation must also take into account the survival rates which are already known from past experience and any likely improvement. Again, clinicians are usually optimistic in guessing the latter: a true improvement in survival of 5% would be an enormous advance in current circumstances; a true improvement of 10% is exceedingly unlikely and an improvement of more than this would demand an entirely new form of treatment. The appropriate numbers required for a trial are shown in Table 5.2.

Regimens and scheduling of chemotherapy for head and neck cancer

Adjuvant chemotherapy

This may be given after, during or prior to definitive treatment, in which case it is termed neoadjuvant therapy. The chemotherapy may be given as a single agent, most commonly methotrexate, or as a combination of drugs. Among the most widely used drug combinations are vincristine, bleomyin, methotrexate and 5-fluorouracil (VBMF), and cisplatin or carbolatin and 5-fluorouracil, with or without folinic acid.

Scheduling of adjuvant chemotherapy

- Before radiotherapy: neoadjuvant; induction; up-front
- During radiotherapy: synchronous; concomitant
- After radiotherapy: Adjuvant; subsequent

Table 5.2 Numbers required in a phase III trial

Known 5-year survival of standard treatment	Anticipated improvement in survival with new treatment	
	5%	10%
30%	1124	300
40%	1248	325
50%	1273	325

Power 80%, $p < 0.05$.

These drugs undoubtedly have biological activity against squamous carcinoma, as objective single agent response rates up to 40% are reported, rising to 75% if combinations are used. It must be recognized that while the 'response rate' is easily measured in relatively small groups of patients, it is clinically irrelevant and is, at best, a rather poor proxy for more significant outcome measures. The important outcomes are, in the adjuvant setting, improvements in local control rates and survival rates, and in palliative treatment, symptom control and possibly improvements in duration of survival.

However, despite the fact that in the 1980s and 1990s, dozens of trials have examined its use, the place of adjuvant chemotherapy remains uncertain. Many of these trials have been too small to detect a modest improvement in survival but it is unlikely that they would have overlooked a major beneficial effect. Observed beneficial effects relate principally to improved local control rather than increased survival. Local control appears to be improved, especially in oropharyngeal carcinoma, by the use of synchronous chemotherapy and radiotherapy. Acute radiation reactions are often enhanced; indeed, in some studies the potential benefit of adjuvant chemotherapy is offset by treatment-related deaths.

Outcome measures for the assessment of adjuvant chemotherapy

- Improvement in local control rates
- Improvement in survival rates

Induction therapy, unlike synchronous therapy, has never been shown to confer a survival advantage overall. Although patients who achieve a complete remission have improved survival times, this may be because response to induction chemotherapy is a predictor of radiotherapy response. The results of further, large-scale studies are awaited. In the meantime, adjuvant chemotherapy should be used only in a trial setting and not considered for the routine management of squamous carcinoma of the head and neck.

Palliative chemotherapy

If other options have been exhausted, chemotherapy should be considered in patients with significant symptoms caused by advanced or recurrent tumour considered to be incurable. This can often produce considerable improvement, but the benefit is usually short-lived. Chemotherapy is toxic. Its safe administration is expensive, requiring considerable expertise and, in a palliative context, frequent hospitalization of a patient whose life expectancy is very limited. It is also difficult to determine whether a patient has benefited in terms of survival and/or symptom relief. Any costly treatment of questionable benefit must be administered only after careful consideration, as its use inevitably means a reduction in available resources elsewhere. Savings made by stopping inappropriate chemotherapy in the terminally ill would increase funds available for consultation time and supportive care.

Psychosocial supportive care and counselling

The diagnosis of cancer of any type comes as a great blow not only to the patient but also to their family and friends. They are faced, not just with a life-threatening illness, but often with complex and prolonged treatment which may be associated with severe short-term and long-term side-effects and possibly permanent disfigurement and loss of essential functions such as speech and swallowing. Not only can there be great practical difficulties coping with loss of a major bodily function, but it will also have tremendous impact on social function.

It can often be difficult for a patient to understand what is being proposed by way of treatment and what the likely probems will be. Things can be made more difficult for some patients when they are offered choices between treatment options or asked to take part in clinical trials.

In recent years, vocal and articulate patient groups, often led by professional women with breast cancer, have protested against their perception of medical arrogance and the paternalism of doctors who decide what is best for their patients. It is quite understandable that people who are used to being in charge of their own lives can feel doubly threatened by the loss of autonomy in addition to the arrival of their cancer. Such people rightly have an aversion to being processed as tumours rather than people by the medical machine, and they seek recognition as individuals and wish for empowerment in making therapeutic choices for themselves.

Not all patients with head and neck cancer, however, are so advantaged. Many are from the underclass, elderly victims of social exclusion with poor educational attainment, compounded by unemployment, homelessness, alcoholism and comorbidity. How often have these typical head and neck cancer patients felt empowered in other aspects of life? Most often they wish for decisions to be made on their behalf: 'just do whatever you think is best, doctor'. Such patients need their doctors to be their advocates. All patients need their doctors need to listen compassionately, explain carefully and act in their best interests. The head and neck surgeon and oncologist needs to treat each patient as an individual, assessing their particular requirements and tailoring information and therapeutic options to their personal needs. 'Just do whatever you think is best, doctor' does not, therefore, give the unscrupulous practitioner *carte blanche* to try out some novel chemotherapy or to practise some new operation. Rather, it is a sensible approach when interpreted ethically: after all, it is the head and neck team's responsibility to be *au fait* with the results of randomized clinical trials and evidence-based consensus agreements.

There are various sources of support and guidance for patients with head and neck cancer. Many hospitals will have clinical nurse specialists in head and neck cancer, and speech and language therapists have essential skills to help in the preparation of patients for treatment and subsequent rehabilitation of speech and swallowing. The diagnosis of cancer often highlights social and financial problems for patients, and access to a social worker can be important. More and more cancer centres have patient support and information centres which integrate social, physical and emotional supportive care.

In addition to hospital-based support, charities such as CancerBACUP and CancerLink provide telephone helplines, information booklets and individual counselling. There are also patient support groups which are often locally based, such as laryngectomee clubs and groups for patients with facial disfigurement.

Useful contacts

■ CancerBACUP
  3 Bath Place, Rivington Street, London EC2A 3JR
  Tel: 020 7696 9002

■ CancerLink
  17 Brittania Street, London WC1X 9JN
  Tel: 020 7833 8898

■ National Association of Laryngectomee Clubs
  in the UK
  Ground Floor, 6, Rickett Street, Fulham,
  London SW6 1RU
  Tel: 020 7381 9993

■ Macmillan Cancer Relief
  Anchor House, 15–19 Britten Street,
  London SW3 3TZ
  Tel: 020 7351 7811

Principles of palliative and terminal care

It has been pointed out earlier that while the treatment of patients with cancer is traditionally divided into radical or palliative categories according to the likelihood of cure, this distinction is not infrequently difficult to make. Initial treatment is most often radical in intent, and even following relapse salvage treatment is usually performed in the hope of cure but with the realization that this goal is less likely to be achieved.

Between one in three and one in four patients with head and neck cancer will die from their disease. In the UK survival from laryngeal cancer is approximately 65% (regional variations are from 60% to 70%). About half of all deaths in this group are due to comorbidity rather than directly caused by the cancer itself. In the USA, reported survival rates are better, with a 5-year cause-specific survival of 75% in laryngeal cancer across the board (59% for subglottic and 85% for glottic cancer).

As the disease progresses it may become apparent that further attempts at potentially curative therapy are not possible, yet active anticancer therapy may still be appropriate in carefully selected cases if this might relieve distressing symptoms or prolong useful life. There usually comes a time, however, when further active palliation is not possible and symptom control measures become paramount.

The palliative care approach

■ is the right of every patient
■ and the duty of every health professional

As the patient progresses along the spectrum from radical primary treatment through salvage procedures to palliative treatment and onwards to terminal care, it can be difficult to decide at which point the transition in therapeutic aim should be made. Continuity of care is important, and while it may be necessary for the surgeon or oncologist to seek the aid of a palliative medicine physician it is also essential for the patient and family to realize that he or she has not been abandoned, and that care will be continued. The proper management of the patient with advanced malignant disease is one of the most demanding aspects of medical practice, requiring experienced clinical judgement, compassion and common sense in equal measure. A display of insensitivity or indifference in this field is never forgotten and rarely forgiven by the bereaved.

Location of terminal care

The aim of terminal care should be to make the patient free of pain, mobile and sufficiently alert so that he or she can spend time in comfort at home with his or her family if possible. Domiciliary care of the terminally ill patient requires a close liaison between the hospital services which have provided care earlier in the course of the illness and the community health service. The latter comprises the general practitioner, nursing support and ancillary help. The care provided by district nurses is often supplemented with help from those with special experience and training in palliative and terminal care, such as Macmillan or Marie Curie nurses. Advice may also be sought from palliative medicine physicians who, although often hospice based, play a greater role in the community than was previously the case. Attendance at a day hospice may enable patients to stay longer at home. Admission to a hospice is not necessarily permanent. It is common practice for patients to be admitted for short periods for convalescence following hospital treatment or to obtain symptom control before returning home. Sometimes hospices will admit patients for a period of respite care to allow their domiciliary carers to take a holiday. If domestic circumstances are not suitable for terminal care, for example patients without immediate family or the socially disadvantaged head and neck cancer patients who live in hostels, institutional care is necessary. Similarly, some patients are well managed at home during the early part of their terminal illness, but require institutional care later on. The options here are either continued care in the hospitals which have looked after the patient earlier, or hospices. The former is particularly appropriate if a strong relationship has developed between the patient and the staff on the ward where the patient has been previously treated and where the staff have the necessary time and skills to provide appropriate care, or if specialized nursing is required, say for a laryngectomee. The appropriate location for terminal care should be decided jointly among the patient, family and medical attendants.

Pain relief

In the minds of many patients and their families, death from cancer is synonymous with pain and anguish. In the past, this fear was well founded, but with modern analgesic techniques intractable pain should be very rare. Unfortunately, many patients with pain which could be alleviated are still left to suffer unnecessarily. For adequate analgesia, more than analgesics are required: the prerequisite of successful pain control is careful assessment of the patient's symptoms.

As pain in the patient with far advanced cancer can affect several areas, and may be completely unrelated to the cancer itself or be caused by its treatment, the site or sites, nature, severity and causes of the patient's discomfort need to be elucidated. In the majority of cases when the pain is rightly attributed to the cancer, it is also important to determine the mechanism underlying it, as the treatment may depend on the cause. For example, the pain of constipation caused by opiates will not be relieved by increasing the dose, but requires the use of laxatives or enemas. It is important to record the details of the pain and to review the patient regularly to monitor the response to changes in therapy, to evaluate any new symptoms and to provide explanations of the pain and the necessary medication to the patient and relatives. As attention to detail is an important ingredient in the recipe for success and polypharmacy is often unavoidable, it is helpful to write out the medication schedule for the patient.

Persistent pain caused by tumour infiltration requires regular therapy to abolish the pain and prevent its recurrence. The pain should not be allowed to recrudesce before the next analgesic dose is due. For this reason, 'as required' or p.r.n. medication is inappropriate as the sole treatment. It is the doctor's responsibility to ensure not only that adequate analgesia is prescribed, but that the patient and carers understand the need for its regular administration. If pain also breaks through before the next dose, it is better to increase the regular dose rather than to increase the frequency of administration or to prescribe small supplementary doses.

Analgesics may be classified according to the severity of pain that they can treat effectively. For mild pain, simple analgesics such as paracetamol may be all that is required. Simple analgesics with some anti-inflammatory effects such as aspirin or ibuprofen may be more effective than paracetamol, especially in the case of bone pain. As a second simple analgesic is unlikely to succeed where a first has failed, the prescriber should use a more powerful analgesic in this case. Moderate pain may call for a simple analgesic–mild opiate combi-

nation such as paracetamol and codeine (cocodamol) or dextropropoxyphene and paracetamol (coproxamol). Some of these combinations are available in different ratios, and it is the prescriber's responsibility to know the exact proportion of the ingredients and prescribe appropriately.

If simple analgesic–mild opiate combinations are inadequate, the pain is by definition severe and strong opiates such as morphine or diamorphine are required. This step on the analgesic ladder is sometimes known as the 'suffering gap' because patients (and sadly sometimes health-care professionals) have unjustified fears about the use of strong opiates. If strong opiate analgesia is necessary, patients should not be denied it by their carers or misguidedly permitted to deny themselves its benefits. Analgesic regimens should be kept as simple as possible and there is no sense in using more than one analgesic of any class, although there is logic in combining analgesics which act through different mechanisms, such as aspirin and morphine.

> **Classes of analgesic**
>
> ■ Simple analgesics, e.g. paracetamol
> ■ Anti-inflammatory drugs, e.g. diclofenac
> ■ Mild opiate combinations, e.g. coproxamol
> ■ Strong opiates, e.g. morphine

Short-acting analgesics such as pethidine should be avoided. Buprenorphine is also best avoided, despite its longer duration of action and potential for sublingual administration, as being a partial antagonist it can precipitate withdrawal symptoms including pain in patients who have been using other opiates.

If possible, oral medication should be used. For patients unable to swallow tablets, liquid preparations of morphine and transdermal patches containing fentanyl are available. For patients who are vomiting, parenteral administration may be required temporarily until effective antiemetic therapy has been instituted. For patients in whom oral therapy is impossible, subcutaneous injections are far preferable to intramuscular injections, especially in those with cachexia. If a patient comfortable with oral morphine becomes unable to swallow, the appropriate parenteral dose is half the oral one. Alternatively, suppositories may be used. Syringe drivers giving a continuous subcutaneous infusion are especially valuable in the dying patient who is bed-bound and semicomatose, as sedatives and antiemetics such as haloperidol may be given simultaneously, but may also be used in ambulant patients. Syringe drivers are not without their own problems and should not be used prematurely in a patient who is quite able to take drugs by mouth. Oral medication is often erroneously deemed inadequate when in reality it is the prescribed dose which is inadequate rather than the oral route which is inappropriate. When injections are necessary, diamorphine is generally preferred to morphine as it is much more soluble and the volume to be injected is therefore smaller.

The principles of successful analgesic therapy can thus be summarized as 'by mouth, by the clock, and by the ladder'.

Two fears, drug dependence and respiratory depression, sometimes limit the proper use of strong opiates in the terminal-care setting. It is often the patient rather than the doctor who is unwilling to commence opiates as they are concerned about becoming addicted. This possibility is, however, of no significance in the patient who is destined to die from malignancy within weeks. Nonetheless, if the patient or the family expresses anxieties about the appropriateness of strong opiates, the health-care professional should be prepared to discuss analgesia in some detail, acknowledging their concerns. It is usually possible to explain why strong opiates are needed and to reassure the patient and family members that they can be given safely.

Pain is a powerful respiratory stimulant and respiratory depression as a result of opiate use is uncommon in terminally ill patients. Nonetheless, it may occur, and antagonists should be available for use if necessary.

When strong opiate therapy is initiated, it is best to use oral morphine solution regularly every 4 h. The dose given can be rapidly titrated to the level required to control the pain. Thereafter, the patient can continue on this schedule, or an equivalent dose as slow-release tablets which are given only once (e.g. MXL) or twice (e.g. MST) a day may be preferred by the patient. Milligram for milligram, the total daily dose of morphine preparations is equivalent, whether they are unmodified preparations (fast-acting, short-duration) or sustained-release formulations.

In this day and age it is increasingly common for unscrupulous drug misusers to steal opiates from their dying relatives either for their own use or for resale, and the prescriber should be alert to this crime.

As all opiates cause constipation which can be very troublesome, it is essential that a laxative is given concurrently. When the patient is reviewed, it is important to enquire whether bowel function is satisfactory and adjust the laxative if necessary.

As well as laxatives, other drugs may be required in combination with opiates. Nausea or vomiting is often a problem following the initiation of opiate therapy and a wide variety of effective antiemetics is now available. These should be prescribed separately from the opiate, so that the dose of each can be adjusted independently.

Tablets which contain combinations of opiates and antiemetics such as dipipanone and cyclizine are available but should not be prescribed, as the fixed ratio of the combination makes it impossible to increase the analgesic level without also increasing the antiemetic. Antiemetics are generally needed only for the first few days after the start of opiate treatment and may then be discontinued. Care should be taken to distinguish vomiting due to opiates from that due to other causes, for example intestinal obstruction or raised intracranial pressure. There is no place for cocaine in dying patients, although this drug was once popular as an ingredient of the 'Brompton cocktail'.

Pain caused by raised intracranial pressure or by nerve compression may be helped by the coadministration of corticosteroids. Superficial dysaesthetic pain which is caused by nerve infiltration or compression may be alleviated by amitriptyline. Sodium valproate or carbamazepine may help sudden lancinating pain which occurs intermittently. Bone metastases are uncommon in patients with head and neck cancer, but radiotherapy should be considered if painful osseous deposits become manifest and, as mentioned above, non-steroidal anti-inflammatory agents may also be of value.

Other symptoms

While psychotropics should not be used routinely, anxiety and depression frequently occur in the patient with pain due to advanced malignant disease. These symptoms may abate when pain control is achieved, but if no improvement is seen despite good analgesia, anxiolytics or antidepressants may be indicated. Insomnia is a frequent problem. Once obvious precipitating factors such as pain have been dealt with on their own merits, benzodiazepines such as temazepam may be used. Restlessness and confusion may occur, especially in the dying patient. Major tranquillizers such as haloperidol are then indicated. Chlorpromazine is an alternative, but causes a greater degree of sedation. Methotrimeprazine is also occasionally useful. Patients complaining of a dry mouth or dysphagia should be examined for signs of oropharyngeal candidiasis, which can be treated with nystatin suspension, fluconazole, amphotericin lozenges or miconazole gel. A dry mouth can also be caused by morphine, amitriptyline or prior radiotherapy to the parotid salivary glands. Patients with intracranial disease or metabolic disturbance may develop epileptic fits. If intermittent these may be controlled by oral anticonvulsants. A prolonged fit may be terminated by intravenous administration of diazepam emulsion. Diazepam may also be administered rectally.

One symptom, generally more distressing for the attending relatives than the sufferer, is the 'death rattle' caused by an accumulation of excessive respiratory secretions in the moribund patient. This may be reduced by the use of an anticholinergic agent such as atropine or hyoscine.

Summary

Terminal care, like most other aspects of medicine, requires experience, careful assessment of the patient's needs and meticulous attention to therapeutic detail, if it is to be practised successfully. Emotional and social factors, as well as physical ones, need to be taken into consideration in tailoring treatment to an individual patient's requirements. Good terminal care requires a large investment by the doctor of both time and effort and should, therefore, not be undertaken lightly or unwillingly.

Further reading

MacDougall R. H., Munro A. J. and Wilson J. A. (1998) Palliation in head and neck cancer, in *The Oxford Textbook of Palliative Medicine* (D. Doyle, G. W. C. Hanks, N. MacDonald, eds.), Oxford Medical Publications, Oxford. Section 9.9, pp. 677–689.

Robertson A. G., Wheldon T. E., and Robertson C. (1996) Applying sound radiobiology principles to the management of carcinoma of the larynx, in *Current Radiation Oncology 2* (J. S. Tobias, and P. R. M. Thomas, eds), Arnold, London, pp. 121–143.

Saunders M. I. (1994) Accelerated fractionation and its applications in clinical radiotherapy, in *Current Radiation Oncology 1* (J. S. Tobias and P. R. M. Thomas, eds), Edward Arnold, London, pp. 160–181.

Syed A. M. N. and Puthawala A. A. (1996) Current brachytherapy techniques, in *Current Radiation Oncology 2* (J. S. Tobias and P. R. M. Thomas, eds), Arnold, London, pp. 88–106.

Tobias J. S. (1994) Chemotherapy–radiotherapy combinations for advanced head and neck cancer, in *Current Radiation Oncology 1* (J. S. Tobias and P. R. M. Thomas, eds), Edward Arnold, London, pp. 231–49.

Wang C. C. (1998) Importance of schedule and fractionation in head and neck radiation oncology, in *Current Radiation Oncology 3* (J. S. Tobias and P. R. M. Thomas, eds), Arnold, London, pp. 131–145.

6 Complications

'If anything can go wrong, it will'
Murphy's Law

Introduction

Complications following head and neck surgery are inevitable. They can be divided into major and minor ones. Major complications such as wound breakdown, fistulae, flap failure and deep vein thrombosis (DVT) will occur in up to 20% of patients in any large series for head and neck cancer surgery. Minor complications such as wound or chest infections or thrombophlebitis around a drip site will occur more often.

It is important to think how complications might best be avoided. Assessment is crucial (see Chapter 2) and the patient's condition with regard to chest and nutritional status should be evaluated prior to surgery. The patient should be in optimum condition for the operation and if help is required from other disciplines, advice should be sought prior to, rather than on, the day of operation.

Classification of complications

These can be classified as early, intermediate and late, local and systemic and those that are specific to the cause. Immediate complications are most often the direct result of technical faults during the operation and manifest themselves within the first 24 h after surgery. Intermediate complications come on during the succeeding days after surgery before the patient leaves hospital and are often due to failure in the healing process. Finally, there are late complications which come on months or years after the operation following the time when the patient has returned home. The surgical team is responsible for the correct identification of all possible complications. Local complications usually require treatment by the head and neck surgeon while general complications may well require advice from other specialists. The specific complications which relate exclusively to one particular operation will be discussed in the chapters relating to that specific tumour site.

Classification of complications

- Major and minor
- Early, intermediate and late
- Local and systemic
- General and specific

Vigilant work-up, meticulous surgery and hawk-like follow-up with early anticipation of problems are necessary to forestall and successfully prevent and treat head and neck complications. Ideally, the preoperative haemoglobin should exceed 11 g/dl and the serum albumin 40 g/l. Murphy's pessimistic law 'if anything can go wrong it will' is a pertinent reminder that unless attempts are made to avoid complications, problems are likely to be encountered.

The potential occurrence of complications is an essential component of preoperative counselling and the obtaining of informed consent.

Immediate local complications

Bleeding

After any major head and neck operation, immediate bleeding manifests itself either from an anastomosis site into the mouth or pharynx or by haematoma formation under the skin flaps. In either case it is usually quite obvious to the trained observer and should be detected long before there are changes in the vital signs.

After resection of a carcinoma in the mouth, pharynx or larynx, bleeding may take place from the suture line. Bleeding into the mouth may also occur after a total maxillectomy if all of the branches of the maxillary artery have not been tied properly or the venous ooze from the pterygoid venous plexus continues following surgery. In either of these events, blood is seen trickling from the mouth and the diagnosis is easy. This complication of bleeding following major head and neck surgery from the oral cavity and pharynx explains why patients require a temporary tracheostomy, and a cuffed tube can prevent interference with the airway by blood and subsequent inhalation into the bronchial tree. It also allows for the patient to be returned to theatre quickly to have the bleeding dealt with without fear of the airway being compromised.

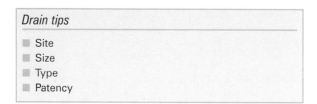

Potential sources of bleeding

- Suture lines
- Skin flaps
- Major vessels:
  - external carotid
  - thyrocervical trunk
  - internal jugular vein

Bleeding may also occur after a neck dissection. This may be from the skin flaps and, in particular, the posterior surface of the bridged flap used in the double horizontal MacFee incision. Other potential sites of bleeding are branches of the external carotid artery, the thyrocervical trunk or the transverse cervical artery and branches of the internal jugular vein following selective neck dissection.

Bleeding in this instance manifests itself by swelling in the neck if the suction drains are unable to cope with the blood or if they become blocked. This is one reason why bandages should not be applied to the neck following surgery so that this complication is easily recognized.

Some disasters happen when too small a drain is used. Following major head and neck surgery, the authors favour using a large drain (i.e. 12 Fr or Surgidene 10 mm). The correct type and number of drains must be used and confirmed to be working at the end of the procedure. Any leaks through the skin should be corrected if possible by further suturing or pressure. If the leak continues, the drain should be attached to a Roberts pump or wall suction.

Drain tips

- Site
- Size
- Type
- Patency

When closing a large wound during which considerable pooling of blood can occur, it can be advantageous to have the drains attached to the suction to maintain their patency and remove the excess blood. Wherever possible, drains should be inserted at inconspicuous sites (e.g. behind the ear or in the hairline) to avoid unnecessary scarring.

The principles of management relating to haemorrhage in these two situations are the same as those after any operation. They are to diagnose the problem, resuscitate the patient, stop the bleeding and treat the cause.

Management of bleeding

- Diagnose the problem
- Resuscitate the patient
- Stop the bleeding
- Treat the cause
- Do not postpone re-exploration

Blood should be cross-matched if not already available. Intravenous access must be adequate for rapid volume replacement if this becomes necessary. Brisk arterial bleeding requires two cannulated access sites. A 14 G cannula (brown venflon) allows a flow rate of 270 ml/min so two are usually adequate. Ideally, a size 7 Fr Swan-Ganz catheter placed in the femoral vein or antecubital fossa is ideal for large volume infusion. In the absence of blood, the most favoured non-blood volume expander is Hespan (modified starch) or Jelofusine (succinylated gelatin). In view of the fact these compounds have no oxygen-carrying ability, only limited amounts (approximately 1 litre) can be used. The haemoglobin should be returned to the preoperative level (11 g/l) but it is paramount that patients with microvascular anastomoses are not overtransfused since a high haemoglobin can lead to sludging, stasis and thrombus formation. The patient should be returned to theatre, any bleeding points should be found and ligated and the blood that has been lost should be replaced by transfusion. Attempts to arrest the haemorrhage by applying pressure dressings to the neck or attempting to pack a bleeding cavity are a waste of time. The bleeding will almost certainly not stop, valuable time is lost, and further exsanguination occurs with a probability of subsequent infection or necrosis of skin flaps. The possibility of major vessel exposure, infection and rupture is also increased by delay. Therefore, a prompt decision must be made to return the patient to theatre, reopen the wound, which should then be cleaned with hydrogen peroxide diluted 1:1 with saline, and then place a swab soaked in warm water in the wound. The bleeding points are then secured, the patient's circulating blood volume is restored to normal, further drains are inserted and the patient is returned to the ward. The anaesthetist may insert a central line to monitor fluid requirements and bladder catheterization with hourly urimetry is also helpful.

Airway obstruction

After extensive resection of tissue within the mouth, pharynx or larynx, there is inevitable oedema of the remaining organ(s) and the airway is often likely to be compromised. Furthermore, if a bilateral neck dissection is carried out (either simultaneously or staged) there maybe associated soft-tissue oedema. In these situations, it is prudent to carry out an elective tracheostomy to prevent airway obstruction and protect the airway. This facilitates control of the airway, so that the patient does not have to go to the intensive treatment unit (ITU), and allows the airway to be suctioned by nursing staff and the physiotherapist. It also prevents a difficult reintubation with undesirable cervical hyperextension, should any problems occur in the immediate postoperative period. Should a tracheostomy not be carried out for any reason, then at the first sign of any airway obstruction it becomes mandatory. A very wise aphorism is that if a tracheostomy comes into one's mind then that is the time to do it. Failure to act then will often lead to more problems later on. The procedure of tracheostomy is described in Chapter 9.

Increased intracranial pressure

The intracranial pressure rises three-fold when one internal jugular vein is divided and five-fold when both are tied, but often returns to near normal levels within 24 h. This rise will seldom cause symptoms, especially if both internal jugular veins are not tied simultaneously (which happens rarely) but may do so when both veins are tied as a staged procedure or if a dominant jugular vein has been tied on one side.

Signs and symptoms of increased intracranial pressure

- Restlessness from headache
- Slowing of the pulse
- A rise in blood pressure
- Gross swelling and cyanosis of the face

If a patient's lips and ears are cyanosed at the end of a head and neck operation, do not presume that they are suffering from peripheral cyanosis due to cardiorespiratory failure before examining the other extremities. If these are found to be pink and warm, the facial cyanosis is due to ligation of the major neck veins.

Reducing the risk of raised intracranial pressure

- Place no dressings around the neck
- Do not allow the patient to hyperextend the neck (particularly after bilateral neck dissection)
- Sit the patient up as soon as possible after surgery

If increased intracranial pressure occurs, the patient should be sat up and given 200 ml of 25% mannitol intravenously as quickly as possible and a urinary catheter passed. If the diagnosis is correct, the results of this are usually dramatic. A diuresis will occur, the condition should reverse within 10–15 min and the patient can be expected to pass 500 ml of urine within the next 2 h. As the intracranial pressure usually falls rapidly to normal with 24 h, mannitol rarely needs to be given again.

Significant facial oedema will occur on its own after extensive facial surgery such as a lip split with a mandibulotomy. This is because the curved extension of the cervical incision divides the superficial lymphatics. This problem can be compounded by a rise in the intracranial pressure as described above. If significant facial

swelling occurs, a short course of postoperative steroids is of particular value and dexamethasone can be prescribed 4 mg three times a day for 5 days, bearing in mind that some patients can develop problems such as an acute confusional state or glucose intolerance secondary to steroid administration. In specific operations such as midfacial degloving or external rhinoplasty, a preoperative stat dose of methylprednisolone (40 mg) can significantly reduce postoperative swelling.

Carotid sinus syndrome

The carotid sinus is a baroreceptor; an increase in carotid arterial pressure normally causes bradycardia and decreased systemic blood pressure. This stimulus is slight compared with the manipulation at operation, which may result in a marked drop in blood pressure and slowing of the pulse. This can be anticipated and dealt with by an experienced anaesthetist, but may be alarming to one more junior. The surgeon can help by injecting 2% lignocaine around the sinus, thereby blocking afferent glossopharyngeal fibres.

Postoperative scarring may leave the sinus in a highly sensitive state so that palpation of the neck or even turning the head from side to side may result in faintness or even loss of consciousness due to hypotension and bradycardia. This hypersensitivity persists indefinitely. These symptoms coming on some months after operation usually indicate recurrent tumour invading the glossopharyngeal nerve or skull base.

Nerve injury

The nerves listed in the following box are at risk during head and neck surgery.

Nerves at risk

- Lower cranial nerves (VII–XII)
- Brachial plexus
- Phrenic nerve
- Recurrent laryngeal nerve
- Superior laryngeal nerve
- Sympathetic chain

These nerves may suffer neuropraxia or may be transected during surgery. The way to avoid any injury is to have a proper awareness of the anatomical relationships in the neck, and the procedures and tips to avoid any nerve damage are discussed in the appropriate chapter which relates to the surgery during which they are placed at risk, i.e. the facial nerve during parotid surgery (Chapter 22), the recurrent laryngeal nerve and the superior laryngeal nerve during thyroid surgery (Chapter 23) and the accessory nerve, brachial plexus and phrenic nerve and marginal mandibular branch of the facial nerve during neck dissection (Chapter 13).

Immediate general complications

Pneumothorax

The cervical pleura may be damaged during any operation low in the neck, especially if the manubrium is removed. The mediastinal pleura is under significant risk of damage during oesophageal resection or mobilization. It is customary following the stomach pull-up procedure to insert bilateral chest drains prophylactically and ventilate the patient on intensive care for 24 h postoperatively. In addition, artificial ventilation may cause pleural rupture, especially in cases of bullous emphysema (or in children, whose inflation pressures must be monitored carefully).

However, in those cases as described above where the pleura is at risk and elective chest drain insertion with postoperative ventilation is not anticipated, then if the patient has been ventilated during the anaesthetic the presence of a pneumothorax may not be appreciated until shortly after the end of the operation. In such patients a portable chest radiograph should be taken in the operating theatre at the end of the procedure. If the patient becomes restless, cyanosed or dyspnoeic after operation he or she probably has a pneumothorax: provided the suspicion enters the surgeon's mind, the diagnosis is made clinically by conventional methods without a chest radiograph. Indeed, if a pneumothorax is extensive, it may not be to the patient's advantage to wait until a radiograph is obtained; it is preferable to introduce a catheter into the second intercostal space in the midclavicular line and connect it to an underwater seal (Fig. 6.1). If this does not restore normal ventilation, it is worthwhile remembering that there may be a pneumothorax on the other side and that, if there has been extensive bleeding, there may even be a haemopneumothorax.

Haemopneumothorax may be difficult to diagnose even by radiography because at the end of the operation radiographs are usually taken with the patient lying supine. In these circumstances, fluid in the pleural cavity will not be shown. If there is a large quantity of fluid in the pleural cavity it can be readily be aspirated, either by applying suction to the underwater seal or by inserting another catheter into the seventh or eighth intercostal space in the midaxillary line and applying suction to that catheter.

> **Clinical features of a pneumothorax**
> - Hyperresonance to percussion
> - Hyperinflation
> - Diminished breath sounds
> - Trachea deviated away (if under tension)

Intermediate general complications

All patients who have undergone major head and neck surgery require a full clinical examination twice a day. Following head and neck examination the chest, abdomen and calves should all be examined. The following complications may be encountered.

Basal collapse

Following extensive surgery, there may be unilateral or bilateral basal pulmonary collapse in the first 48 h. Initial treatment is with vigorous physiotherapy and if coincidental infection is suspected, then the appropriate antibiotic cover should be prescribed. Many patients will already be on 72 h prophylactic antibiotic cover.

Bronchopneumonia

This is a common complication following major head and neck surgery and relates to coexistent smoking-related lung disease, associated tracheostomy and lengthy operations. Treatment is in the conventional manner with physiotherapy and appropriate antibiotic therapy when sputum culture is obtained. When infections are unusual or do not respond to standard therapy, the advice of a microbiologist is recommended.

In those patients who undergo major surgery, and in particular those having the abdomen opened, an ileus may develop. If this is the case, then feeding via the nasogastric tube or PEG is delayed until the condition improves. Similarly some patients may develop urinary retention and because of this, those patients with prostatic hypertrophy and any patient undergoing surgery for longer than 4 h require a urinary catheter. Patients are at risk of peptic ulceration and because of this should receive prophylactic H_2 antagonist therapy. If haematemesis and/or melaena develops, this should be treated conventionally.

In patients with established infection, septicaemia may ensue and, if the temperature rises over 38°C, with associated rigors and hypotension, then blood cultures are mandatory. Treatment is directed towards the cause.

Deep vein thrombosis

Some patients undergoing major head and neck surgery will develop a DVT and unfortunately, although

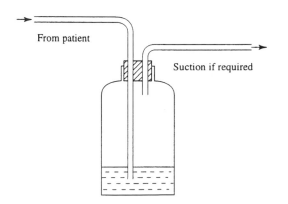

Figure 6.1 Underwater seal drainage.

From patient

Suction if required

Table 6.1   Risk groups for deep vein thrombosis (DVT) and pulmonary embolism (PE) in ear, nose and throat surgery

Risk group	Factors
(I) **Low risk**	(a) Surgery lasting less than 45 min. No risk factor other than age (b) Surgery lasting more than 45 min. Aged under 40 years and no other risk factor (c) Minor medical illness not requiring prolonged bed rest
(II) **Moderate risk**	(a) Surgery lasting more than 45 min and aged over 40 years. (b) Low-risk surgery plus risk factors for thromboembolism (other than age) (c) Surgery lasting less than 45 min in patients with a history of DVT, PE or thrombophilia
(III) **High risk**	(a) Major surgery (including the neck), trauma or illness in a patient over 60 years, or who has a history of DVT, PE or thrombophilia (b) Lower limb paralysis (c) Trauma involving a fracture of the pelvis, hip or lower limb

Table 6.2   Guidelines for prophylaxis against deep vein thrombosis (DVT) and pulmonary embolism (PE)

Risk group	Guidelines
(I) **Low risk**	Early mobilization
(II) **Moderate risk**	Early mobilization Graduated compression stockings until fully mobile
(III) **High risk**	Perioperative and postoperative subcutaneous heparin (tinzaparin 3500 units once daily) until mobile Graduated compression stockings until mobile Perioperative intermittent pneumatic compression

History of DVT/PE	(a) Is operation necessary?
	(b) **Low risk** becomes **moderate risk**
	     Consider subcutaneous low molecular weight heparin (tinzaparin 3500 units once daily)
	(c) **Moderate risk** becomes **high risk**
	     Consider full anticoagulation
	(d) If heparin or warfarin are contraindicated then use graduated compression stockings and intermittent pneumatic compression
	     Consider postoperative heparin if feasible
	(e) Consider haematological advice regarding alternative anticoagulants

rarely, some will succumb to the fatal complication of a pulmonary embolus. In the past, the incidence of DVT and fatal pulmonary embolism (PE) in patients undergoing major head and neck surgery was thought to be extremely uncommon and, because of this, patients have not usually received antithromboembolic prophylaxis. However, recent reports (Hargreaves, 1993; Gallimore *et al.*, 1997; Dawes, 1997) have suggested that the incidence of DVT is higher than originally thought and some patients can subsequently succumb to fatal pulmonary emboli. Because of this patients are now categorized into low, intermediate and high risk groups and depending on their category should receive the appropriate combination of thromboembolic deterrent (TED) stockings, pneumatic stockings during surgery and subcutaneous heparin. Various regimes are in use but what is important is that each unit or centre has a departmental policy. Most large centres around the world now adopt a similar regime to that shown in Tables 6.1 and 6.2 for patients undergoing major head and neck surgery. The risk factors associated with thromboembolism are shown in Table 6.3.

Table 6.3 Thrombosis risk factors*

- **Age (greater than 60 years; high risk)**
- **History of DVT/PE (high risk)**
- Oral contraceptive pill
- Malignancy
- Anticipated bed confinement over 72 h
- Varicose veins
- Obesity (>20% of ideal body weight)
- History of previous major surgery
- Previous immobilization (>72 h)
- Myocardial infarction
- Congestive cardiac failure
- Stroke
- Crystalloid infusion (>5 l/24 h)
- Severe chronic obstructive airways disease
- Trauma
- Confining travel, air/rail/road (>4 h within week of admission)
- History of pelvic or long bone fracture
- Leg oedema, ulcers or stasis
- Pregnancy or postpartum (<1 month)
- Inflammatory bowel disease
- Severe infection
- Hormone replacement therapy
- Hypercoagable states

*Note that smoking is not a risk factor.

Intermediate local complications

These occur later than 24 h after surgery and before the patient leaves hospital. They are listed below.

Intermediate local complications

- Chylous fistula
- Seroma
- Skull-base syndrome
- Wound infection
- Failure of skin healing
- Carotid artery rupture
- Flap failure
- Fistula formation

Chylous fistula

If a chylous leak is allowed to continue, the skin flaps will not sit properly, leading to subsequent neck infection, and the patient rapidly becomes emaciated within the first 24 h. There is no disgrace in damaging or cutting a thoracic duct whilst operating low on the left side of the neck. Indeed, it may often be necessary to do so when carrying out radical surgery low in the neck or the mediastinum. What is disastrous, however, is failing to recognize this complication at the time of surgery, since this may have serious consequences.

If a chylous fistula is suspected, it should be searched for and every attempt made to seal it at the time of surgery. The patient may be positioned head down and the leak exaggerated using a modified Valsalva manoeuvre instigated by the anaesthetist. This means that in an intubated patient, the ventilation circuit is changed to manual, the expiratory valve closed and the pressure in the circuit increased to about 30 mmHg.

Operating loupes may be helpful in this situation to identify a leaking vessel which should be oversewn using silk, as it excites a vigorous inflammatory reaction. Sometimes, because the patient has fasted, it may not be obvious that the duct has been cut because the fluid from the duct is clear and in small amounts.

If an injury is overlooked, it does not usually manifest itself until the patient is subsequently fed and at this time the suction drainage increases dramatically in volume. A bar chart should be constructed to show the leakage level over time and the amount of leakage documented per 24 h. Many small leaks (less than 400 ml/day) will settle with conservative treatment to include nil by mouth, a low-fat enteral diet and pressure on the supraclavicular fossa.

When the drainage reaches 600 ml a day (particularly early on), it is wise to return the patient to theatre, reopen the lower part of the neck, find the injured duct and oversew it with silk. This is often quite easy to do using magnifying loupes and can be achieved by careful dissection up to 10 days following surgery.

It is also possible for significant lymphatic leaks to occur not only from the jugular lymph duct on the right side of the neck but also from its communicating branches across to the left side with the thoracic duct, and these can give rise to large amounts of clear lymph as opposed to chyle. Treatment is similar.

Seroma

A collection of fluid under a neck flap can be prevented by using suction drainage. A seroma may occur in the first 48 h after the drainage tubes have been removed. Serum always collects in the supraclavicular fossa, the most dependent part of the neck.

Part of the routine daily care should be to ask the patient to hunch the shoulder, whereupon the fossa should form a pronounced dip. If the dip is absent, then serum is present and must be aspirated.

A wide-bore needle is used and the fluid aspirated daily until no more serum collects. It may be necessary to do this for up to 2 weeks in order to stop serum accumulating and thus lifting the neck flaps. After each aspiration, pressure may be applied to prevent further accumulation of serum via this low-pressure system.

Skull-base syndrome

In those patients who undergo surgery to the skull base and, in particular, where there is retraction in an upward direction at some time during a procedure, i.e. modified radical/radical neck dissection or superficial/total conservative parotidectomy, then there may well be some temporary paresis and dysfunction of the lower cranial nerves. This may manifest itself in a number of ways such as a temporary facial paresis or changes in the voice with some difficulty in swallowing. It is important to be aware of these problems following such surgery and to be able to advise accordingly. They will usually improve with conservative treatment.

Infection

Wound infection following simple, clean head and neck surgery is uncommon and prophylactic antibiotics are not usually indicated. With extensive surgery, revision surgery or lengthy operations and with those operations that are composite in nature and include entry into, or resection of part of the upper aerodigestive tract, prophylactic antibiotics are mandatory.

Despite this, some degree of wound infection is inevitable. This often settles with appropriate antibiotic care but, if not, then the antibiotics need to be changed. There may be some degree of wound breakdown (discussed below) and very rarely patients develop systemic infection as previously described.

Failure of skin healing

Some degree of minor wound breakdown with major head and neck surgery is not uncommon and should be treated conservatively. It is best prevented by the use of meticulous surgical technique and appropriate incisions, prophylactic antibiotics where appropriate and the use of postoperative surgical drains to prevent haematoma formation. Established infection should be treated in a conventional manner but inevitably there will often be some degree of wound breakdown. Minor wound dehiscence in the early postoperative period in the absence of significant infection and with minimal wound tension may be resutured primarily.

Full wound dehiscence may be treated similarly but it is often wise in the presence of infection and tension to exercise caution with regard to rushing in since many of these wounds are best left to heal by secondary intention. If there is wound dehiscence where major vessels are exposed, these should be covered with either a musculocutaneous flap or muscle-only flap with a skin graft for external cover. However, it is more common that this is not the case and such wounds should be cleaned, packed and allowed to heal by secondary intention.

Open, infected wounds should have swabs taken for culture and sensitivity purposes and then be cleaned with saline (or chlorhexidine in the presence of gross infection). Shallow wounds can be then packed with a hydrocolloid dressing, i.e. Granuflex or Intrasite (Hydrogel). Deep wounds can be packed with Granuflex paste or Sorbisan (biodegradable alginate dressing). Such dressings maintain a high wound humidity, remove excess exudate, keep the wound clean and facilitate granulation and healing by secondary intention. They may require changing once or twice daily depending on the size of the wound and the degree of infection.

Necrosis of the skin of the neck is a disaster that is fortunately much less common than it was 25 years ago. It is caused by many factors and may be fatal. Even when it is non-fatal, the patient is in discomfort because the neck flaps need to be débrided regularly, the resulting raw area may have to be repaired with skin grafts, the hospital stay is prolonged and the resulting scar is often cosmetically unacceptable.

As discussed previously in the section on incisions (Chapter 4), surgery in the neck differs markedly from surgery in the abdomen or chest because to gain access to the neck structures, large skin flaps need to be elevated. These flaps are usually so large that their viability may be marginal and may be compromised by the use of unsuitable incisions, particularly in a patient who has been previously irradiated.

When wound infection does occur (as discussed previously), treatment is conventional with antibiotics whilst swab results are awaited. Provided there is no known necrosis of tissue, infection is usually due to Gram-positive cocci and treatment is with a cephalosporin or coamoxiclav.

Several metabolic factors mitigate against good wound healing and these include both local and general factors. Local factors have been discussed and general factors include poor nutrition, cachexia, uncontrolled diabetes, renal failure and anaemia.

If flap necrosis is about to occur, the circulation in the skin is poor and there is congestion so that finger pressure produces blanching and rapid refilling. Within the first 24 h, the flap will be dark blue or black and at this stage it must be excised back to healthy, 'breathing' skin. If this is done before infection supervenes, the resulting defect can be covered with a split-thickness skin graft but if excision of dead tissue is not carried out at this stage, infection will inevitably supervene and healing by granulation must then be awaited. If infection occurs, culture of the discharge will usually reveal a mixture of Gram-negative organisms such as *Pseudomonas, Proteus* or *Escherichia coli*. In this situation where there is poor blood supply to the infected tissues, use of systemic antibiotics should be avoided and treatment should be conservative with local toilet and débridement to allow healing by secondary intention and skin grafting some weeks later. This is outlined in Chapter 7.

Recently, methicillin-resistant *Staphylococcus aureus* (MRSA) has become a significant problem in hospitals and, in particular, on head and neck wards. On admission to the hospital, patients should be checked for carrier status and if they are positive, should be treated prophylactically during surgery with vancomycin. Any persistent and atypical wound infections should be regarded as suspicious and this organism looked for and, in the presence of established infection, the patient should be nursed in isolation and treated conventionally along with specific intravenous antibiotics (to include vancomycin) which attack this organism.

Carotid artery rupture

Rupture of one of the major blood vessels of the neck is usually the culmination of several complications: the skin wound breaks down, usually because an improper incision has been used in an irradiated patient (a vertical component and a three-point junction are often the culprits); infection supervenes, particularly if the patient is in a poor metabolic state and has an infected mouth to begin with; the carotid arteries are then exposed and gangrene of their walls occurs because infection leads to thrombosis of the vasa vasorum. Finally, the artery ruptures and the patient often dies, or at best survives with a hemiplegia.

This disaster can be prevented by attention to all of the points of preparation and operative technique (Chapters 2 and 4). In particular, the carotid arteries in all patients at risk (i.e. those who have been irradiated) may be protected by a muscle graft. One must not deprive the arteries of the vasa vasorum, derived from the branches of the thyrocervical trunk, and the adventitia of the carotid sheath should not be stripped during neck dissection unless absolutely necessary.

Despite all precautions, some wounds break down and some patients develop fistulae so that the carotid sheath is exposed from without or within. Rupture virtually never occurs unheralded; in the 48 h before rupture there is always a small prodromal bleed and this must be respected. The airway is protected with a cuffed tracheostomy tube, a drip is set up and 4 units (approximately

Table 6.4 Clinical assessment of flap circulation

Clinical parameter	Normal circulation	Venous occlusion	Arterial occlusion
Colour	Pink	Blue/purple hue cyanotic	Pale, mottled blue
Capillary refill time	1–2 s	Increased, fast <1 s	Decreased, slow >2 s
Temperature	Warm	Warm–cold	Cooler
Tissue turgor	Full	Distended, swollen, tense	Hollow, 'prune-like'
Dermal bleeding (on doctor's orders)	Bright red blood	Blood changes from dark red or bluish hue to eventually pink. Bleeds briskly. Bleeds for a long time (artery is throbbing to push blood past venous occlusion)	Minimal bleed to absence of blood. Only serum = dead tissue.

2 litres) of blood are cross-matched. All dead tissue is excised and keep the artery covered by frequent moist soaks.

All personnel must be warned that massive rupture may occur and instructed as follows: control bleeding with immediate finger pressure, secure the airway by inflating the cuff on the tracheostomy tube, and give blood immediately.

The patient is taken to theatre; if possible, blood volume should be restored before anaesthesia is induced. It might be necessary to remind the anaesthetist to keep the head down, the blood pressure up and the arterial carbon dioxide tension normal, as carbon dioxide retention predisposes to decreased cerebral blood flow. Then each end of the carotid artery is isolated under a healthy piece of skin and tissue, and tied off with a transfixion stitch. If an attempt is made to repair it or tie it off in the middle of any infected area – it will blow again the next week.

At least one-third of patients on whom this tragedy falls will die; of those who survive, half will have a hemiplegia.

Flap failure

All flaps performed in the head and neck should be monitored postoperatively (see Chapter 7). Local flaps should be observed in the immediate postoperative period. One can often push a local flap within the head and neck to its limits and there is very rarely a problem, so it should be remembered that 'white flaps on the face and neck are safe flaps – they become pink'. If a local flap becomes blue and congested, the pedicle and base may well be under tension and some sutures may have to be removed to reduce this.

Pedicled flaps, e.g. pectoralis major and latissimus dorsi, should again be observed in the postoperative period. There is often no problem with these and since the microcirculation of many of these flaps undergoes significant changes in the first 24 h, their colour may vary from white through to a congested mottled colour. They should be left well alone unless obviously under severe vascular embarrassment, and most will settle down. Very few of these flaps fail completely and, if there is loss of the skin paddle, this can often débrided and the underlying muscle allowed to heal by secondary intention.

In the case of free tissue transfer, any flap needs to be monitored very carefully in the first 48 h following surgery when many of the major complications will occur. This is because problems need to be recognized immediately so that the patient can be returned to surgery for salvage. The patient should be checked so that there is no evidence of wound haematoma or infection and the flap monitored with a chart (Chapter 7). The flap needs to be checked for its colour, temperature, the presence or absence of capillary refill and its texture. The parameters listed in Table 6.4 may be helpful.

In the presence of arterial occlusion, flaps will become pale, the capillary refill time will be decreased and tissue turgor is reduced. On pin-prick there is no bleeding. In contrast, outflow venous occlusion results in a congested blue/purple cyanosed flap with increased capillary refill time and increased temperature. A pin-prick test produces dark blue blood. The presence of either arterial or venous occlusion suggests that the flap is under threat and the patient should be returned to theatre immediately for inspection of the anastomosis and revision as appropriate. In some cases where there is venous congestion but no occlusion, the use of leeches should be considered.

Methods of flap monitoring

- Direct inspection in the presence or absence of dermal bleeding
- Flexible endoscopy
- Jejunal skin pedicle
- Serial photography

Fistula

An orocutaneous or pharyngocutaneous fistula can occur after any operation on the oral cavity, pharynx or larynx to remove a tumour. There are three aspects of such a fistula that need to be considered: prevention, management in the immediate postoperative period and treatment of an established fistula.

Prevention of fistula formation

The most important causative factors are previous radiotherapy and inadequate control of nutritional status, diabetes and anaemia in the preoperative period, poor operative technique, including a poorly made suture line, and allowing a seroma, haematoma or abscess to proceed untreated or altered nutritional factors (e.g. anaemia or hypoalbuminaemia) to go uncorrected postoperatively.

Early management of a fistula

A fistula may form because a suture line gives way or because tissue becomes necrotic. With suture failure there is no loss of tissue as there is with necrosis. A fistula on a suture line almost always closes spontaneously, particularly if the patient has not previously been irradiated. All that is required, therefore, is to prevent epithelium forming along the edges of the tract and to keep the fistula covered and packed with a dressing such as Sorbisan to promote healing by secondary intention. Where further surgery is planned, the fistula can be kept clean by packing with ribbon gauge covered with Metronidazole jelly (Metrotop). Any dressing must be anchored externally to avoid it disappearing into the upper aerodigestive tract. In the presence of excessive saliva, it may be necessary to apply a suction catheter to remove this and there are now custom-made tracheostomy tubes available with specially designed suction points above comfortable foam cuffs for long-term inflation. However, in some cases where the fistula is associated with exposed vessels or is in continuity with the stoma causing chronic aspiration, then early planned repair is advisable.

Loss of tissue occurs in the patient who has been irradiated; if not too much tissue has been lost, the fistula may close spontaneously but before it can begin to do so all dead tissue must be cut away to allow healing to begin. A long time is often needed to control local infection and at least 8 weeks should be allowed for a fistula to close spontaneously. In some instances, local availability permitting, healing rates can be improved by using hyperbaric oxygen. If the fistula at that time is stable and established, it is often necessary to close it surgically.

> Established fistulae must be closed in such a way as to provide a lining both on the inside of the mouth or pharynx and on the outside

Technique of closure of an established fistula

In closing an established fistula, several important factors need to be noted. Closure needs to be obtained both internally and externally and the gap filled in between with vascularized tissue. Because of this, one normally requires a flap with bulk and the technique will now be described to close the most common type of fistula which often occurs in head and neck surgery, which is the neopharyngocutaneous fistula which follows total laryngectomy. This often occurs after previous radiotherapy and results in loss of most of the anterior wall of the pharynx and the overlying neck skin. This method could be used for any large hole which has resulted following surgery on the oral cavity, oropharynx or hypopharynx.

While free tissue transfer may have a role to play in closing established fistulae, there is often infection present and the donor vessels may lie in the infected area and have often been irradiated. Moreover, in some patients the fistula has occurred because a free flap has failed.

One of the most reliable ways of closing the established fistula described above is therefore to use a pedicled myocutaneous pectoralis major or latissimus dorsi flap. These techniques are quick and reliable, and the latissimus dorsi is particularly useful because it does not violate the breast area in a female.

The flap is designed as described in Chapter 7. The skin paddle is outlined to close the fistula and the paddle of muscle designed in a different plane to close the soft-tissue defect because often this is at a different angle to the pharyngeal fistula.

The flap is delivered into the neck and turned upon itself, avoiding any tension; to achieve this it may be necessary to island the flap vessels on the remaining muscle by dividing the musculotendinous pedicle. The edges of the fistula are mobilized, freshened and separated from the trachea. The skin paddle is sewn to the fistula edge using Vicryl or polydioxanone sutures (PDS) (Fig. 6.2)

It is wise to use some blanket sutures at this point to increase stability and promote healing. The muscle is then sewn around the edge of the cutaneous part of the fistula (Fig. 6.3) using absorbable sutures such as Vicryl and covered with a split skin graft. This is best taken at the time of surgery but laid on the following day using the technique of delayed open grafting (Fig. 6.4).

In cases where the flaps are not visible, they may be inspected via the nasopharyngoscope, e.g. free jejunum or radial free forearm for pharyngeal repair. Alternatively, with free jejunal transfer, some surgeons favour isolating a separate pedicle of jejunum and sewing it to the outside skin wound to allow inspection. This technique is not widely used because false positives and false negatives can occur. The best way to monitor a free flap is with clinical assessment and dermal bleeding by instruction. The experience of the nurse performing the observations is crucial and consistent handover is also important. Photographs may help to monitor sequential change and should be taken immediately postoperatively and thereafter as required.

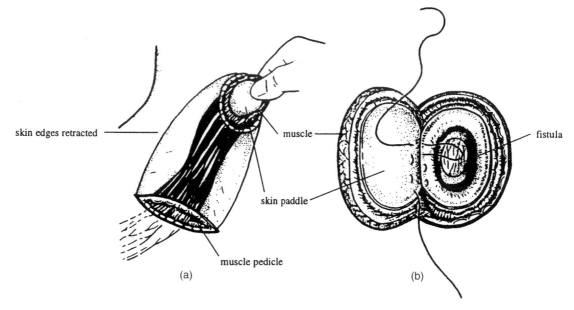

skin edges retracted

muscle

fistula

skin paddle

muscle pedicle

(a)

(b)

Figure 6.2 (a) Latissimus dorsi flap brought through supraclavicular tunnel with the myocutaneous skin paddle facing inwards; (b) suturing of skin paddle to edge of fistula.

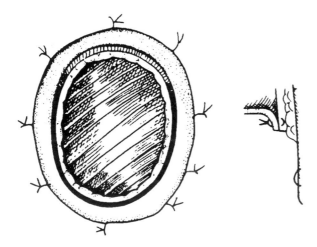

Figure 6.3 Fixation of muscle of flap to the edge of the cutaneous part of the fistula.

Late complications

Late complications can be classified into physical and functional and are outlined below. The functional and psychosocial complications are dealt with in Chapter 5.

Physical complications
▪ Recurrence: primary/nodal/distant
▪ Thyroid/parathyroid failure
▪ Parotid tail hypertrophy
▪ Lymphoedema
▪ Hypertrophic scars

Primary recurrence

If tumour excision was initially complete, subsequent recurrence at the primary site should be uncommon; however, when it does occur it is often incurable and untreatable. There are sometimes occasions when a recurrence at the primary site may be treatable either by radiotherapy or by resection, extensive reconstruction and postoperative radiotherapy as appropriate.

The cure rate for this sort of salvage surgery is below 10% and so careful consideration needs to be given to what one is offering the patients with regard to palliation, cure and quality of life before embarking on such an enormous resection.

Because recurrence at either the primary site or the cervical lymph nodes is most common within the first 2 years following initial treatment, intensive follow-up is mandatory during this time.

Lymph-gland metastases

Following treatment, some patients with head and neck cancer may later develop lymph-node metastases either in the midline or in the contralateral neck. This is particularly common in those suffering from carcinomas of epithelial sites with bilateral lymphatic drainage such as the aryepiglottic fold, the epiglottis, the hypopharynx and the tongue base. When this situation arises, these patients should usually be treated by further radical surgery. However, as the ipsilateral neck has often been previously dissected, these patients are at increased risk of raised intracranial pressure and facial oedema which may cause respiratory obstruction similar to that in patients undergoing bilateral neck dissection. In view of

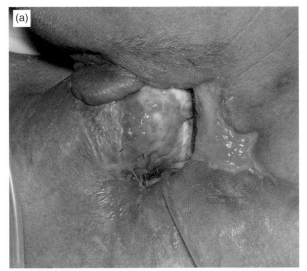

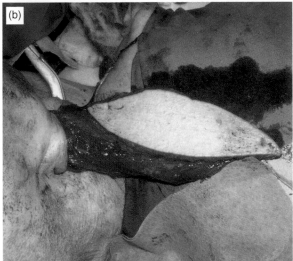

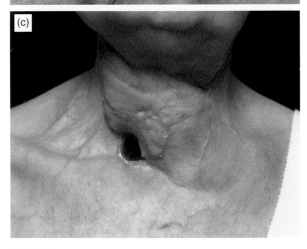

Figure 6.4 Final result following repair of a pharyngo-cutaneous fistula (a) following salvage laryngectomy and partial pharyngectomy after radiotherapy for carcinoma of the larynx. A pedicled latissimus dorsi flap was used (b) with a delayed skin graft on the muscle pedicle. The final result is shown in (c).

this, a temporary tracheostomy is usually mandatory in the immediate postoperative period. The risk of these complications is reduced by the use of conservation neck surgery.

Occasionally, small, infiltrating lymph nodes occur following radical neck dissection, especially in some of 'the corners of consternation' at the lower part of the posterior triangle, under the trapezius, the root of the neck and the skull base. These should be treated by local excision and postoperative radiotherapy if possible, but they usually carry a gloomy prognosis.

Recurrence in the ipsilateral neck is often deep seated, and because of this often is associated with attachment to vital structures such as the brachial plexus and the common carotid artery. Such a situation is usually not salvageable so before heroic surgery is undertaken, careful assessment is mandatory to avoid embarking on the impossible.

The place of chemotherapy and radiotherapy in palliation in these situations is discussed in Chapter 5.

Distant metastases

Distant metastases in sites such as lung, liver and bone should be assessed clinically at each postoperative visit and the patient asked about any significant symptoms. The lungs are also the most common source of second primary tumours outside the upper aerodigestive tract. A chest X-ray may be performed once a year.

Failure of the thyroid and parathyroid glands

As part of laryngectomy and pharyngolaryngectomy, the thyroid and parathyroid glands may be resected on one or both sides of the neck. Furthermore, subsequent fibrosis on the contralateral side may develop so that the blood supply to the remaining thyroid and parathyroid glands may be compromised and, in particular, parathyroid failure may occur. Postoperative radiotherapy is a further cause of late failure of these glands.

The development of hypothyroidism is often slow and insidious, but is usually avoided following total thyroidectomy because the patients are immediately put on thyroxine. When patients have undergone partial thyroidectomy, it is important to check their thyroid function every 6 months to detect subclinical hypothyroidism. In this situation, a persistently raised thyroid-stimulated hormone (TSH) level (>10 mU/l) in the presence of a normal T_4 6 months following surgery should be treated with replacement therapy (100–150 mg of thyroxine is the usual dose). Hypoparathyroidism may begin immediately after the surgery when all parathyroid glands have been resected and the symptoms of hypocalcaemia are usually obvious (see below). Slow insidious failure of the parathyroids is more difficult to detect but it is important to ask patients about intermittent peripheral numbness and tingling.

All patients undergoing major head and neck surgery which involves resection of part or all of the thyroid gland should have their calcium checked on the first post-operative day. Usually there is no problem with the calcium in patients who have had a lobectomy or near-total thyroidectomy and, even if the calcium does fall, it inevitably returns to normal very soon afterwards. If it does not, the patient should be treated with calcium supplements (see below).

Patients who are at greatest risk of suffering post-operative hypocalcaemia are those who have undergone a total thyroidectomy either as a lone procedure or as part of a pharyngolaryngectomy. Even in this situation, it is often surprising how many patients following what is presumed resection of all parathyroids are able to maintain a normal blood calcium level postoperatively. This is presumably because ectopic parathyroid tissue is left behind in the neck or mediastinum. All attempts should be made at the time of surgery to preserve the parathyroid glands but this should only be done within the limits of oncological safety.

Hypocalcaemic patients who are assumed to have no effective parathyroid function owing to damage or removal of the parathyroids will be resistant to the effects of vitamin D. Hence, oral calcium will not be effective in combating their hypocalcaemia. The total serum calcium and albumin should be checked on the first post-operative day and daily thereafter. There is no need to check it before or replace calcium as the remaining circulating parathormone will be adequate. The patient should be monitored daily for symptoms of hypo-calcaemia, i.e. circumoral tingling, paraesthesia and Chvostek's sign. If the patient becomes symptomatic (confirmed on serum calcium measurement) then intra-venous calcium replacement should be instigated (10 ml 10% calcium gluconate given slowly IV over 5–10 min) until symptoms subside and vitamin D replacement should be commenced. If the patient's corrected calcium falls below 1.8 mmol/l this places them in potential danger of fitting secondary to low calcium (even if they are asymptomatic) and they should be given an infusion of calcium gluconate and commenced on vitamin D replacement [1α-hydroxycholecalciferol (alfacalcidiol) 2 μg daily]. This is activated in the liver to 1,25-dihy-drocholecalciferol. This increases serum calcium by increasing gut uptake and reabsorption from the kidney. An alternative to vitamin D is the newer preparation of Calcichew D3, which contains both 1α-hydroxycholecalciferol and calcium. Once the patient is stabilized on oral alphacalcidol or Calcichew D3, then the calcium should be checked weekly as the dose may need reducing since patients can become hyper-calcaemic. On replacement therapy the aim is to keep the total corrected serum calcium level between 2 and 2.3 mm/l and the dose of replacement therapy should be reduced if the corrected serum calcium is above 2.5 mm/l. Usually it is possible to wean patients off treatment as parathyroid function returns so that only a small proportion of patients having total thyroidectomy (less than 5%) have permanent hypoparathyroidism.

Parotid gland tail hypertrophy

In a small proportion of patients after radical neck dissection there may appear, after a few weeks, a swelling at the amputated tail of the parotid gland. This resembles a recurrent cancer and, naturally, causes a lot of worry both to the patient and the surgeon. It should be recognized as a reasonably common complication and the patient should be reassured. Fine-needle aspiration cytology provides further reassurance to both patient and surgeon that all is well. Unless there is an obvious localized hard swelling indicating a recurrence, surgery should not be performed on the tail of the gland because further hypertrophy will merely occur higher up. Its importance lies in recognizing it and doing nothing about it apart from reassuring the patient.

Lymphoedema

When both internal jugular veins are tied, lymphoedema often follows, owing to interruption of the lymphatic drainage channels from the head, especially those in the lateral aspect of the neck. Lymphoedema is particularly marked when neck dissection is combined with excision of a midline structure such as the larynx or pharynx. If all steps are taken to minimize oedema, such as forgoing dressings, sitting the patient upright, treatment with steroids and using mannitol, it often subsides within a month. If it becomes established the patient can have a grotesquely oedematous head for a long time after surgery. The condition is untreatable. Lymphoedema may also follow splitting of the lip to gain access to the mouth or an incision under the eyelid during maxillectomy.

Hypertrophic scars

Following neck dissection using the utility or Schobinger incision, a band-like formation in the lower limb of the scar with hypertrophy leads to contracture which patients often complain about as it limits neck movement. This may be due, in part, to contracture of the platysma muscle.

In the small group of patients who complain, this problem may be easily dealt with by excision and Z-plasty repair to achieve good cosmetic results, even in those patients who have had previous radiotherapy where the scar overlies the common carotid artery.

Acquired immunodeficiency syndrome

Acquired immunodeficiency syndrome (AIDS) and human immunodeficiency virus (HIV) are of considerable importance to the head and neck surgeon for several reasons. First, several clinical forms of AIDS and AIDS-related diseases regularly present in the head and neck. For example, in one series of 150 AIDS patients attending a San Francisco oral medicine clinic, 80% had Kaposi's sarcoma (53 with oral involvement), seven had oral squamous cell carcinoma, three had oral non-

Hodgkin's lymphoma and candidiasis was almost universal. These clinical aspects are discussed in Chapters 11 and 25. Secondly, the allied immunodeficiency may compromise the host response to surgical trauma. Finally, as in any surgical procedure, there is a risk of cross-contamination of the surgeon and also the patient. Percutaneous injuries which could result in cross-infection occur in 2–15% of surgical procedures, although higher rates of cross-infection with HIV or hepatitis B occur with conjunctival rather than stick injury.

Analysis of the nucleotide sequence of HIV provirus from an infected dentist in 1991 showed an unusual degree of similarity with specimens obtained from five of his patients and this was probably the first reported case of a health-care worker infecting his patients. Some argue for the testing of patients suspected of being at high risk and, by inference, of the medical, dental and allied professions. Others advocate a policy of universal and anti-infective precautions for all workers and all patients: heterosexual contact is the only exposure category in 10% of AIDS cases in the UK. Moreover, surgeons' awareness of patients' seropositivity or high-risk status does not appear to affect their exposure to blood or body fluids.

The positive measures which can be taken to reduce the risk of cross-infection include universal vaccination of medical personnel against hepatitis B, which is much more readily acquired from a carrier following percutaneous injury (6–30% incidence of seroconversion) than HIV (0–4% seroconversion). In one USA series, 60% of HIV carriers were also hepatitis B positive. It is important to be aware of any breaches in integrity of the hand skin, and always to avoid cutaneous contact with blood or saliva, not only in the operating theatre, but also in the clinic, where the wearing of gloves for indirect or flexible laryngoscopy is recommended. Intraoperative precautions include the use of goggles for conjunctival protection by all scrubbed theatre personnel and a face visor during heavily contaminating procedures (e.g. the use of drills or saws). A safe technique should be developed for the exchange of sharp instruments among operating theatre personnel and a no-touch method of inserting sutures used later.

Complications of radiotherapy

The fact that radiotherapy can cause side-effects has already been mentioned in Chapter 5, where it was stated that the therapeutic ratio between the dose required to cure squamous cancer and the dose at which unacceptable morbidity occurs is small. In this section, the complications of radiotherapy and their management are discussed in more detail. In general, side-effects can be divided into **acute** effects which occur during or immediately after a course of treatment, and **late** effects, which may come on in the subsequent months or years. Acute effects, although they may be severe and consequently dose limiting, usually settle spontaneously after treatment.

Late effects, however, are usually permanent and may be gradually progressive.

Complications of radiotherapy

- Acute effects
  - Occur during or immediately after treatment
  - Usually settle spontaneously
- Late effects
  - Occur months or years after treatment
  - May be progressive and irreversible

Acute side-effects of radiotherapy

The most commonly seen acute complications of radiotherapy for head and neck cancer are on the skin and mucosa.

Skin reaction

Cutaneous erythema develops in the irradiated area after 2–3 weeks of conventionally fractionated radiotherapy, and may progress to peeling of the skin or dry desquamation. If the skin receives the full dose, blistering or moist desquamation will ensue, but the skin-sparing quality of megavoltage radiation makes this uncommon unless the dose to the skin surface is enhanced by natural or artificial build-up material such as the pinna, the treatment shell or added bolus. The acute reaction usually settles over 2–4 weeks. Hyperpigmentation, like suntan, may develop in the treated area. This is more common in dark-skinned people. Hair loss will occur in the treated area after about 3 weeks of treatment. At doses of up to about 50 Gy this is temporary, with hair regrowth starting about 3 months after the end of treatment. At higher doses, permanent alopecia may result. To diminish the severity of the skin reaction, patients are advised to avoid the use of soaps and cosmetics in the treated area and to wash with warm water only. Wet shaving is not advised, although use of electric razors is permitted. For cutaneous erythema, which may be itchy, the use of aqueous cream or E45 cream twice daily may be soothing. Hydrocortisone cream is often used, but there is no evidence to show that the use of topical steroids limits either the severity or the duration of the reaction. Areas of moist desquamation should be kept clean and free from abrasion. Dressings such as 'second skin' or 'intrasite gel' may be helpful. Secondary infection may occur over areas of moist desquamation, but the use of topical antibiotics is not recommended. Gentian violet lotion was once effective and popular in this setting, but its use has fallen out of favour.

Mucosal reaction

The mucosa undergoes a series of changes similar to skin when irradiated. In the first place erythema occurs, then a fibrinous exudate may form. The exudate at first is not uniform and the appearance is described as a patchy membranous reaction. Subsequently, it may involve the whole of the treated area and forms a confluent membranous reaction. The mucosal surfaces are also prone to develop *Candida*, and this can resemble a membranous radiation reaction. The difference is that patches of *Candida* are easily rubbed away with a tongue depressor, whereas fibrous membrane is not easily displaced.

In the oral cavity xerostomia, due to loss of function of irradiated salivary gland tissue, can make the acute mucosal reaction more unpleasant for the patient. Chewing and swallowing become both painful and difficult. The sense of taste is altered and virtually all foods may become unpalatable. If large volumes of mucosa, especially in the pharynx, are affected the patient may no longer be able to take solid food and have to move on to a diet of soft food, purées and oral nutritional supplements. Patient should be weighed weekly during treatment and input from a dietician before nutrition is compromised is essential. Previously, it was common practice to rest patients midway through treatment to allow the acute mucosal reaction to settle. It is now recognized that this adversely affects outcome in squamous cancer. The likelihood of cure falls by 0.5% for each day that the overall treatment time is prolonged, so a 2-week break may reduce the chances of success by 5–7%. Nowadays, the majority of patients having wide-field treatment for head and neck cancer should have a percutaneous gastrostomy fitted prior to the start of radiotherapy to enable treatment to proceed without delays. Adequate analgesia is essential. In the early stages compound analgesics such as coproxamol are often sufficient, but not infrequently oral morphine may be required as the reaction progresses.

In the larynx, mucositis can lead to hoarseness if that was not already a feature. Sometimes the oedema associated with an acute mucosal reaction may prejudice an airway already narrowed by tumour. The current practice of laser debulking of large laryngeal tumours prior to radiotherapy makes this less common. Nonetheless, as it remains possible, the airway should be carefully monitored throughout treatment as a tracheostomy is sometimes called for.

Late effects of radiotherapy

Although the division of the complications of radiotherapy into early and late effects is simple and convenient, sometimes the two are interrelated. For example, even when apparently complete recovery from acute effects has taken place, the stem cell pool of rapidly dividing tissues is often depleted. This may mean that the tissue in question is prone to subsequent damage by relatively trivial insults. For example, a biopsy of soft tissue in a previously irradiated area can lead to an area of localized necrosis which may not readily heal.

Dental and bone effects

Another example of the interrelationship of acute and late effects concerns the domino effect of xerostomia on the teeth and mandible. One of the principal functions of saliva is dental protection, and rapid caries can result from radiotherapy-induced xerostomia unless meticulous attention is paid to dentition and to oral hygiene. For this reason, most patients who are not already edentulous prior to radiotherapy should be assessed by a restorative dentist who should either repair initially carious teeth or perform a dental clearance if conservative treatment is not possible. In the radical treatment of oral and pharyngeal tumours it is often impossible to avoid incidental irradiation of a substantial proportion of most of, if not all of the salivary glands. These glands are exceptionally sensitive to irradiation, and relative if not absolute dryness of the mouth comes about during treatment and so must be classed as an early effect. It is usually persistent, however, and substantial improvement is unusual. When dental extractions become necessary after radiotherapy, problems can arise. Even the trauma of simple dental extraction to the irradiated mandible can give rise to osteoradionecrosis which can be difficult to treat and will take a long time to heal, and sometimes may never heal at all.

With modern megavoltage radiotherapy, where the absorption of radiation is no greater in bone than in other tissue, spontaneous osteoradionecrosis is much less common than it was in the days when low-voltage treatments, with differential absorption in bone and calcified cartilage, were the main type of radiotherapy available. None the less, trauma and infection can initiate osteoradionecrosis in previously irradiated bone. Similarly, laryngeal cartilage necrosis is rare nowadays. This is also because surgery is the preferred treatment for advanced laryngeal cancer. However, where residual or recurrent tumour, or even a deep biopsy of an oedematous larynx, opens up a pathway for infection, necrosis may ensue.

Skin and soft-tissue effects

The late effects of radiotherapy on skin and mucosa include telangiectasia, atrophy, hypopigmentation and fibrosis. Apart from the cosmetic changes, the disrupted vasculature in the skin may lead to problems with wound healing if subsequent surgery is required. This can be helped by the use of vascularized flaps to repair the defects resulting from salvage surgery.

Neurological effects

It is sometimes difficult to irradiate a head and neck tumour adequately without also irradiating part of the brain or spinal cord. Symptomatic brain necrosis is, however, very rare and should be avoided by careful treatment planning. Sometimes, for example in the retreatment of a recurrent nasopharyngeal carcinoma when there are no alternatives, the oncologist will knowingly exceed recognized levels of tolerance, accepting that there may be a substantial risk of normal tissue damage. The optic chiasm is a radiosensitive structure and great care has to be taken in the treatment of tumours in this area to avoid the administration of an excessive dose.

The spinal cord is also recognized to be a sensitive structure. L'Hermitte's syndrome is characterized by shooting pains down the arms and legs on neck flexion. It is an uncommon symptom caused by demyelination in the cervical spinal cord which may occur about 12 weeks after radiotherapy to the neck. Recovery occurs spontaneously and the occurrence of L'Hermitte's syndrome does not herald permanent cord damage. With careful planning and dosimetry, permanent cervical myelopathy should be encountered in fewer than 0.5% of patients treated with radiotherapy for head and neck cancer.

Hypothyroidism

Hypothyroidism can develop years after radiotherapy to the neck in up to 25% of patients treated. The likelihood is greater if there has also been some surgical intervention which has removed part of the thyroid gland. It is wise to check thyroid function routinely in patients at risk. Thyroid hormone replacement therapy should be started if the TSH level is elevated, even if the free thyroxine level is normal, as compensated hypothyroidism can easily lead on to overt myxoedema.

Visual problems

The eyesight can be affected by radiotherapy in a number of ways. The risk to the visual pathways behind the eye (the optic nerves and chiasm) has already been mentioned. The retina can also be damaged by radiotherapy, but it is a relatively radioresistant structure and problems are unusual. The cornea and conjunctiva are normally protected by a film of tears. The lacrimal glands are sensitive to irradiation, although to a lesser extent than the salivary glands, and care should be taken to shield them from the radiotherapy field if at all possible. Dry eyes are not only unpleasant, but can lead to corneal ulceration and thence to blindness. The lens of the eye is one of the most radiosensitive structures in the human body and cataracts can result from doses as low as 6 Gy. Care should therefore be taken to minimize the dose to the eye, but if it is inevitable that the dose to the eye is such that cataracts may result, the patient should be warned during the consenting discussion. If cataracts occur this is not a disaster as they can be dealt with surgically. It is far better for a patient to end up with cataracts than to die because tumour has been shielded in a misguided attempt to protect the eye. In radiotherapy, as in surgery, there is sometimes a trade-off between the likelihood of cure and the possibility of severe treatment-related problems. Loss of vision is unlikely to be the price of cure of head and neck cancer with radiotherapy, but exceptionally it is necessary to make the decision to sacrifice an eye in the treatment of sinonasal tumours invading the orbit.

Complications of chemotherapy

All chemotherapeutic drugs are toxic to both normal and malignant cells. For successful treatment, the effect on cancer cells needs to be greater than on normal cells. There is some generic toxicity, common to most cytotoxic agents. This is usually due to damage to the stem-cell pool of a tissue which is turning over rapidly, such as the bone marrow or the gut mucosa. Some drugs have unique toxicities. The dose of an individual drug, or of a combination, which can safely be given is limited by its toxic effects. Before prescribing chemotherapy, or even talking about it to a patient, the doctor needs to know about these side-effects and what measures can be undertaken to minimize them.

Acute side-effects of chemotherapy

- Neutropenia and infection
- Thrombocytopenia
- Nausea and vomiting
- Alopecia
- Diarrhoea
- Soft-tissue necrosis with extravasation

Myelosuppression

Almost all cytotoxic drugs have an effect on the bone marrow and can cause anaemia, leucopenia and thrombocytopenia. In general, leucopenia, especially neutropenia, is most important. This is partly because it is more common, and partly because it can be life-threatening. Patients who are likely to become neutropenic as a result of chemotherapy should be warned that they must seek medical attention immediately if they become unwell, especially with pyrexia, around the time of the anticipated haematological nadir, which is usually 10–14 days after chemotherapy. An elective nadir blood count is helpful. A fever or flu-like symptoms can herald the development of neutropenic sepsis which, if untreated, can rapidly prove fatal. Patients need, at the least, an urgent blood count and if neutropenia is confirmed then hospital admission for further investigation and intravenous antibiotics are mandatory.

Patients who are repeatedly neutropenic after each cycle of chemotherapy should be considered for a dose reduction, or possibly for support with growth factors such as granulocyte-macrophage-colony stimulating factor (GM-CSF).

Patients who become thrombocytopenic will need platelet transfusion. In the absence of bleeding, or complicating factors such as sepsis or invasive procedures, the platelet count can usually be allowed to fall as low as 10×10^9/l before prophylactic platelet transfusion is required. Some drugs such as carboplatin seem to have a more profound effect on the platelets than on other blood components.

Anaemia is not a common problem with chemotherapy, although some drugs, such as cisplatin, seem to have a disproportionately greater effect on red cells than on other blood components. Many patients may have concurrent factors which make them anaemic. If anaemia occurs, transfusion of packed red cells is a simple remedy.

Myelosuppression can be dose limiting and this may be one reason why responsive tumours are not always cured by chemotherapy. The cure rate might be improved if higher doses of chemotherapy could be given safely. One way of achieving this is to harvest some of the patient's haemopoietic progenitor cells prior to the administration of high-dose (myeloablative) chemotherapy and reinfuse them afterwards. The use of autologous bone marrow has now been superseded to a large extent by the use of circulating haemopoietic stem cells from the peripheral blood. The patient is primed with either GM-CSF alone or GM-CSF in combination with a cytotoxic agent such as cyclophosphamide, which causes haemopoietic stem cells to leave the bone marrow and enter the peripheral circulation. The peripheral blood stem cells (PBSC) are then harvested by leucopheresis and stored. Following high-dose chemotherapy and PBSC reinfusion, the patient is likely to be profoundly myelosuppressed requiring in-patient supportive care for at least 3 weeks before reconstitution occurs. High-dose chemotherapy and PBSC autografting are now firmly established as a successful treatment for some patients with high-grade non-Hodgkin's lymphoma and Hodgkin's disease. This treatment is being evaluated experimentally in some common tumours such as breast cancer.

Gastrointestinal toxicity

The management of nausea and vomiting, formerly among the most feared side-effects of chemotherapy, has been revolutionized in recent years with the introduction of new and powerful antiemetics such as ondansetron and granesetron which act on the 5-hydroxytryptamine-3 receptor (5-HT-3 antagonists). These are usually given prophylactically in conjunction with dexamethasone before severely emetogenic chemotherapy such as cisplatin. 5-HT-3 antagonists are less good at treating the delayed nausea which sometimes follows chemotherapy. Traditional antiemetics such as metoclopramide can be helpful here and are often sufficient for use with less emetogenic chemotherapy schedules. Premedication with lorazepam can be helpful for some patients who develop severe anticipatory symptoms prior to chemotherapy.

Some drugs, particularly 5-fluorouracil, have an effect on the stem cells in the bowel, leading to diarrhoea. Other drugs seem to have a greater effect on the mucous membranes. Mucositis can be a particular problem with methotrexate. The mucosal toxicities of chemotherapy and radiotherapy can be synergistic.

Extravasation damage

The majority of cytotoxic drugs are given by intravenous injection, although some, such as bleomycin, can be given intramuscularly, and others are occasionally given orally. If, during intravenous administration, the cytotoxic leaks

out into the perivascular soft tissues, local damage can result. At its mildest this may just be pain and erythema at the site of injection, but at the other extreme there may be tissue necrosis which may need a plastic surgical repair procedure. The drugs most likely to cause these problems are the vinca alkaloids and anthracyclines. With care, extravasation should be unusual. If it does occur, damage can often be limited if appropriate action is taken promptly.

Hair loss

Hair loss is common with chemotherapy, although it is not associated with some drugs such as bleomycin and cisplatin. Most head and neck cancer patients are older men for whom hair loss is not a problem. Nonetheless if it is a possible consequence of a proposed treatment schedule, it should be mentioned during the consenting process. Wigs can be ordered in advance of hair loss for patients who require them, as this does not usually occur until about 3 weeks after chemotherapy.

Kidney and urinary tract toxicity

Renal damage can be associated with drugs such as cisplatin, ifosfamide and high-dose methotrexate. Baseline renal function should be assessed by glomerular filtration rate (GFR) estimation. Hydration is necessary to promote rapid renal excretion. As methotrexate can precipitate in renal tubules if the urine is acidic, care must be taken to ensure alkalinization of urine when high-dose methotrexate is used. Knowledge of the renal function is also required to determine the dose of some drugs such as carboplatin which have complex pharmacokinetics and are largely renally excreted. Various types of nephrotoxicity can be produced, and both cisplatin and ifosfamide can cause renal tubular leakage of elements such as magnesium.

Metabolites of ifosfamide and cyclophosphamide are renally excreted and can damage the urothelium, leading to haemorrhagic cystitis. For this reason ifosfamide should always be given with the drug mesna, which protects the urothelium. Mesna is sometimes necessary when cyclophosphamide is used, particularly if at the higher end of the dose range.

Late side-effects of chemotherapy
■ Nephropathy
■ Cardiomyopathy
■ Pulmonary fibrosis
■ Ototoxcity
■ Peripheral neuropathy
■ Infertility
■ Second cancers

Neurotoxicity

Vincristine can lead to a peripheral neuropathy which often manifests as tingling and numbness in the fingers and toes, and loss of reflexes. There may be a slow but often incomplete recovery after treatment. It can cause transient jaw pain and also an autonomic neuropathy with constipation or even ileus. Vincristine should only ever be given intravenously. Inadvertent intrathecal use is fatal.

Cisplatin can also produce peripheral neuropathy and in addition it is ototoxic, producing high-tone deafness. Patients should have a baseline audiogram and undergo regular monitoring throughout treatment.

Cardiotoxicity

The anthracycline drugs such as doxorubicin can produce both acute arrhythmias during administration and potentially fatal cardiomyopathy. This side-effect is related to the cumulative dose. Baseline tests of cardiac function including electrocardiography (ECG) and some measure of ejection fraction (either a multiple-gated arteriography (MUGA) scan or an echocardiogram) are sensible precautions and are mandatory if there is a history of pre-existing cardiac disease. A cumulative dose of $450 \, mg/m^2$ should not usually be exceeded in adults. The safe limits for children are lower than this. Some sparing of cardiotoxicity without impairing the likelihood of disease control may be achieved either by fractionating the dose per course over 2–3 days or by administering the drug as an infusion rather than a bolus. Liposomal formulations are available which may similarly be less cardiotoxic.

Pulmonary toxicity

Alkylating agents, particularly busulphan, may cause pulmonary fibrosis after prolonged use. Bleomycin can cause pulmonary infiltrates which can lead to fibrosis. Although idiosyncratic responses can occur at low doses, the likelihood of occurence is usually dose related, and the cumulative dose should not exceed $300 \, mg/m^2$. Care should be taken in patients with pre-existing lung disease and pulmonary function should be measured both before and during treatment. Overoxygenation during anaesthesia in patients who have received bleomycin previously, especially within recent months, can lead to respiratory failure.

Infertility

Many cytotoxic drugs, especially alkylating agents, can lead to infertility in both men and women. Most patients with head and neck cancer will be too old for or have no wish for further children. The infrequent younger patients must, however, be warned appropriately about the loss of reproductive potential and young men offered the opportunity to store sperm before treatment starts.

Second malignant neoplasms

It is well recognized that patients who have the aetiological lifestyle for head and neck cancer have a propensity to develop second tumours in the head and neck and lung if they survive the first tumour. It is also known that there is a small possibility that radiotherapy may induce a cancer years after treatment, which is one reason for trying to avoid irradiating patients with benign disease where possible. Chemotherapy also has the ability to damage DNA, and chemotherapy-related second malignancies are seen especially in younger patients who have been treated for cancers such as Hodgkin's disease, where there is a high likelihood of cure. Alkylating agents and etoposide are the drugs most often implicated. Leukaemia is one of the more common malignancies after chemotherapy.

References

Arcelus J. I., Candocia S., Traverso C. I., Fabrega F., Caprini J. A. and Hasty J. H. (1991) Venous thromboembolism prophylaxis and risk assessment in medical patients, *Semin Thromb Haemost* 17: 313–18.

Dawes P. J. D. (1997) Thromboembolic prophylaxis and ENT surgery (Editorial), *Clin Otolaryngol* 22: 1–2.

Drugs and Therapeutic Committee UBH NHS Trust, December 1998.

Eisle D., ed. (1992) *Complications in Head and Neck Surgery*, Mosby, St Louis, MO.

Grubb N. R., Bloomfield P. and Ludlam C. A. (1998) The end of the heparin pump? (Editorial), *British Medical Journal* 1540–1542.

Gallimore S. C., Hoile R. W., Ingram G. S. and Sherry K. M. (1997) *The Report of the National Confidential Enquiry into Perioperative Deaths 1994/5.*

Hargreaves S. P. and Watkinson J. C. (1995) Thromboprophylaxis in head and neck surgery (Abstract). *Clin Oncol* 7: 336.

Shaheen O. H. (1984) *Problems in Head and Neck Surgery*, Baillière Tindall, London.

7 Reconstruction

'Thou shalt provide thyself with a lifeboat'
Sir Harold Gillies

Introduction

Defects following head and neck surgery can often be closed by direct suture. This applies to both the skin and mucous membranes. This technique is used when the defect is small, and where local conditions dictate that there is enough lax tissue. However, for larger defects or in situations when direct suture is not applicable, surgical defects may be filled by free grafts, local skin flaps, with pedicled flaps which may be either axial cutaneous or musculocutaneous, or by using free tissue transfer.

Question: When is a hole half a hole?

Answer: There is no such thing as half a hole!

Any surgeon can perform head and neck **destructive** surgery. The test of skill comes in performing head and neck **reconstructive** surgery and the size of a defect should never be underestimated. The care and skill that go into the planning of the reconstruction will usually pay off in terms of long-term functional outcome.

There are some simple rules to head and neck reconstruction. These are well summarized by some of the commandments of Sir Harold Gillies (1968), which relate to reconstruction in general.

Gillies' principles of reconstructive surgery

'Losses must be replaced in kind'
'Treat the primary defect first'
'Thou shalt provide thyself with a lifeboat'
'Thou shalt not throw away a living thing'
'Replace things into their normal position by recreation of the defect'

Reconstructive techniques can be used effectively as building blocks, either singly or in combination to reconstruct the defect. However, before they are described in detail, it is important to understand in general terms how they work. The many and varied clinical situations in which they may be used will be discussed in those chapters that relate to the resection of the specific tumour in question.

Free grafts

A skin graft is something that is potentially dead and its subsequent survival depends on how it is treated, whereas a flap is a graft that remains attached at one or more points by its pedicle which provides an arterial blood supply with venous and lymphatic drainage. It is alive at the time of harvesting and how it is subsequently treated determines whether or not it may live or die.

The following free grafts have been described:

- Split-thickness skin grafts (free skin grafts)
- Full-thickness skin grafts (free skin grafts)
- Composite full-thickness skin and cartilage grafts
- Pinch grafts (free skin grafts)
- Dermal and fat grafts
- Fascial grafts
- Chondromucosal grafts

The first four receive their blood supply from the recipient site; the last three are avascular.

Free skin grafts

Free skin grafts consist of the entire thickness of the epidermis and a variable amount of the dermis. They are designated according to their dermal component, as either whole skin grafts which consist of the entire thickness of the dermis, or split skin grafts which contain all of the epidermis and only part of the dermis. Split skin grafts may be further subdivided into thin, medium or thick according to the amount of dermis harvested. The various constituents of thin, medium and thick skin grafts, and a whole skin graft are shown in Fig. 7.1.

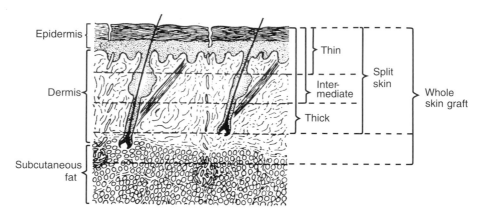

Figure 7.1 Various constituents of thin, medium and thick skin grafts, together with a whole skin graft.

> 'The thinner the graft, the better the take; the thicker the graft, the better the result'.

These different types of skin grafts are not strictly distinct from one another. They really represent reference points on a gradation scale of increasing thickness from a graft which consists of little more than the epidermis through to the whole full-thickness skin graft. The main difference in practice is that a full-thickness skin graft is harvested using a scalpel, whereas a split skin graft is taken with either a dermatome or a Humby knife.

A split skin graft is the most commonly used graft in head and neck cancer surgery. It may be used to cover donor sites or secondary defects, to line flaps, to cover muscle when flap pedicles are exposed or rotated and to replace small areas of skin loss. Thinner grafts take more readily in difficult circumstances, such as inflammation, but thicker grafts give a better cosmetic result in the long term. This is because they contract less. The thinner the graft the better the take, the thicker the graft, the better the result. Therefore, each graft should be cut according to the requirements of the particular situation.

The whole skin graft, once cut, leaves behind no epidermal structures to allow resurfacing in the donor area and therefore must be closed primarily. This limits the size of the graft that can be used in clinical practice. In contrast, the split skin graft leaves adnexal remnants of pilosebaceous follicles or sweat gland apparatus which act as foci from which the donor site can resurface. Because of this, the donor area requires little more care than is usually given to any raw surface and, therefore, much larger areas of a skin graft may be taken.

During its transfer from donor to recipient site, a free skin graft is completely, albeit temporarily, detached from the body and therefore is potentially a dead piece of tissue. Its lifespan while detached depends on the ambient temperature but when wrapped in gauze, moistened in saline and stored in a fridge at 4°C, it may live for up to 3 weeks. To survive permanently, it must be planted, become reattached and obtain a new blood supply from

its new surroundings, and the various processes involved in achieving this are called 'take'.

A skin graft adheres to its new bed by fibrin. This diffuses from the plasma bed and supplies the immediate nutritional requirements in the form of 'plasmatic circulation'. This is enhanced by the outgrowth of capillary buds such that a circulation of blood in the graft can be demonstrated at 48 h. At the same time, fibres grow into the fibrin, which convert the adhesive clot into a more definite fibrous tissue attachment that increases over the ensuing days so that, by 5 days, reasonable anchorage has occurred.

Graft 'take'

- Is by fibrin and capillary budding
- Vascular bed is required
- Good apposition essential
- Well-covered bone is needed
- Bone of palate, maxilla and zygoma. 'Take' can be improved by drilling
- Crane principle can help
- Is threatened by prior radiotherapy
- Can be destroyed by fibrinolysing bacteria

The speed and effectiveness of this process depend on the provision of a non-infected vascular bed, good apposition of the graft to the underlying bed without any intervening haematoma and the application of pressure to allow the process to take place. The graft bed must have a rich blood supply to enable this process to occur.

Surfaces that take a graft well are:

- granulation tissue
- the soft tissues of the face
- muscle fascia and fat cartilage
- bone covered with perichondrium and periosteum

Bare cartilage does not usually take a graft but if the area is small, the surrounding tissues may supply enough blood supply to facilitate a take.

Bare bone is a complex issue. In principle, it does not take a skin graft, e.g. the bare cortical bone of the outer table of the skull and the mandible. However, the bone of the hard palate, maxilla, the walls of the orbit and the zygoma can all take a graft. In addition, if the bone is drilled to expose vascular diploe, this will take a graft or the Crane principle may be applied. This involves using a vascularized flap to cover the bone to promote a vascular bed. The flap is then transferred back to its donor site after 3 or 4 weeks, leaving a new vascular bed which will then take a skin graft. This technique is particularly applicable on the forehead, where a bipedicled scalp flap may be advanced down for a period of 3 or 4 weeks and then transferred back later and skin grafting effected.

When tissue has received previous radiotherapy, it may take a graft less well. As a general rule, previous radiotherapy is not a contraindication to grafting but the tissue in question should be assessed at the time of surgery. Extensive induration and fibrosis with small amounts of bleeding indicate that grafting may not be successful, whereas the converse would suggest that a graft will take. The surgeon should use his or her own assessment and experience to decide which tissues may or may not take a graft following radiotherapy.

The adherence of a graft depends on fibrin anchorage and any surface which is considered suitable for grafting has fibrinogen together with the enzymes which can convert it into fibrin to facilitate adhesion. It is important to realize that some organisms can destroy fibrin and prevent this mechanism taking place, the main one being the β-haemolytic *Streptococcus pyogenes* which produces fibrinolysin. Other organisms that can do this, but to a lesser extent, include *Pseudomonas aeruginosa* and methacillin-resistant *Staphylococcus aureus* (MRSA). The presence of these organisms within the recipient bed requires that the process of grafting be deferred until they are eliminated.

Sites for grafting

Split skin can easily be taken from the thigh, the upper arm and the flat surface of the abdomen (Fig. 7.2). The site is dictated by the size of the graft required, the presence or absence of hair, the desirability of avoiding the leg, thereby increasing postoperative mobility, and access to various donor sites during extensive surgery.

Instruments to take the graft

A considerable amount of training and practice is required to acquire the skill of judging the thickness of a split skin graft properly when using the Humby knife. An alternative technique is to use the electric dermatome. The Humby knife is set depending on the thickness of the graft required but most grafts average around 12/1000 of an inch (0.3 mm).

Arm   Leg and Abdomen

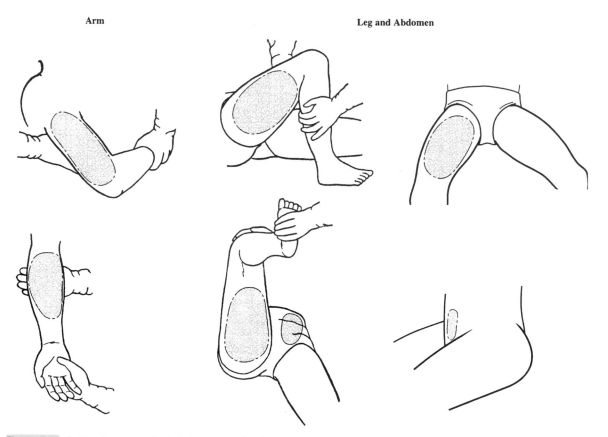

Figure 7.2 Split skin can easily be taken from the thigh, the upper arm and the flat surface of the abdomen.

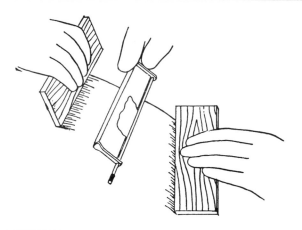

Figure 7.3 Technique of taking a split-skin graft.

Technique of taking the graft (Fig 7.3)

A non-hair bearing area is used, such as the inside of the thigh, and prepared well using either a non-staining disinfectant such as chlorhexidine or, if necessary, povidone iodine.

An assistant holds the limb in such a position that the muscles are relaxed, a hand is placed round the underneath of the leg to tighten the muscle forward, and the skin stretched so that the maximum flat area is available for grafting. The dermatome blade is set to obtain the required thickness of graft. As explained before, most grafts will be of intermediate thickness (0.3 mm). The thickness may be assessed by holding the knife up to the light, a technique which comes with practice. The dermatome blade must be able to move smoothly and not drag on the skin, so that both it and the skin of the leg are lubricated with liquid paraffin. The skin surface is held steady and flat with two boards; the upper board is not lubricated, to maintain its fixation, but the lower board is held at the starting end of the donor site by the operating surgeon, is lubricated, moves down just in front of the dermatome and maintains skin taughtness. Firm pressure is now applied to the dermatome and cutting is achieved with a continuous movement and plenty of side-to-side action. The skin graft is collected on to the blade. When enough skin has been raised, the end of the graft is cut and placed on tulle gras to keep it moist. If there is excessive bleeding from the donor site, swabs soaked in adrenaline or hydrogen peroxide may be applied to reduce this and, when the bleeding has stopped, the wound is dressed using a dressing such as Opsite. Another useful dressing is calcium alginate to which 0.5% Marcaine with adrenaline is applied to reduce postoperative pain and ooze. The area is then covered with gauze dressing, cotton wool and a crêpe bandage, and left covered for 10 days before being removed.

Grafts may also be taken with electric dermatomes which are easier to use and able to provide grafts of predetermined and fixed thickness, but are expensive. Local availability and experience will dictate which method is used.

Application of a graft

The graft may be applied immediately (primary) or as a delayed procedure.

- **primary:** healthy, non-bleeding recipient site
- **delayed:** often exposed, i.e. scalp, forehead, neck
- **pressure:** wool, cotton or foam bolster. Large grafts need peripheral clips or sutures; always use sutures for full-thickness grafts
- **exposed:** good for large, immobile, delayed grafts. Use if excessive bleeding.

Whether the graft is applied immediately or delayed depends upon a number of factors but where the recipient site is healthy, not bleeding excessively and not infected, grafts are usually placed primarily. In this situation, pressure is usually applied, which provides immobility for the graft and holds it in place with the bed until take is effected.

When applying a split skin graft to a recipient site, it is usually laid over the wound and allowed to drape over the edges and then trimmed at the first dressing. It is covered with tulle gras. Various bolus materials may be used to apply pressure, e.g. proflavine wool, cotton wool moistened with saline or liquid paraffin, or foam. Pressure may be maintained by the application of a tie over to the pressure bolster or, in the case of the foam, this may sewn or stapled to the skin. The split skin graft is not usually sewn in place but some form of movement prevention is sometimes helpful and, in this situation, either sutures or staples may be used. Where large areas of graft are used, easily removed absorbable tacking sutures (plain cat gut) may be placed across the area of the graft to keep it in place.

Pressure methods are preferable when a graft is small and should always be used for a full thickness skin graft. They are also preferable where a cavity is being filled or the defect is irregular in contour, such as the orbit or around the ear.

If the area to be grafted is in a suitable position where movement will not be a problem, i.e. the top of the scalp where pressure may be difficult to apply over a curved surface, then the graft may merely be covered with tulle gras until the patient wakes up and then exposed.

The larger and less mobile the area to be grafted, the more likely it is to be suitable for delayed exposed grafting. This is particularly true on the scalp, the forehead and the anterior neck. Where there is excessive bleeding, e.g. the muscle pedicle of a latissimus dorsi flap exposed after repair of a neopharyngeal fistula, the technique of delayed exposed grafting is preferable. The recipient site is covered with tulle gras and moist saline dressings which should be changed every 4 h and moistened with saline in between. At 24–48 h, these may be removed and the stored skin applied to cover the defect.

Secondary skin grafting

This method is used when neck skin has died and the lost skin and underlying tissue must be replaced. In this situation, if there are exposed blood vessels, immediate reconstruction is required with vascularized tissue using either pedicled or free flaps to cover the vessels, since any delay and subsequent infection will lead to a carotid blow-out.

As long as vessels are not exposed, the exposed area is kept clean and moist, is dressed regularly and allowed to granulate, and at the appropriate time may be repaired with a split skin graft. Experience is needed to know when a granulating bed is ready for skin grafting, but the following points are helpful.

Signs of readiness for secondary grafting

- Flat red granulation
- No slough
- Marginal healing
- Débride or clean off necrotic areas first
- Swab for and eradicate bacteria
- Deep wounds may require Sorbisan or Granuflex

The granulations ought to be flat and red and not raised, and should not bleed unduly, although they should exhibit the appropriate vascularity. The area should be totally free of slough and there should be evidence of marginal healing, defined as a thin blue rim growing in at the edge of the defect. It is unwise to promote granulation by the use of caustic agents such as silver nitrate and other 'stimulating' agents. They kill tissue locally and cause more slough, and there is no evidence to show that they improve the speed of granulation. The necrotic area is initially infected, and must be disinfected and regularly dressed and cleaned and not grafted until a healthy bed of granulations has formed, which usually takes at least 2–3 weeks. In this situation, it is wise not to rush in and it is amazing how the body heals with time.

General principles of wound care apply. Granulations that are sloughing, gelatinous or oedematous will not accept a skin graft because they are often infected with *Streptococci* which eat the graft. Swabs should be taken regularly and if *Streptococci* are grown, the appropriate systemic antibiotic (which is usually penicillin based) should be administered until the wound is free of infection. Other organisms that are significant and require treatment include *Pseudomonas* and MRSA and are treated accordingly. Oganisms such as *Escherichia coli* and the *Proteus* group should be regarded as opportunists and not as a contraindication to grafting.

One of the main causes of infection is slough and dead tissue and these should be removed and débrided widely so that the defect may be closed from the bottom up. The wound is dressed daily with ribbon gauze soaked initially with a local antibiotic such as Metronidazole gel but, as the wound becomes clean, saline-soaked dressings are appropriate. These should be changed regularly. For deep, narrow wounds, granulation-promoting preparations such as Sorbison or Granuflex may be useful. Once the area is clean and granulating properly, the defect is covered with stored split skin using delayed exposed grafting.

Oronasal cavity

In areas such as the mouth, and oral and nasal cavity, pressure methods to apply a split skin graft are required.

Bolus grafting

The technique of applying a skin graft draped around a bolus 'sausage' is rarely used nowadays because the bolus rapidly becomes soaked with saliva and secretions and then becomes infected. The best material to use is polyurethane and a larger bolus than originally thought is usually required. In addition, it is particularly difficult to maintain the pressure on certain areas within the oral cavity, such as the lateral tongue border. For defects within the maxillary sinus and nasal cavity, the skin is laid over the recipient site and then the pressure applied with a prosthetic appliance which is fixed into place to maintain the pressure. An alternative reconstructive technique in this situation is to reduce the cavity size using free muscle transfer e.g. rectus abdominus.

At other sites, the newer technique of graft quilting has now superseded bolus pressure methods in the mouth. The graft is lain on the recipient site, then sewn in around the edge and also quilted over the bed to maintain fixation. This works extremely well.

Full-thickness skin grafts

Under ideal conditions, the full-thickness skin graft provides a surprisingly good form of reconstruction and is often the technique of choice for small areas after removal of tumours in areas such as the nasal tip, parts of the pinna and the lower eyelid par excellence. The success for grafting is often not quite as good as that for split skin thickness grafting because the plasmatic circulation takes longer to establish itself and, during this time, factors such as movement, infection and haematoma can delay the take. The other reason is that the number of cut capillary ends exposed when a thick split skin graft or full-thickness skin graft is cut is less than with a thin graft and therefore vascularization is slower. To combat this, the head and neck donor sites have a rich blood supply which allows their vascular characteristics to be compared favourably with split skin grafts. The take is usually much better than for full-thickness grafts taken from non-head and neck sites.

Common head and neck full-thickness skin graft donor sites

- Postauricular
- Preauricular
- Lower neck

A full-thickness skin graft must have a freshly cut vascular bed and therefore it cannot be used on granulating surfaces. It will not take in the presence of infection or haematoma at the recipient site. Moreover, the size of the graft is limited because the donor site will have to be

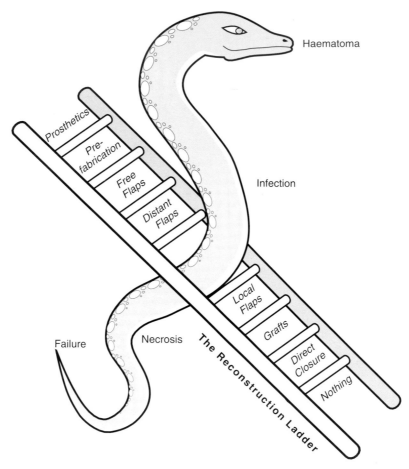

Figure 7.4 Reconstruction ladder.

closed by undermining and primary closure. However, the full-thickness skin graft has several advantages. It is one of the simplest methods of reconstruction, is low on the reconstruction ladder (Fig. 7.4) and therefore leads to fewer complications than with more complicated techniques. It usually provides a good colour match on the face and neck and contracture is minimal (Fig. 7.5). In the presence of failure, which may be partial or complete, subsequent healing by secondary intention may still give a reasonable long-term result. Alternatively, another technique such as a local flap may be used which will provide the appropriate lifeboat and get the surgeon out of trouble.

Within the head and neck, the best donor sites are either the postauricular or preauricular areas. If larger areas of skin are required, the lower neck may be used but the supraclavicular skin does not give as good a colour match and shows up obviously on the face as a graft. Although the postpostauricular and preauricular areas are limited in size, the skin is usually hairless and gives an excellent match to facial skin in colour, appearance and texture. The best way to replace the skin of the face is with the skin of the face.

Advantages of full-thickness skin repair

- Simple
- Low complication rate
- Good colour match
- Minimal contracture
- Lifeboats for failure – healing by secondary intention
  – local flap repair

A full-thickness skin graft should be accurately fitted to the recipient defect (Fig. 7.6) and it is common practice to use a template of the defect to facilitate the taking of the graft. One simple way of doing this is to apply a piece of paper or the back of a suture packet to the recipient site and then cut out the appropriate 'blood tattoo'. The graft is marked out on this template. It is wise to take more than is required because if the graft taken is too small, then a further graft will have to be harvested.

After the graft has been marked out, it is injected with saline and excised, carefully leaving any fat behind. During elevation, the graft may be rolled over the finger and stretched with a skin hook so that the knife dissects on

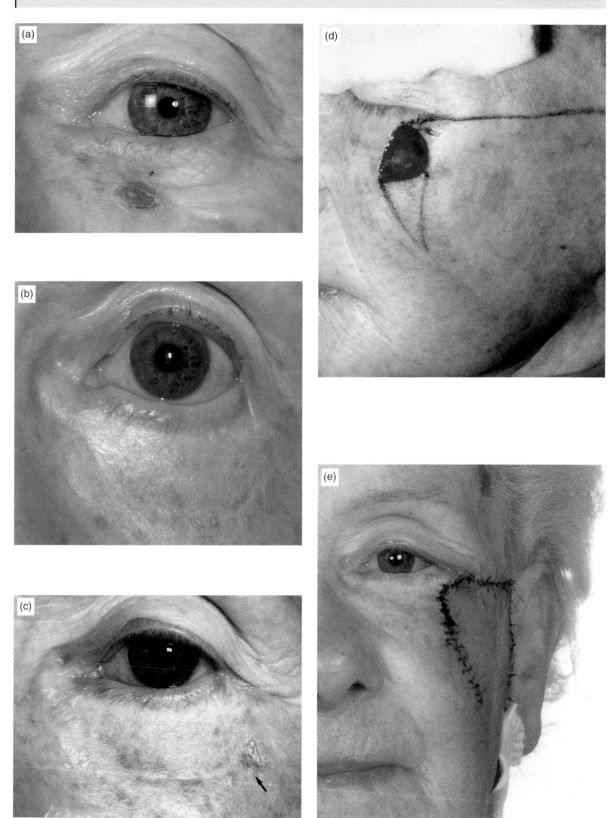

Figure 7.5 (a) Patient with a radiorecurrent basal cell carcinoma on the skin of the lower eyelid. (b) Treatment was with wide excision and repair with a pre-auricular full thickness skin graft. (c) Two years later, a recurrence was noted at the lateral edge of the resection. (d, e)This was widely excised under local anaesthetic and repaired with a simple transposition flap. There was no further recurrence.

Whole skin graft

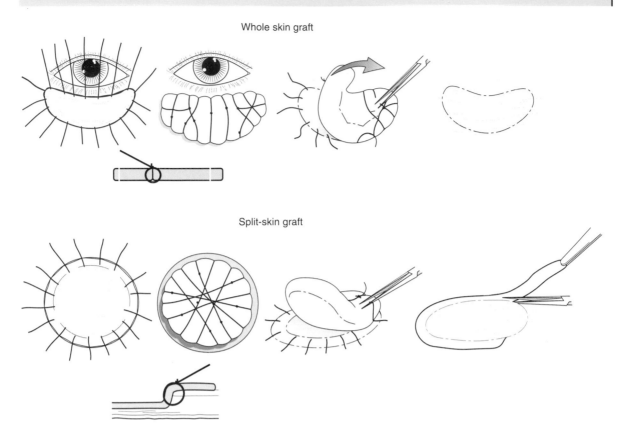

Split-skin graft

Figure 7.6 Technique of full-thickness skin grafting showing the pressure method and the use of a tie-over bolster dressing. Note that with a whole skin graft, the graft edge is sewn to the edge of the defect. When split skin is used, any excess is allowed to over lie the edge of the defect to allow for contracture. This can be trimmed later.

to the underneath of the dermis and hair follicles are seen, and to ensure that no fat is left on the graft. An alternative technique is to take the graft, roll it over the finger afterwards and remove any excess fat with sharp pointed scissors, remembering that the less the fat there is, that the better the take. Although taking the fat after the graft has been harvested is a tedious process, it is probably easier to do for the inexperienced surgeon. To take a graft without fat requires both skill and care, since buttonholing can easily occur with excess vigour.

The donor site is closed by direct suture using either subcuticular Ethilon or Prolene, or an interrupted non-absorbable or absorbable suture. The advantage of using an absorbable suture is that in a young child it does not have to be removed. Probably the ideal alternative in that situation is a subcuticular absorbable suture. In the postauricular region, it may be wise to apply a pressure head bandage for 24 h.

Full-thickness skin and cartilage (composite) grafts

Composite grafts consisting of a full-thickness skin graft with underlying cartilage may be taken from the auricular region and used to reconstruct small and moderate sized defects where tissue loss indicates that skin and underlying cartilage are required for reconstruction. Usually this technique is indicated to reconstruct areas in the nasal tip or the alar rim and, in certain instances, the skin loss may be extended up to include the whole of the lateral side of the nose. The take rate is unpredictable and many of these grafts go blue in the first few weeks, but their ultimate outcome is surprisingly good. They may also be used to reconstruct defects in the contralateral ear.

Pinch grafts

These are small full-thickness grafts taken by pinching skin in a pair of forceps and a layer of skin being sliced off using a no. 10 scalpel blade. The pinch graft leaves depressions in the donor site and elevations in the recipient site. Its one role in head and neck surgery is in the lining of a mastoid cavity following radical mastoidectomy, where it is used by some surgeons as a form of cover in preference to either split skin, fascia or no graft at all.

Dermal and fat grafts

These are rarely used in head and neck surgery today. They were formerly used for sunken defects around the orbit and maxillary sinus following surgery. As they are avascular and difficult to position, and as some absorption and gravitational drop occurs with time, it is probably preferable to use vascularized flaps in this situation such as a fascial radial forearm flap or de-epithelialized groin flap.

Dermal grafts may be either pure dermis or dermis and fat. To take a pure dermal graft, the steps are similar to taking a split skin graft. The dermatome is first set to 10/1000 inch (approximately 0.254 mm) and the epidermis is shaved off but left attached at one end. The dermatome set to 22/1000 inch (approximately 0.5 mm) and a strip of dermis is then taken as the graft. Once bleeding as been stopped with adrenaline soaks, the original epidermis is replaced and sewn in place and the donor site closed as for a split skin graft with a pressure dressing.

If a plumper graft is required, then the area is marked out as appropriate on the thigh and the skin is de-epithelialized with either a scalpel blade or a dermatome. A rectangular or ellipse area of dermis is then cut with a scalpel to include the underlying fat and this is used as the free graft. The donor site is then closed primarily.

Fascial grafts

These may be used as free grafts to cover the carotid arteries, e.g. temporalis fascia, which may now be taken as a free flap based on the superficial temporal vessels. However, simpler methods are now available to perform this technique using pedicled or free muscle only or myocutaneous flaps. Tensor fascia lata remains particularly useful for the creation of fascial slings and this is described in detail later.

Chondromucosal grafts

These are avascular grafts consisting of nasal septum and mucosa which are particularly useful for providing internal lining to replace the conjunctiva following total lower eyelid reconstruction. The nasal septal cartilage supplies replacement for the tarsal plate, with the appropriate support and replacement for the tarsal plate,while the mucosa replaces the conjunctiva.

Flaps

The types of flap used in head and neck reconstruction are shown below.

Flaps in head and neck reconstruction

- Local flaps – Random
  - – Axial pattern
- Distant axial – Deltopectoral
  - – Cervical
  - – Occipitomastoid
- Myocutaneous
- Free

Local flaps

In essence, a local skin flap consists of a tongue-like protrusion of tissue which is made up of skin and a variable amount of the underlying subcutaneous tissue. It remains attached at one or more points by its pedicle, which provides an arterial blood supply with venous and lymphatic drainage. This is then moved with its blood supply in order to reconstruct the primary defect and this procedure will leave a secondary defect which may be closed by either a split skin graft or direct closure. Flaps that are moved from the area close to the defect are called local flaps and those that involve movement over a considerable distance from the defect site are called distant flaps. By convention, a flap that is transferred into the head and neck region from below the mandible is defined as a distant flap.

When movement of local tissue occurs, it happens in one of two ways. The tissue may be marched or advanced in a forward direction using advancement techniques or moved laterally using the pivot principle when there is movement round a pivot point. The techniques of transposition and rotation rely on this principle. When a flap is designed, it remains attached to the body, usually by its distal end, which is referred to as the base, and it is through this area that the blood supply enters. The arteries, capillaries and veins together with all of the local networks of communication are in the base. Sometimes the whole of the skin may be isolated as an island with the blood supply coming in from the subcutaneous component and this is referred to as an island flap. Occasionally, flaps may be bipedicled, with bases at either end, to facilitate better blood supply and when larger areas of tissue are to be transferred. Examples include the 'bucket-handle' scalp flap and the upper to lower eyelid 'Tripier' flap.

When distant flaps are transferred they may be single, pedicled and transferred straight into the defect or, as in the past, where the distance to be travelled by the flap was considerable, the technique of 'waltzing' was used. This involved taking two pedicles from the abdomen or thoracic wall to create a bipedicled flap. Over the ensuing months the pedicles were waltzed up one at a time and planted sequentially until the head and neck was reached. Such techniques are seldom used in the Western world today. In a case of named axial cutaneous flaps where the flap needs to be extended, it is possible to extend the design of the flap to add a random pattern flap on the end of the axial flap. An example of this is extending the deltopectoral flap beyond the anterior axillary fold on to the shoulder region. In this situation, the technique of delay may be used. The flap is outlined and elevated and then sewn back into place for a period of 2–3 weeks to promote and facilitate circulation through the base prior to transfer.

Many criteria can help a surgeon decide which form of reconstruction to use. Local flaps require expertise in design and any mistakes will show up in the form of undesirable scarring and possible flap failure. When dealing in tumour surgery, the flap may hide recurrence and sometimes a graft may be better. Where the recipient bed will not take a skin graft, a flap of some sort will have to be used.

Random pattern flaps

Most local skin flaps within the head and neck are random pattern flaps. They may be not only random in their blood supply, but also random in their design, although some do follow a particular design pattern, e.g. the rhomboid flap.

Local vascular physiology dictates that there are strict rules to be obeyed in the design of a random flap. As a general rule, the height of a random flap should not exceed 1.5 times the length of the base. This is because there is no named specific vascular supply, so that blood supply via the base is random. Blood supply to the flap apex is thus inversely proportional to its height. Outside the head and neck this rule must be adhered to but within the head and neck there is an extensive subdermal vascular plexus, where it is possible to relax some of these rigid constrictions and push local flap design to its limits, so that random flaps may be designed where the length is up to three or four times the base (Fig. 7.7).

Even within the head and neck, there are variations in the blood supply. On the face below the level of the zygomatic arch, there is a very rich subdermal plexus in the fatty layer between the skin and the muscles of facial expression fed from the deeper facial vessels which emerge from the facial musculature. Above the zygomatic arch, the vascular anatomy is different, with the blood vessels running horizontally between the skin and fascia in the deep connective tissue with no deep vascular connections.

The vessels that enter this area from below include the superficial temporal artery and vein, the posterior auricular and occipital vessels and the supraorbital and supratrochlear vessels. In particular, the superficial temporal vessels, the supraorbital and supratrochlear vessels may all be used in axial arteriovenous flap design. Elsewhere on the scalp, there is extensive communication

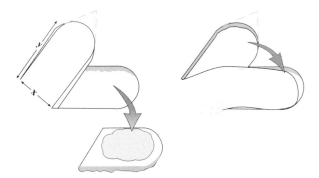

Figure 7.7 Technique of local random flap design using the transposition technique. As a general rule, the distance *Y* should only be 1.5 times the distance *X* but in the head and neck region, it is sometimes possible to exceed this so that *Y* can be up to three times *X*.

across the midline such that it is possible to design large flaps crossing the midline despite the absence of a named axial vessel.

Design of random pattern flaps

- Height 1.5 (up to 3) times base width
- Zygomatic watershed: more vascular inferiorly
- Forehead vasculature allows extension across midline

Planning considerations

The following considerations are considered important:

- the anatomy and physiology of the skin, including colour, texture, appearance and amount
- local muscle anatomy: vascular supply, nerve supply and lymphatic drainage
- the aesthetics of the area
- possible sites for incision placement
- areas of local tissue availability in relation to the area to be reconstructed.

Any one flap has advantages and disadvantages, indications and contraindications.

When excising a tumour on the face, clearance is paramount but it is also important to consider the concept of cosmetic units (Fig. 7.8) and that lines of excision are designed with these in mind. It is often preferable to excise the whole cosmetic unit to give the optimum reconstruction. When areas of resection extend beyond one cosmetic unit, then more than one flap may be necessary to reconstruct the defect and it is important to realize that complex reconstruction is often a series of building blocks combining a number of simpler techniques.

In the design of any local flap, it is crucial to assess what areas of tissue are available. The flap should be designed and marked out, and then elevated, transferred, inset and monitored. If any mistakes are made in the design, elevation or transfer, then the subsequent outcome will usually be less than favourable. Anybody can raise the flap, it is the marking out which is the difficult part. Flap loss is a devastating complication which usually results from either a design fault (flap too small, appropriate blood supply not included) or a technical error (damage to blood supply, too narrow a pedicle, sutures too tight, no backcut or a haematoma).

There is nothing magic about the movement of tissue on the face. You do not get something for nothing! The principle of a local flap works because skin is elastic and stretches, and it is possible to take tissue and move it from areas where it is redundant into an area where it is needed.

The stretching of skin is a mechanical property which relates to the viscoelastic properties of the collagen bundles. It is time dependent, i.e. the longer one pulls, the more it stretches and initially a small increase in load produces a rapid and significant increase in length. However, a point of compromise is soon reached where, despite an increase in load, little more movement is achieved and

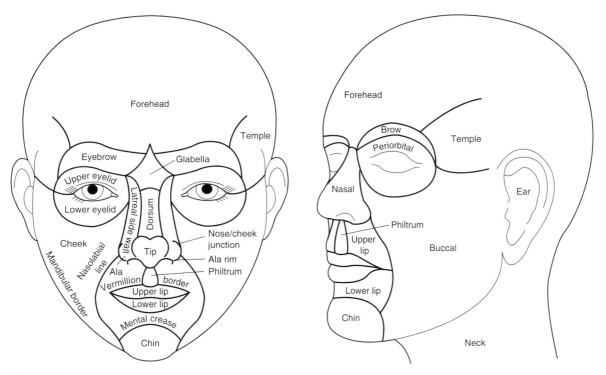

Figure 7.8 Concept of facial cosmetic units.

vascularity is severely compromised. This will lead to blanching and distal flap necrosis. In essence, tension and vascularity are friend and foe and the flap surgeon must balance the two to obtain optimum results.

Particular areas on the face not only facilitate direct closure but also provide lax skin for transfer (Fig. 7.9).

They include the glabellar and temporal areas, the nasolabial area and the mandibular–masseteric region where the lower face joins the upper neck. The surgeon decides where the flap is going to come from by a pinch test which identifies lax tissue. The flap is then drawn out bearing in mind the size of the primary defect, the lines

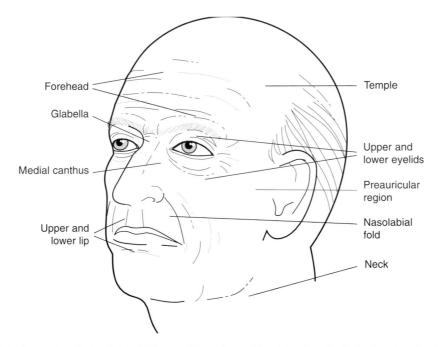

Figure 7.9 Possible donor sites for both full-thickness skin grafts and local flap transfer in the head and neck region. They include the glabellar and temporal areas, the nasolabial area and the mandibular/masseteric region as well as the neck.

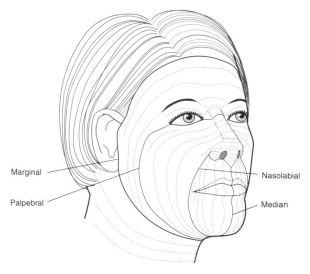

Figure 7.10 Relaxed skin tension lines.

of election on the face and closure of the donor site. Relaxed skin tension lines are those skin tension lines that follow the furrows formed when the skin is relaxed. They are not visible features of the skin, such as wrinkle lines. Rather, they can be found by pinching the skin and observing the furrows and ridges that are formed. These relaxed skin tension lines are the same in all people (Fig. 7.10) and where possible incisions in the head and neck should follow these lines. The Langer's lines are important from a historical point of view. They represent the skin tension in rigor mortis. The relaxed skin tension lines and Langer's lines do not correspond in many areas of the body.

Planning in reverse is usually used where mock transfer is carried out using a piece of thread around the pivot point; if the flap is not big enough, it is redrawn as appropriate. Excision of a tumour should always be complete without any consideration of skimping on the reconstruction, since it is better to have a large scar than a small tombstone!

In certain areas on the face, particularly on the cheek and in the neck, it is wise to think big and use large flaps that heal well. Big is beautiful in this area, since small flaps such as rhomboid or bilobed flaps placed injudiously on the cheek can lead to awful scarring, pincushioning and subsequent disfigurement with unhappiness for both the patient and the surgeon. Head and neck surgeons are usually lucky in that the majority of patients are elderly and thus often have plenty of lax tissue.

The movement of tissue on the face is either by advancement or by the pivot principle using rotation or transposition. In order to achieve this, the length of the flap is crucial. These techniques are described below.

Advancement

> **Tissue may be advanced on the face using the following techniques**
>
> - Burow's triangles
> - V-Y advancement
> - Panthographic expansion
> - Transposition Z-plasty

Burow's triangles. This technique relies on a single pedicled rectangular flap which is raised and advanced to close the defect. This is facilitated by the excision of Burow's triangles at either side of the base of the flap, which facilitates the movement of tissue. The longer the flap, the more precarious the blood supply at the base; however, on the face (where this flap has its major application), the ratio of length:breadth can be between 3:1 and 4:1. Movement of tissue is facilitated by laxity in the surrounding skin, which makes the advancement appear greater than it actually is (Fig. 7.11).

V-Y advancement. This elegant technique is ideally suited to lesions in the medial cheek at the alar base (Fig. 7.12). Once the defect is made, a flap is outlined as shown and is pedicled deeply or sometimes supe-

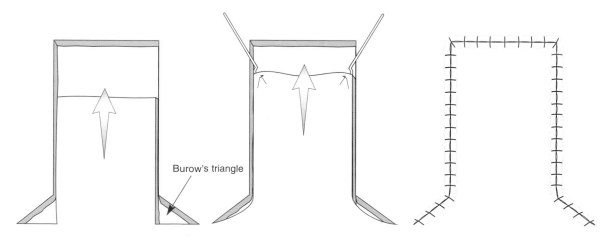

Figure 7.11 Skin advancement using Burow's triangles.

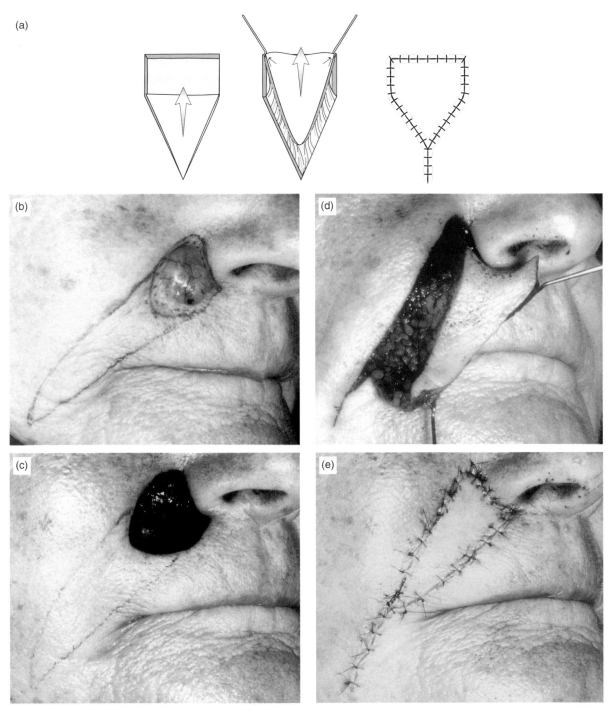

Figure 7.12 Skin advancement using V to Y advancement. (a) Outline of the technique (b) lesion at the right alar base. (b) The flap is outlined, (c) the lesion excised, and (d, e) the flap elevated and transferred to close the defect.

riorly on the subcutaneous tissues (Herbert flap). Advancement occurs and the donor site closes primarily. Quite large defects in and around the alar base region can be closed with this technique and the scars are well camouflaged in the lines of election on the cheek.

Panthographic expansion. This is a variation of advancement where instead of the flap being designed as a rectangle, the limbs of the flap are designed at 120° with back cuts at the bottom so that it looks like an inverted tumbler. The flap is then advanced (Fig. 7.13) so that the donor site closes primarily. This is an ingenious technique

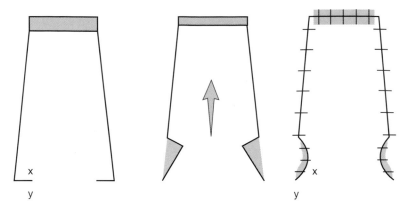

Figure 7.13   Technique of advancement using panthographic expansion

which uses the same principle as the anglepoise lamp on one's desk. It is particularly useful on the cheek and neck.

Advancement Z-plasty. One of the problems with skin advancement is that once the tissue has been advanced, unless it is stopped where it is, it tends to return whence it came. One way to prevent this is to break up the scar with a Z-plasty (Fig. 7.14). This technique is ideally suited to reconstruction of the defects in the lower eyelid which are excised as a triangle, and tissue is advanced laterally (see Chapter 21). The addition of a Z-plasty as described by McGregor not only enhances the upward lift on the scar to prevent any ectropion, but breaks up the suture line to prevent any movement of tissue back from whence it came.

Pivot principle

Rotation flap. In its ideal form (Fig. 7.15), the flap is defined as the large arc of a semicircle where the triangular primary defect represents a small arc approximately one-eighth the size of the flap. The flap is elevated and then the difference in lengths of the two sides of the defect

is made up by suturing with a degree of differential tension. It should be recognized that the larger the flap, the less the differential tension (Fig. 7.16). In general, the larger a rotation flap the better, but this should be coun-

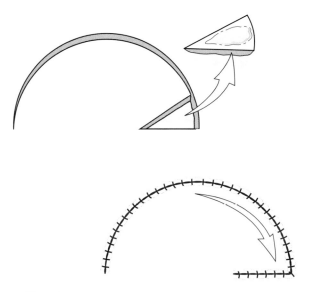

Figure 7.15   Technique of a rotation flap based on the pivot principle.

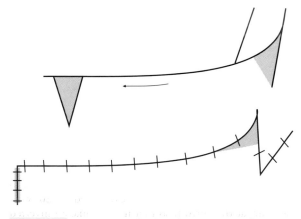

Figure 7.14   Technique of skin advancement using transposition 'Z' plasty.

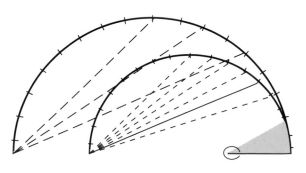

Figure 7.16   Note the differential tension when closing the defect using the technique of rotation. It is better to make a rotation flap larger rather than smaller.

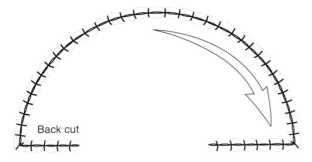

Back cut

Figure 7.17 If the closure is a little tight using the rotation flap, a back cut may be necessary.

terbalanced by the anatomical restraints within the head and neck region. Certainly, it is better to make a rotation flap larger rather than smaller.

If closure is a little tight, rotation may be facilitated by a back cut (Fig. 7.17), which will leave a small secondary defect that may be sutured directly or closed with a skin graft. If excess skin is left in the form of a dog ear this may be excised. Rotation flaps work well on a convex surface and are ideally suited on the cheek, the submandibular area extending into the upper neck and the scalp.

Crescentic advancement is an ingenious method which has its main use in the alar base, perialar regions and upper lip. It involves incising two areas (A and B), and the tumour may be in either area (Fig. 7.18). Either way, advancement occurs medially and the reconstruction is completed. This method is particularly useful in reconstructing large defects in the upper lip when the technique can be used bilaterally.

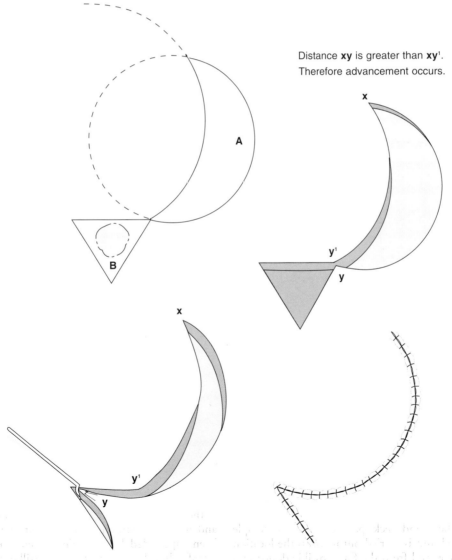

Distance **xy** is greater than **xy**¹.
Therefore advancement occurs.

Figure 7.18 Technique of perialar crescentic advancement. The lesion excised may be in A or B.

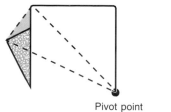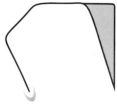

Pivot point

Figure 7.19 Pivot principle using a simple transposition flap. Note that the flap has a well-defined and precisely positioned pivot point.

Transposition flap. Conventionally, a transposition flap is a rectangle (little more than a square) which is designed, raised and elevated into a triangulated defect (Fig. 7.19). This inevitably leaves a donor site (which is at least as large as the defect) to be closed. Therefore, in its true form, the technique has little application in the head and neck. It is ideally suited on the scalp when a surgical defect will not take a skin graft but can be covered with a transposition flap and the subsequent donor site covered with a skin graft, which may be hidden in the hair-bearing region.

However, modifications to the transposition flap allow it to have major uses within the head and neck region. The properties of skin and head and neck tissue laxity, particularly on the face, allow the design of transposition flaps which may be routinely raised with an abundant skin circulation so that they are much longer than they are wide, with ratios of between 3:1 and 4:1. The donor sites that are left with these flaps can usually be closed by direct suture (Fig. 7.7) and therefore they produce excellent results. There is considerable pleasure to be gained in the correct design, elevation and execution of a local transposition flap on the face.

Great care is needed in the design of a transposition flap and it is important that it is drawn correctly and that a practice transfer is carried out before any cuts are made, to ensure that the appropriate movement will take place. Each flap has a well-defined and precisely positioned pivot point (Fig. 7.19), which is on the side of the flap away from the direction of movement of the flap so that the length of the flap will always have to be greater than is anticipated. This problem is made even more problematical by the fact that the further the flap rotates through 90°, the shorter it becomes, so that if a flap is rotated 180°, its length is considerably reduced and vascular flow through the base is compromised. For this reason, transposition flaps are not normally designed to rotate more than 90°.

Some transposition flaps are named based on their design. A classic transposition flap is the rhomboid (Fig. 7.20) which, when correctly executed, gives an excellent result in the head and neck, particularly in the temple region. A pinch test is carried out to assess the location of the lax tissue, and from the four possible donor sites (Fig. 7.20) the appropriate one is chosen which will give

the best result with minimal secondary deformity and scarring. As Borges said 'let the limbs of the flap follow the relaxed skin tension lines'. The excision is designed as a rhomboid and the flap is designed as shown and transposed into the defect. The donor site is closed primarily. Rhomboids can also be designed as a double or even triple flaps ('swastika flap') to close larger defects.

The bilobed flap is a double transposition flap which masquerades as a rotation flap and has its major role in the head and neck on the nose. It provides an elegant way of reconstructing defects in the lower half of the nose by designing two transposition flaps in the arc of a circle, where the larger of the two flaps will close the surgical defect, the smaller flap closes its donor site and the donor site for the smallest flap closes primarily. This is a difficult flap to design and execute properly, but can give excellent results (Fig. 7.21). The best way to reconstruct the nose is with the skin of the nose.

A commonly used transposition flap on the face is the nasolabial flap. Whilst it is usually described as a random flap, anatomical studies have shown there is an arteriovenous pedicle arising in the region of the alar base, based on branches of the facial artery which allow flaps in this area to be designed with an axial component (see below). Quite long flaps are possible which may be transposed to reconstruct defects on the nasal tip and alar rim, columella and upper lip. When islanded, they may be transposed into the oral cavity, and when combined with a similar contralateral flap, they may be used to reconstruct defects in the anterior floor of mouth.

Random transposition flaps may be islanded. An example of this is the glabellar island transposition flap which may be tunnelled through to reconstruct defects in the upper medial canthal region. Although, in principle this technique sounds advantageous, such flaps are often unreliable. In practice, the glabellar island flap often pincushions and a surgeon's large flap series will usually feature only one. There are also named axial island transposition flaps where islands of tissue may be islanded on a main vessel, e.g. the temporalis island transposition flap, which may be transposed from the temple downwards to reconstruct cheek defects, and the donor site then covered with the skin graft (Fig. 7.22).

Axial flaps

An axial flap is based on a named arteriovenous pedicle that runs within the skin superficial to the underlying muscle layer, parallel to the overlying skin (Fig. 7.23). Axial flaps have an extremely good blood supply which is determined not only by their length and breadth ratio but also by the vascular territory of the vessels that supply them. Because of this, they can generally be raised to a much greater length than random flaps and can therefore be used to move skin over a greater distance. The use of these flaps in the 1960s was the first major step in head and neck reconstruction. Their routine use has largely been superseded by musculocutaneous and free tissue transfer, but the deltopectoral flap still has a role in head and neck surgery.

(a) The rhomboid flap

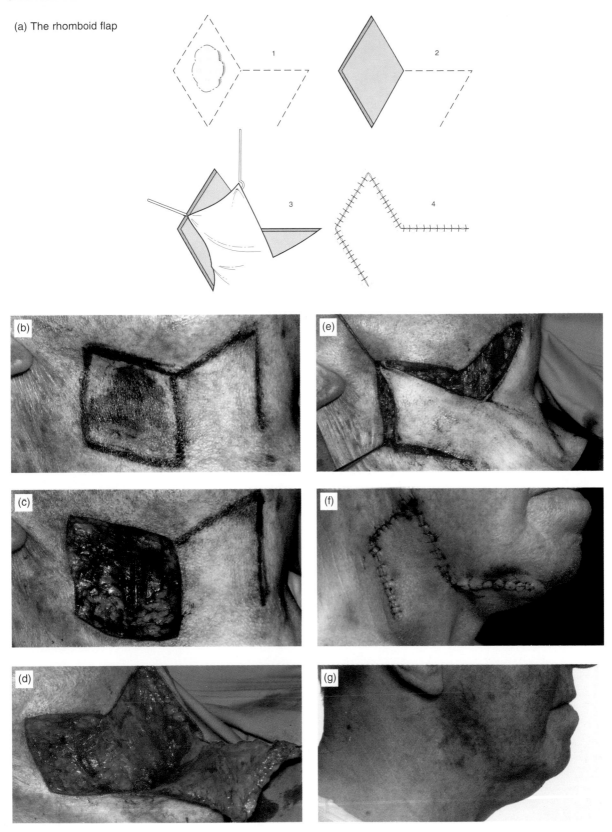

Figure 7.20 (a) Example of a named classic transposition flap: the Rhomboid or Limberg flap. (b) Patient with a lentigo maligna of the left upper neck. (c) The excision is marked as a rhomboid, the lesion is excised and (d) the flap raised and (e, f) transposed into the defect. (g) The final result.

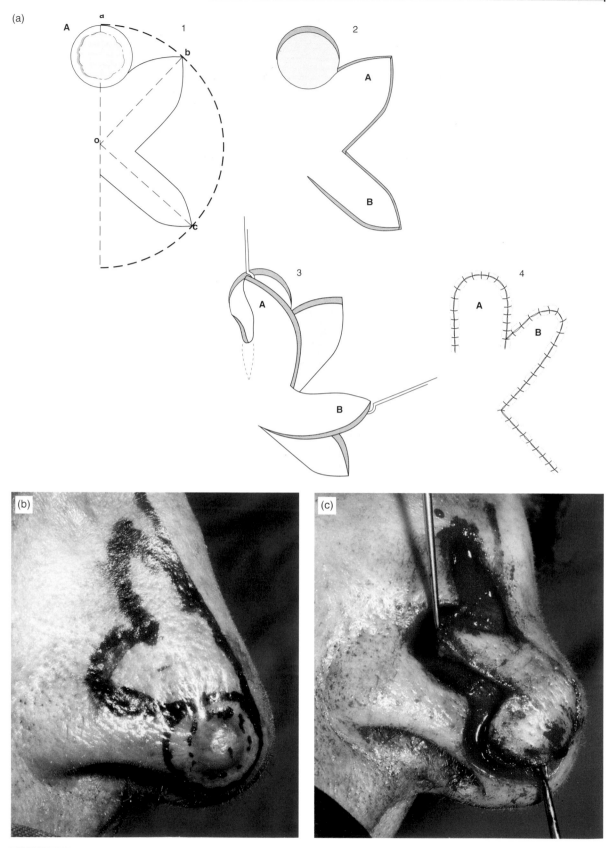

Figure 7.21 (a) Principle of a bilobed flap. (b) Patient with a basal cell carcinoma on the lower lateral aspect of the nose. (c) The lesion is excised with a 6 mm margin, and repair was with a bilobed flap. (d) The final result (*shown opposite*).

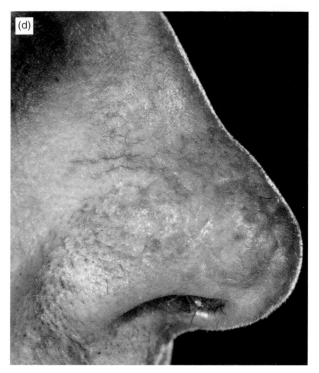

Figure 7.21 (d) The final result.

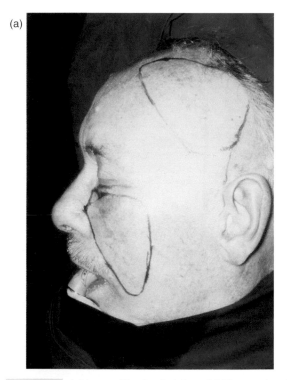

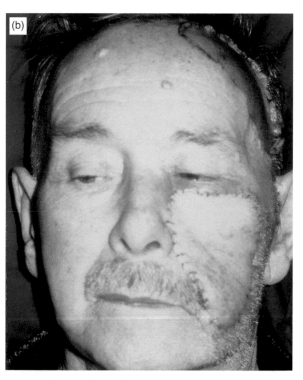

Figure 7.22 (a) Large skin cheek defect, (b) The repair using a temporalis island flap. The donor site has been skin grafted

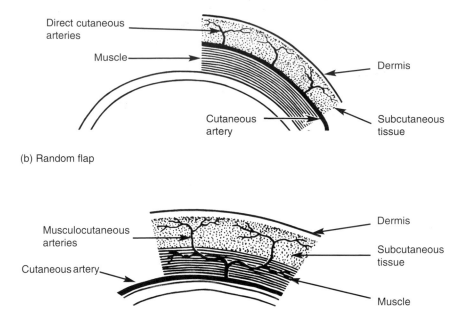

(a) Axial flap

Direct cutaneous arteries

Muscle

Dermis

Cutaneous artery

Subcutaneous tissue

(b) Random flap

Musculocutaneous arteries

Cutaneous artery

Dermis

Subcutaneous tissue

Muscle

Figure 7.23 Blood supply of axial and random flaps. (a) Note that the axial flap is based on an arteriovenous pedicle which runs within the skin superficial to the underlying muscle layer and parallel to the overlying skin. (b) This differs from a random flap.

Forehead flaps

The forehead flap is an axial flap which provides large areas of skin and subcutaneous tissue which may be used to reconstruct defects below the level of the eyes. In its original form (as described by McGregor), the axial forehead flap based on the anterior branch of the temporal artery was one of the first flaps used in intraoral reconstruction. It is rarely used nowadays since it leaves a horrendous donor site and there are better alternatives, but it may be used occasionally. If a radial forearm flap fails in the mouth and an immediate, reliable 'lifeboat' is required, the forehead flap may be quickly raised to get the surgeon out of trouble! It is passed into the oral cavity medial to the zygomatic arch. The temporalis muscle tendon must be divided from the coronoid process to facilitate access.

The most commonly raised forehead flap is the cutaneous axial median forehead flap, based on the supratrochlear artery. It can be raised and transposed to reconstruct areas in the upper medial cheek region and the lower half of the nose and alar rim (Fig. 7.24). The donor site will close primarily and the cosmetic result is excellent. Where larger areas of tissue are required, for example in complete nasal resurfacing, larger forehead flaps may be designed (e.g. Millard flying seagull flap), which may be facilitated by prior tissue expansion to ease donor site closure. Otherwise, a skin graft is required, which makes the cosmetic result less favour-

able. These techniques are best suited in patients with high foreheads with some lax tissue to facilitate primary closure.

Other cutaneous axial flaps such as the nasolabial flap have already been mentioned.

Distant axial flaps

Deltopectoral flap

This flap was described by Bakanjian in 1965 and is an axial pattern flap designed on the anterior chest wall between the line of the clavicle and the level of the anterior axillary fold. It is based medially on the upper part of the chest in the upper three or four perforating branches of the internal mammary artery which emerge through the medial end of the intercostal spaces (Fig. 7.25). Its boundaries are the clavicle superiorly, the acromium laterally and a line running through the anterior axillary fold to above the nipple inferiorly. The flap will extend to any site in the neck and occasionally up to the level of the zygoma. This flexibility is explained first by the fact that it retracts from side to side after it has been elevated, and not from end to end, so that it may elongate slightly over time, particularly in those patients over 60 years of age. Secondly, its flexibility is due to an anomalous pivot point (see below).

The basic flap design is safe over the skin territory that has been described, but when attempts are made to

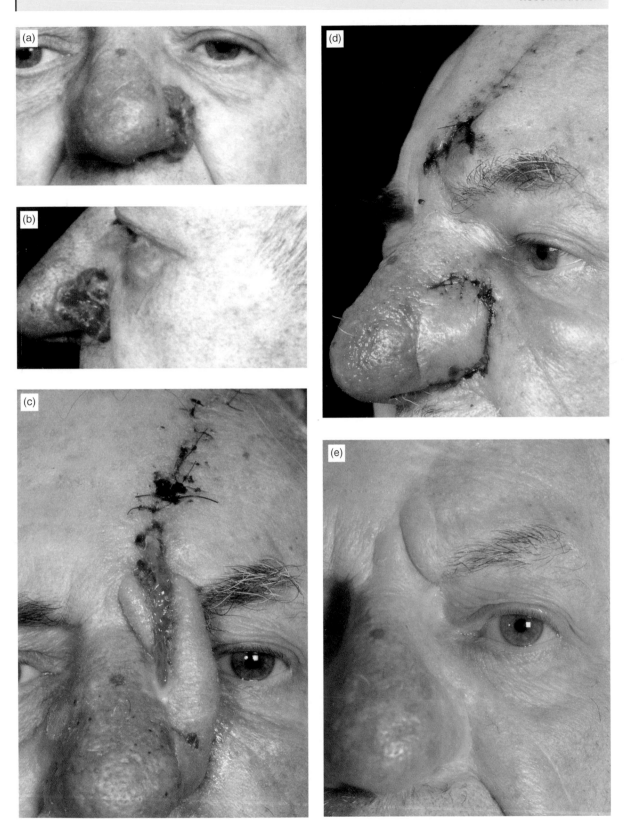

Figure 7.24 Use of a midline forehead flap to repair a defect in the left lower aspect of the nose and cheek. (a, b) A patient with a T_4 basal cell carcinoma of the lower aspect the nose and medial part of the cheek. (c) Wide excision was achieved, repair of the lateral side of the nose was with an infolded delayed forehead flap and the cheek repaired using V to Y advancement. (d) The forehead flap was divided 3 weeks later. (e, f) The final result (*shown overleaf*).

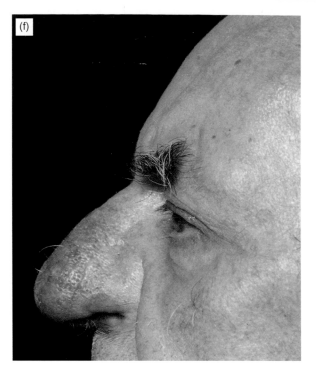

(f)

Figure 7.24 Use of a midline forehead flap to repair a defect in the left lower aspect of the nose and cheek. (f) The final result.

increase its length beyond this as a straight extension round the shoulder and a random segment applied on to the axial component, then flap survival may be compromised. Problems with necrosis arise because the extension allows the branch of the acromiothoracic axis to be formally divided and this is the only other vessel of note other than the axial perforators to enter the deep surface of the flap. The territory of the perforator vascular system has been shown to extend as far as the groove separating the deltoid from the pectoralis major. Any extension of the flap beyond this should not be regarded as an axial pattern flap. One must be aware that any extension of the flap beyond this area may result in failure of the tip of the flap.

The flap is marked out using the landmarks described above and then elevation begins laterally. The pectoral fascia is left on the flap, leaving the muscle fibres below absolutely bare. Any branches of the acromiothoracic axis that are encountered should be tied and ligated. Diathermy should not be used on either flap or the muscle, as this could damage the flap and any diathermy marks on the muscle may compromise the subsequent take of any skin graft. When raising the flap, retraction is upwards by an assistant using skin hooks; it must not be doubled back on itself as this could lead to buttonholing.

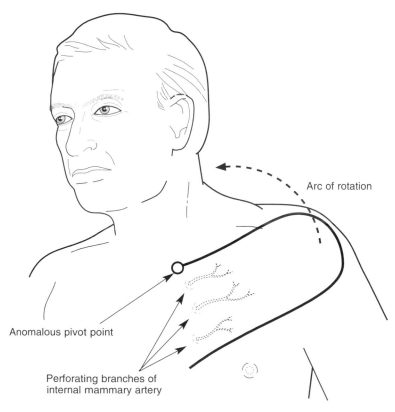

Arc of rotation

Anomalous pivot point

Perforating branches of internal mammary artery

Figure 7.25 Design and planning of the deltopectoral flap. Note the position of the anomolous pivot point at the upper medial end of the flap.

Planning the transfer. The deltopectoral flap has an anomalous pivot point. There is considerable slackness in the skin on the anterior axillary fold when the arm is abducted. This means that the lower border of the flap is considerably longer than the upper part. The pivot point on the flap is thus at the medial end of the upper limb and not the lower limb. This needs to be taken into account when planning the flap (Fig. 7.25).

The donor site is covered with a split skin graft. The subsequent uses of a deltopectoral flap are:

- to cover the whole anterior neck skin without any subsequent revision
- to reconstruct a defect by passing as a bridge over normal tissue where conventionally the pedicle may be tubed. Once take has occurred over a period of 3 weeks, the pedicle is divided and the remaining part of the flap may be returned to the donor site or discarded
- to reconstruct large defects on the lower face and upper neck. The pedicle may be inserted into part of the defect to facilitate take and then the pedicle is divided inferiorly and the flap inserted into the rest of the lower defect. This is analogous to 'waltzing'. The deltopectoral flap may also be used in the repair of a pharyngeal fistula but usually muscle bulk is required with the skin, and therefore other flaps are preferable.

Other distal axial cutaneous flaps

These include cervical skin flaps and occipitomastoid-based flaps.

Cervical skin flaps of varying shape, size, site and direction may be designed to make good use of lax neck skin for reconstructive purposes. In general, they make use of the side of the neck and those that are usually used are in the occipitomastoid region. They may be used occasionallyfrom time to time to reconstruct defects in certain situations, particularly for salvage procedures. The nape of neck (Mütter) or posterior scalp flap is a random pattern skin flap which exploits the neck skin over the trapezius muscle and can be raised on the occipital vessels and extended downwards to the spine of the scapula. It may be swung on its upper pedicle to reconstruct areas in the lower face and submandibular region.

Very rarely in patients with lax neck skin and a low forehead, a tubed cervical skin pedicle flap may be used to repair lower nasal defects.

Myocutaneous and muscle only axial distant flaps

One of the most important discoveries in the last 20 years is that the skin over most parts of the body receives its blood supply by small musculocutaneous arteries that enter it from the underlying muscle, perpendicular from its surface (Fig. 7.26). It subsequently became apparent that an obvious way to move a large area of skin for reconstructive purposes was to transpose the skin with its underlying muscle from which it receives its nutrient blood supply.

Myocutaneous and muscle-only axial distant flaps
Pectoralis major
Latissimus dorsi
Sternomastoid
Trapezius
Platysma

The pectoralis major and the latissimus dorsi flaps represent the workhorses for many head and neck reconstructions and will satisfy requirements in approximately 90% of cases.

The muscles are supplied ultimately by segmental vessels that have similar perfusion pressures to the aorta. They run deep within the muscle and give off perforators that enter the muscles and provide communication between the segmental vessels and the musculocutaneous vessels in the skin. There may be several arterial pedicles. The artery is usually accompanied by two venae commitantes that unite after leaving the muscle to drain into a major regional vein. Five types of muscular arterial supply have been described (Table 7.1).

The blood supply to the muscles may also be random or axial in pattern. Most of the round muscles, for example the sternomastoid, have a random supply: perforators penetrate the belly at one end and immediately break up into small branches. The flatter muscles such as pectoralis major and latissimus dorsi have an axial supply: the major

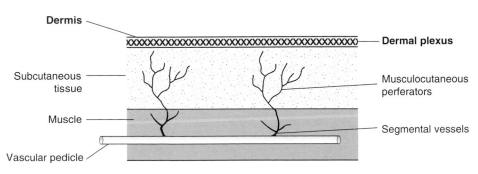

Figure 7.26 Blood supply to a myocutaneous flap.

Table 7.1 Patterns of vascular anatomy

Vascular pedicle	Examples used in head and neck surgery
I One pedicle	None
II Dominant pedicle and minor pedicles	Sternocleidomastoid Trapezius Platysma
III Two dominant pedicles	Temporalis
IV Segmental pedicles	None
V One dominant pedicle plus secondary segmental pedicles	Pectoralis major Latissimus dorsi

arterial supply runs the whole length of the deep surface of the muscle, giving off perforators as it goes.

Essential surgical points

- With the axial muscular flaps, although the blood supply to the muscle is axial, the blood supply of the skin upon the muscle is random.
- There is a minimum size of skin paddle that should be taken to ensure that a number of random perforators are entering the skin from below.
- For pectoralis major and latissimus dorsi flaps, this usually means a skin paddle measuring 5×3 cm (the size of the palm of an adult's hand).
- Smaller skin paddles may not survive.

Pectoralis major flap

This flap was first described by Aryian in the late 1970s. The muscle arises from the clavicle, from the sternum and by slips from the upper seven ribs. There is also a variable origin from the aponeurosis of the external oblique which is variable in size. It is inserted into the bicipital groove of the humerus. The muscle has three major segmental sub units: clavicular, sternocostal and an external segment (the most lateral part of the muscle), which originates from the ribs.

The main arterial supply, which provides the vascular basis for this flap, comes from the pectoral branch of the acromiothoracic artery which arises from the first part of the axillary artery (Fig. 7.27). The pectoral branch of the acromiothoracic axis emerges from the clavipectoral fascia, along with the lateral pectoral nerve, medial to the insertion of pectoralis minor on the coracoid process, a bony prominence that can be felt below the clavicle near the junction of its middle and outer thirds. The point, 2–3 cm medial to the coracoid process, represents the surface marking of the vascular hilum of the muscle. The vessels do not enter the muscle belly immediately, but run on its deep surface in a downward and medial direction giving off its branches. The acromiothoracic artery gives off a superior (clavicular) branch to the clavicular segment of the muscle and a main pectoral branch which then gives off an inferior thoracoacromial branch to the sternal segment and a lateral thoracic trunk to the external segment.

In approximately 50% of cases, the external segment of the muscle may be supplied exclusively by the lateral thoracic vessels which arise from the second part of the axillary artery and descend along the lateral border of the pectoralis minor. In one-third of cases, this external segment receives a dual supply from both the lateral thoracic and the thoracoacromial vessels. The sternocostal segment also receives a supply immediately from a perforating branch of the internal mammary artery, which may account for significant bleeding during the raising of the flap. The pectoralis major flap has a type V vascular pedicle.

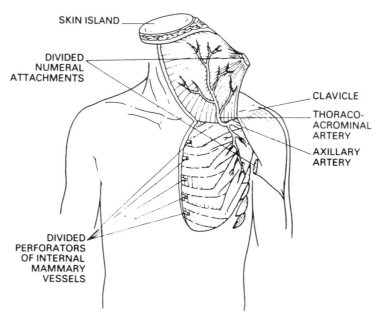

Figure 7.27 Blood supply to the pectoralis major myocutaneous flap.

The major advantages of this flap are that it has a large skin territory (the whole of the skin overlying the muscle may be raised), it has a rich vascular supply and it can be transferred without prior delay. It has a large arc of rotation and can be transferred up to the upper aspect of the ear to the level of the zygomatic arch. It can be harvested in the supine position, and can be transferred as either a muscle only, skin and muscle paddle, or indeed as two epithelial surfaces for inner and outer lining with a de-epithelialized segment between them. Primary donor site closure is easily achieved. However, it is a large bulky muscle which is relatively immobile and, therefore, is suited best to providing well-vascularized tissue to fill large defects where mobility is not of paramount importance, as in the repair of fistulae. It violates the breast in the female and, in this situation, the latissimus dorsi flap provides an appropriate alternative.

Technique. The whole of the skin overlying the pectoralis major muscle may be raised if required. However, this will leave a large defect which will require filling with a skin graft and so the flap is usually designed to facilitate primary closure.

With the patient in the supine position, the surface markings of the acromiothoracic artery are outlined. A dotted line is marked from the acromium to the xiphoid process and a further dotted line is dropped to join this line in a perpendicular direction from the sternal notch. The point at which line bisects the first line represents the place where the vascular pedicle meets the first line (Fig. 7.28), which then runs in the direction of the first line from the acromium towards the xiphisternum. The clavipectoral fascia is then marked by a point two-thirds of the distance along the clavicle from the sternal notch to the coracoid process. The vascular pedicle runs in a curved direction downwards to meet the bisection point already described. A skin island of the appropriate size and shape may be drawn over the distal part of the artery, to facilitate a suitable arc of rotation. The borders of the skin paddle should lie between the lateral edge of the sternum medially and the nipple laterally. The incision for access should be extended into the axilla. The technique described by McGregor, i.e. the raising of a defensive deltopectoral flap incision, is not required nowdays unless this latter flap is to be used at the same time in the reconstruction.

Unless the arc of rotation needs to be increased, it is advisable not to extend the lower part of the skin paddle beyond the inferior edge of the muscle. This part of the flap is random and, although the survival of this segment can be increased by taking part of the rectus sheath, this is not wholly reliable and should not be done unless absolutely necessary. Remember that the flap will retract by 10% in all directions when the skin is cut and this should be allowed for in planning, although some expansion will occur when the muscle is sewn in under tension.

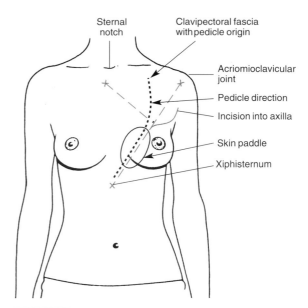

Figure 7.28 Landmarks for raising the pectoralis major myocutaneous flap.

Elevating the pectoralis major flap

- Start the dissection inferiorly
- Incise the skin down to the underlying muscle
- Define the lower limits of the pectoralis major muscle
- Incise the lower muscle to gain access to the subpectoral plane which is relatively avascular
- Divide the inferior muscle attachments from the ribs or rectus sheath
- Mobilize in an upward direction
- At this point the pectoralis minor muscle will be visualized
- If the paddle is too thick, suture the muscle to the skin edge with absorbable sutures to prevent shearing
- Combine mobilization in an upward direction first laterally and then medially.
- Identify the lateral border of the external segment of the muscle
- Identify and ligate the major branch of the lateral thoracic artery to increase the arc of rotation
- Continue the dissection upwards
- Divide the clavicular head of the muscle and remember to continue in an upward direction
- Do not curve the scissors medially **or you may cut the pedicle – the ultimate disaster**
- The muscle will be now rotated and the vascular pedicle will be clearly identified

Once the clavicular head of the muscle has been divided, the flap may be easily elevated by blunt dissection in the subpectoral fascial space between pectoralis major and minor. The vascular pedicle is now clearly seen and the sternal edge of the muscle may be divided up to the level of the clavicle with the pedicle in clear view. There is often a lot of bleeding at this stage. If there is any lateral muscle mass left (which is making up the anterior axillary fold), this is divided at this point, bearing in mind that the axillary vein is extremely close. The flap is now fully raised and mobile and if further mobility and arc of rotation are required, it may be islanded on the vessels by dividing the remaining muscular pedicle.

As a teaching aid, it is prudent to observe the neurovascular pedicle of the pectoralis minor muscle at this point, which is now visible and easily accessible. This muscle may be raised on its own as a free flap and used in facial reanimation techniques (see later).

Whilst the flap is being sewn in at the recipient site, the donor site can usually be closed at the same time. Haemostasis must be carefully achieved, two large drains are inserted and the defect is closed primarily using a two-layer closure. If closure is anticipated to be difficult, a one-layer blanket Nylon or Ethilon stitch is an elegant technique of closing the wound as it takes up the tension gradually in the same way as a mastectomy wound is closed. Large defects may require a skin graft.

Modifications of the flap include harvesting of muscle alone when, for example, closing large lower neck wounds which require bulk with no skin paddle. A subsequent skin graft can be applied to the raw muscle surface. Access is achieved along the lateral border of the muscle and primary closure easily achieved. The incorporation of vascularized bone has been described where part of either the fifth rib or the sternum can be transferred with the flap to provide composite soft tissue and bony reconstruction. The vascular supply to these bony segments is at best precarious and in the majority of instances non-existent. Newer techniques for composite soft-tissue and bony reconstruction are now available. Double skin paddles may be used with de-epithelialized islands in between them to provide inside and outside cover but, again, in this situation, the muscle is very bulky and newer techniques such as double-paddled radial forearm flaps are probably better. Where the excessive bulk of the pectoralis major is a problem, then harvesting over the thinner, parasternal area has been described, e.g. to tube the flap for reconstruction in the hypopharynx. Although this sounds attractive, practical experience has shown that it is virtually impossible to tube a pectoralis major myocutaneous flap. This should be avoided at all costs since better techniques are currently available.

When the above guidelines are followed, there are very few potential pitfalls with this flap. It is highly reliable and even when the skin paddle fails, the underlying muscle will usually survive and can be allowed to granulate and heal by secondary intention, or covered subsequently with a skin graft. It is always worth checking for congenital absence of the pectoralis major, although it is extremely rare with an incidence of 1:11 000. Congenital absence of the sternocostal head is part of Poland's syndrome.

When a conventional flap is used, the skin paddle is below and medial to the nipple, at about the level of the sixth rib. In this area, the skin which precisely overlies the muscle is quite small but the skin paddle may be extended inferiorly beyond the confines of the muscle. The variable extent of this inferior extension is not entirely clear but depends on age, gender, the presence of intervening adiposity and the musculature and the size of the muscle. The extension should not be beyond 3–4 cm of the abdominal skin below the inferior part of the muscle. If the flap is raised to this extent, part of the rectus abdominus aponeurosis together with the rectus sheath should be raised with the flap. In this situation, the survival of the lower part of the flap is unpredictable. The size of the flap may be extended by including the nipple/areolar complex, particularly in a male, but this should be avoided in females unless absolutely necessary.

Latissimus dorsi flap

This flap represents the first myocutaneous flap described in the medical literature (Tanzini, 1896). It was repopularized by Olivari in 1976 for the repair of local defects. Further work by Quillen in 1978 described its use for head and neck reconstruction, where it remains a reliable and versatile fundamental component of the surgeon's repertoire.

The muscle is large and triangular in shape and arises from the sacrum and lumbar vertebrae, thoracolumbar fascia, the posterior iliac crest and the lower six thoracic vertebrae. In addition, some slips arise from the lower three ribs and the muscle converges to have a narrow insertion into the intertubercular groove of the humerus. Hence, it forms the posterior wall of the axilla. It is a type V muscle which receives a significant but smaller blood supply from the perforating vessels through the lumbosacral fascia, and a pedicled flap can be based on this to repair defects in the buttock region.

Its major vascular supply arises from the thoracodorsal vessels, which have their origin in the subscapular artery (Fig. 7.29a). This latter artery arises from the axillary artery, gives rise to the circumflex scapular artery about 4 cm from its origin (Fig 7.29b) and then continues as a thoracodorsal artery to enter the latissimus dorsi about 10 cm from its humeral insertion. Just before its insertion, it gives off a branch which accompanies branches from the lateral thoracic artery (which also arises from the subscapular artery) and carries on to supply the serratus anterior. Within the latissimus dorsi muscle, the thoracodorsal vessels divide into superior and lateral branches which allow the muscle to be split into two. Either two flaps can then be taken or just one flap, thereby leaving some muscle behind.

Venous drainage is by the venae commitantes, which accompany the thoracodorsal artery and drain into the axillary vein. The nerve supply is via the thoracodorsal nerve, which is a branch of the posterior cord of the brachial plexus.

(a)

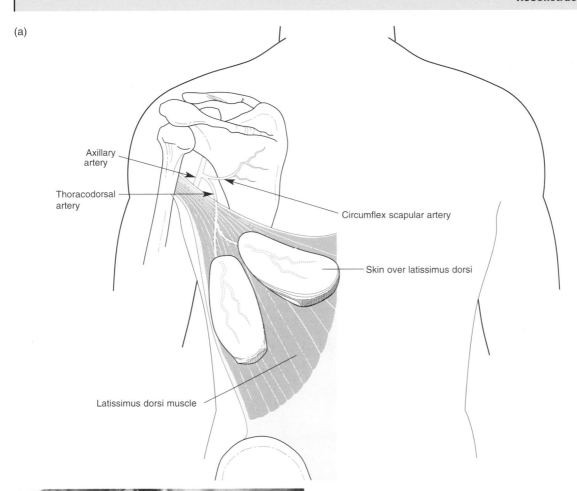

Axillary artery

Thoracodorsal artery

Circumflex scapular artery

Skin over latissimus dorsi

Latissimus dorsi muscle

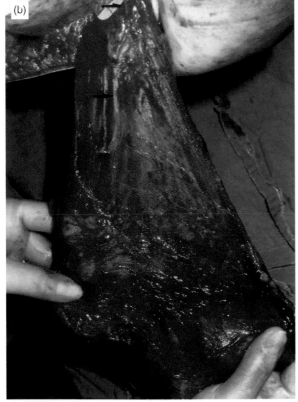

(b)

Figure 7.29 Blood supply to the lattissimus dorsi flap. (a) The thorocodorsal artery is a continuation of the subscapular artery which comes directly off the axillary artery. (b) The circumflex scapular artery (upper arrow) and the thorocodorsal artery with its branches on the muscle (lower arrow) are shown during flap elevation.

Large amounts of tissue are made available using this flap. Flaps measuring 10×8 cm are easily harvested and subsequent primary closure is easily achieved. Even larger amounts of tissue may be taken as a musculocutaneous flap measuring 40×20 cm but this requires skin grafting of the donor defect and may lead to problems with healing on the back.

A latissimus dorsi flap may not only be raised as a myocutaneous pedicled flap but also used for free tissue transfer. It is totally reliable with a long pedicle which is longer than 10 cm and can be lengthened by dividing the circumflex scapular artery. The diameter of the subscapular artery at this point is at least 3 mm and the veins are of similar size.

By designing the flap low down on the back, the arc of rotation allows transfer into the head and neck region up to the zygomatic arch and flaps can be made to reach the top of the head (particularly if only muscle is used). The other advantages of this flap are that it does not violate the breast and because it is a large flat muscle, it is possible in extreme circumstances to tube it for total pharyngeal reconstruction. In addition, the subscapular artery offers a variety of flaps which may be used either singularly or in combination. Therefore, a scapular flap along with a latissimus dorsi flap and serratus anterior flap may all be raised on the same pedicle.

Advantages of latissimus dorsi flap

- Large amounts of tissue transferred
- Pedicled or free tissue transfer
- Cosmetic advantage, especially females
- Versatile: may be tubed/multiple/osseous components
- When pedicled, can reach the upper face and scalp

Despite these advantages, it still remains a musculo-cutaneous flap with thick skin and is therefore more bulky than, for example, a radial free forearm flap. Its use tends to be in filling larger holes in the head and neck and for the repair of neopharyngeal fistulae rather than use within the oral cavity, unless required to repair defects following total glossectomy. Serious donor site problems are rare but dehiscence can be a problem. Congenital absence of the muscle should be checked for prior to surgery, and in athletes and those who do manual work the flap should be raised from the non-dominant side. In addition, raising the flap usually involves turning the patient, but this is not a problem when the surgeon and the theatre staff are thoroughly conversant with the procedure and, in some instances, turning the patient to 45° allows raising of the flap and neck surgery to be carried out simultaneously.

Disadvantages of latissimus dorsi flap

- Very bulky
- Occasional donor site dehiscence
- Reduction in upper limb power
- Need to move patient to harvest

Raising the flap. Small flaps may be raised with the patient supine, but larger flaps require the patient in a lateral thoracotomy position with the upper arm abducted and prepared so that it may be moved around.

Skin may be raised over the whole area of the muscle, although the vascular supply from the thoracodorsal artery decreases as one approaches the lumbosacral fascia. Additional muscle may be harvested at this time to fill a large defect once the skin has been inserted internally (e.g. into a neopharyngeal fistula). A skin graft may then be applied to the muscle externally. The posterior axillary fold is marked out and this represents the anterior edge of the muscle. The posterior iliac crest is also marked, together with the tip of the scapula. The skin flap is designed to the appropriate size and shape, with particular reference to the length of pedicle, if an arc of rotation is required to facilitate transfer to the head and neck via a pedicled myocutaneous flap (Fig. 7.30). This will usually mean an oblique design, but if a free flap is required the flap may be harvested in a horizontal direction, which gives a more acceptable scar in young women since it can be hidden behind the bra strap. Men and older women do not mind a longer oblique scar in this posterior location.

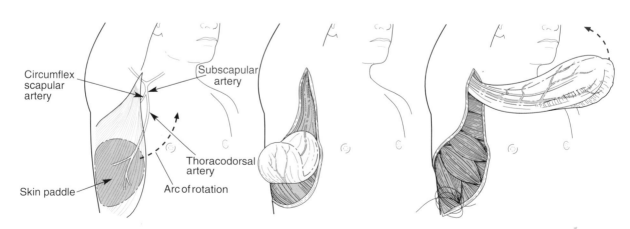

Figure 7.30 Technique of raising the latissimus dorsi flap. When designing for pedicled transfer, an oblique incision is used to allow maximal length to the flap. The dissection begins low down and then the pedicle is identified more proximally as the dissection approaches the axilla.

Elevation of latissimus dorsi

- Outline the flap
- The initial incision exposes the anterior edge of the latissimus dorsi muscle
- Dissect round inferiorly, cutting through the muscle
- Identify the serratus anterior
- Do not go **deep** to serratus anterior here: this places the pedicle under jeopardy
- Recognize serratus anterior as its fibres run at right angles to those of the latissimus dorsi
- Divide latissimus dorsi inferiorly
- The muscle flap may be extended in an anteroposterior direction to provide the covering additional muscle flap for the fistula closure. Remember at this point that if one is low and on top of the latissimus dorsi, the pedicle is not in jeopardy. Elevate the flap in the submuscular plane
- Identify the pedicle running down the muscle, usually in its central portion (Fig. 7.29b). Divide the vessels to serratus anterior
- Continue the dissection up towards the tip of the scapula
- The junction of the thoracodorsal vessels with the circumflex scapular vessels to form the subscapular artery can be clearly seen at the upper anterior end of the muscle in the axilla.
- If only a small flap is required, take the thoracodorsal pedicle here
- If a longer pedicle is required (as is usual), ligate the circumflex scapular vessels now
- Follow the subscapular vessels into the axilla.

At this point, it is usual to island the flap if a free transfer is required. This also facilitates an easier arc of rotation for a pedicled flap. The surgeon may insert a pair of scissors under the latissimus dorsi tendon above the vessels and then cut the muscle to complete the islanding. Further finger dissection into the axilla completes the flap dissection and, if a free flap is needed, the vessels may be clearly isolated and ligated.

If a pedicled transfer is to be completed, the arm is held in the abducted position and dissection takes place from above and below. The axillary artery and vein are very close and care needs to be taken to avoid damage to these two structures. Dissection from above is facilitated by a concomitant neck incision (usually part of a neck dissection), which is extended over the clavicle to give access to the clavipectoral fascia region and the clavicular head of pectoralis major but, if not, a horizontal incision may be made under the clavicle in this region to deliver the flap. Blunt finger dissection in the axilla proceeds on top of the pedicle, going over pectoralis minor and under pectoralis major. Dissection from above is started laterally, goes through the clavipectoral fascia, lateral to the acromiothoracic pedicle, and is facilitated by dividing some of the lateral part of pectoralis major where it attaches to the clavicle. Finger dissection in this region allows

completion of a tunnel to join the dissection from below. By opening up the tunnel from above and below using finger dissection, it is possible to deliver the flap. The tunnel may be widened by dividing the fascial bands that exist under the skin using a scalpel.

Delivery of the latissimus dorsi flap

- Ligate the circumflex scapular artery and vein
- Follow the subscapular vessels into the axilla
- Use blunt finger dissection going on top of the pedicle
- Remember to go 'over pectoralis minor – under pectoralis major'
- Dissect from above through the clavipectoral fascia, dividing some of the lateral fibres of pectoralis major
- Open and widen the tunnel
- Deliver the flap

Some rotation of the pedicle is inevitable but kinking should be avoided. The donor site is closed primarily in two layers using two large drains, one of which should be left for up to a week to avoid a seroma, which can occur following such a large dissection. This can be avoided by suturing the muscle remnants to the chest wall prior to closure. If a free flap is required, then the pedicle may be left attached to the patient while the wound is closed almost to the end. Then the flap may be taken, the wound closed and flap transfer completed. With a pedicled flap, the muscle should be denervated by dividing the nerve. If a free flap is being used, the thoracodorsal nerve may be preserved and used for reinnervation procedures such as anastomosis to a cross facial nerve graft for facial reanimation, or following total glossectomy when postoperative movement has been noted following anastomosis to the hypoglossal nerve.

For very large defects within the head and neck, a pedicled latissimus dorsi may be raised in continuity with a free groin flap, which is then transferred to the head and neck as a pedicled flap, and free tissue transfer completed to the epigastric vessels to revascularize the groin flap.

Sternomastoid flap

The sternocleidomastoid muscle, unlike the previously described muscles, does not have a localized vascular hilum. It is supplied segmentally by vessels which enter the muscle at intervals along its length. There are two principal vessels in its upper half, which consist of two branches of the occipital artery, and in its lower half, a branch from the superior thyroid artery. Further minor arterial branches enter in between. Its use has been described as a myocutaneous flap raised as a composite skin muscle flap, as a myocutaneous skin island flap taking a skin island based over the lower aspect of the muscle (Fig. 7.31) or as a composite muscle–bone flap used for mandibular reconstruction taking a segment of clavicle. Its routine use is not recommended as it has a number of distinct disadvantages.

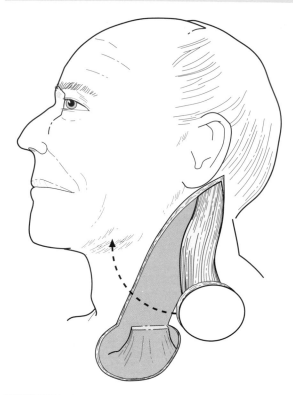

Figure 7.31 Sternomastoid flap.

Disadvantages of the sternomastoid flap

- The upper sternomastoid composite skin muscle flap is poorly viable
- The blood supply to the skin paddle based over the lower third of the muscle is similarly unreliable
- The upper and lower ends of the muscle are areas of oncological significance
- The inclusion of clavicle for mandibular reconstruction is usually no longer required as superior flaps are available

---

The sternomastoid flap is therefore rarely used but it may still have a role to play in two situations. First, it can be particularly useful as a muscle only-flap pedicled superiorly to fill small defects in the pharynx and oral cavity, and second, when split along its length and rotated anteriorly, it may be used to cover vessels in the compromised neck.

Trapezius flap

Three basic myocutaneous flaps have been described which make use of trapezius: the upper trapezius, the lateral trapezius and the lower trapezius flaps. These may be pedicled into the head and neck area and, in addition, descriptions of the upper and lateral trapezius flaps to include transfer of the spine of the scapula have been described for mandibular reconstruction. The vascular supply of these flaps comes via the dominant pedicle supply from the transverse cervical artery.

Although these flaps are reasonably reliable and may play a role particularly in the repair of the posterior aspect of the head and neck, such areas are easily reached with a pedicled latissimus dorsi flap. The possible donor site problems related to the trapezius flap mean that it has almost no role to play in current head and neck reconstructive practice. Its role is principally to salvage, e.g. as a lifeboat when other flaps have been exhausted.

Platysma flap

The platysma flap was first described in 1978. It is really one half of the myocutaneous apron flap and the skin transferred can either be at the level of the hyoid or in the supraclavicular region, after which the donor site is closed primarily. The blood supply to the upper part of the flap comes from the submental branch of the facial artery and to the lower part from a branch of the transverse cervical artery. Although initially attractive as a simple way of providing a method of intraoral reconstruction, this flap has a number of distinct disadvantages and is rarely used today.

Disadvantages of the platysma flap

- Blood supply can be unreliable
- There may have been previous surgery which has violated the neck and therefore precludes its use
- When based on the submental branch of the facial artery, this requires preservation of muscularity in an area of oncological significance which may have to be addressed in the resection
- By and large, the neck should be avoided as a source of reconstruction for the oral cavity
- Removal of the platysma interferes with the blood supply to the overlying skin, which can have disastrous results

---

Stomach transposition

Mobilization of the stomach based on the preservation of the marginal vessels arising from the right gastroepiploic artery and subsequent mobilization into the neck is, in effect, a stomach transposition pedicled flap. Its use in pharyngeal and oesophageal reconstruction is discussed in Chapter 17.

Free tissue transfer

This technique has been introduced into routine head and neck reconstructive clinical practice over the last 10–15 years, but has already revolutionized the approach to filling major surgical defects in this area. Following Seidenberg's first free tissue transfer in

1959 using a revascularized segment of jejunum to reconstruct the cervical oesophagus, there was a gap of some 15 years during which the techniques of microsurgery expanded following the joining of small vessels to enable reimplantation of amputated limbs to take place.

In 1973, a number of descriptions were made of free tissue transfers involving microvascular anastomosis. These included the groin flap which became one of the standard flaps used in the head and neck until the 1980s when a variety of other free flaps were described.

A wide variety of designer flaps are now available to facilitate major tissue transfer to the head and neck. The principle is the reanastomosis of the donor artery and vein to the recipient site to transplant, either singly or in combination, skin, fascia, muscle, tendon, nerve and bone. A transplanted free jejunal graft forms the ideal solution for pharyngeal reconstruction in many cases of hypopharyngeal cancer.

No form of surgery can be learnt only from books and microvascular surgery is no exception. It is technically demanding and requires the appropriate apprenticeship. Having first read it up, one must practise on artificial models and then on animals at one of the various practical courses that are now available. To maintain their expertise, surgeons should practise regularly in the microsurgical laboratory by reanastamosing vessels from fresh placentae, varicose veins obtained at surgery or the vessels of a chicken wing bought from the supermarket. It is important to realize that one has a false sense of security on successful completion of a microvascular course, having joined up vessels on a rat with healthy vessels of similar diameter, at 90° to the hands and plane of vision, and at a preset distance from a fixed microscope head. This is a long way from joining up and reanastamosing an artery behind the mandible when access and vision are less than ideal.

Many beginners, having been full of enthusiasm following many successful anastomoses in the rat, have learnt that in humans the technique is more difficult and that practice makes perfect, particularly with these techniques. Some of the special problems which relate to these issues, including exposure, how to deal with the vascular problems of suturing vessels, and monitoring vessel patency, can to some extent be learnt by assisting someone more experienced. Microvascular surgery is an all-or-none phenomenon. If it works all is well, but if it does not things go wrong very quickly.

Principles of microvascular surgery

Preoperative assessment

The anaesthetist will assess patient suitability for a prolonged general anaesthetic. Many free flaps can now be performed in under 3 h, but some require

longer and this time is at least partly additional to the resection and other elements of the repair. Most operations involving free tissue transfer, e.g. floor of mouth (radial forearm) or hypopharynx (jejunum), can be completed in 6–8 h. Although age is not a contraindication to free tissue transfer, it is an important consideration. The vascular status of both donor and recipient sites should be assessed during the physical examination. The peripheral pulses are carefully palpated and a check made to ensure that pulsation remains when the vessel is occluded distally to prevent backflow. In certain instances such as fibula transfer, a preoperative angiogram may also be required. In addition, further information can be obtained both preoperatively and at operation using Doppler ultrasound. Previous radiotherapy to the head and neck is not a contraindication to free tissue transfer. Ideally, free tissue transfer should be avoided on patients who smoke (as they usually have significant vascular disease) but within the realms of head and neck cancer surgery, this counsel of perfection is usually unrealistic.

Criteria for selecting a free flap

- The length and diameter of the vascular pedicle available
- The type, thickness and colour match of the skin required
- Whether associated tendon, fascia or nerves are needed
- Whether a large composite free flap is required, e.g. vascularized skin with bone
- The morbidity caused by harvesting the flap should be considered

---

Operative assessment

Position

It is uncommon for microvascular free transfer to be carried out without an initial major head and neck resection and, therefore, the surgery time is often lengthy and operative techniques are complex, so that a great deal of skill and patience is required. Microvascular surgery should not be rushed. The surgeon should be well rested and relaxed and a good rapport established among the surgeon, the anaesthetist and all members of the theatre staff. Usually there will be two teams working, one involved with the resection and the other with the reconstruction, since it is usually possible to carry out this type of surgery simultaneously. It is important to take regular breaks and if possible to consider relief staff who can take over from teams who have been operating for longer than 6 h.

In many theatres it is now possible to relay the operation to a television monitor, both in the operating theatre and beyond, so that all members of the team can be involved and visitors can be taught new techniques.

Anaesthetic considerations

Vital anaesthetic considerations in free flap harvest
■ Temperature of
– ambient theatre environment
– operating table
– non-operated parts of the patient
– infused fluids
■ Pain control
■ Blood pressure
– early hypotensive anaesthesia
– pressure restored to perfuse flap

It is important that the anaesthetist is aware of the special techniques related to free tissue transfer and anaesthesia. The maintenance of body temperature is vital if blood flow through a flap is to be maintained. When a free skin flap is raised, this may cause the temperature of the skin to drop by 10°C and such a drop can reduce blood flow dramatically. Steps have to be taken to keep the patient warm and these include keeping the ambient temperature of the operating room as warm as possible; the operating table should be warmed and areas of the patient not involved in surgery should be kept warm with a space blanket. Intravenous fluids and irrigating fluids should be prewarmed and the anaesthetist should monitor the patient's core and peripheral temperature. The control of pain is important since increased adrenaline output may cause spasm of small vessels. The use of hypotensive anaesthesia may be important in the early part of the operation, but as the microvascular anastomosis is completed, the blood pressure should be well maintained to maintain blood flow through the flap. In addition, a fall in the circulating fluid volume will cause reflex vasoconstriction and contribute to variations in blood pressure and temperature. It is important that fluid loss is measured and replaced with warmed fluid, and the central venous pressure and urine output are monitored sequentially. In principle, the blood volume should be maintained and the haemoglobin kept at around 11 g/dl. This results in a high-volume bounding pulse and reduces any sludging of blood cells, which may precipitate thrombosis if the patient is overtransfused.

Surgical technique

Position. It is important that surgeons carrying out microvascular surgery are comfortable in both mind and body, as well as suitably rested and happy with their technique. If possible one should try to sit down both during the raising of the flap and when performing the anastamosis. Whilst this is usually possible when raising, for example, a radial free forearm or a fibula flap, one will usually have to stand when raising a rectus, deep circumflex iliac or latissimus dorsi flap. The most comfortable and the most stable position for prolonged sitting is to have the major joints at right angles to each other. In other words, the feet should be flat on the floor, and the hips and knees should be approximately at right angles,

as should the elbows. The forearm and hands or wrists should at least be supported if at all possible by resting on the patient or a roll of towels, but occasionally this is not possible, particularly if one is standing, and this has to be accepted.

Fogging of the microscope eye pieces or loupes can be reduced by placing adhesive tapes at the top of the mask and by tying the lower strings of the face mask loosely, or allowing it to hang just below the nose so that only the mouth is covered. Microvascular instruments should be held like a writing pen in a pincer grip, with the middle finger supporting the tip, which facilitates the fine and delicate movements that are required to carry out this form of surgery.

Equipment. Otolaryngologists are ideally suited to microvascular surgery, having used the operating microscope (Fig. 7.32a) since it was introduced in 1921 by the otolaryngologist Nylen for the treatment of otosclerosis. Recent developments have further facilitated the ease with which this surgery can be carried out under magnification with the introduction of foot-pedal zoom magnification and X and Y movement control, making the instrument more flexible so that surgeons can keep their eyes on the work and their hands on the instruments, and control the microscope independently with the feet. Coaxial illumination has improved vision and the use of a double-headed microscope, which allows simultaneous vision of the same operating field by the assistant, greatly enhances the performance of the procedure.

Some surgeons prefer to operate under magnification using loupes (Fig. 7.32b). There is no hard and fast rule, but using loupes on larger vessels (greater than 2 mm) appears to speed up the surgical operating time. Results show that for vessels greater than 2 mm in diameter, patency rates and flap survival are no different using either loupes or the microscope. One of the advantages of using loupes is that every time the field of vision needs to be changed, all that is required is a movement of the head rather than having to shift the microscope. In addition, loupes can be used to raise the flap, to isolate and prepare recipient donor vessels and perform the anastomosis. They are available in a number of magnification sizes ranging from × 2.2 up to × 4.5. The most expensive part of equipment for this sort of surgery is the microscope and if loupes are used this reduces the cost even further. However, most theatres have an operating microscope for use in otology and skull-base surgery and these can usually be easily adapted for microvascular surgery.

The instruments that are required are quite simple and a standard set includes jewellers' forceps, vessel-dilating forceps and microvascular clamps, along with the appropriate needle holders and microscissors. These can be obtained commercially for around £3000 per set. Single or double clamps may be used. Single clamps are labelled with an A or a B for use on either arteries or veins and vary in size depending on the vessel in question. Double clamps are used when the surgeon is operating alone and have the advantage of supporting the two ends of the anastomosis, but have the disadvantage of obscuring the amount of tissue tension present and also can prolong the anastomosis time. If possible, it is preferable for the assistant to hold the sutures rather than using a double clamp. The sutures used are usually 8/0, 9/0 or 10/0 monofilament Nylon or Ethilon with a three-eights of a circle tapered-point atraumatic needle, which measures less than 100 μm in diameter.

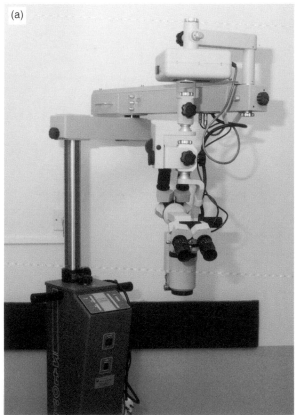

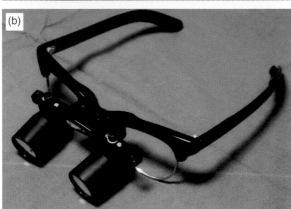

Figure 7.32 (a) Operating microscope (courtesy of D. P. Medical) and (b) a pair of operating loups ×2.2 (Design for Vision).

Basic principles

- A good assistant is essential.
- There must be meticulous atraumatic dissection of both the donor and recipient blood vessels and of any vein grafts that are taken.
- The vessel wall and intima at the site of the anastomosis must be normal under magnification and if there are any abnormalities, it should be resected back until this condition is achieved.
- Normal blood flow must be restored and adequate proximal flow demonstrated.
- Vessels of similar diameter should be used for end-to-end anastomosis.
- End-to-side anastomosis is preferable since it provides for better patency rates.
- The anastomosis should be performed carefully, under no duress without any tension, kinking or tension, with the surgeon in a comfortable position with adequate vision.
- All local overhanging adventitia should be removed. Sutures should be placed without grasping the intima at the appropriate intervals. They should be neither too tight, too close nor too few to facilitate a good anastomosis without any leaks. Vessels may be reanastomosed using either end-to-end or end-to-side anastomosis.

End-to-end anastomosis. End-to-end anastomosis is probably the simplest, most reliable and most widely used method of vascular anastomosis. As this repair is the most basic of all vascular techniques, it must be totally mastered by the budding microvascular surgeon. Blood vessels smaller than 2.5 mm in size should always be anastomosed using this technique since continuous suturing will invariably result in some degree of constriction due to purse-stringing. In smaller vessels, this can make all the difference between success and failure.

The vessels to be anastomosed are adequately mobilized, and excess perivascular connective tissue trimmed under magnification using jewellers' forceps and dissecting scissors. There is no need to do this to excess. Adventitia trimming is necessary to prevent the adventitia being caught in the lumen during the anastomosis, which may lead to thrombosis, and the distal 2–3 mm of the media and intima of the vessel should be exposed and clearly visible.

The vessels are clamped using either single- or double-applicator clamps and are irrigated with heparinized Ringer's solution in a 1 or 2 ml syringe attached to a 22 gauge angiocath. This needs to be repeated intermittently to keep the ends of the vessels clean and free of blood. Excess fluid is removed by microirrigation, which may be controlled by a foot pedal or by using specially designed microswabs.

The vessel walls are then dilated, and the needle is held in the needle holder perpendicular to the edge of the vessel, grasped just beyond the middle portion of the needle shaft and placed 1–2 mm back from the tip of the needle holder. Depending on the position of the patient and the anastomosis, these positions may have to be modified to facilitate suturing. The ends of the vessels are then assessed under magnification and the usual way to proceed with an anastomosis is to use the triple-suture technique described by Correl in his Nobel prize-winning paper in 1905. The anastomosis consists of placing guide sutures 120° apart. The surgeon visualizes their placement and begins by placing two sutures 120° apart, which effectively lift the front wall of the anastomosis away from the back wall. These two sutures are then held either by an assistant or by a cleat on the double approximator clamp, a suture is placed half way between them and the line of the anastomosis between A and B is completed. The vessel is then rotated or the double clamp rotated and the third suture (C) placed at 180° on the back wall of the vessel. At this point the front wall of the anastomosis may be inspected. Using a similar technique as described previously, the vessel wall between B and C is then halved with a suture and the vessel may be rotated by suture traction and the anastomosis completed. The same is done between C and A so that about eight or nine sutures are placed in the vessel wall (Fig. 7.33).

Needle placement is a precise action. The needle should pierce the full thickness of the vessel wall perpendicularly. Oblique passage with the needle should be avoided since it will lead to inversion and interruption of the intima when the knot is tied. The needle entry point should be twice the thickness of the vessel wall away from the edge, equal bites should be taken from each side and the sutures should be an equal distance apart. Suture placement requires both hands and the vessel wall should be manipulated with jeweller' forceps either by holding the adventitia on the outside or by opening the forceps slightly, placing them in the vessel wall and elevating and splaying the vessel wall to allow needle placement, but the intima should not be handled. When the suture has been placed, the thread should always be pulled through right to the end and the needle placed at a reference point from which it can be easily retrieved. The knot is then tied and cut by the assistant. The usual suture length is 10 cm and the shorter the thread becomes, the easier it is to handle. A long suture tail must not be left dangling from a vessel, since it will be difficult to find under magnification. If the microscope is being used, it is common practice to insert the suture under high magnification (×20–30) and then zoom down (×8–16) for tying knots. This flexibility is not available using loupes. Knots are thrown as a double throw for the first knot and a second reverse throw for guide sutures. Regular square knots will normally suffice for the other sutures.

In some situations where access is difficult, it will prove impossible to rotate the vessel, and in this situation the back wall of the anastomosis should be completed first by placing the first 180° suture in the posterior wall and the anastomosis completed in reverse fashion. The same microsurgical technique as described above applies to veins, except that in general the venous anastomosis is more difficult because their walls are thinner and are more

challenging. Whereas the arterial wall is self-supporting, the venous wall collapses and tends to float around in the physiological fluid being used, and placement of the first suture can be very difficult. However, great care should be taken because the placement of the first two or three sutures is crucial to the success of the anastomosis. In general, fewer sutures are needed to complete a venous than an arterial anastomosis.

End-to-end anastomosis

- Mobilize vessels
- Clamp and irrigate
- Trim adventitia
- Perpendicular sutures
- Guide sutures at 120°
- Enter 2 × wall thickness from edge
- Use short threads
- Reduce magnification for tying
- Venous anastomoses are more difficult, but require fewer sutures

---

Releasing the clamps and patency tests. Both arterial and venous anastomoses should usually be completed before the clamps are released. It is uncommon for anastomoses that have been completed successfully completed and that run well at the time of surgery to cause any problems postoperatively. There is no real order to the way in which the anastomosis is completed. The arterial anastomosis is often completed first but, in general, it is better to perform the difficult one first as any problems will be encountered early. Once all of the sutures are inserted, the clamps are removed (the venous one first) and the anastomoses inspected. Blood will flow slowly across the venous anastomosis, dilating the vessel lumen, and invariably there will be some modest leakage which can be controlled with a small swab. Following this, the clamp on the donor artery is released, followed by the recipient artery, and the vessel should dilate completely with pulsation distal to the anastomosis. Minor initial leakage from the anastomosis will usually stop, particularly when a moist swab is placed on it. If there is a significant leak, further suture placement will be required and this is best done, by using the original guide sutures and placement of a further suture whilst leakage continues. This avoids further application of the clamps, which may lead to vascular stasis within the flap. Any significant bleeding from the anastomosis requires formal reapplication of the clamps, reinspection and resuturing as appropriate.

Patency tests. It is important to assess the patency of the anastomosis prior to closure of the surgical wound. The flow in the veins may be assessed by direct observation, and within the thicker walled veins, techniques applied to arteries will apply. Within the arterial system, longitudinal and expansile pulsation maybe observed distal to the arterial anastomosis. The presence of expansile pulsation indicates a patent anastomosis but longitudinal pulsation may be present with partial or complete obstruction to

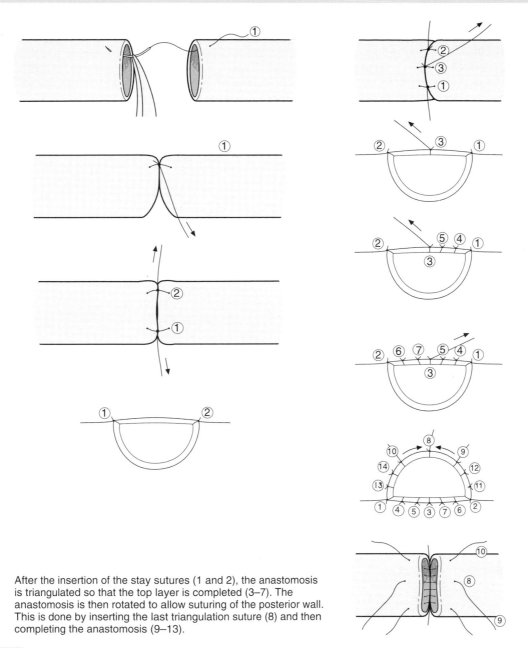

After the insertion of the stay sutures (1 and 2), the anastomosis is triangulated so that the top layer is completed (3–7). The anastomosis is then rotated to allow suturing of the posterior wall. This is done by inserting the last triangulation suture (8) and then completing the anastomosis (9–13).

Figure 7.33 Triple suture technique for end-to-end anastomosis.

blood flow. However, more than observation is required to assess an arterial anastomosis. This is done by the flicker test and the strip test, both of which may be traumatic and should only be done if there is concern about the anastomosis. In the flicker test, a pair of closed forceps is placed beneath the artery distal to the anastomosis and gently raised to stretch the vessel. As the artery is gradually occluded then alternate collapsing and filling of the vessel can be seen when pulsatile flow is present.

The strip test or milking patency test is a more reliable method but can be very traumatic to the vessel endothelium and should only be used if there is significant concern. The artery is occluded with forceps distal to the anastomosis, a second pair of forceps is placed distal to the first and the vessel is stripped for several millimetres in the direction of blood flow. As a result of this, the lumen of the vessel between the two pairs of forceps should contain no blood. Removal of the first pair of forceps should allow the vessel to fill, indicating patency of the anastomosis. However, as described previously, this puts some pressure on the anastomosis and should only be used in extreme circumstances.

Vessel mismatch. There will often be discrepancy between the two ends of vessels. Minor discrepancy will be assessed under magnification and may be dealt with by dilating both ends of the vessels, and appropriate suturing, which takes a little less on the side of the smaller vessel to facilitate dilatation. Where discrepancies approach 2:1, the end of the smaller vessel may be spatulated giving the resultant anastomosis a V shape. Alternatively, the end of the smaller vessel may be cut obliquely to increase the anastomotic circumference. Bevelling of one vessel end results in an angulated anastomosis and the oblique angle should not exceed 30°, as this may lead to excess turbulence. Once the discrepancy between the vessel ends approaches 3:1, then an end-to-side anastomosis should be used (see below).

Vascular spasm. One of the problems with microvascular surgery is that small peripheral arteries often go into spasm when they are resected. This phenomenon explains why, in some circumstances, an end-to-side anastomosis is better than an end-to-end one, as it can overcome this problem. This is seen, for example, if the renal artery is transected following nephrectomy. It is possible (although not recommended) that following transection, a hot swab can be placed on the artery and a coffee break taken, since spasm in the renal artery prevents excessive bleeding. If a major artery is partially transected with an oblique cut, then a significant haemorrhage will happen since spasm does not occur.

Management of spasm

- Careful handling
- Gentle irrigation
- Antispasmodics
- Take down anastomosis
- Abandon flap

Where minor spasm takes place close to the anastomosis site, this may be overcome with gentle dilatation of the vessel ends. Gentle irrigation of the vessel with heparinized Ringer's solution under some pressure may also help, but the technique of forced ram-rodding these solutions under considerable pressure should be avoided since it can cause damage to the intima distally with changes in the microcirculation, which can lead to the no-reflow phenomenon. The gentlest way to avoid spasm is by careful handling of the tissues under the appropriate temperature, but if it does occur it may be dealt with as previously described and the use of local spasmolytic agents such as Verapamil hydrochloride may help. In its absolute form, the no-reflow phenomenon may be observed. In this, despite completing a successful anastomosis, when the clamps are released there will be arterial input into the flap but no venous outflow. In this situation, when temperature, patency and blood pressure are at an optimum and there is still no reflow, then the anastomosis should be dismantled, the flap perfused with heparinized Ringer's solution and spasmolytic agents, and the anastomosis redone. This may solve the problem, but in certain instances if no reflow still persists, then the flap will have to be abandoned and an alternative one used.

End-to-side anastomosis. In head and neck reconstruction, some of the larger free flaps have quite big vessels and many of these require end-to-side anastomosis. As described previously, the basic difference between the two techniques is one of haemodynamic principles, since blood flow is in either a laminar or a turbulent pattern. Laminar flow, as in end-to-end anastomosis, retains kinetic energy but if there is an irregular or angulated flow then this may dissipate energy, which will result in decreased flow rate, thus enhancing platelet aggregation and thrombus formation.

Turbulence is created by any sudden alteration in the direction, velocity or magnitude of blood flow. Therefore, the angle of the union and the size and shape of the recipient vessel orifice are critical to successful end-to-end anastomosis. Normal vascular bifurcations are common in the head and neck and an end-to-side anastomosis performed under ideal conditions with an optimum result may be more reliable than an end-to-end anastomosis. General principles are that the angle of the union between donor and recipient vessels should be as small as possible. Angles of less than 60° are recommended. The size and shape of the recipient vessel are assessed under magnification and the vessel is cleaned. The appropriate arteriotomy or venotomy is then made in a recipient vessel. The anastomosis is often made around a natural bifurcation site, e.g. the junction of the common facial vein with the internal jugular vein, or the origin of the facial artery with the external carotid artery. Depending on the siting of the anastomosis and whether the vessels may be rotated, assessment will dictate whether or not the back wall or the front wall is sutured first. Vessels less than 2 mm in size should be sutured using an interrupted technique but larger vessels (e.g. cephalic vein to internal jugular vein) may be sutured using a continuous suture.

There is no need to have an occlusive clamp on the recipient vessel and if the internal jugular is being used a right-angled vascular clamp is placed to occlude blood flow. The first suture is placed at one end of the anastomosis (Fig. 7.34) and then the back wall may be completed using a running suture and then locked at the other end. Alternatively, two end sutures are placed and the anastamotic line in between completed with interrupted sutures. The anastomosis is then rotated, the posterior suture line inspected and the front wall completed using a similar technique. As the vein walls are flimsy, a good assistant is crucial since with the sutures under tension the two vessel walls may be kept well apart, thus making suturing easy. Interpositional vein grafts are performed as multiple end-to-end anastomoses.

Postoperative care

This is complex surgery and high standards of general postoperative care are required. Patients undergoing free tissue transfer do not automatically need to go to intensive care and can often be cared for on the ward using a dedicated area with one-to-one nursing.

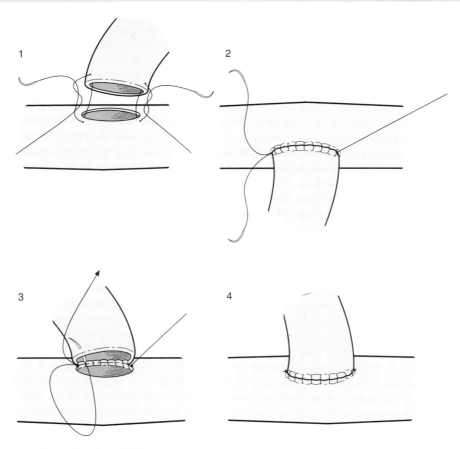

Figure 7.34 The technique of 'end to side' anastomosis.

One of the important deciding factors as to whether or not the patient goes to intensive care is the length of the operation. Once this exceeds the normal working day, i.e. 8 h, the seepage of anaesthetic agents into body fat, along with other mitigating factors, often dictates that the patient will fare better in intensive care overnight. However, nowadays with two teams working this is uncommon.

Monitoring free tissue transfer

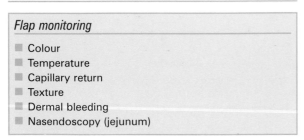

Flap monitoring

- Colour
- Temperature
- Capillary return
- Texture
- Dermal bleeding
- Nasendoscopy (jejunum)

All free flaps require monitoring in the postoperative period. There should be a standard protocol (Fig. 7.35) and, in general, flaps are best assessed by inspection. The colour, temperature and texture, along with the capillary refill time, should all be recorded sequentially and depending on the observations obtained, subsequent clinical assessment guidelines indicate a normal circulation or evidence of either venous or arterial occlusion. There is some debate as to how long these recordings should be undertaken, but certainly all flaps should be inspected regularly up to 48 hours and then intermittently until discharge. This is because if a flap is going to develop any problems, it usually does so within the first 48 hours. Although there are many sophisticated techniques described to monitor free flaps such as using plethysmography, temperature differences or the Doppler principle, these often lead to an increase in false positives and false negatives.

Nowadays, in most units, the above parameters based on clinical observation are used. These can be combined with the technique of dermal bleeding performed by the medical staff where a 20 Fr (green) needle is pricked into the flap to assess the colour of the blood within the flap circulation. Another technique is to make a scalpel mark on the flap at the time of surgery on the flap which may then be wiped by the nursing staff postoperatively and the colour of the ensuing blood assessed. These flap observations are usually made by the nursing staff and if

HEAD AND NECK FLAP CHART

Patient's Name:	Name of Flap:
Registration no:	
Date of Birth:	Recipient site/dressings:
Consultant:	
Surgery Date:	Donor site/dressings:
Medical Instructions:	
	Light source:

DATE														
TIME														
INITIAL														

COLOUR

White														
Pink														
Mottled														
Blue														
Purple														

TEMPERATURE

left/right side	L	R	L	R	L	R	L	R	L	R	L	R	L	R	L	R	L	R	L	R	L	R	L	R	L	R	L	R	L	R
Cold																														
Cool																														
Warm																														
Hot																														

TEXTURE

Soft														
Full														
Tense														
Bulging														

CAPILLARY REFILL TIME

No blanch														
<1 second														
1-2 seconds														
>2 seconds														
No refill														

Figure 7.35 Flap chart (*continued opposite*).

there is any deviation from the norm, the medical staff should be asked to inspect the flap. If there is any worry about the state of the flap, it is wise to return the patient to theatre for assessment of the anastomosis. Free jejunal transfer should be inspected using the nasoendoscope. This is because early arterial failure of this flap may be missed unless a jejunal window is placed externally in the neck wound. Venous occlusion of a free jejunal transfer should be noticed early owing to the high metabolic rate of the small bowel mucosa which sloughs within 24 h leading to the production of large amounts of dark red, frothy sputum.

Commonly used free flaps in head and neck reconstruction

- Latissimus dorsi
- Rectus abdominus
- Jejunum
- Scapula
- Deep circumflex iliac flap
- Fibula

The commonly used free flaps in head and neck reconstruction are discussed in turn.

CLINICAL ASSESSMENT GUIDELINES

Clinical parameter	Normal circulation	Venous occlusion	Arterial occlusion
Colour	Pink	Blue/purple/cyanotic	Pale/mottled blue
Capillary refill time	1-2 seconds	Increased, fast <1 second	Decreased, slow, >2 seconds
Temperature	Warm	Warm-cold	Cool
Tissue turgor	Full	Distended, swollen , tense	Hollow, "Prunelike"
Dermal bleeding (By medical staff instruction only)	Bright red blood	Blood changs from dark red or blue coloured to eventually pink. Bleeds briskly	Minimal blood / absence of any blood. Only serum indicates dead tissue

INFORM MEDICAL STAFF OF ANY CHANGES OUTSIDE THE NORMAL PARAMETERS

POST OPERATIVE RECORDINGS

* Hourly recordings for 2 h

* Two-four hourly recordings for a further 24 h

* Four-six hourly recordings until discharge

(Further recordings to be taken as appropriate)

AFFIX PHOTOGRAPHS BELOW (One to be taken 1 h post operatively to be used as a guide)

PHOTOGRAPH

Figure 7.35 Flap chart (*continued*).

Radial free forearm flap

The radial free forearm flap is a fasciocutaneous flap (Fig. 7.36a) based on the radial artery which was first developed by Drs Yang, Guofan and Gao Yuzhi in 1978. It is sometimes known as the Chinese free forearm flap. Its use in head and neck reconstruction was popularized in the UK by David Soutar's group in Canniesburn, Glasgow.

It is one of the workhorses for head and neck reconstruction, providing pliable skin which may be used to reconstruct three-dimensional defects, particularly within the oral cavity. It can provide skin and fascia and, if required, vascularized tendon, nerve and bone may be combined in the flap. It may be used as a fascial flap for recontouring.

The radial artery sits in a condensation of the deep fascia known as the lateral intermuscular septum. Lying subcutaneously for much of its length in the forearm, it gives off branches to the deep fascia and much of the underlying flexor muscles, and supplies the skin of the forearm

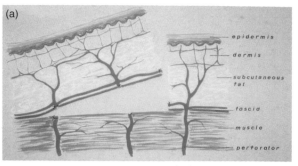

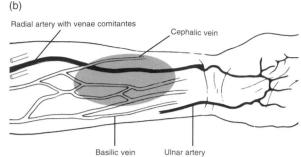

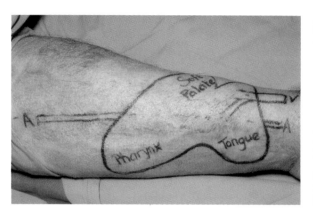

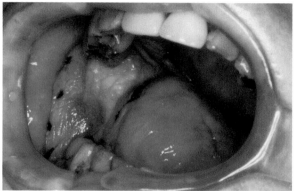

Figure 7.36 (a) Principles of a fascial flap; (b) blood supply to the forearm. (c) The flap may be designed to provide three-dimensional reconstruction to (d) the tongue base, soft palate and tonsillar fossa.

from the elbow to the wrist. In addition, it gives a periosteal blood supply to the underlying radius. Venous drainage is provided both by two venae comitantes which accompany the artery and by a variable pattern of subcutaneous forearm veins which drain into cephalic, basilic and median cubital veins. The nerve supply to the overlying skin is provided by the medial and lateral cutaneous nerves of the forearm (Fig. 7.36b).

A very large amount of tissue may be made available using this flap. The whole of the skin from elbow to wrist may be harvested apart from a narrow strip on the subcutaneous ulnar border. In addition, very small flaps can safely be raised provided a large fascial component is included in the flap. The donor paddle may be placed anywhere on the forearm but in general the further down the forearm, the longer the vascular pedicle and the thinner the flap.

The day before surgery, the patency of the radial artery should be assessed using Allen's test and the result written in the notes. It is wise to use the non-dominant hand. In Allen's test, the patient is asked to open and close his or her wrist rapidly 10 times while the radial and ulnar arteries are occluded with the surgeon's fingers. The patient then opens the fist and the skin of the hand will

be white. The finger is then released over the ulnar artery and if it is patent, the skin of the palm will become pink. This test is usually reliable but if there is any doubt about ulnar artery patency, further assessment may be necessary such as Doppler arteriography or the advice of a vascular surgeon. If the flap cannot be used, then the contralateral forearm should be investigated or an alternative option sought.

Once the surgical defect has been assessed, the flap is marked out and it is usual for a separate team to begin work synchronously with the excisional team. It is wise to use a tourniquet, which should be applied prior to preparing the patient. The arm is then preped, the wrist wrapped in a separate crêpe bandage, the arm elevated for 5 min and the tourniquet inflated to a level approximately twice the blood pressure. It should not be left inflated for longer than 90 min. The arm is then laid out on a support board. The flap is outlined, together with the markings of the radial artery and subcutaneous forearm veins if they are to be used. These may be mapped on the day before surgery by using Doppler to identify the arteries and applying a tourniquet to identify the veins. This procedure may be facilitated by placing the patient's hand in some warm water for 10 min.

Dissection is begun by incising the ulnar border of the flap, dividing skin and subcutaneous tissues and taking the fascia on the flap by removing it from the underlying muscle. The epimysium over the muscle should be left. Dissection is best performed using magnifying loupes (× 2) and haemostasis achieved using bipolar diathermy or ligaclips. The dissection is continued, distally and laterally, until the condensation of deep fascia surrounding the radial artery and venae comitantes is reached. It is important to take care at this point because this is where one of the common mistakes in raising the flap can be made. The radial artery sits in a condensation of the intermuscular septum in a trench in between the brachioradialis and flexor carpi ulnaris, and flap elevation must allow the artery to be raised with the septum. If the dissection is carried across horizontally to the lateral edge at this point over the top of the intermuscular septum the artery will be separated from the undersurface of the flap. At this point either the lateral or medial cutaneous nerves of the forearm may be identified and preserved and a piece of palmaris longis tendon taken if needed. The radial artery in its intramuscular septum is then identified lying between the flexor carpi ulnaris and brachioradialis.

Elevation of the flap then continues proximally following the vascular pedicle up and preserving the superficial venous system as required. As the flap is reliable using the superficial venous system and the vessels are quite large (the cephalic vein is sometimes 1 cm in diameter) they can be used, but it is advisable that if bone is being taken, the venae comitantes should be used as well as or instead of the superficial system. When raising the flap proximally, the perforators between the radial artery and the radius should be ligated, but if bone is being taken they should be preserved. Up to 10 cm of bone may be taken with the flap between pronator teres and pronator quadratus. It is important that the attachment of the lateral intermuscular septum to the periosteum and the radius be preserved intact and a boat-shaped segment of bone taken, being harvested first in pronation and then in supination. The thickness of bone that can be taken with safety is less than half the cross-section of the radius. Any greater resection will lead to inevitable fracture. Once the flap is raised and the arterial and venous pedicles have been identified, the tourniquet is deflated and the flap left to perfuse for 20–30 min when its vascular viability can be assessed prior to transfer.

If very small flaps are taken or if only a fascial flap is used, the donor site may be closed primarily. In elderly people, larger areas may be closed primarily using an ulnar transposition flap (Fig. 7.37). Otherwise, the donor site is closed using either a split or full-thickness skin graft and take is usually satisfactory as long as the epimysium of the muscles and the paratenon over the tendons have been left intact. If not, skin grafting may be unsuccessful and a rotation flap required. The arm should be wrapped in a crêpe bandage and elevated in a Bradford sling for a week. Where bone is removed, it should be protected in plaster of Paris for about 3 weeks.

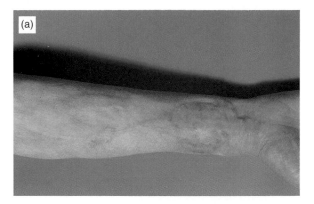
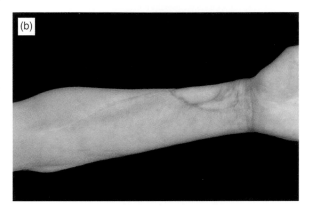
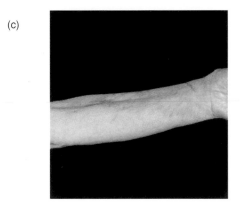

Figure 7.37 Postoperative result of the radial forearm donor site. Note that the defect can be repaired using either (a) split skin graft, (b) a full-thickness skin graft, or (c) the use of an ulnar transposition flap.

This flap has several important advantages. Its vascular anatomy can be assessed preoperatively, it is highly reliable and easy to raise, and provides thin, pliable skin which is well suited to three-dimensional intraoral reconstruction. In addition, it offers the possibility for reinnervation via the two cutaneous forearm nerves to provide a sensate flap. Vascularized tendon can also be transferred in the form of palmaris longus, and short segments of bone as part of an osteocutaneous flap are also possible. The vessels are large (approximately 2–3 mm diameter) and a long pedicle is possible. It has few disadvantages. The major one is that a graft may be required to the donor site; however, the take rate is good and the subsequent defect can be well hidden. It is an excellent flap.

Advantages of radial free forearm flap

- Preoperative assessment is possible
- Easy to raise
- Reliable
- Thin, pliable skin
- Long pedicle
- Good sized vessels
- Versatile

Latissimus dorsi flap

This has been described already in this chapter. A free latissimus dorsi flap is exactly the same as a pedicled one, except that detachment provides greater manoeuvrability.

Rectus abdominus flap

This flap has a type III vascular supply with two dominant vascular pedicles entering at either end of the muscle.

The muscle extends from the pubic tubercle and pubic crest up to the fifth, sixth and seventh costal cartilages. It is a paired muscle representing a strategic part of the anterior abdominal wall.

The blood supply is via the superior and inferior epigastric vessels which run on its undersurface and anastomose freely with each other (Fig. 7.38). The larger pedicle includes the inferior epigastric artery (and vein) which arises directly from the external iliac artery and passes from lateral to medial to lie on the undersurface of the rectus muscle. It lies between this muscle and the peritoneum below the arcuate line and between the muscle and the posterior rectus sheath above this point. Branches supply the muscle and perforators supply the skin, and there is an area of dominant perforation in the para-umbilical area supplying the skin around this area. It is possible to take a small amount of muscle containing two or three perforators which will supply a large amount of skin in this area.

The rectus abdominus can be raised either as a muscle flap or more commonly as a myocutaneous flap. Transfer may be completed either as a pedicled flap to the sternal area or more commonly as free tissue transfer. Pedicled transfer can be based on the superior epigastric vessels when muscle-only flaps in particular can be used to repair sternal defects but, more commonly within the head and neck, a flap is transferred as a free one based on the inferior epigastric vessels. The amount of tissue that is available can be huge. Flaps in lax individuals can be

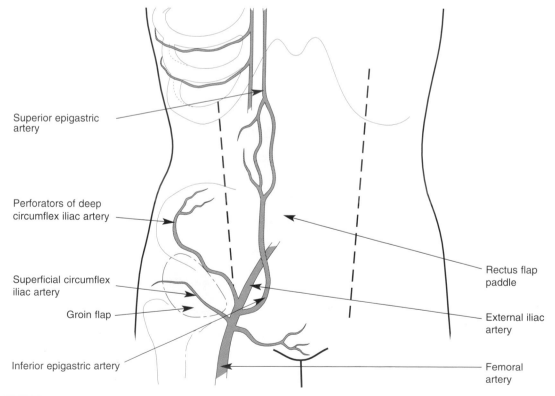

Figure 7.38 Blood supply and position of the skin paddle for the rectus abdominus myocutaneous flap.

raised measuring 45 × 15 cm. Primary closure should always be achieved and as there is no posterior rectus sheath below the arcuate line, postoperative herniation should be avoided by using some Marlex mesh which can be sewn to the surrounding fascia or used to repair the posterior abdominal wall. Alternatively, a contralateral rectus abdominal anterior sheath flap may be used.

One of the main advantages of this flap is that it can be raised in the supine position and can be harvested by a second team while the primary surgical team is working in the neck. Further advantages include greater variation in size, shape and design and it is extremely reliable. It has a constant and reliable vascular pedicle with large sized vessels (3 mm), and when the flap is designed transversely an associated effective abdominoplasty may be completed. Its disadvantages are that it may be bulky and, unless care is taken in closing the abdominal wall, ventral herniation can be a problem. However, in experienced hands it provides a useful alternative to the latissimus dorsi myocutaneous flap.

Raising the Rectus abdominus flap

If muscle alone is being raised, then this may be done rapidly through a paramedian incision. The inferior epigastric pedicle enters the muscle on the posterolateral aspect. The rectus sheath is identified and opened and the muscle mobilized to the appropriate size, beginning superiorly, then followed down so that the vessels are identified and the pedicles isolated.

The design of the musculocutaneous flap requires careful consideration. Small flaps may be designed overlying one rectus muscle. The flap is outlined (Fig. 7.38) and dissection completed through skin, subcutaneous tissue and down to the anterior rectus sheath. This can be done rapidly through a paramedian incision. The rectus sheath is entered laterally, the flap is raised from lateral to medial and the appropriate amount of rectus abdominus muscle taken, which will include the perforators to supply the skin paddle. In this situation in the paraumbilical area, the skin paddle can safely be extended 3–4 cm across the midline. Following isolation of the muscle, it is raised as described previously. Larger areas of skin (30 × 15 cm) may be obtained by making use of the paraumbilical perforators so that a transverse flap (tram flap or large oblique flap) may be designed. Meticulous closure is required. Care is taken to approximate each layer of the closure and repair of the posterior abdominal wall performed with Marlex mesh as required.

Free jejunal flap

The free jejunal transfer is the reconstruction of choice, oncological conditions permitting, for repairing large pharyngeal defects created by the resection of tumours in the hypopharynx and cervical oesophagus. Its advantages are that segments of small bowel can be removed without functionally impairing either absorption or digestion, a length of jejunum in excess of 20 cm can be obtained and

the process repeated two or three times in the unusual event of flap failure. In the elective situation, the risks from this surgery are minimal and it has the added advantage that the chest is not violated.

The 10–16 arteries to the small intestine arise from the superior mesenteric artery. They pass between the layers of the mesentery, each dividing into two branches that anastomose with the adjacent artery to form a series of arcades that give off secondary branches to supply the gut. The upper jejunal branches form only one to two arcades, but the process of division is repeated three or four times in the ileal arteries, forming four or five arterial tiers. Venous drainage accompanies the arteries and while it is usually possible to isolate any segment of jejunum on a suitable arcade of vessels, in practice the second or third loops of jejunum have proved consistently reliable.

The abdomen is prepared and opened through an upper transverse or paramedian incision, the jejunum identified and a suitable loop of adequate length chosen. The vessels can be identified by holding up the mesentery against the light. The artery and vein are then followed to their attachments at the superior mesenteric artery and vein and the mesentery is divided into a V shape, dividing any lateral branches (Fig. 7.39).

Bowel clamps are placed across the bowel at the proximal and distal ends. The proximal and distal ends of the jejunal loop to be used are isolated by either using a stapling device or clamp, or simply oversewing them. The bowel is divided and the loop allowed to perfuse while a jejunojejunal anastomosis is performed to restore intestinal continuity. The vascular pedicle of the jejunum is isolated using loupes and, when the recipient vessels have been prepared in the neck, they are clamped and ligated and the transfer completed.

The operation is performed under the cover of prophylactic antibiotics, the abdomen is closed in layers with no drain, and in high-risk patients a jejunostomy may be performed. In the authors' practice, the jejunal loop is then placed in ice-cold Ringer's solution for approximately 10 min and transferred to the neck, where the vascular anastomosis is completed. The artery varies in size from 1 to 3 mm as does the vein, but particular care needs to be taken with the latter as it is often flimsy. The jejunum is sewn in to ensure an isoperistaltic anastomosis and it is important not to put in too long a loop

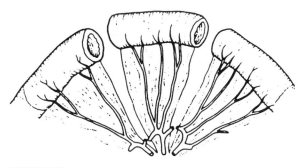

Figure 7.39 Free jejunal flap.

length, which can lead to functional dysphagia. A one-layer anastomosis with continuous 3/0 prolene is completed at the upper and lower ends, and a nasogastric tube is inserted prior to completion. Depending on the size and shape of the oropharyngeal defect, the jejunum may be left closed in its proximal part and an end-to-side anastomosis fashioned to accommodate the greater oropharyngeal diameter. One of the other advantages of this flap is that it can be raised simultaneously using two teams. Whilst some authors have suggested monitoring the flap by isolating a separate loop and bringing it out on to the neck skin as a window, this is not always reliable, there are inevitable false-positives and false-negatives, and the flap can easily be monitored daily using flexible nasopharyngoscopy. Failure should be treated where possible (when salvage is not feasible), by another immediate free jejunal transfer.

Scapular flap

The scapular flap is principally a cutaneous flap based on the cutaneous branch of the circumflex scapular artery which arises from the subscapular artery (Fig. 7.40). This artery passes posteriorly through the triangular space formed by the long head of triceps laterally, teres minor above and the teres major below. The cutaneous branch supplying the skin runs more or less horizontally and the skin paddle is usually designed in this direction, although it is possible to take a parascapular flap which runs in a more oblique direction along the lateral border of the scapula. Venous drainage is by the venae comitantes that accompany the artery. It is also possible to take bone from the lateral border of the scapula (up to 14 cm) as long as some of the teres muscles are left on the bone.

Raising the flap

The patient is turned to the prone position and the arm abducted. The flap is marked out and its size depends on the laxity of skin, since primary closure should always be achieved. It is possible to take large flaps measuring 25 × 12 cm.

The flap is raised from medial to lateral and this ensures that the cutaneous artery is preserved when the triangular space is identified. At this point the pedicle is short and the arterial vessel size between 1 and 2 mm. The pedicle may be lengthened by dividing the circumflex scapular artery and tracing it anteriorly to the subscapular vessels. This increases the pedicle length to around 14 cm and the vessel diameter up to 3 mm.

The advantage of the scapular cutaneous flap is that it is safe and reliable. As a pure cutaneous flap it has few advantages over other skin flaps such as the radial free forearm flap, but may be of use where thicker skin is required. Its major advantage is in that it can provide a combination of both scapular and parascapular skin flaps which can be used for inside and outside cover and combined with a length of bone from the scapula for composite transfer. This therefore makes it useful in oral reconstruction. The bone may be used for complete hemi-mandibular reconstruction or, when osteotomized, for defects in the anterior mandibular arch. Its main attraction is the combination of bone with double skin flaps to provide versatile three-dimensional reconstruction.

The donor site is closed directly which can give a good linear scar but may, over time, separate. With bone removed from the lateral border, the remaining teres muscles which have been divided should be sutured in layers. The main disadvantage of the scapular flap is that the patient has to be turned, but this is outweighed by the versatility described, although the skin element is not a candidate for sensate reinnervation.

Three-dimensional flaps are possible using the unique anatomy of the subscapular arterial tree combined with the latissimus dorsi and serratus anterior muscles, along with overlying skin and adjacent segments of rib. In addition, two separate segments of bone from the scapula are possible. The scapula consists of cortical and cancellous bone similar to the iliac crest, it is suitable for osseointegration, but can be a little thin in females.

Deep circumflex iliac flap

This is a composite groin flap based on the deep circumflex iliac artery (DCIA) which arises from the external iliac artery just above the inguinal ligament (Fig. 7.41). Venous drainage is via the venae comitantes which unite to form a large, single vein that drains into the external iliac vein. This vascular pedicle gives an excellent blood supply to the iliac crest and a somewhat variable supply to the skin situated over the iliac crest, which is posterior and lateral to the anterior iliac spine.

It permits both osseous and osseocutaneous free tissue transfer and its main use is in oromandibular and maxillary reconstruction.

Raising the flap

The anterior superior iliac spine, the public tubercle and the line of the inguinal ligament are all marked. The femoral vessels are palpated, the course of the iliac vessels is noted and a point 1 cm above the inguinal ligament in the line of the iliac artery acts as a surface marker for the origin of the deep circumflex iliac vessels. A line is then drawn parallel to the iliac ligament towards the anterior superior iliac spine to mark the course of the pedicle and, if skin is required, the appropriate skin paddle is marked out at this time.

A transinguinal approach over the external iliac artery allows identification of the inferior epigastric artery which acts as a marker for the origin of the deep circumflex iliac artery. The pedicle is identified and followed, and as the anterior superior iliac spine is approached the ascending branch of the deep circumflex iliac artery is identified. This pierces the transverse abdominus muscle and the internal oblique, and supplies both of these muscles. The main branch continues on the iliacus in a groove between it and the transversalis fascia. Both of these branches need to be preserved and once they have been identified, the inguinal dissection is complete and the lateral dissection

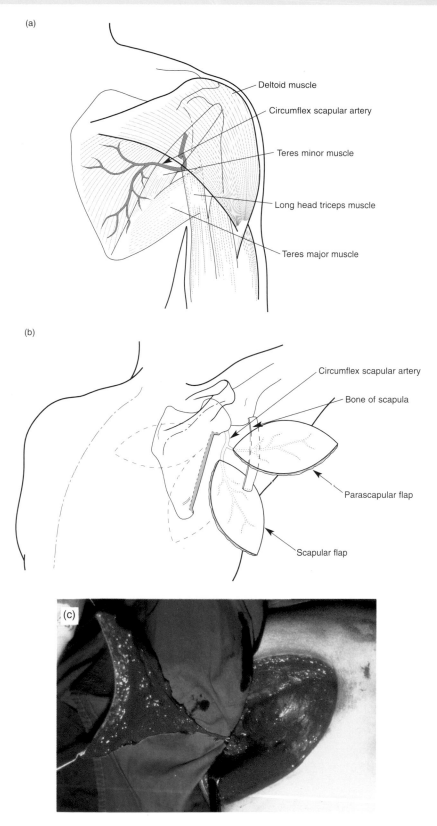

(a)

- Deltoid muscle
- Circumflex scapular artery
- Teres minor muscle
- Long head triceps muscle
- Teres major muscle

(b)

- Circumflex scapular artery
- Bone of scapula
- Parascapular flap
- Scapular flap

(c)

Figure 7.40 Blood supply to the scapula flap. (a) Note that the circumflex scapular artery and vein emerge from the lateral aspect of the scapula through a muscular triangle which is usually palpable 2 cm superior to the posterior axillary crease. (b) It is possible to use the horizontal as well as the descending branch of the circumflex scapular artery to supply a skin flap accompanied by a segment of scapula. (c) The elevated flap.

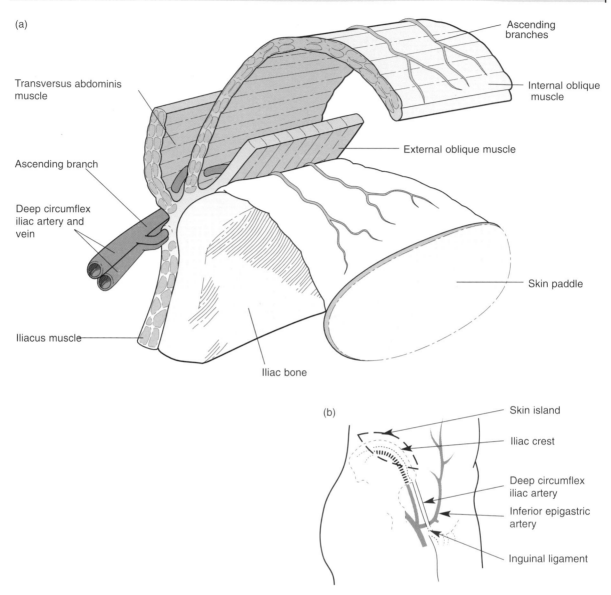

(a)

Ascending branches

Transversus abdominis muscle

Internal oblique muscle

Ascending branch

External oblique muscle

Deep circumflex iliac artery and vein

Skin paddle

Iliacus muscle

Iliac bone

(b)

Skin island

Iliac crest

Deep circumflex iliac artery

Inferior epigastric artery

Inguinal ligament

Figure 7.41 Blood supply to the deep circumflex iliac (DCIA) flap. (a) Cuffs of the iliacus and external oblique muscles are harvested with the internal oblique muscle to protect the skin perforators. (b) Blood supply and positioning of the skin island.

completed by dividing the origin of tensor fascia lata and the attachment of the gluteal muscles to reach the outer plate of the iliac bone. Medially, the skin is incised down to the external oblique fascia and the external oblique incised parallel to the iliac crest along with the internal oblique and transversus muscle. The vascular pedicle lies attached to the iliacus and the inner plate of the iliac bone.

Once both sides of the iliac bone have been exposed, the appropriate bony cuts can be made to remove the bone and flap as required.

The advantages of this flap are that it provides larger segments of vascularized bone which may be used for hemimandibular or maxillary reconstruction. The patient does not require turning, the vascular pedicle is moderate (at least 6 cm) and the vessels are of average size (3 mm). The disadvantages are that it is difficult to raise,

and gives rise to significant morbidity since an abdominal hernia is a distinct possibility following closure of the surgical defect. In addition, the skin paddle lacks mobility on the bone and can be unreliable. This can be overcome by not taking skin and replacing it with a large part of internal oblique which can then be skin grafted. The iliac crest is capable of reconstructing defects in the mandible as short as 6 cm or as long as 18 cm.

It is ideally suited for bone-only defects since the natural curvature of the pelvis facilitates hemimandibular reconstruction using either the contralateral or ipsilateral hip. It is also ideal for large composite defects of the mandible and maxilla where excessive flap bulk is not a problem. For smaller mandibular defects, the scapular composite or radial free forearm flaps are better choices. Sensate restoration of the skin paddle to an iliac crest composite flap has not been reported and the problem with the poor blood supply to the overlying skin paddle may be overcome by using the tripartite flap, as described by Urken *et al.* (1995). This includes the external oblique, internal oblique and transverse abdominus, as well as iliacus, which improves the blood supply to the skin paddle, or not taking a skin paddle at all and taking a large portion of internal oblique which can then be skin grafted. The iliac crest composite flap has been used in the reconstruction of mandibular, maxillary and hard palate defects as well as defects in the skull. In addition, the iliac bone is composed of a thick layer of cancellous bone sandwiched between two layers of cortical bone, which on cross-sectional area is greater than either the fibula, scapula or radius. It offers a wide range of bony orientations and is suitable to receive endosteal osseointegrated dental implants.

Fibula flap

The fibula provides a superb donor site for vascularized bone, which may be used to reconstruct large mandibular defects from angle to angle. It is also useful for maxillary reconstruction. It has a tubular shape with thick cortical bone, which renders it one of the strongest bones possible for free tissue transfer and can be used for endosteous dental implants. Up to 20 and even 25 cm of bone can be harvested and an ellipse of the overlying skin may also be taken to provide an osteocutaneous flap.

The fibula is supplied by a nutrient artery arising from the peroneal artery (Fig. 7.42a). This enters the medial surface of the bone just above its midpoint and it is this artery that is used for subsequent anastomosis. The pedicle is usually up to 8 cm in length. Venous drainage is via the venae comitantes. The skin paddle is a fasciocutaneous flap centred on the peroneal intermuscular septum and therefore the deep fascia must always be included when the flap is raised (Fig. 7.42b).

Preoperative assessment will usually include angiography to assess the vascular supply. There is some uncertainty in the blood supply to the skin of the fibula osteocutaneous flap. This must be accepted and postoperative injury to the common peroneal nerve is possible. Minor functional deficits such as weakness in dorsiflexion of the great toe along with scarring and weakness of flexor hallucis longis have all been described.

The flap is raised with the patient supine and the knee flexed. A tourniquet may or may not be applied. The fibula is palpated under the skin and a line is drawn from the head of the fibula to the lateral malleolus. The segment of bone to be used is based on the midportion of the fibula (Fig. 7.42) and at this point the flap of skin is marked as appropriate. Where a skin paddle is to be used, a wide fringe of deep fascia centred over the bone is included, as well as the peroneal muscles at the posterior edge of the fibula. This means that a cuff of tibialis posterior and flexor hallucis longus must be included.

The dissection begins by mobilizing the skin paddle and preserving a cuff of attached muscles posteriorly so

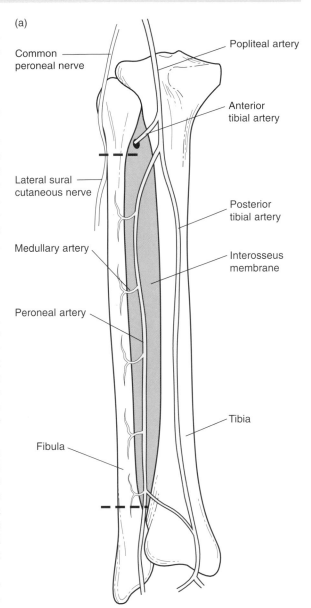

(a)

Figure 7.42 (a) Posterior view of the left leg showing the position of the perineal artery and the blood supply to the middle two-thirds of the fibula. Note the position of the common perineal nerve. (b) and (c) are overleaf.

that the integrity of the peroneal vessels is preserved. The key to dissection is early division of the bone which allows easy identification of the peroneal vessels. The pedicle is first identified distally and the artery and venae comitantes are divided. This allows elevation of the fibula proximally and the pedicle can be dissected up to the trifurcation of the popliteal artery. The bone is divided using either a reciprocating or Gigli saw.

The pedicle is short, and for head and neck reconstruction it may be necessary to take a saphenous vein graft and perform an arteriovenous fistula within the neck, i.e. joining the external carotid artery or one of its branches to the internal jugular vein with the graft and

(b)

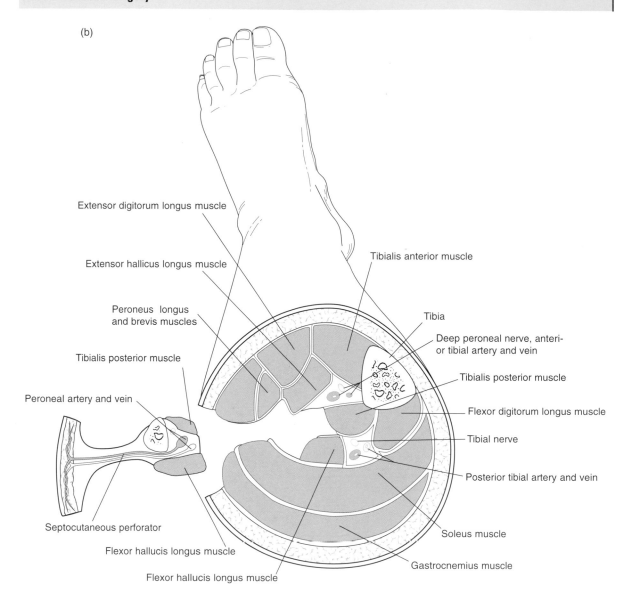

Extensor digitorum longus muscle

Extensor hallicus longus muscle

Peroneus longus and brevis muscles

Tibialis posterior muscle

Peroneal artery and vein

Septocutaneous perforator

Flexor hallucis longus muscle

Flexor hallucis longus muscle

Tibialis anterior muscle

Tibia

Deep peroneal nerve, anterior tibial artery and vein

Tibialis posterior muscle

Flexor digitorum longus muscle

Tibial nerve

Posterior tibial artery and vein

Soleus muscle

Gastrocnemius muscle

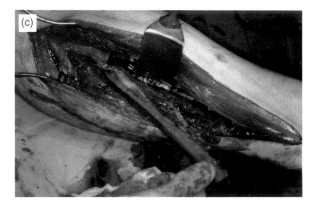

(c)

Figure 7.42 *Continued.* (b) Cross-section of the lower leg showing the elevation of a free fibula osseocutaneous flap. (c) Free fibula osseous-only flap being raised. The pedicle with a cuff of tibialis posterior muscle is arrowed.

allowing this to function. Following inset of the flap, this fistula may be divided to give arterial and venous pedicles which may then be anastomosed to the vascular pedicle of the flap.

The fibula flap (bone only) provides good strong cortical bone which is reliable (Fig. 7.42c). The donor defect will usually close primarily but when large amounts of skin are taken, skin grafts may be required. Its major disadvantage is that the skin paddle may be unreliable, but in experienced hands this is not usually a problem since a second flap (such as the radial free forearm) may be used to provide skin cover. The fibula flap is ideally suited for the reconstruction of angle-to-angle mandibular defects (Shpitzer *et al.*, 1997).

Occasionally used free flaps in head and neck reconstruction

- Lateral arm flap
- Pectoralis minor flap
- Temporoparietal flap
- Groin flap
- Gracilis flap
- Serratus anterior flap
- Omentum flap

Lateral arm flap

This was described in 1982 and is a fasciocutaneous flap. It is based on the profunda brachii artery and, if required, a segment of humerus, triceps tendon and two nerves, one of which can act as a sensory supply and the other as a vascularized nerve graft, can be transferred with skin. It is a plumper graft than the radial free forearm, and the donor defect can be closed primarily.

The profunda brachii vessels are approximately 2.5 mm in size, and there is a superficial and deep venous system drainage. The superficial system drains through the cephalic vein while the deep system drains through paired venae commitantes, which are around 2.5 mm in diameter. The nerve that supplies the sensation to the skin of the lateral arm flap is the posterior cutaneous nerve of the arm, a branch of the radial nerve. In addition, branches of the posterior cutaneous nerve of the forearm can be used where a vascularized nerve graft is required.

The profunda brachii artery arises from the brachial artery and curves around the posterior aspect of the humerus and the spiral groove to reach the lateral intermuscular septum, where it divides into two branches, the anterior and posterior radial collateral arteries. The posterial radial collateral artery is the artery of the lateral arm flap. During its course through the lateral intermuscular septum, it supplies the skin of the posterior lateral aspect of the distal half of the upper arm and gives a periosteal blood supply to segments of the underlying humerus. The artery may be harvested without any concern for loss of function.

The flap elevation begins posteriorly with an incision through the deep fascia and the flap is elevated subfascially over the triceps. The neurovascular pedicle is identified, and anterior radial collateral artery together with the radial nerve are identified passing between the brachioradialis and brachialis muscles. The radial nerve should be isolated and preserved and the anterior radial collateral vessels ligated and divided. A long vascular pedicle of 6–10 cm can be gained by dissecting up into the spiral groove. If humerus is required, then segments of the lateral head of the triceps and brachioradialis should be included with the lateral intermuscular septum.

Pectoralis minor flap

The pectoralis minor is a flat, triangular muscle arising from the second, third, fourth and usually the fifth ribs and is inserted by a flat tendon into the coracoid process (Fig. 7.43). It is supplied by the pectoral branch of the thoracoacromial artery and venous drainage is through the venae commitantes. The nerve supply is the medial pectoral nerve.

The flap is raised by retracting pectoralis major, and sometimes this muscle has to be divided to gain access. The short vascular pedicle to the pectoralis minor is identified and the muscle removed along with its neurovascular pedicle. The artery is approximately 2 mm in size but the pedicle is short.

This muscle may be used for facial reanimation. A cross-facial sural nerve graft is taken from the buccal branch of the facial nerve on the patient's good side and placed across the lip into the ipsilateral face. Growth along the graft is plotted using the Tinel sign.

After 6–12 months, a pectoralis minor free tissue transfer graft is placed *in situ*. Microvascular anastomosis can be completed to either the superficial temporal or facial vessels. The medial pectoral nerve is anastomosed to the sural nerve graft and the slips of pectoralis minor are placed appropriately in the upper and lower lip, nasolabial fold and lateral canthal region.

Temporoparietal flap

The temporoparietal fascial (TPF) flap is based on the superficial temporal artery and accompanying vein and both the anterior and posterior branches of the artery can be included. The extent of the fascial flap conforms to the outline of the temporalis muscle and can be extended to include up to 2 cm of pericranium. The vessel size is in the order of 1.5–2 mm and the pedicle length is short, measuring no more than 3 cm. The flap can be used as a transposition flap to repair defects on the ear, temple and parotid region and can then be skin grafted. Alternatively, it can be used as a free flap in, for example, hemilaryngeal reconstruction where it is used to envelop a neocord created from a free cartilage graft from the contralateral thyroid ala.

Groin flap

This was the first free cutaneous flap to be used in head and neck reconstruction. It is an axial pattern flap and was described by McGregor and Jackson in 1972. It is based

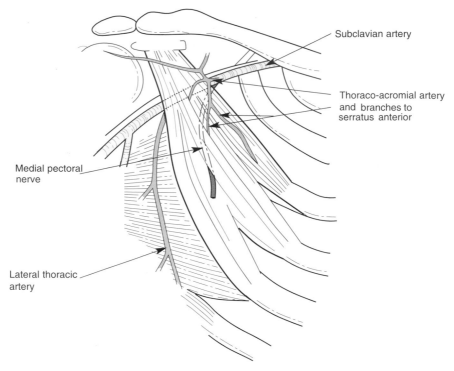

Figure 7.43 Blood supply to the pectoralis minor flap.

on the superficial circumflex iliac artery which arises from the femoral artery. Occasionally, it may have a common origin from the latter artery with the superficial epigastric artery. The artery runs laterally parallel to the inguinal ligament and the medial border of the sartorius muscle, where it gives off a deep branch before continuing superficial to this muscle. Venous drainage is via the superficial circumflex iliac vein and a deep system consisting of venae commitantes, which usually accompany the artery and drain into the femoral vein. Flaps up to 20 cm long and 10 cm wide can be safely harvested and the donor site closed primarily. The flap is drawn out using a number of surface markers. The anterior superior iliac spine and pubic tubercle are palpated and the inguinal ligament is drawn between them. A point 1 inch below the inguinal ligament is marked on the skin overlying the femoral artery and this is the surface marking of the origin of the superficial circumflex iliac artery (Fig. 7.41). A line drawn laterally marks the course of this artery and acts as the central axis for the flap.

Flap dissection begins medially by identifying the origin of the superficial circumflex iliac artery. Superficial and deep veins are identified and variations in anatomy noted. Flap dissection then continues laterally, superficial to the deep fascia and medial to the anterior superior iliac spine. The deep fascia should be included as this corresponds to the lateral border of sartorius and subfascial dissection at this point ensures that the superficial circumflex iliac artery is included.

This flap has a short pedicle (3 cm) and the average diameter of the artery vessels is 1.5 mm. It is not used very often in head and neck reconstruction because of this

short pedicle and its variable vascularity. However, once de-epithelialized, it provides a very good bulking flap with dermis, fascia and fat which can be used as a vascularized plumping graft to fill in hemifacial defects following surgery, such as following previous maxillectomy. The dermis allows placement of nonabsorbable sutures and the graft can be fixed in position so that it does not prolapse with time.

Gracilis flap

The gracilis muscle may be used as a free muscle transfer. It is a thin strap-like muscle which arises from the pubic symphysis and inserts in the medial tibial condyle. It has a type II vascular pattern with a dominant pedicle and a number of minor pedicles. The dominant pedicle is a branch of the medial circumflex femoral artery, which enters the muscle 10 cm from its origin. This is a branch of the profunda femoris artery. Venous drainage is via venae comitantes which accompany the arteries and the nerve supply is from the anterior branches of the obturator nerve which enter the muscle with the dominant vascular pedicle.

The flap is raised along an incision line drawn from the pubic tubercle to the medial tibial condyle. The muscle is mobilized, the medial circumflex femoral artery with accompanying veins and nerve identified and the artery may be followed back to the origin of the profunda femoris to obtain a pedicle length of around 8 cm. The vessel diameters are around 2 mm.

It is transferred in a similar manner to pectoralis minor for facial reanimation, but is a bulkier muscle and does not have the flat, slip-like morphology of the pectoralis minor. This problem may be overcome by raising only part of the muscle and performing a fascicular nerve dissection, removing only those fibres supplying a part of the muscle.

Serratus anterior flap

The serratus anterior muscle is a broad flat muscle which arises in slips from the outer surface of the superior borders of the upper 8–10 ribs and inserts on to the costal surface of the medial border of the scapula.

Its blood supply is via the thoracodorsal artery (Fig. 7.29) and is innervated by the long thoracic nerve of Bell. It is raised by an incision made in the posterior axillary fold. By retracting the latissimus dorsi muscle, both serratus anterior and its pedicle will be identified as described previously (see latissimus dorsi flap). A vascular pedicle of up to 15 cm in length with 3 mm diameter vessels can be achieved. Serratus anterior can be used as either a muscle flap for facial reanimation, or a musculocutaneous flap or as a composite flap including a segment of rib.

It is not used very often but its main advantage is that based on the subscapular vessels, it is possible to raise bilobed or trilobed flaps using the latissimus dorsi and overlying skin on one paddle, the serratus anterior with either skin plus or minus rib on another pedicle, as well as a scapular flap based on the circumflex scapular vessels.

Omentum flap

The omentum hangs like an apron from the greater curvature of the stomach on a vascular pedicle formed by the right and left gastroepiploic vessels. It may be taken as a free flap on a single vascular pedicle (usually the left gastroepiploic vessels). The vessel size is 2–3 mm.

The advantage of this flap is that it enables large areas of tissue in a three-dimensional plane to be harvested, which can be used for resurfacing the whole of the scalp and to augment soft-tissue defects in facial deformity. Its disadvantages are that a laparotomy is required.

Although it is a useful flap to have in one's armamentarium, its use in the filling of soft-tissue defects is not as good as with the groin flap since it tends to fall with time, and total scalp resurfacing may be done with either a free or pedicled muscle latissimus dorsi flap and subsequent skin graft.

Alternative methods and adjunctive techniques

Prosthetics and osseointegration

Following a head and neck resection, there are some areas where reconstruction by conventional methods is inappropriate and the best results are achieved using an alternative method such as a prosthesis. This is demonstrated par excellence in areas such as major auricular reconstruction, and the defects that follow both total rhinectomy and orbital exenteration. They may also be appropriate for areas such as the alar base when reconstruction would be inadvisable, e.g. following resection of recurrent basal cell carcinoma.

The patient is seen both preoperatively and postoperatively by a maxillofacial technician who is experienced in prosthetics, so that a temporary prosthesis may be fitted at or soon after surgery.

Prosthetic planning prior to surgery

- Meet patient before surgery, establish rapport, give patient information on prosthetics and expected time scale of treatment
- Take impression of area to be resected, e.g. ear or nose, and take photographs for reference
- Take intraoral impression and construct surgical plate. If defect is to extend into the mouth, carry out any routine dental work.
- Prosthetist to be present at resection to advise on placement of fixtures. Provide template if necessary
- Prosthetist to advise during reconstructive procedure to help to produce defect that will give the best possible prosthetic result

---

These silastic prostheses may be held in place using adhesive; more common nowadays is the use of osseointegration (usually performed at the time of resection), which will facilitate a bolt-on prosthesis held by magnets (Fig. 7.44). The subsequent prosthesis is then tailormade during a series of fittings with the patient and suitable skin matches are obtained for both winter and summer wear. Osseointegration should not be performed in patients who have had previous radiotherapy without prior administration of hyperbaric oxygen.

Principles of osseointegration

- The direct and intimate association between living bone and an implant surface
- Implants predominantly made of titanium and titanium alloy
- Inserted using a meticulous surgical technique to avoid thermal bone damage
- Implant site developed with burrs and taps to ensure maximum stability
- Implants can be buried under skin or left exposed
- Implants allowed to osseointegrate for 3–6 months before loading
- Irradiated bone should be pretreated with hyperbaric oxygen
- Osseointegrated implants are used to reconstruct form and function. Teeth and the supporting tissues as well as extraoral applications such as ears, nose, eyes and composite defects can all be replaced.
- Both reconstructs and rehabilitates patients back into the community
- Team approach required, assuming a common purpose between surgeon, prosthodontist and technician

---

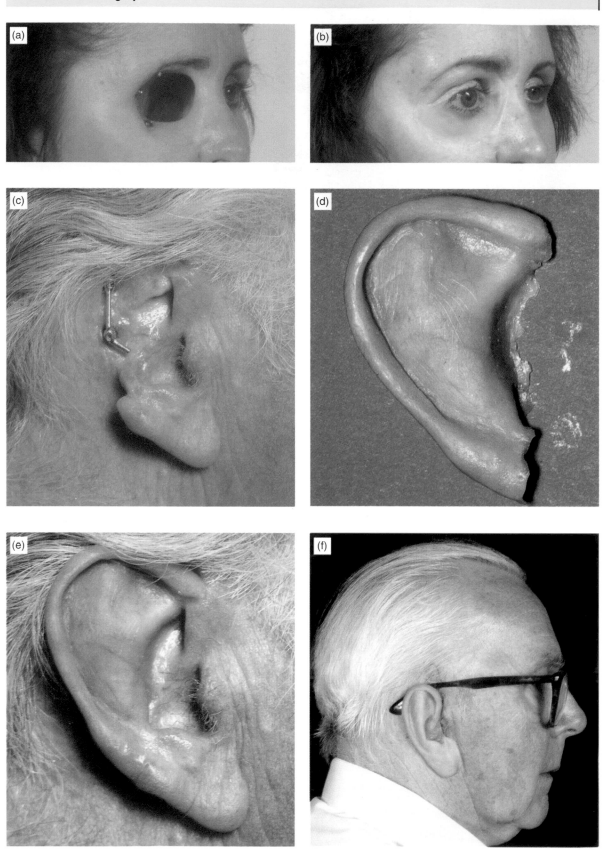

Figure 7.44 Prostheses may be used to repair defects following surgical resections that involve (a, b) the eye or (c–e) the ear. (f) Glasses may be attached to the auricular prosthesis. (g)–(k) continued overleaf.

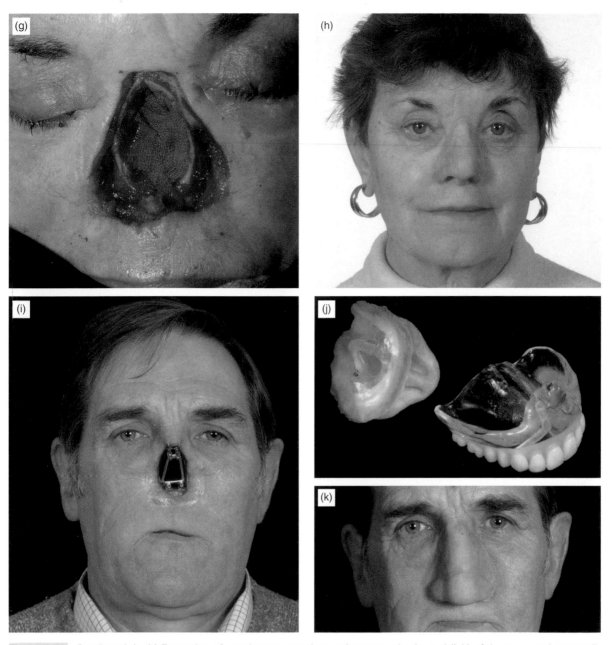

Figure 7.44 *Continued.* (g, h) Examples of nasal reconstructions using a prosthesis, and (i–k) of the nose and premaxilla. The latter patient also had a two-thirds upper lip reconstruction using bilateral perialar crescentic advancement.

Surgery for facial palsy (Fig. 7.45)

In some patients following surgery to the facial nerve with or without resection and nerve anastomosis, there may be long-term residual deficits in facial nerve function. Patients learn to live with minor deficits but for complete facial palsy following surgery, many patients request that something is done to improve their appearance.

In the young, patients complain of lack of movement of the face and in appropriate cases they may be considered for dynamic improvements using facial reanimation.

A number of techniques is available and they take the form of either pedicled muscle transfer such as tempo-

ralis or free tissue transfer using the pectoralis minor, gracilis or serratus anterior muscles. The most common technique used today is free tissue transfer of the pectoralis minor muscle, which involves a cross-facial sural nerve graft from the buccal branch of the contralateral normal facial nerve and subsequent free tissue transfer of the pectoralis minor muscle, with microvascular anastomosis, transplantation of the muscle slips into the mouth, nasolabial fold and eyelid and a nerve anastomosis to the medial pectoral nerve.

In the elderly patient, the problem is not so much lack of dynamic movement but the static appearance of the

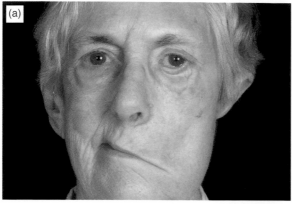

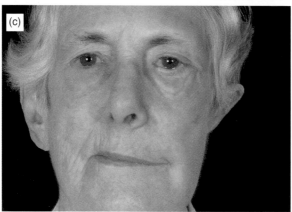

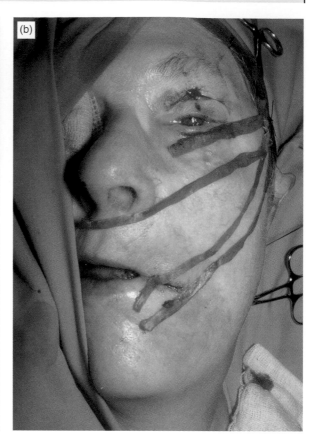

Figure 7.45 (a) Patient with a left total facial nerve palsy following extended radical parotidectomy. (b) A fascia lata sling was used to provide support to the face following surgery and postoperative radiotherapy. (c) The patient remains alive and well 3 years later.

face at rest, with significant drooping on the affected side. These problems may be addressed by performing a fascia lata sling taken from the thigh, suspended from the zygomatic arch and attached to the lateral part of the upper and lower lip (Fig. 7.45). At the same time, a middle-third face lift may be performed with submental liposuction.

In these circumstances (and often as a localized problem), the otolaryngologist has to deal with a paralysed eyelid. Often at the time of surgery a temporary lateral tarsorrhaphy will have been performed and if recovery is not expected this may be done as a permanent technique. In addition, other adjunctive techniques can improve the appearance of the eyelid. A browlift may be considered necessary, which can be combined with an upper lid blepharoplasty to improve the aperture of the eye. Eyelid closure may be facilitated using a gold-weight implant to the upper eyelid. This is inserted using a similar incision to a blepharoplasty and is laid over the tarsal plate. Where there is a specific problem in the elderly with paralysis to the lower eyelid combined with excess tissue and significant ectropion, a lateral canthal sling should be considered. This detaches the lateral canthal tendon, which is then reattached with a non-absorbable suture more laterally to the lateral orbital margin or zygoma. This may be done in combination with a medial tarsorrhaphy.

When using a fascial sling, it is important to overcorrect as some settling will take place. An alternative to this technique is the temporalis muscle transfer, which has the rehabilitative advantage in that its attachment is to the temporal bone and the coronoid process of the mandible, and carries with it some dynamic function. However, it is very difficult to control, is a bulky technique and is seldom used nowadays since, as stated previously, where movement is important, the best results are obtained with free tissue transfer.

Facelift

The facelift forms an important part of reconstruction. Not only may it be used to improve the appearance of the face in those patients with a facial palsy (Fig. 7.45), but it may act as a form of reconstruction where, for those skin tumours or parotid tumours that involve the preauricular skin, wide resection may be carried out and a facelift used to reconstruct the defect (Fig. 7.46).

Liposuction

This technique may be used to revise flaps and is particularly useful, as described previously, in combination with other adjunctive procedures to rehabilitate the paralysed face.

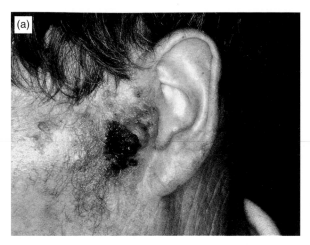
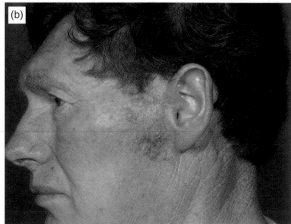

Figure 7.46 (a) Patient with a T$_4$ basal cell carcinoma overlying the left parotid. (b) Treatment was with wide excision, superficial parotidectomy and repair with skin advancement using the facelift technique.

Tissue expansion

In certain instances, where oncological conditions permit, tissue expansion may be appropriate to facilitate the reconstruction. This technique involves the insertion of a subcutaneous expander with a buried portal to facilitate serial weekly expansion using saline. It requires time and therefore its use may be precluded in those situations where urgent resection and immediate reconstruction are of the essence, but there are occasions when it may be of value.

Where total resurfacing of nasal skin is required, the use of the forehead is usually indicated and tissue expansion will facilitate primary closure of the donor site with improved postoperative cosmetic appearance. In addition, it is now possible to prefabricate radial free forearm flaps by tissue expansion to allow increased areas of skin to be transplanted that would otherwise be available from the conventional donor site. Using this technique, the whole skin from one side of the face may be replaced.

Scar revision

Despite all of these efforts to achieve optimum reconstructive results, there are times when scars result with which both the surgeon and patients are unhappy. Like good wine, scars mature over time. It is important not to rush in and do anything foolish but to analyse carefully any scar and allow it a maturation period of at least 12 months before coming to any decision regarding revision. The surgeon should remember that: 'by your scars you will be judged'.

A small hypertrophic or keloid scar may be injected with a steroid such as triamcinolone and then subsequent pressure applied with tape for a period of up to 6 months. Larger scars require surgical excision, remembering to keep the excision just within the edge of the keloid. This is combined with steroid injection and then pressure applied as before. The procedure should be repeated for recurrences and radiotherapy considered for difficult

problems, when it should be given immediately postoperatively since it has no role in treating established keloid scarring.

Where a scar is unacceptable in either its width or position, then revision may be appropriate. For thin scars near facial landmarks, excision is appropriate with careful resuturing. For those away from facial landmarks, the scar should be assessed in respect to relaxed skin tension lines. Where scars are wide, they can be serially excised and then subsequently assessed with respect to relaxed skin tension lines. Following excision, some will require additional tissue in the form of a local flap or graft.

Depressed scars are treated with collagen injection. Small scars with little effacement may be treated by shave excision, but for significant effacement treatment is with geometric broken line closure combined with dermabrasion as appropriate.

Where a scar lies outside the relaxed skin tension lines (greater than 35°), it may be revised, with or without repositioning. If the scar is not contracted and it is on a flat surface, then geometric broken line closure with dermabrasion is appropriate. On convex surfaces, such as the cheek or the forehead, a W-plasty can be used with dermabrasion. If the scar is contracted, then it may be repositioned and a Z-plasty is particularly useful.

In addition to providing an increase in length and a change in direction, a Z-plasty in the head and neck can be used to close defects, to supplement closure in scar tension and to realign distorted anatomical areas such as the corner of the mouth or eye. The classic Z-plasty has a 60° angle and mathematically the larger the angle, the larger the increase in length but more undermining is required and greater tissue areas are involved. Angles of 60° give a theoretical gain of 75% (Fig. 7.47) and the Z-plasty may be used as a single procedure or as multiple Zs. Practically speaking, Z-plasty angles between 30/35° and 70/75° work well, since angles below 30° may result in tip necrosis and those above 75° may cause excessive dog-ear formation.

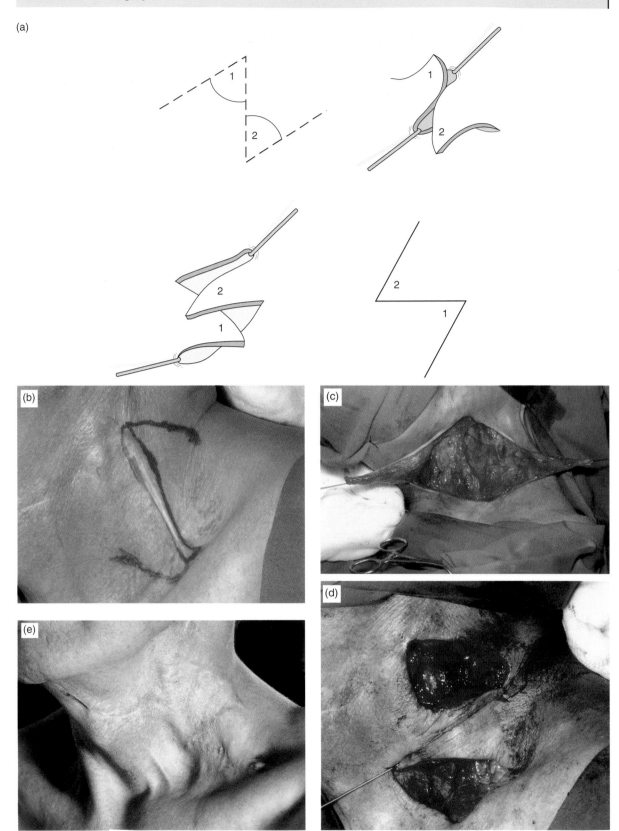

Figure 7.47 Principles of a Z-plasty. (a) In its simplest form it is the transposition of two equal triangular flaps. (b) Patient with a hypertrophic scar following neck dissection. (c, d) The scar is excised and repaired with a transposition Z-plasty. (e) The final result.

References and further reading

Baker S. ed. (1989) *Microsurgical Reconstruction of the Head and Neck*, Churchill-Livingstone, London.

Borges A. F. (1973) *Elective Incisions and Scar Revision*, Little, Brown and Co., Boston, MA.

Gillies H. D. (1968) In Fitzgibbon G. M. The Commandments of Gillies, *Br Journal of Plastic Surg* **21**: 226.

Gillies H. D. and Millard D. R. (1957) *The Principles and Art of Plastic Surgery*, Little, Brown and Co., Boston, MA.

Jackson I. T. (1985) *Local Flaps in Head and Neck Reconstruction*, CV Mosby Co., St Louis, MO.

Last R. J. (1968) In Fitzgibbon G. M. The Commandments of Gillies, *Br J Plastic Surg* **21**: 226.

McGregor I. A. and McGregor F. M. (1986) *Cancer of the Face and Mouth. Pathology and Management for Surgeons*, Churchill-Livingstone, Edinburgh.

Shpitzar T., Neligan P. C., Gullane P. J. *et al.* (1997) Oromandibular reconstruction with the fibula free flap. Analysis of 50 consecutive flaps, *Arch Otolaryngol Head Neck Surg* **123**: 939–44.

Soutar D. S. and Tiwari R. ed. (1994) *Excision and Reconstruction in Head and Neck Cancer*, Churchill-Livingstone, Edinburgh.

Stepnick D. W. and Mesin J. J. (1997) The increased use and applicability of the fibula osteocutaneous flap in mandibular reconstruction, *Curr Opin Otolaryngol Head Neck Surg* **5**: 245–50.

Thomas J. R. and Holt G. R. (1989) *Facial Scars Incision, Revision and Camouflage*, CV Mosby Co., St Louis, MO.

Urken M. L, Cheney M. L., Sullivan M. J. and Biller H. F. (1995) *Atlas of Regional and Free Flaps for Head and Neck Reconstruction*, Raven Press, New York.

Webster M. H. C. and Soutar D. S. (1986) *Practical Guide to Free Tissue Transfer*, Butterworths, London.

8 Treatment outcomes

*'Patients' best interests: phrase doctors
use to justify pursuing their own'*
Michael O'Donnell, 1997

Introduction

Health care resources are now rationed throughout the world. All clinicians therefore share a responsibility to ensure that their treatment is

- effective
- efficient.

Efficacy implies that a treatment actually achieves what it sets out to do, e.g. cure a given proportion of patients of their disease. Efficiency incorporates concepts of cost efficiency, i.e. could it be obtained more cheaply? The costs include not only the health care resources required to provide the treatment but also the costs to the patient in terms of treatment-related morbidity and the opportunity cost of not treating another condition because of the expenditure.

The measurement of outcomes of treatment is compounded by the fact that patients and carers, and patients and healthy observers have different opinions as to what constitutes the most favourable outcome.

Mortality

For most cancers, the reporting of mortality remains the cornerstone of outcomes assessment. None the less, it must be accepted that, despite the many advances in the method of cancer treatments, there are many cancers, including most head and neck cancers, where these treatment developments have not been mirrored in changes in mortality rates, which have remained static since the 1960s. It is important, however, not to let a lack of improvement in mortality obscure the value of a genuine therapeutic advance. For example, modern techniques of head and neck resection with skilful reconstruction often result in a far superior cosmetic and functional outcome and quality of life, even if the cure rate is no greater than with older, more morbid procedures. Much of the recent modest survival improvement observed in certain other

cancers relates to prevention programmes or earlier diagnosis by screening.

Advantages of death as an outcome

- It is undeniably the most important outcome to both doctor and patient
- There are only two categories: alive or dead
- The distinction cannot be fudged

Disadvantages of death as an outcome

- Insensitive in diseases with low mortality
- Usually a delay before manifest
- Inaccuracies in recording the cause of death
- Disregards functional outcome and quality of life

Survival analysis

- Disease-specific survival
- Actuarial survival
- Median survival time
- Kaplan–Meier survival curve
- Log-rank test

Quality-of-life outcome measures

- General factors
- Disease- or site-specific factors
- Patient-generated instruments
- Health care professionals' measures

Karnofsky in 1948 made the first attempt to quantify the performance status of patients with advanced cancer. Most of the general quality-of-life measures used regularly in head and neck cancer now include at least a regionally specific symptom checklist. Typically, this focuses on functions such as speaking, swallowing and body image which are traditionally affected by head and neck cancer and its treatments. The sum of aspects of patients' subjective well being is known as 'quality of life', a concept that incorporates not only an individual's functioning, but also their degree of satisfaction with that functioning. The acute impacts of surgery or radiotherapy on patient well-being are obvious, but long-term survivors of head and neck cancer also report a high level of disease and treatment-related symptoms.

Quality of life

- Multidimensional: elements of emotional, social and physical well-being
- Subjective: relies principally on patient's own judgements
- Non-static: subject to change over a patient's lifetime

Applications of quality-of-life measures

Treatment decisions involve choosing a management plan that offers the best survival with least side-effects. Unfortunately, all treatments currently available (radiotherapy, surgery and chemotherapy) produce physical, functional and psychosocial problems. Significant technological advances, e.g. hyperfractionated radiotherapy, laser surgery and titanium implants, may not have produced comparable improvements in either survival or quality of life. The systematic collection of quality-of-life data using validated instruments is extremely important to establish a database of information about the effects of treatment, to enable better decision making by doctor and patient and to assist in the evaluation of efficacy of treatment in clinical trials. Quality-of-life assessment will also help to identify patients who might benefit from psychosocial interventions such as counselling and to evaluate the efficacy of supportive interventions. Finally, quality data are necessary to help to inform economic evaluations and health-care decisions.

Uses of quality-of-life measures

- Assist clinical decision making, including trial recruitment
- Assess rehabilitation needs
- Help to understand patient preferences
- Policy making

The World Health Organization has categorized the impact of a disease state as one of three types:

- impairment: limitation of functioning of a body part, e.g. restricted tongue movement
- disability: restriction in daily activities, e.g. speaking or eating, as a result of the impairment
- handicap: impact on the individual's social activity, e.g. employment, as a result of the disability.

A further category of psychosocial outcome has recently been added:

- distress: relates to the psychological reaction to a disease state and its impact.

Outcome domains

- Mortality
- Functional morbidity: impairment of function
- Psychosocial consequences:
  Disability
  Handicap
  Distress

Head and neck cancer quality-of-life measures

A number of disease-specific outcome instruments are available, which generally show good correlation. There is a less good correlation with general quality-of-life measures, however, and thus general and disease-specific instruments each give unique information. Several head and neck measures also include, or have evolved from, general health-status measures, the EORTC and FACT questionnaires (see box).

Head and neck cancer disease-specific quality-of-life measures

- Functional Assessment of Cancer Therapy: Head and Neck Scale (FACT–H&N)
- University of Washington Quality of Life Scale (UW QoL)
- EORTC Quality of Life Questionnaire (EORTC–QLQ)
- Performance Status Scale for Head and Neck Cancer Patients (PSS–HN)

To date, there have been 10 published head and neck quality-of-life scales. Most scales cover a combination of functional outcomes: eating/swallowing and speech, with scales for pain, xerostomia and taste. Appearance and social contact are the two regular psychosocial variables. The EORTC (European Organization for Research and Treatment of Cancer) study group on quality of life was founded in 1980. European and Canadian researchers spent a decade developing a core quality-of-life measure (EORTC QLQ-C30) to assess the outcome of cancer patients in international trials. The EORTC head and neck module to supplement the QLQ-C30 is still under development (the EORTC QLQ-H+N37). The University of Washington Quality of Life Head and Neck Questionnaire has the option of open responses and may have advantages in some research settings. The Performance Status Scale for Head and Neck is a clinician-rated instrument consisting of three subscales: normality of diet, understandability of speech and eating in public.

The Functional Assessment of Cancer Therapy – General (FACT-G) is a self-report instrument with 28 general items each rated 0 to 4. Items are then combined to describe patient functioning in five areas.

The FACT–H&N includes an additional module for head and neck cancer patients, which is effectively a symptom checklist. The total score for the list of symptoms can be used as a single item: the higher the score, the better the quality of life. Each subscale can also be analysed separately and includes a weighting item to reflect the relative importance of different aspects of a patient's quality of life, e.g. 'How much would you say your physical well being affects your quality of life'?

Impact of head and neck cancer on quality of life

Although there is some improvement over time, both functional and psychosocial deficits persist in up to 50% of patients. Early data also point to a consistent lack of relationship between functional and psychosocial adjustment. Social distress and social avoidance tend to peak immediately after surgery, and caregivers should anticipate this reaction and help to support the patient through to the later phases of adjustment. The severity of quality-of-life impact relates both to T-stage (with larger tumours obviously having a greater impact) and to the site of the primary. For example, following combined therapy with surgery and radiation, patients with base of tongue tumours have lower functional scores than those with oral cavity or tonsillar oropharyngeal primaries.

Comparative impacts of treatment modalities

Treatment decisions in head and neck cancer are typically made by weighing up survival outcome (cure rate) and functional/cosmetic outcome. It is only more recently, however, that any hard quality-of-life data have been published to indicate just how devastating is the impact of major head and neck surgery on daily life, especially if the patient has a permanent stoma. Several papers now confirm that quality-of-life scores are lower following total than partial laryngectomy, and suggest that single

modality primary radiotherapy has a minimal impact (De Santo *et al.*, 1995; List *et al.*, 1996; McDonough *et al.*, 1996; Moore *et al.*, 1996; Deleyiannis *et al.*, 1997). Quality-of-life scores are higher and social distress/avoidance is lower in non-surgically treated patients. For surgically treated laryngeal cancer patients, the overall life adjustment appears to be less successful than for non-laryngeal cancer patients. The former group reports more work problems, changes in spouse and family interaction, reduced sexual interest and performance, and financial concerns. For advanced (stage III–IV) oral cancer patients, surgical treatment is associated with a higher rate of worsening of appearance and speech, and a 67% incidence of pain, compared with only 29% in the primary radiotherapy group. These findings (Deleyiannis *et al.*, 1997) were based on small numbers, however, and until such quality-of-life data are collected routinely, it is impossible to weigh these factors objectively against the improved survival from primary surgery.

The findings from Gainsville (Moore *et al.*, 1996) showed the functional results of tongue base cancer treatment to be similar after external beam radiotherapy and external beam plus iridium implant. Both were superior to the results of surgery. In the long term, patients with no or minor surgery have better emotional outcomes than those who have had major surgery (Bjordal *et al.*, 1994a, b).

Whose outcome is it anyway?

The term quality-adjusted life year (QUALY) refers to a unit used in early attempts to compare the health benefits of, for example a hip replacement versus a renal transplant. The QUALY acknowledges a difference in types of measurable outcome among different diseases and treatments. Sometimes, however, there are also marked differences between what the patient and the care-giver regard as the important outcome measures. Several studies have now addressed this difference in perception of outcome within the head and neck.

An early classic paper (McNeil *et al.*, 1981) on the cost utility analysis of the treatment of advanced laryngeal cancer by radiotherapy and laryngectomy presented a trade-off of quality of life (retention of laryngeal speech) versus quantity of life (improved survival after primary laryngectomy) to a group of healthy (non-medical) volunteers. In order to maintain natural speech, approximately 20% of those questioned would have chosen radiation instead of surgery. In a later paper by De Santo *et al.* (1995), 20% of patients expressed themselves willing to accept a reduced lifespan in order to preserve their larynx and quality of life. In contrast, 46% of the health-care professional questioned felt that the patients would accept this trade-off.

There are also differences in the perception of the relative importance of different categories of symptom between patients and carers. Mohide (1992) demonstrated that carers ranked impaired communication and self-image/self-esteem as the two most important quality-of-life outcome domains following laryngectomy. The patients ranked the physical symptoms such as tracheal mucus production, and interference with social activities as the two most important items. It is important to bear this lack of correlation between patient and carer priorities in mind when counselling patients about treatment options.

Function-specific outcome measures

The assessment of speech and swallowing following head and neck cancer therapy is discussed fully in Chapter 18. Two scoring systems for swallowing which may supplement the swallowing times in the head and neck quality of life scales are worthy of mention here. The first, the 30 ml water swallow test is one of a number of timed liquid swallow tests to have been described (DePippo *et al.*, 1992). The principal value of this test is in the detection of aspiration. A detailed swallow questionnaire, supplemented by a performance score for a test meal, has the potential to evaluate a larger number of abnormalities than simply aspiration (Dakkak and Bennett, 1992). In particular, the meal tests swallow function with a number of different consistencies. These measures may be used to supplement the essentially qualitative swallow assessments: bedside clinical assessment, videofluoroscopy and videoendoscopic swallow study.

Summary

There are few clinical situations in which the analysis of treatment outcomes is more challenging than in the patient with head and neck cancer. As mortality remains, unfortunately, a relatively insensitive barometer for treatment advances, so qualitative issues must have a crucial role in the selection and health economic analysis of treatment options. The scale and scope of some of the consequences of head and neck cancer to the sufferer call for the use of a range of different quality of life and functional measures to appreciate fully the impact of the disease and of our 'treatments'.

References and further reading

Bjordal K., Kaasa S. and Mastekaasa A. (1994) Quality of life in head and neck cancer patients, *Int J Radiat Oncol Biol Phys* **28**: 847–56.

Bjordal K. *et al.* (1994b) Development of a European Organisation for Research and Treatment of Cancer (EORTC), questionnaire module to be used in quality of life assessments in head and neck cancer patients, *Acta Oncol* **33**: 879–85.

Campbell M. J. and Machin D. (1993) *Medical Statistics: A Commonsense Approach*, John Wiley and Sons, Chichester.

Cella D. F. (1993) The Functional Assessment of Cancer Therapy Scale: development and validation of the general measure, *J Clin Oncol* **11**: 570-9.

Cella D. F. (1994) *Manual for the Functional Assessment of Cancer Therapy (FACT) Measurement System (Version 3)*, Rush Medical Center, Chicago, IL.

Dakkak M. and Bennett J. R. (1992) A new dysphagia score with objective validation, *J Clin Gastroenterol* **14**: 99–100.

D'Antonio L. L., Zimmerman G. J., Cella D. F. and Long S. A. (1986) Quality of life and functional status measures in patients with head and neck cancer, *Arch Otolaryngol Head Neck Surg* **122**: 482–7.

Deleyiannis F., W., Weymuller E. A. and Coltrera M. D. (1997) Quality of life of disease-free survivors of advanced (stage III or IV oropharyngeal cancer), *Head Neck* **19**: 466–73.

DePippo K. L., Holas M. A. and Reding M.J. (1992) Water swallow test, *Arch Neurol* **49**: 1259–61.

De Santo L. W., Olson K. D., Perry W. C. *et al.* (1995) Quality of life after surgical treatment of cancer of the larynx, *Ann Otol Rhinol Laryngol* **104**: 763–9.

Enderby P. and John A. (1997) *Therapy Outcome Measures – Speech and Language, Therapy.* Singular Publishing Group.

Harrison L. B., Zelefsky M. D., Armstrong J. G. *et al.* (1994) Radiation versus surgery for base of tongue cancer, *Int J Radiat Oncol Biol Phys* **30**: 953–7.

Hassan S. J. and Weymuller E. A. (1993) Assessment of quality of life in head and neck cancer patients, *Head Neck*, **15**: 485–96.

Karnofsky D. A., Abelman W. H., Cravel L. F. and Burchenal J. H. (1948) The use of nitrogen mustards in the palliative treatment of carcinoma, *Cancer* **1**: 634–56.

McDonough E. M., Varvares M. A., Dunphy F. R., *et al.* (1996) Changes in Quality of Life Scores, *Head and Neck* **18**: 487–93.

McNeil B. J., Weichselbaum R. and Pauker S. G. (1981) Speech and survival. *N Engl J Med* **305**: 982–7.

Mohide E. A. (1992) Post laryngectomy quality of life dimensions identified by patients and health care professionals, *Am J Surg* **164**: 619–22.

Moore G. J., Parsons J. T. and Mendenhall W. M. (1996) Quality of life outcomes after primary radiotherapy for squamous cell carcinoma of the base of tongue, *Int J Radiat Oncol Biol Phys* **36**: 351–4.

Morton R. P. (1995) Evaluation of quality of life assessment in head and neck cancer, *J Laryngol* **109**: 1029–35.

Morton R. P. (1997) Laryngeal cancer: quality of life and cost-effectiveness, *Head Cancer* **19**: 243–50.

Muir Gray J. A. (1997) *Evidence-based Healthcare*, Churchill Livingstone, New York.

Otto R. A. (1997) Impact of a laryngectomy on quality of life: perspective of the patient versus that of the health care provider, *Ann Otol Rhinol Laryngol* **106**: 693–9.

Zelefsky M. J., Gaynor M. D., Kraus D. *et al.* (1996) Functional outcome for oral and oropharyngeal carcinoma, *Am J Surg* **171**: 258–62.

9 Tracheostomy

'For this relief, much thanks'
William Shakespeare, 1604

Introduction

The procedure of tracheostomy appears to have been performed in ancient times, but was considered hazardous, for obvious reasons, and was then rarely performed until the early nineteenth century. Modern approaches to open tracheostomy still draw on the classic descriptions of Chevalier Jackson. In recent years, however, more and more airway problems are managed with either endotracheal intubation, or percutaneous endoscopically guided tracheostomy. Conversely, the minitracheostomy procedure, which enjoyed brief popularity for tracheal toilet in the mid-1980s, is now performed relatively infrequently.

Not only have the indications for tracheostomy evolved of late, but the range of tracheal appliances has also expanded. The performance of percutaneous procedures in intensive care units by non-otolaryngologists means that larger numbers of personnel need to be familiar not only with tracheostomy care but also with the techniques of decannulation.

Indications for tracheostomy: the five Rs

- Respiratory obstruction
- Respiratory failure
- Respiratory paralysis
- Removal of retained secretions
- Reduction of dead space

Cricothyrotomy

In the emergency situation, any medical or paramedical worker may on occasion find themselves confronted with the need to alleviate acute upper airway obstruction, either in hospital or out in the community. The two dilemmas for the health-care worker confronted with a possible need for cricothyrotomy are:

- whether to perform it
- how to perform it.

Cricothyrotomy: whether to perform it

- Suspicion of acute upper airway problem
- Worsening stridor
- Reducing self-ventilation

Cricothyroidotomy: how to perform it

- Extend the neck
- Palpate the cricoid arch: enter just above it
- Enter larynx just above the cricoid
- Midline incision using either blade or IV cannula
- Knife may be rotated through 90° to keep the incision open
- Convert to formal tracheostomy as soon as possible

The complications of cricothyrotomy include perichondritis, subglottic oedema and stenosis.

Open tracheostomy (Figs 9.1–9.3)

Open tracheostomy

- Collar incision 2 cm > suprasternal notch
- Elevate Platysma; divide strap muscles in midline
- Thyroid isthmus may be avoidable. Otherwise divide
- Palpate and expose the trachea
- Alert anaesthetist; suction ready
- Child – insert two stay sutures; vertical incision
- Adult – horizontal incision, third tracheal space – may need to excise part of one tracheal ring
- Insert tube: connect to anaesthetic circuit
- Tape stay sutures to the chest in a child
- Loose sutures on skin
- Suture and tape tube

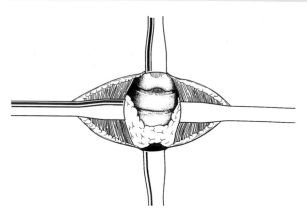

Figure 9.1 Horizontal skin flaps separated and infrahyoid strap muscles separated.

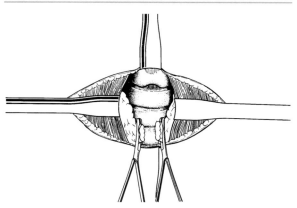

Figure 9.2 Division of the thyroid isthmus.

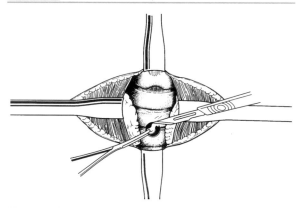

Figure 9.3 Opening the anterior tracheal wall.

Anaesthesia for tracheostomy

> *Anaesthesia for tracheostomy*
>
> - Local anaesthesia
>   - Avoid injecting the trachea (cough reflex)
>   - Avoid paratracheal gutter (recurrent laryngeal nerve (RLN) palsy may exacerbate obstruction)
> - General anaesthesia
>   - Gas induction
>   - Never give any muscle relaxants until airway secured

Tracheostomy tubes

> *Tracheostomy tubes*
>
> - Inner tube
> - Cuffed/uncuffed
> - Fenestrated/unfenestrated
> - Speaking valve

A great deal of confusion can arise, particularly on non-otolaryngological wards, from the large number of tracheostomy tubes which is now available (Fig. 9.4). Tubes are made of either metal or plastic. Metal tubes are becoming less fashionable as some of the synthetic material tubes may now be left in position for a considerable time. Metal tubes may not be used in patients undergoing CT scans or radiotherapy. It is convenient for nursing staff if a patient has an inner tube which can be removed for cleaning. Otherwise, crusting may build up on the end of the tube, necessitating a full tube change. The presence of an inner tube slightly reduces the available area for ventilation. For spontaneously breathing patients, a cuffed tube is usually adequate. An exception is a patient with a tendency to aspirate during deglutition. Sometimes in this situation a cuffed tube may be used particularly during rehabilitation swallow therapy manoeuvres. It should always be kept in mind that the presence of a tracheostomy handicaps swallow performance and sometimes in this situation it is possible to remove the tracheostomy tube rather than convert the patient to a cuffed tube, with infinitely preferable results.

If the patient has a functioning larynx it is helpful to use a fenestrated tube so that expired air may be blown up between the vocal cords for phonation. Some patients become very adept at occluding their tracheostomy tube manually in this situation in order to phonate. Others find a speaking valve more convenient and such valves are available even on disposable non-metal tubes. They are either mounted on a special inner tube or applied to the opening of the outer tube, and used only intermittently throughout the day and removed at night.

Tracheostomy care

> *Tracheostomy care*
>
> - Nursing
> - Fixation of the tracheostomy tube
> - Removal of secretions
> - Humidification
> - Changing the tracheostomy tube
> - Care of the inflatable cuff
> - Breathing exercises
> - Dressings
> - Nursing

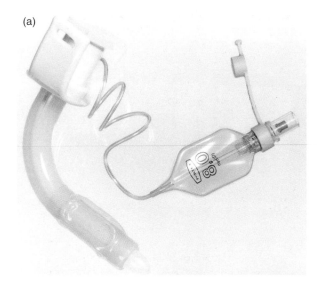

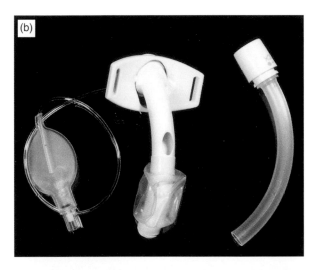

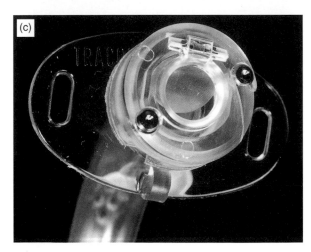

Figure 9.4 Tracheostomy tubes; (a) cuffed unfenestrated Portex tube; (b) cuffed fenestrated Shiley tube with inner tube; (c) Tracoe fenestrated tube with speaking valve on the inner tube (Kapitex Healthcare Ltd).

A trained nurse should be in attendance at all times for the first 24 h after a tracheostomy. They should be acquainted with all complications of the operation and the principles of sterile suction and humidification, and also be able to replace the tube if necessary. The patient should be told before the operation that he or she will not be able to speak until the tracheostomy is closed. He or she should be given a 'magic slate' on which to write and a bell with which to summon assistance.

Fixation of the tracheostomy tube

A tracheostomy tube can be very difficult to replace if it is dislodged within the first 48 h. Therefore stitch the tube to the skin. These stitches must be cut out when the tube is changed for the first time, and tapes are then applied to the second tracheostomy tube. The tapes are tied so that they are doubled over, with the head in the neutral position; if they are tied in the extended position they will be too loose when the head is in the neutral position. A reef knot is used and the knots are placed so that there is one on each side of the neck. The tapes should not be tied so tightly that they obstruct the lymphatic drainage, causing oedema of the skin flaps above the ties. The tapes ideally should never be taken across a pedicled skin flap from the chest.

Removal of secretions

Excess secretions are inevitable after a newly created tracheostomy because the tube acts as a foreign body and stimulates secretions, and the trachea has never before been exposed to cold dry air; there may also be some oozing of blood from the operation site. Secretions should be removed by suction every 30 min, or more often if indicated. After the first 48 h, this period may be lengthened but suction will always be required at least every 4 h. The nurse should wear sterile gloves and use the special suction tubes that minimize tracheal and bronchial trauma.

Humidification

The normal channels for warming and humidifying the air have been bypassed, so artificial humidification is required to prevent crusting of secretions. Humidification is provided by hot water bath humidifiers or by nebulizers delivering cold droplets. An alternative is heat and humidity exchangers. The humidified air is delivered by a mask or a T-tube applied to the tracheostomy tube. A satisfactory alternative to prevent crusting is the instillation of saline into the trachea. The Tracoe is well suited to long-term use as it is soft and, being transparent, relatively inconspicuous.

Changing the tracheostomy tube

Normally for the first 48 h a cuffed plastic tube is used, or occasionally a silver tube, in which case the inner tube is cleaned at hourly intervals. The tracheostomy tube is changed after 48 h and a smaller one inserted. Thereafter, it is changed every 2–3 days in order to avoid wound infection or crusting. After a tube is inserted into the trachea, one must establish with absolute certainty that it is actually in the tracheal lumen, as it is easy to place the tube in the mediastinum anterior to the trachea. The patient is asked to take deep breaths so that the surgeon can feel the air coming out of the tube. A foolproof method of changing the tube at 48 h is to insert a sterile catheter into the old tube, which is then withdrawn over the catheter. The new tube is then threaded over the catheter into the trachea. There is always a risk of failure of reintubation and this can result in unnecessary death. A pair of tracheal dilators should always be taped to the head of the bed, and a tracheostomy set, a battery laryngoscope and bronchoscope should be available on the ward in case of dire emergencies.

Care of the inflatable cuff

When a cuff is inflated to occlude an airway, the area of the tracheal wall with which it is in contact is in danger of ischaemic necrosis. The tube is left inflated for the first 12 h after operation, and the cuff deflated for 5 min every hour and then let down. New low-pressure cuffs on most makes of tubes minimize the risk of tracheal damage but the above procedure is still good practice.

Breathing exercises

The patient almost always needs postoperative breathing exercises from the physiotherapist. If secretions are excessive, more vigorous treatment by intermittent positive-pressure breathing triggered by the patient is used. If this is not available the patient's lungs can be inflated with an Ambu bag after suction has been performed. This gives greater ventilation than deep-breathing exercises and can be done more often. After sucking out the trachea the Ambu bag is fitted on to the tracheostomy connection, the cuff of the tracheostomy tube is inflated and the patient is ventilated for 3 min. The Ambu bag is then taken off and the cuff let down. They should be changed regularly.

Dressings

Waterproof squares are used in the care of tracheostomies; they have a slit on their top surface that is passed around the edges of the tube and secured above it with a safety pin.

Decannulation

Sometimes a patient who has been established on a tracheostomy with a large-bore tracheostomy tube does poorly when other parameters would suggest decannulation to be possible. The most common of this difficulty

is that no attempt has been made to reduce the size of the tube prior to occlusion. If there is very little room for air passage round the tube and it is effectively occluded the patient has a large plastic airway obstruction *in situ*. Thus, prior to decannulation, the tube size should be decreased in order to allow ventilation around the tube. Once the tracheostomy tube has been removed according to the protocol below, various modern dressings, such as Comfeel, provide an effective semiwaterproof seal. Alternatively, a traditional gauze dressing with overlying waterproof tape may be used.

Principles of decannulation

- Tube size reduced before decannulation
- Tube is corked off for increasing periods
- Self-ventilating for at least one full night
- No further need for tracheal suction
- Remove tube; plug tracheostomy site

Percutaneous tracheostomy (Figs 9.5–9.8)

Percutaneous tracheostomy had been described decades before it gained acceptance in the mid-1980s, owing to the development of graded tracheal dilators by Ciaglia's group. Tracheostomy is a common procedure in the intensive care unit (ICU): approximately 13% of ICU patients will have a tracheostomy at any one time.

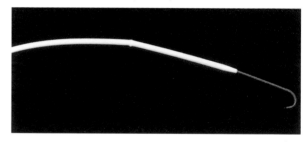

Figure 9.5 Percutaneous Tracheostomy: J-shaped guide wire and guarded guide catheter.

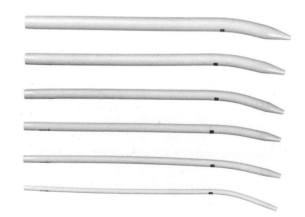

Figure 9.6 Radio-opaque dilators. In this kit, the 24 FG dilator is required for the 8 mm tube.

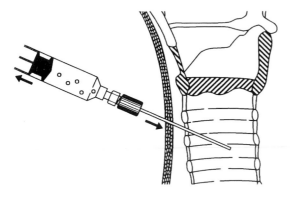

Figure 9.7 Air aspiration into a syringe confirms the position of the Teflon sheath. The guide wire is inserted through the sheath and the sheath withdrawn.

Advantages of tracheostomy in the ICU

- Lower doses of sedation
- Preservation of cough reflex
- More efficient pulmonary toilet
- Reduced duration of ventilation
- Less laryngeal trauma

Advantages of percutaneous tracheostomy in the ICU

- No need to book theatre time
- No patient transport hazards
- Comparable complication rates to open

Unfortunately, the mortality in the ICU remains high at around one in three, and so the long-term effects of percutaneous tracheostomy have only recently been addressed. Percutaneous tracheostomy is more hazardous in those with short, thick necks and goitres, but may still be undertaken by those experienced in the technique, preferably with endoscopic control.

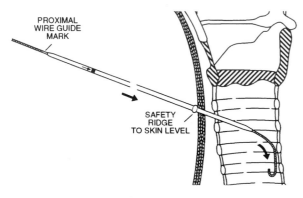

Figure 9.8 Guiding catheter inserted over a guide wire. The two are advanced as a unit until the safety ridge is at skin level.

Percutaneous tracheostomy

- (Seldinger) puncture of tracheal wall
- Pass dilators over the guide wire
- Insert lubricated tube
- Variants: one-stage tracheal spreader; endoscopic control

The most popular method of percutaneous tracheostomy currently in use is to carry out a Seldinger type puncture of the tracheal wall, and insert a guide wire over which the tube can be passed. A number of commercially available kits for percutaneous tracheostomy are now available.

Contraindications to percutaneous tracheostomy

- Children
- Bleeding diathesis
- Previous surgery
- Infection
- Enlarged thyroid

The procedure requires two trained personnel, one to perform the procedure and the other to maintain the patient's airway and circulation, and to provide anaesthesia. Because the procedure is frequently performed in an ICU, pulse oximetry, capnography, electrocardiography and blood pressure monitoring are routine. The patient is ventilated on 100% oxygen and the neck extended with the pillow under the shoulders. The endotracheal tube is withdrawn to the laryngeal inlet, the cuff deflated and the pharynx suctioned under direct vision. The cuff is reinflated to stabilize the tube at this higher level. The head must be kept strictly in the midline. The suprasternal notch and the surface markings of the laryngeal framework structures are marked. The skin incision should approximate to the first and second, or second and third tracheal rings.

Equipment for percutaneous tracheostomy

- Scalpel
- 14 G intravenous needle and cannula
- 10 ml syringe
- Flexible Teflon-coated guide wire
- Plastic dilator
- Pair of tracheal dilating forceps
- Tracheostomy tube with a hollow obturator to slide over the guide wire

Tracheal forceps have a groove in the jaws to allow their passage around the guide wire. The tracheostomy cuff must be fully deflated prior to insertion. Then, 3 ml of saline should be drawn into the 10 ml syringe via the 14 G cannula. As indicated above for open tracheostomy, 10 ml of 1% Lignocaine with 1:200 000 adrenaline is used to infiltrate locally. A difference here is that because the procedure is being carried out under general anaesthesia in an ICU, the trachea may be directly infiltrated at the outset. A 1.5–2 cm incision is made at the midpoint of the distance between the lower border of the cricoid and the sternal notch. After some blunt dissection the anterior tracheal wall may be palpated. A 14 G cannula with the syringe attached is inserted in the midline and as the surgeon passes more deeply he or she should aspirate on the syringe. Successful tracheal puncture is indicated by a sudden air entry; at this point the syringe and needle are removed, and a guide wire inserted through the plastic cannula (Fig. 9.5). The cannula and the guide wire introducer are then removed.

Next, using a gentle oscillation motion to help advance it, the surgeon inserts the dilator into the anterior wall of the trachea. He or she must always ensure that the guide wire is not kinked because if a bend occurs in the wire it is possible to create a false passage anterior to the trachea. The dilating forceps are locked on to the wire and used in a movement to dilate the soft tissues by being inserted as far as the tracheal wall, opened and withdrawn. They are then reclosed around the guide wire and reinserted into the tracheal wall; this time, the tracheal wall is dilated.

The surgeon confirms free movement of the guide wire, opens the forceps and withdraws them. The more forcibly the jaws of the forceps are opened, the larger the eventual stoma size. Finally, the obturator and tracheostomy tube are fed over the guide wire (Fig. 9.6), the obturator and guide wire removed and suction performed on the trachea. The tracheostomy cuff and fixation are managed

in the usual way. The anaesthetist confirms the position of the tube by auscultation and withdraws the endotracheal tube from the pharynx. Note: percutaneous tracheostomy should be undertaken very cautiously in patients whose airway is not maintained by an endotracheal tube, in whom there is an increased risk of creating a false passage between the tracheal mucosa and the cartilaginous rings.

References and further reading

Ciaglia P. and Graniero, K. D. (1992) Percutaneous dilational tracheostomy: results and long-term follow-up, *Chest* **101**: 464–7.

Fisher E. W. and Howard D. J. (1992) Percutaneous tracheostomy in a head and neck unit, *J Laryngol Otol* **106**: 625–627.

Friedman Y., Fildes J., Mizock B., Samuel J., Patel S., Appavu S. and Roberts R. (1996) Comparison of percutaneous and surgical tracheostomies, *Chest* **110**: 480–5.

Hill B. B., Zweng T. N., Maley R. H., Charash W. E., Toursarkissian B. and Kearney P. A. (1996) Percutaneous dilational tracheostomy: report of 356 cases, *J Trauma Injury Infect Crit Care* **40**: 238–43.

Jackson C. (1909) Tracheotomy, *Laryngoscope* **19**: 285–90.

Jeannon J. P. and Mathias D. (2000) Percutaneous (Portex) tracheostomy: an audit of the Newcastle experience, *Ann R Coll Surg Engl* **82**: 137–140.

Law R. C., Carney A. S., and Manara A. R. (1997) Long-term outcome after percutaneous dilational tracheostomy, *Anaesthesia* **52**: 51–6.

Milner S. M. and Bennett J. D. C. (1991) Emergency cricothyrotomy, *J Laryngol Otol* **105**: 883–5.

10 Trauma and stenosis of the larynx and cervical trachea

'A neck God made for other use than strangling in a string'
A. E. Houseman, 1896

Acute laryngeal trauma

Because cervical spine fractures are commonly associated with laryngeal injury, the neck must be manipulated carefully until cervical spine X-rays have been obtained. The cricoid is the most important part of the laryngeal skeleton. It is the only complete ring in the upper or lower respiratory tract. The thyroid and the hyoid and tracheal rings are all U-shaped with soft tissue attachments posteriorly. If the cricoid is disrupted, then it will constrict. Even a linear fracture in the cricoid will cause some resorption of cartilage and reduction of the calibre of the airway at the level of the cricoid. This has severe effects on airflow as a consequence of Poiseuille's law, which relates the airflow indirectly to the fourth power of the radius of the airway. This is probably why high tracheostomies have such a deleterious effect on the airway. There is nothing magic about the first ring, but a tracheostomy tube here is contiguous with the cricoid cartilage and may result in enough resorption of that cartilage for it to stenose.

As a general rule, acute injuries to the cricoid cartilage pose the most immediate airway threat to the airway, as there is no room for expansion of a subglottic haematoma. Injuries to the thyroid present with delayed airway compromise from expanding haematoma, and hyoid injury may even be overlooked altogether. The subglottic space in children is very much more susceptible to internal soft-tissue injury than it is in the adult.

Causes of laryngeal injury

■ Penetrating wounds: knives, bullets, wires and agricultural implements.
■ Blunt injuries
  – High-velocity: usually road traffic accidents or injuries at work. The velocity may be so high that the wound becomes compound.
  – Low-velocity: blunt injuries rarely become compound and result from ligature or manual strangulation, blows with fists and sports injuries. Similar injuries may arise from inhalation of smoke and fumes

---

As with nasal injuries, most laryngeal injuries in the West are related to fighting or sports. The sports that are particularly associated with laryngeal injury are snow-mobile racing, motorcycle racing, basketball and karate; injuries have even been reported from contact with golf balls and cricket balls, and to the practice of garroting with ice-hockey sticks. Thus, young males are particularly at risk.

Epidemiology

All emergency-room personnel must maintain a high index of suspicion of laryngeal trauma as the incidence is low, estimated at <1/30 000 emergency-room attenders. In North America and western Europe, the condition of laryngeal trauma was first associated with road traffic accidents. Nowadays, the incidence in these continents of laryngeal damage from road traffic accidents has been massively reduced by the cross-over seat belt, enforcement of speed limits and other safety features in cars, such as collapsible steering wheels and air bags. In countries where driving by a large number of people is a relatively new development, laryngeal injuries as a result of road traffic accidents present a significant otolaryngological problem. World-wide, improved delivery of immediate medical care allows more survivors from road traffic accidents to reach hospital.

Mechanics of injury

Classification of laryngeal injury

■ Sites
  – supraglottis
  – glottis
  – subglottis
  – mixed
■ Tissues
  – laryngeal framework: hyoid, thyroid, cricoid, tracheal rings
  – internal soft tissues

Penetrating wounds tend to bounce off the laryngeal skeleton and enter either the thyrohyoid membrane with bleeding in the paraglottic space and airway obstruction, or the cricothyroid membrane when air escape predominates with surgical emphysema in the neck. The voice is not affected in any way. A little bleeding or oedema will be absorbed. More significant bleeding will be organized to cause some degree of stenosis of the supraglottis.

The penetrating wound, however, may be covered with thyroid tissue. The bleeding may fill the subglottic space causing respiratory obstruction, but it is more likely to run down the trachea through a clean cut and cause coughing.

Low-velocity blunt injuries: soft tissue

Low-velocity blunt injuries (e.g. sport) may fracture the hyoid but most of the related injuries are to the soft tissues.

Soft-tissue injury

- Oedema
- Haematoma
  - supraglottic
  - paraglottic space
  - Reinke's space
- Web: abrasions at anterior commissure
- Glottic incompetence
  - arytenoid fixation
  - resorption of the thyroarytenoid muscle
  - atrophy of the cord
  - recurrent laryngeal nerve paralysis (subglottic injuries)

Any injury to the larynx will result in soft-tissue oedema. Swelling of the tongue base may cause dysphagia, but the only permanent effects are in Reinke's space: permanent oedema of the vocal cord or laryngeal polyp. Far more important is the effect of organized haematoma, most marked in the supraglottic space or interarytenoid area, where there is the most scope for expansion of soft tissue and obliteration of the airway.

High-velocity blunt injuries: skeletal framework

If cartilage has prolonged contact with blood, then the blood is absorbed. This is especially important in the trachea, where loss of the U-shaped rings may cause no observable abnormality in the airway until the patient takes exercise or a deep breath. The increased velocity of airflow pulls in the weakened tracheal walls and the patient will have dyspnoea on exercise due to tracheomalacia. If cartilage is left denuded of mucosa and is in contact with secretions, then the surface of the cartilage will become inflamed. This will result in the formation of granulations and is most frequently seen in intubation granuloma of the vocal process of the arytenoid. Less often, use of an oversized endotracheal tube may split the anterior commissure, with granuloma formation.

The hyoid, the only bone in the respiratory tract, may be fractured and may well heal without the patient knowing that anything has happened apart from a few days of discomfort. Sometimes, however, swallowing is exquisitely painful. On rare occasions, the fractured ends of the hyoid bone form a bursa, which results in continual movement of the fractured edges together. This is treated by excision.

Thyroid cartilage and arytenoids

- Injury depends on degree of calcification and, thus, on patient age
- If pushed backwards over the cervical spine, then it splays apart
- Minimal injury: no fracture as inherent elasticity lets it spring back
- Greater force: fracture down the thyroid prominence – elastic cartilage: pre-epiglottic space bleeding, posterior displacement of epiglottis calcified cartilage: detachment of the tendon of the anterior commissure and the petiole of the epiglottis (rare) (Fig. 10.1).

The epiglottis falls backwards and the vocal cords literally roll up on themselves towards the arytenoid. Alternatively, the cartilage may shatter like an egg, with loss of the thyroid prominence (Fig. 10.2). The arytenoids become sandwiched between the thyroid and the cervical spine, with either displacement or at least bleeding into the interarytenoid space and consequent swelling. The fractured thyroid cartilage will heal with fibrous tissue; provided it is in a good position, this is just as satisfactory as wiring or stitching it together. A compressed, calcified thyroid cartilage has to be reconstituted and stented.

Cricoid cartilage

It is rare that acute injuries damage the soft tissue within the cricoid but if a high-velocity acute injury damages the integrity of the cricoid cartilage, then there will be a very difficult defect to repair. Rehabilitation of this area must involve widening the cricoid cartilage and keeping the edges apart with non-resorbable material.

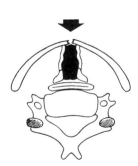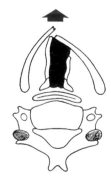

Figure 10.1 Compression of an uncalcified cartilage leads to a linear thyroid fracture and possible detachment of a vocal cord and/or epiglottis.

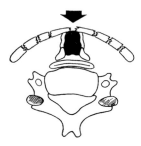

Figure 10.2 Compression of a calcified thyroid cartilage causes flattening of the neck due to shattering.

Cricotracheal separation

The final soft-tissue injury from high-velocity blunt injuries takes the form of separation of the trachea from the cricoid. This usually results in death at the roadside, but enough lumen may remain to allow the patient to reach hospital. Several tracheal rings can be damaged with this sort of injury and the cricotracheal membrane may be sheared off.

Investigations

History and examination

With obstruction above the level of the larynx the stridor is likely to be of lower pitch, with indrawing of the cheeks during inspiration and blowing out during expiration. Stridor from the laryngeal level is high pitched and there may be suprasternal retraction and, indeed, reduced respiratory drive. Once the airway is re-established, e.g. by intubation, there is a risk of persistent respiratory depression.

Symptoms

- Awareness of the possibility in every upper body trauma victim
- Dyspnoea
- Dysphonia
- Dysphagia
- Pain
- Cough
- Haemoptysis

Signs

- Stridor
- Cervical bruising
- Surgical emphysema confined to the neck: almost pathognomonic
- Loss of thyroid prominence is also diagnostic
- Be aware of risk of associated damage
  - Great vessels
  - Cervical spine
  - Chest: haemothorax/pneumothorax; emphysema; distant oesophageal tears abdomen
- Abdomen: gastric dilatation

The chest is palpated and auscultated; an intrapleural tracheobronchial laceration gives a massive pneumothorax. If the laceration is mediastinal, then emphysema results. Signs of gastric dilatation in the abdomen may complicate either tracheostomy or the laryngeal injury and require prompt decompression by nasogastric intubation.

Radiology

A computed tomographic (CT) scan should be obtained if a fracture is suspected but not clinically obvious.

A plain cervical X-ray is helpful in some emergency situations. Deep cervical or prevertebral air may be the principal findings in a patient who arrives at the hospital already intubated.

A chest X-ray may show:

- incomplete bronchial transection: the apex of the collapsed lung sits at the level of the hilum
- deep cervical emphysema: a radiolucent line along the prevertebral fascia
- peribronchial air
- sudden obstruction along the course of an air-filled bronchus
- fracture of the first rib, scapula or sternum: suggests severe injury and the possibility of airway trauma.

Flexible laryngoscopy should be performed in all patients. Direct laryngoscopy, in contrast, adds little and may exacerbate the effects of injury.

Treatment policy and principles

Protection of the airway

- If there is merely oedema present, with no suggestion of intraluminal bleeding or tracheal damage, then the patient can be kept on bed rest with or without steam inhalations. A sitting posture with the jaw kept forward is said to favour the clearing of secretions.
- If there is bruising and oedema but no major mucosal laceration, and no displacement of the arytenoids and the tracheal lumen can be visualized, the patient should be intubated, perhaps passing the tube over a bronchoscope.
- In the first-aid situation, a tracheostomy may be needed, e.g. in the presence of significant subcutaneous emphysema and a large laryngeal laceration, especially if cartilage is visible in the wound or if the tracheal lumen cannot be visualized. The operation is, however, much less favourable than immediate intubation. Cricothyroidotomy should be avoided as it may exacerbate late stenosis.
- If there is associated bronchial injury, flexible bronchoscopy with elective intubation of one bronchus allows the patient to be stabilized prior to emergency thoracotomy.
- Associated great vessel damage may indicate emergency thoracotomy as part of the resuscitation process.

At intubation, there will be contusion and perhaps bleeding in the throat. It is quite impossible, with the equipment and time available to an anaesthetist in this situation, for them to characterize the precise nature of the laryngeal injuries. The arytenoids will be swollen in almost every moderately severe laryngeal trauma, and so the patient should be fed with a nasogastric tube to stop inhalation from glottic incompetence for at least a few days.

Although an endotracheal tube is not much smaller than many of the stents that are used in the later reconstruction of a larynx, neither they nor the stents do anything to stop intraluminal bleeding, especially in the supraglottic area, or to prevent fibrosis or webs in either the posterior or anterior glottis. An inflated endotracheal cuff can however prevent aspiration of blood. The role of stents is only to scaffold a reconstituted skeletal structure. The best method to control bleeding and fibrosis is to open the spaces and obliterate them with quilting sutures. Any significant degree of endolaryngeal bleeding should be approached by a midline laryngofissure and the spaces evacuated and quilted with 3/0 Vicryl sutures. Inserting drains into the spaces is quite useless.

Protection of laryngeal function

The functions of breathing and speaking take priority.
A successful breathing outcome may be classed as:

- no requirement for a permanent tracheostomy tube
- patient undertakes normal daily activities
- minimal or no dyspnoea.

A successful phonating outcome depends on the type of injury. If there has been vocal cord damage, a normal speaking voice is unlikely. Success, therefore, may include not only normal voice but indeed any non-whispering phonation.

Laryngeal Framework Damage

The principle is of minimal débridement. There is not very much cartilage in the larynx; therefore, excision of any tracheal rings, and certainly of the cricoid cartilage, has grave consequences. It is important to remember in this situation the words of Sir Harold Gillies – 'Thou shalt not throw away a living thing'. Although much damaged cartilage may resorb in any case, it is better to cover it with mucosa and see whether it forms a scaffold for firm fibrous tissue. The worst that can happen is what would be achieved with débridement.

Treatment

General supportive measures

- Bed rest and voice rest
- High humidity atmosphere
- Oxygen may be given
- Antibiotic therapy is usually helpful
- Maximum dose parenteral steroid therapy: said to slow granulation formation and reduce fibrosis

Penetrating injuries

Sharp penetrating injuries with bleeding into the supraglottic area almost all require the larynx to be opened and the supraglottic area drained and quilted. It is usual for patients with supraglottic injury to end up with a reasonably good voice and no tracheostomy.

Bullet wounds most certainly require exploration and débridement of cartilage, which will probably also be fractured, and exploration of the neck vessels and nerves. On occasion the injuries as the result of bullet wounds are so severe that total laryngectomy is necessary. In this situation, perhaps, the excision should be carried out bearing in mind the recent developments in laryngeal transplantation so that the relevant nerves are tagged.

Low-velocity blunt injuries

The majority of patients require only overnight observation in hospital, in cases of laryngeal oedema and airway obstruction. If either the airway or the voice is clearly disturbed, however, then the larynx should be intubated and perhaps later explored and reconstructed.

Many patients will ultimately have a poor voice if the glottis has been damaged, because there may well be later minor web formation or arthrodesis of an arytenoid. It is unusual, however, for these patients to require a permanent tracheostomy.

High-velocity blunt injuries

About half of the patients who have laryngeal injuries as a result of road traffic accidents require laryngeal exploration and reconstruction:

- skeletal damage: may be repaired by reconstitution, usually using stents
- soft-tissue injuries: bleeding must be reduced, spaces evacuated and quilting sutures inserted
- cricoid injury: primary repair is attempted. If it should fail, one of the many techniques for chronic cricoid stenosis is applied
- separation of the cricotracheal membrane: this unusual injury may be approached by dropping the larynx in the neck, freeing the trachea down to the carina with end-to-end anastomosis and excising any damaged tracheal rings.

Most high-velocity blunt injuries will result in combined injuries to the glottis and subglottis. If only the glottis is involved then the results with regard to breathing should be good, but if the subglottis is involved, then the patient faces future surgery for chronic subglottic stenosis.

Technique of operations for laryngeal trauma

Fractured hyoid

- Treat minimally displaced fractures without pharyngeal lacerations conservatively.
- Small pharyngeal lacerations with displaced fractures may be managed by endoscopic reduction and suture.

- If there is comminution or gross displacement, an external exploration is performed. Removal of bone on either side of this fracture line will not result in disability and prevents the jagged ends rubbing against each other and causing pain.

Fractured thyroid cartilage and internal soft-tissue injuries

Fractures of the thyroid cartilage with greater than 15–20° degrees angulation between the fragments should be reduced as even minor displacement alters glottic configuration.

- A collar incision is made and the skin flaps elevated.
- The strap muscles are retracted and the thyroid prominence displayed. A fracture line extending obliquely down the front of the thyroid cartilage will probably be seen; the cricoid cartilage should be examined carefully to ensure that the fracture line has not extended lower.
- A laryngofissure through the fracture line is performed with scissors.
- The vocal cords are resutured to the vocal processes or the anterior commissure, depending on from where they are detached.
- The mucosal lacerations are sutured with 3/0 chromic catgut or 4/0 Vicryl.
- The epiglottis is fixed in position by two sutures of silk, which are placed so as to hold the epiglottis forwards by anchoring it to the hyoid bone.
- The cartilage fragment may be fixed directly, e.g. by 24–26 G stainless-steel wires. Alternatively, if the cartilage is mostly unossified, titanium miniplates may be more appropriate.

If the anterior commissure has been damaged, simple wiring of the thyroid cartilage will not suffice to prevent the formation of an anterior web. A McNaught keel may be fashioned using 0.18 mm thick tantalum sheeting, cut to the appropriate size with Mayo scissors, and placed in the laryngofissure with the external flanges sutured to the thyroid perichondrium with 3/0 chromic catgut (Fig. 10.3). An alternative to this is to put a sheet of rolled-up silastic in the lumen of the larynx and to hold it

with two transfixion sutures, fastened on the outside with silastic buttons.

The wound is closed in layers without drainage and the patient started on perioperative antibiotics. After 4–6 weeks the neck is reopened and the keel or silastic removed. There will almost inevitably be some exposed bare cartilage at the anterior commissure, over which granulation tissue will form. This tissue may need to be removed several times via an endoscope before the larynx is fully healed. The tracheostomy tube can be withdrawn when the patient can breathe normally again.

Shattered thyroid cartilage with internal soft-tissue injuries

There is a marked flattening of the thyroid prominence and when the thyroid cartilage is exposed instead of a single fracture line, multiple stellate fracture lines are seen. The external perichondrium is usually intact but the internal perichondrium is invariably breached with pieces of cartilage lying in the laryngeal cavity. A laryngofissure is carried out and the internal derangements sutured as before. In this case a more solid splinting is required with an internal laryngeal stent.

Laryngeal stents

A stent may be used as long as 3 months postinjury. There is no ideal laryngeal stent available, as evidenced by the multiplicity of designs that have been tried in the past. Although the patient is able to whisper through a hollow stent on closing off the tracheostomy tube, it causes aspiration on swallowing. It is better to use a solid laryngeal stent made of some inert material, such as one of the various silicone rubbers. In an emergency, a finger-cot filled with sponge may be used as a temporary measure.

Indications for laryngeal stenting

- To maintain the shape of the cartilaginous framework:
  - posterior displacement of the base of the epiglottis
  - dislocation of the arytenoids
  - depressed fracture cricoid
  - markedly displaced thyroid fracture
- To separate mucosal lacerations

The stent is fixed with two no. 26 stainless-steel wires passed through the neck from side to side, passing, in order, through skin, thyroid cartilage, stent, thyroid cartilage and skin. The two free ends on either side of the neck are threaded through buttons and tightened (Fig. 10.4). Further tightening at daily intervals will be required as the swelling settles.

The stent remains in the larynx for at least 3 months; when the time comes to remove it, the wires are cut flush with the skin on one side and pulled through from the other side of the neck. A thread attached to the stent allows endoscopic removal. The thread is attached to a piece of stainless-steel wire inside the laryngeal stent, to prevent it loosening from the stent.

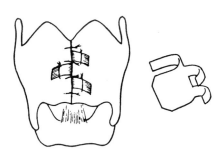

Figure 10.3 McNaught keel (right) shown in position between the vocal cords with the flanges sutured to the thyroid cartilages.

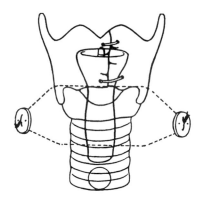

Figure 10.4 Fixation of a solid laryngeal stent.

Fractured cricoid

This injury is invariably associated with a fracture or shattering of the thyroid cartilage with internal damage. It is vital to recognize it when the thyroid cartilage is fractured. Chevalier Jackson stated that 'loss of the cricoid cartilage practically always precludes the possibility of eliminating the wearing of a tracheal cannula'. This is not completely true, but any loss of cricoid cartilage must be very skilfully repaired, as will be seen later. The fracture is usually anterior and direct suture of the muco-perichondrial tears is difficult because of poor access. Therefore, the chief goal is to realign the cartilage fragments. As much cartilage as possible must be retained and a laryngeal stent used for 3 months, especially in the event of posterior fracture.

Tracheal injuries

Simple injury

Operation is recommended for a laceration greater than one-third of the trachea or a major bronchus. The principle is one of mucosa-to-mucosa closure if at all possible, e.g. with Vicryl.

Major injury

Transection of the trachea or major bronchus involves adequate débridement and mucosa-to-mucosa apposition (3/0 Vicryl). A pericartilaginous suture is used on the cartilage trachea and simple interrupted sutures on the membranous portion. For a complete severance of a major airway, the site should be intubated with an endotracheal or endobronchial tube.

Tracheal avulsion

In a severe injury the trachea may be avulsed from the larynx by a tear through the cricotracheal membrane. Most such injuries are fatal at the site of the accident from respiratory obstruction, but a surviving patient occasionally arrives at the hospital. An immediate tracheo-stomy is performed and the larynx explored. It is usually possible to suture the first tracheal ring to the cricoid cartilage using 2/0 Nylon sutures. All of the sutures should be in place before being tied, as it is very difficult to insert extra sutures once any are tied. There is no need to use a stent, which may cause infection and subsequent breakdown of the anastomosis.

Postoperative care

Careful maintenance of ventilation and oxygenation is clearly necessary. Bronchorrhoea will follow most major injuries. There is also aspiration of blood, and thus vigorous tracheobronchial toilet is needed.

Chronic laryngeal stenosis

Chronic stenosis may be said to be established if the airway is unsatisfactory 4 weeks after the injury. It is an important condition which interferes with speech, breathing and the ability to clear secretions from the lower respiratory tract. This section will be confined to chronic laryngeal stenosis in the adult. The condition is quite different if it manifests itself in childhood.

Causes

> **Causes of chronic laryngeal stenosis**
>
> - Failed treatment or non-recognition of acute trauma
> - As a complication of
>   - tracheostomy
>   - intubation
>   - partial laryngectomy
> - Scleroma: most common cause in the Middle East
> - Wegener's granuloma
> - Polychondritis
> - Autoimmune thyroiditis

Supraglottic and glottic stenosis may occur, but the most common site is the subglottic area. The main cause is, therefore, disruption of the supporting cricoid and tracheal skeleton. The associated soft-tissue narrowing usually reflects the lack of integrity of the supporting structures.

The soft-tissue damage is due to:

- mucosal loss
- mucosal adhesions
- organization of haematoma in the paraglottic, pre-epiglottic and interarytenoid spaces

Glottic competence is affected by:

- web formation anteriorly
- arthrodesis of the arytenoid posteriorly
- recurrent laryngeal nerve injury either at the time of the initial trauma or in the ensuing treatment.

Arytenoidectomy or cordopexy almost always forms part of the treatment of chronic laryngeal stenosis.

An important factor in the correction of chronic laryngeal stenosis is that of tissue memory. A disrupted cartilaginous framework heals with fibrous tissue compromising fibrocytes with a directional memory. Thus, merely incising and separating scar tissue will lead to replacement of the tissue in its original scarred state. Even with removal of as much scarred tissue as possible, the danger of repositioning will be ever present. This is most important in the cricoid, where the interruption of the ring causes narrowing. The forces within the cricoid are altered, probably permanently, from this narrowing, and excision of the scarred area and separation of the cricoid ends, with support from intervening tissue, is probably the single most difficult problem in the management of chronic stenosis.

Excision of scarred soft tissue is easier. Wide excision of scarred tissue with grafting by split skin or mucosa usually gives good results. It must be re-emphasized, however, that satisfactory soft-tissue healing will not take place if the skeletal framework is disrupted or resumes its scarred altered position. Stents are useful in supporting a reconstituted laryngeal framework and, to an extent, in separating mucosal surfaces that have been adherent.

Investigations

History

■ The cause of the chronic stenosis is obviously important. If it is a result of systemic disease or of an excessively zealous partial laryngectomy, then it is unlikely that enough tissue will be found to augment the lumen of the larynx.

■ Both the surgeon and the patient must realize what is and what is not possible with surgery. Both should realize that the dynamics of tissue healing can alter any result and this should be taken into account in timing the operation.

■ No attempts should be made to increase the laryngeal lumen until 18 months have passed from the time of the initial injury.

■ The patient's objectives from surgery should be clarified in respect of the importance of good voice and the desire to be rid of the tracheostomy tube. More minor cases should also realize that the additional scarring of surgery could, rarely, culminate in permanent tracheostomy.

Examination

■ Flexible endoscopy is performed to gauge the extent of the stenosis.

■ An assessment is made of the length of the neck and how much cervical trachea is available for mobilization

Radiography

■ CT scanning should, if possible, be carried out in all instances.

■ Only where the subglottis cannot be evaluated should laryngography be used.

■ Magnetic resonance imaging may be required to delineate all the soft-tissue features.

Rigid endoscopy

■ The extent of laryngeal damage can be confirmed.

■ The lower extent of subglottic stenosis is shown.

■ The tracheal cartilages are examined from as high as possible without creating any splinting and with the anaesthetist blowing high airflows into the lungs using a Venturi system. In this way, tracheomalacia can be assessed.

■ The state of the arytenoids must be ascertained to determine whether they are fixed or not.

■ Oesophagoscopy should be carried out in every case.

Treatment policy

Most patients presenting for the treatment of chronic laryngeal stenosis will already have a tracheostomy. Warn the patient that

■ the results are unrewarding and the tracheostomy may be permanent

■ postoperatively a nasogastric tube will be required, at least for some days, until the oedema settles

■ it is unlikely that the postoperative voice will be normal.

There is almost universal dissatisfaction with the surgical treatment of the systemic conditions that cause laryngo-tracheal stenosis, such as a scleroma, Wegener's granuloma and polychondritis. These patients should perhaps not be treated other than by occasional dilatations.

Supraglottic stenosis

There are two options:

■ a laryngeal widening procedure: the larynx is opened in the midline and as much as possible of the submucosal scarred tissue removed. The remaining mucosa is stitched back against the laryngeal framework with quilting sutures, or areas of scarred tissue are grafted with either skin or buccal mucosa

■ laser excision allows the patient to keep the tracheostomy tube and to evaluate the effect of serial excisions.

Glottic stenosis

Anterior stenosis can be dealt with by

■ laser excision

■ repeated endoscopic excision.

If the webbing is limited to the glottis, then one of the above options is probably best in the first instance.

■ external excision and separation of the anterior glottis with a silastic or tantalum keel (McNaught keel) for at least 5 weeks. It can then be removed with minimal reopening of the neck wound. The external approach is probably the preferred one when there is also a stenosis of the anterior parts of the false cords.

Posterior stenosis of the glottis is more difficult to treat as it lies between the cartilaginous arytenoids, usually with fixation of at least one arytenoid. The posterior web is easy to excise, but will recur if the posterior commissure is not covered by a mucous membrane. Usually, the arytenoids are also separated by a modified keel with silastic stenting on its end to keep the posterior glottis open. For this to succeed, both arytenoids must be mobile and capable of achieving glottic competence when the keel is removed. A superiorly based mucous membrane flap is obtained from the interarytenoid space above the stenosis. If the arytenoids are not mobiles then one should be removed by a laryngofissure and the cord stitched laterally with stenting applied to stop further adhesions, which should remain in place for 2 weeks.

Complete glottic stenosis is best dealt with by free mucosal grafts, e.g. from the buccal region, combined with local mucosal flaps.

Cricoid stenosis

- A cricoid graft must keep the area open permanently and adhere to the cartilaginous ends.
- Free bone or cartilage grafts, taken from ribs, are unlikely to achieve this objective in a satisfactory and regulated manner.
- Allografts have no place.
- The body of the hyoid bone can be swung down on a muscle pedicle of sternohyoid. When wired into the arch of the cricoid, this may offer the best chance of keeping the cricoid ring open. The soft-tissue scarring must also be removed and replaced with a skin graft and a stent applied either in the form of rolled-up silastic above a tracheostomy tube, or in a modified tracheostomy tube. If a Montgomery T-tube is used for this, then the greatest care must be taken to ensure that it does not crust.
- For greater degrees of cricoid stenosis, where the ring cannot realistically be reconstituted, the cricoid is removed, leaving part of the posterior lamina supporting the arytenoids. The larynx is then dropped and the trachea pulled up and joined to the lower end of the thyroid lamina anteriorly and to the arch of the cricoid posteriorly. This one-stage procedure tends to produce a lump in the back of the immediate subglottic space, but it is fairly reliable and usually allows extubation.

Tracheal stenosis

The more minor degrees of tracheal stenosis are best treated with dilatation. Very often the problem is one of tracheomalacia, rather than true stenosis. No stenosis is seen on endoscopy or X-ray. Very often these patients are frustrated by the lack of a medical diagnosis when they

know full well that they are dyspnoeic on exertion. If a tracheal stenosis is severe enough to warrant the wearing of a tracheostomy tube, then it is a relatively easy matter to excise up to 4–5 cm of trachea to drop the larynx and to join the trachea on the cricoid or first tracheal ring. For a patient dyspnoeic only on exertion, however, surgery to excise the weak area of trachea must be weighed against the high risk of damage to one or both of the recurrent laryngeal nerves and subsequent phonosurgery. Attempts to strengthen the tracheal wall with Marlex mesh, or other external devices, are not often successful.

A very extensive stenosis may be approached via a right thoracotomy and removal of the right mainstem bronchus from the carina, closing the hole at the carina and joining the right mainstem bronchus on the left mainstem bronchus at a lower level (Grillo procedure). This gives several more centimetres of length to the trachea and does not result in stenosis further down. If localized stenosis occurs further down the trachea, then laser excision can be used.

Results

The results from supraglottic or glottic stenoses are usually good, i.e. extubation with a reasonable voice. It is usually possible to remove the tracheostomy tube and leave the patient with a reasonable voice. The results of the treatment of subglottic stenosis, however, are universally poor. The key to the subglottis is the cricoid, and in adults no satisfactory solution has been found to restoring the dynamic elastic forces necessary to preserve the integrity of the only complete ring in the respiratory tract.

Technique of operations for chronic laryngeal stenosis

Laryngeal widening operation for supraglottic stenosis

- Anaesthesia is continued via the tracheostomy.
- The neck is opened with a horizontal collar incision half way between the thyroid notch and the cricothyroid membrane, and the skin flaps are elevated.
- The scarred strap muscles are retracted, exposing the thyroid cartilage and cricoid.
- The larynx is opened in the midline up to the hyoid using a no. 10 blade (with or without an oscillating saw).
- The lumen is entered: an opening usually appears just below the anterior commissure, but if not, entry is at the cricothyroid membrane level, or even lower in very extensive stenosis.
- The thickened scar tissue between the remaining mucosa and the thyroid cartilage is excised from both the paraglottic space and the pre-epiglottic space.
- Multiple 3/0 Vicryl quilting sutures are inserted, pulling the remaining mucosa against the external skeleton of the larynx (Fig. 10.5).

The danger from this operation on the larynx is incompetence of the protective laryngeal sphincter, but the risk

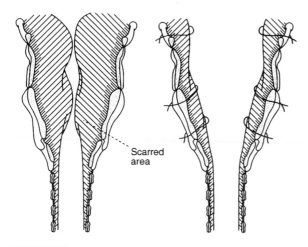

Figure 10.5 Quilting of supraglottic stenosis via a laryngo-fissure.

of aspiration is not excessive, as sensation is usually preserved. There is no need to remove the sutures, but revision procedures may be required at later dates. Closure is in two layers without a stent, but an anterior silicone keel may be inserted.

Tracheal resection and end-to-end anastomosis

■ Anaesthesia is continued via the tracheostomy.
■ A horizontal incision is made and skin flaps are elevated from above the level of the hyoid down to the suprasternal notch. A Joll's clamp is applied.
■ The larynx is freed as in a narrow-field laryngectomy and the entire hyoid dissected free so that a finger can be placed behind the greater horn on each side.
■ The posterior lamina of the thyroid cartilage is freed and a finger placed behind it.
■ An attempt is made to find the recurrent laryngeal nerves in the tracheo-oesophageal grooves, but this is often impossible.
■ The normal trachea is located, the pretracheal fascia is entered and a dissection is made down to the carina on the tracheal wall.

The trachea acts as a concertina and, although it will apparently come well up into the neck, its normal tension will pull it back down into the thorax.

The most important part of this operation is to drop the larynx (see Fig. 10.7).

■ The superior cornu of the thyroid cartilage is cut off on both sides, thus releasing the pull of the stylopharyngeus, salpingopharyngeus and palatopharyngeus muscles.
■ The thyrohyoid membrane is divided as close as possible to the upper lamina of the thyroid cartilage to minimize risk to the superior laryngeal nerves, and the pre-epiglottic space is entered.

The pharyngeal constrictors are removed from the posterior lamina of the thyroid cartilage. This allows the thyroid cartilage to be detached from the hyoid and several centimetres of downward displacement. Additional length can be obtained by:

■ flexing the patient's neck
■ freeing up the trachea within the mediastinum. This must be done carefully and one should try to confine blunt finger dissection to the anterior and posterior planes, as the blood supply enters laterally from intercostal and bronchial arterial branches.

The trachea is joined together or to the cricoid with 2/0 Vicryl sutures. It is important that these sutures do not enter the mucosa of the trachea. All of the sutures should be in position before being tied, in order to distribute the tension correctly. The surgeon starts trying on the posterior wall first and gradually come forward to the anterior part of the anastomosis. It is probably better not to use a stent and to remove the tracheostomy tube at the earliest opportunity.

Management of inadequate glottic opening associated with subglottic stenosis

If the recurrent laryngeal nerves have not been found, or if it is strongly suspected that the nerve is divided on one side, then it is probably advisable to carry out a Woodman's operation or other lateralization procedure on the affected side during the operation. (Some authorities reserve arytenoidectomy for bilateral vocal cord paralysis.) An alternative to widening the glottis where the mucosa is healthy is to carry out vertical posterior cricoid plate division. The edges are separated by 5–7 mm and kept apart by a periosteal or perichondrial graft in the bed of the division. As with any procedure which alters glottic diameter, the right balance must be found between an adequate airway for breathing and sufficient closure to allow acceptable voice quality.

One-stage tracheal resection combined with resection of the cricoid ring (Couraud *et al.*, 1996)

Where there is upward extension of the tracheal stenosis towards the glottis (Fig. 10.6), one-stage tracheal resection with laryngeal drop (Fig. 10.7) can be extended to the subglottic area after resection of the anterior cricoid arch and a rim of the cricoid plate (Fig. 10.8). It is best to avoid attempted identification of the recurrent laryngeal nerves and, if possible, not to perform tracheostomy. Mobilization of the trachea aids mucosal repair (Fig. 10.9). Thus, dissection is right on the tracheal wall. The perichondrium protects the nerves and gives support for tracheal implantation. With heavy steroid cover (up to 80 mg of methyl prednisolone daily for up to one week) extubation is usually possible before the second postoperative day.

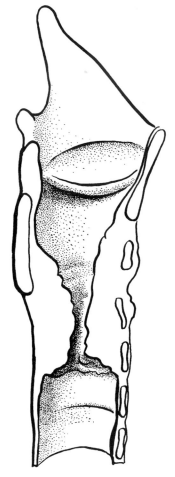

Figure 10.6 Extensive high subglottic stenosis.

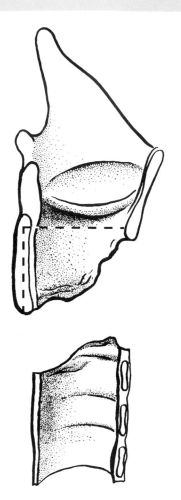

Figure 10.8 Excision of subglottic scar and thinning of the posterior plate of the cricoid.

Microtrapdoor flap repair

The CO_2 laser can be used to develop a microtrapdoor flap which preserves mucosa in the posterior glottis, subglottis and trachea. The stenotic scar is removed and following completion of the procedure the micro-

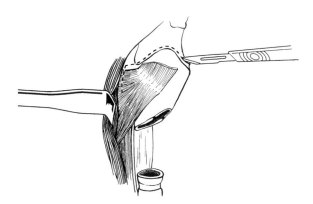

Figure 10.7 Laryngeal drop by division of the thyrohyoid muscles and membrane in the management of extensive subglottic stenosis.

trapdoor flap can provide mucosal coverage to prevent recurrent stenosis. The flap needs to be thin enough to manipulate but not so thin that the blood supply is compromised. An alternative is to perform endoscopic radial laser incisions and dilation using both CO_2 and neodymium:yttrium–aluminium–garnet (Nd:YAG) lasers.

Cricoid expansion

If the stenosis involves the anterior glottis, as is commonly encountered in post-tracheostomy stenosis, then a segment of the hyoid bone can be inserted as a free graft or as a pedicled flap. In the latter procedure the larynx and trachea are exposed through a midline vertical incision and the central part of the hyoid bone is freed up as a pedicle attached to the sternohyoid muscle. The stenosed segment of the cricoid is wedged open by the pedicled flap, the attached soft tissues of which are sutured into place. This technique may not be adequate, however, for posterior or circumferential subglottic stenosis, which may require a procedure to graft both anterior and posterior portions of the cricoid ring.

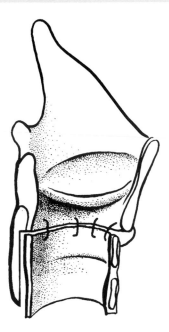

Figure 10.9 Upward mobilization of the trachea allows suture of the posterior wall to the remaining subglottic mucosa. The anterior tracheal wall is sutured to the inferior borders of the thyroid ala.

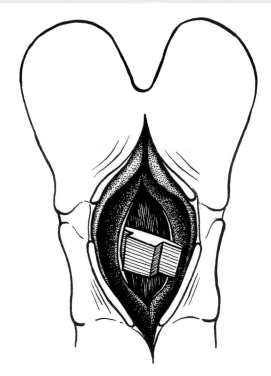

Figure 10.10 Exposure of the cricoid plate through a laryngofissure and insertion of a cartilage splint graft.

Cricoid expansion with cartilage grafts

The insertion of anterior and posterior rib cartilage grafts to splint open the thyroid and cricoid framework is shown in Figs 10.10 and 10.11.

Cartilage for grafting is obtained from the fifth or sixth costal cartilage with its perichondrium attached. The cartilage is shaped into an anterior and a posterior graft. The posterior graft is T-shaped with phlanges which fit under the body of the cricoid cartilage. The anterior graft is spindle-shaped and bevelled towards the interior of the larynx to prevent interior displacement. The posterior cricoid lamina is split and an anterior incision is made from the midpoint of the thyroid notch down to the inferior margin of the first tracheal ring to receive the spindle-shaped wedge.

Controversies in management

Is there any evidence to support early surgical intervention in acute laryngeal trauma?

Data suggest that recognizing and treating the severe injuries early gives a 40% better chance of a good voice and three times less chance of permanent tracheostomy.

Should a patient with chronic laryngeal stenosis be advised to have an operation?

The patient with no tracheostomy should be advised to manage without surgery if at all possible. This may result in a restriction of energetic activity but any surgery on a previously injured area can promote scarring, leading to a tracheostomy. The patient with a tracheostomy has little to lose from surgery. Because the surgery will be confined to the neck, there is a minimal mortality and about a 50% chance of patients being able to discard their tracheostomy tube.

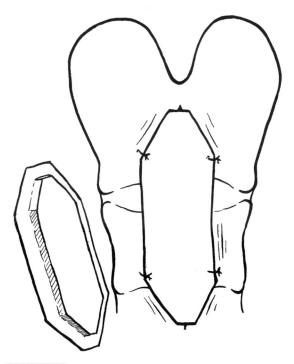

Figure 10.11 Insertion of a spindle-shaped anterior cartilage graft.

How should a patient with persistent restenosis be managed?

Patients who have persistent and increasing scarring are best advised not to have more surgery. Even laser excision seems to be ineffective in these patients.

References and further reading

Austin J. R., Stanley, R.B. and Cooper D. S. (1992) Stable internal fixation of fractures of the partially mineralised thyroid cartilage, *Ann Otol Rhinol Laryngol* **101**: 76–80.

Bent J. P., Silver J. R. and Porubsky E. S. (1993) Acute laryngeal trauma: a review of 77 patients, *Otolaryngol Head Neck Surg* **109**: 441–499.

Beste D. J. and Toohill, R. J. (1991) Microtrapdoor flap repair of laryngeal and tracheal stenosis, *Ann Otol Rhinol Laryngol* **100**: 420–3.

Chagnon F. P. and Mulder D. S. (1996) Laryngotracheal trauma, *Chest Surg Clin North Am* **6**: 733–48.

Couraud L., Jougon J. B. and Ballester M. (1996) Techniques of management of subglottic stenoses with glottic and supraglottic problems, *Chest Surg Clin North Am* **6**: 791–809.

Grillo H. C., Mathisen D. J. and Wain J. C. (1992) Laryngotracheal resection and reconstruction for subglottic stenosis, *Ann Thoracic Surg* **53**: 54–63.

Grillo H. C. (1996) Management of idiopathic tracheal stenosis, *Chest Surg Clin North Am* **6**: 811–18.

Last R. J. (1968) In Fitzgibbon G. M. The commandments of Gillies, *Br Journal of Plastic Surgery* **21**: 226.

Lusk R. P., Gray S. and Muntz H. R. (1991) Single-stage laryngotracheal reconstruction. *Arch Otolaryngol Head Neck Surg* **117**: 171–3.

McCaffrey T. V. (1991) Management of subglottic stenosis in the adult, *Ann Otol Rhinol Laryngol* **100**: 90–4.

McCaffrey T. V. (1992) Classification of laryngotracheal stenosis, *Laryngoscope* **102**: 1335–40.

Muntz H. R. and Lusk R. P. (1990) A comparison of the cartilaginous nib graft and Evans–Todd laryngotracheoplasties for subglottic stenosis, *Laryngoscope* **100**: 415–416.

Schaefer S. D. (1991) The treatment of acute external laryngeal injuries: 'state of the art', *Arch Otolaryngol Head Neck Surg* **117**: 35–9.

Schaefer S. D. (1991) Use of CT scanning in the management of the acutely injured larynx, *Otolaryngol Clin North Am* **24**: 31–36.

Snyderman C., Weissman J., Tabor E. *et al.* (1991) Crack cocaine burns of the larynx, *Arch Otolaryngol Head Neck Surg* **117**: 792–795.

Stolovitzky J. P. and Todd N. W. (1990) Autoimmune hypothesis of acquired subglottic stenosis in premature infants, *Laryngoscope* **100**: 227–230.

Yen P. T., Lee H. Y., Tsai M. H. *et al.* (1994) Clinical analysis of external laryngeal trauma, *J Laryngol Otol* **108**: 221–225.

Chapter 11

Benign neck disease

'Knowing the name of a thing gives power to those who know it'
Michael O'Donnell, 1997

Introduction

Most of the benign neck conditions discussed here present as a cervical mass (Fig. 11.1). Half of all neck masses seen in a general hospital are of thyroid origin (see Chapter 23).

Neck masses

- Congenital: lymphangiomas, dermoids, thyroglossal duct cysts, branchial cysts and branchial fistulae, thymic cysts, haemangiomas
- Acquired: ranulas, laryngoceles, pharyngeal pouches
- Infective: bacterial, viral, tuberculous
- Tumours of the parapharyngeal space
- Neurogenous tumours: paragangliomas, peripheral nerve tumours

Congenital neck masses

Lymphangiomas

The lymph system arises from two jugular sacs, two posterior sciatic sacs and a single retroperitoneal sac. Endothelial outbuddings from these extend centrifugally to form the peripheral lymphatic system.

The probable cause of cystic hygroma is that endothelial fibrillar membranes sprout from the walls of these cysts, penetrate the surrounding tissue, canalize it and produce more cysts. The pressure of the cysts forces the tumour along the lines of least resistance into planes or spaces between large muscles or vessels.

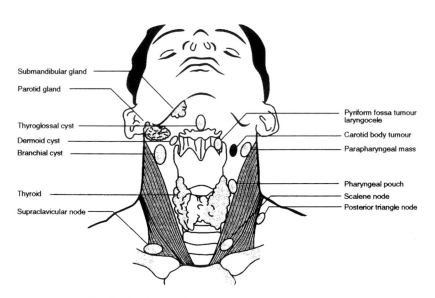

Figure 11.1 The most common sites for benign neck masses.

Submandibular gland
Parotid gland
Thyroglossal cyst
Dermoid cyst
Branchial cyst
Thyroid
Supraclavicular node

Pyriform fossa tumour laryngocele
Carotid body tumour
Parapharyngeal mass
Pharyngeal pouch
Scalene node
Posterior triangle node

Simple lymphangiomas and cavernous lymphangiomas occur in the lips, tongue, cheek and floor of the mouth, where the tissue planes are relatively tight. A cystic hygroma arises mainly in the neck, where it has more space to expand into, and where the tissue planes are more lax. It may then spread into the cheek, floor of mouth, tongue, parotid and ear canal.

Treatment

The treatment of cystic hygroma and the other lymphangiomas is excision. Sclerosant injection, and incision and drainage, are worthless. Only one of numerous cysts can be dealt with and incision can provoke life-threatening infection.

No operation should be conducted without a preoperative chest computed tomographic (CT) scan to rule out mediastinal involvement. Damage to the facial, hypoglossal and accessory nerves may be difficult to avoid and so a nerve stimulator should be used. Because of the enormous skin stretching and interference with the mandibular branch of the facial nerve, a good cosmetic result is difficult to achieve. Excision of excess skin will usually be needed. Multiple excisions may be needed over several years.

Intraoral lymphangiomas should be removed by an external approach because they will almost certainly be more extensive than expected. The recurrence rate after excision of a cystic hygroma is 10–15% and usually becomes obvious within 9 months. Recurrence of cavernous lymphangiomas is more common than that of cystic hygromas.

Problems

Intraoral lymphangiomas can be confused with ranulas, of which there are two types. The simple ranula is a retention cyst arising from a minor salivary gland in the floor of the mouth. It is unilocular and relatively thick walled; it is therefore easy to excise. The plunging ranula is probably part of a cystic hygroma. It is very thin walled and invades the upper part of the neck, penetrating between the muscles. It is very difficult to excise completely.

Midline dermoids

Approximately 7% of dermoid tumours occur in the head and neck. The most common locations are the orbit, oral cavity and nasal region. Oral-cavity lesions tend to present in the second to third decade.

Clinical features

Dermoid tumours present as solid or cystic painless masses in the midline of the neck between the suprasternal notch and the submental region. Obstructive symptoms are rare. Treatment is complete local excision.

Thyroglossal duct cysts

Embryology

The thyroid anlages arise from the floor of the primitive pharynx between the first and second pharyngeal pouches. In addition to the major median anlage, there are smaller paired lateral anlages, which contribute the parafollicular or calcitonin-secreting C cells. The median anlage loses its lumen at 5 weeks' gestation and breaks into fragments, the lower end dividing into two portions that become the thyroid lobes. Thyroglossal cysts form when epithelial cells cease to remain inactive. The stalk should atrophy at the sixth week but if it persists it becomes the thyroglossal duct in which cysts can develop. It runs from the thyroid gland behind, through or in front of the hyoid bone and ends deeply at the foramen caecum of the tongue. The origin of the cystic changes is not fully understood (Todd, 1993). A fistula is usually caused by an attempted drainage of a mis-diagnosed abscess or to an inadequate excision leaving the hyoid bone intact.

Presentation of thyroglossal cysts

- Male:female 1:1
- Mean age: 5 years (range 4 months to 70 years)
- 90% midline
- 10% lateral, of which 95% left and 5% right side
- Most common midline neck cyst
- Three times more common than branchial cysts
- Mostly painless, mobile on swallowing or protruding the tongue
- 75% prehyoid
- 25% at the thyroid cartilage, the cricoid cartilage or above the hyoid
- Mobile in all directions
- Can usually be transilluminated
- 5% have tenderness and rapid enlargement due to infection
- 15% have fistulae at presentation
- Rare familial variants: mostly autosomal dominant in prepubertal girls

---

Investigation

The clinically euthyroid patient with a midline infrahyoid thyroglossal cyst should have a thyroid-stimulating hormone (TSH) estimation. If normal, it is likely that no other tests are required. If, however, the presumptive cyst is suprahyoid, preoperative tests should include TSH and an isotope [technetium-99m(^{99m}Tc)] scan to exclude a lingual thyroid, the inadvertant removal of which would render the patient hypothyroid. Magnetic resonance imaging (MRI) scanning may also be considered: the cyst will have a very high-intensity signal on T_2 weighted images.

Treatment

Treatment is by excision, the operation having been popularized by Sistrunk (Fig. 11.2). Removal may require the division of the sternohyoid and thryohyoid muscles, and should include the body of the hyoid bone between the lesser horns, after the duct has been dissected to this area. Above the hyoid, Sistrunk recommended the removal of a core of tissue including the raphe joining the mylohyoid muscles, a portion of each genioglossus muscle and the foramen caecum, without any formal attempt to identify a tract at this level. To reach the area of the foramen caecum, the dissection must be angled upwards and backwards at an angle of 45°. In a fistula or revision operation, the mouth of the fistula is excised in an ellipse. A double Z-plasty often gives a better cosmetic result than simple closure.

Even with good technique, 7–8% recur and it has been suggested that in addition to a 2 cm suprahyoid core,

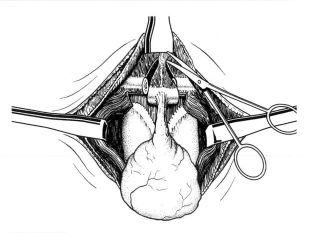

Figure 11.2 Excision of a thyroglossal cyst.

attempts should not be made to trace out a tract in the lower neck either, but to remove 2 to 4 cm of central strap muscles, usually down to the thyroid cartilage and thyrohyoid membrane (Howard and Lund, 1986).

Thyroglossal duct carcinoma

The lining epithelium of a thyroglossal duct cyst is columnar, cuboidal or, more frequently, non-keratinizing stratified squamous epithelium. Fine-needle aspiration cytology (FNAC) thus shows mucoid material with benign squamous cells from the lining of the cyst (Bardales *et al.*, 1996). About 150 cases of thyroglossal duct carcinoma, mostly of papillary thyroid type, but including most other variants, have been described. Most cases have presented as benign cysts and the diagnosis was made histologically, but carcinoma may be suspected if the cyst is hard or irregular, or has recently undergone changes. Histological confirmation requires the presence of malignant cells mixed with normal thyroid cells in the cyst wall. Up to 40% of papillary thyroid cancers show areas of squamous metaplasia. Cytological diagnosis may be problematic; the presence of large, atypical squamous metaplastic cells and/or psammoma bodies in the aspirate of an anterior cystic neck mass should suggest this as a possible diagnosis.

There is no gender predominance and the peak age incidence for women is the fourth decade and for men the sixth decade. Only 10% of those reported had evidence of metastatic disease, compared with 50% of those with carcinoma arising in an ectopic thyroid. Treatment is by local excision followed by suppressive doses of thyroxine. Alternatively, consideration may be given to adjuvant thyroidectomy and iodine-131(^{131}I) ablation (see Chapter 23). Prognosis is better than for papillary carcinoma arising in the thyroid gland (Ferreiro and Weiland, 1994).

Branchial cysts

Branchial anomalies account for up to 17% of all paediatric cervical masses (Choe and Zalzal, 1995).

Theories of origin of a branchial cyst

The branchial apparatus theory: branchial cysts represent remains of pharyngeal pouches or branchial clefts, or a fusion of these two elements. The development of the branchial apparatus extends from the third to the eighth week of gestation. By this theory, more cysts should be present at birth, whereas the peak age of incidence is in fact the third decade.

Arch of origin of branchial anomalies*

- 5–25% first
- 40–90% second
- 2–8% third and fourth

*Tertiary centres report more of the first, third and fourth variants

---

The cervical sinus theory is an extension of the above: branchial cysts represent remains of the cervical sinus of His, which is formed by the second arch growing down to meet the fifth. The second arch mesoderm almost covers the neck and forms platysma. Origin from the branchial apparatus remains the most popular theory.

The thymopharyngeal duct theory suggests that cysts are remnants of the original connection between the thymus and the third branchial pouch from which it takes origin. However, a persistent thymic duct has never been described and no branchial cyst has ever been reported deep to the thyroid gland.

The inclusion theory suggests that the cysts are epithelial inclusions in lymph nodes: most branchial cysts have lymphoid tissue in the wall and they have been described in the parotid gland and pharynx. This theory also explains why branchial cysts have no internal opening.

Pathology

Branchial cysts are usually lined by stratified squamous epithelium, and 80% have lymphoid tissue in the wall. They contain straw-coloured fluid in which cholesterol crystals are found.

Clinical features of branchial cysts

- Male:female 3:2
- Peak age: third decade (range 1–70 years)
- 2/3 left and 1/3 right side; 2% bilateral
- 2/3 lie anterior to the upper third sternomastoid
- 1/3 middle and lower neck, the parotid, the pharynx and the posterior triangle
- Persistent swelling; (80%) intermittent swelling (20%)
- Pain (30%); infection (15%)
- 70% clinically cystic; 30% feel solid

First-arch anomalies are of two types: dorsal and ventral. The dorsal type runs medial to the conchal cartilage, extending posteriorly to the retroauricular scalp. The ventral type presents as a sinus, cleft or fistula, inferior to the cartilaginous ear canal. The lesions are variably related, medially or laterally to the facial nerve. Congenital preauricular pits or sinuses occur in nearly 1% of newborns in the USA, but it remains debated whether they are first-arch defects.

Investigations

The diagnosis of branchial abnormalities is straightforward, but misdiagnosis rates may approach 20% and are higher for lesions originating from the first, third and fourth arches. FNAC yields acellular fluid, in which cholesterol crystals may be seen.

Treatment

Treatment is by excision, particularly in view of the tendency to secondary infection (Roback and Telander, 1994). A 5–7 cm transverse incision is made through the platysma and the flaps elevated superiorly and inferiorly keeping platysma in the skin flap (Fig. 11.3). The fascia is divided on the anterior border of the sternomastoid and retracted laterally. The cyst is identified and care taken to avoid rupturing it, as removal after this accident is rather difficult. It is freed anteriorly, inferiorly, superiorly and medially with a knife and the tail of the parotid gland elevated if necessary. If the lower pole of the gland has to be elevated, then it is best to find the mandibular branch of the facial nerve and follow it backwards through the gland substance to preserve it. Then the cyst is removed *in toto*; there is no need to look for an associated tract as these do not occur.

The principal complication is recurrence, up to 20% in some series.

Branchial fistulae

A branchial fistulae is an entirely different entity from a branchial cyst. It is of congenital origin and consists of a skin-lined track, opening internally as a slit on the anterior aspect of the tonsillar fossa, if it is of second-arch origin. The external opening is at the anterior border of the sternomastoid muscle, at the junction of its middle and lower thirds. It almost always presents in young infants as a discharging sinus, which may or may not have an internal fistulous communication. Those from the first arch open at the junction of the cartilaginous and bony meatus, while third or fourth arch sinuses have internal openings at the level of the piriform sinus or below. A complete fistula of the third pouch and cleft has yet to be reported. The fistula would route caudal to the glossopharyngeal nerve, over the superior laryngeal nerve, posteromedial to the internal carotid artery, piercing the thyrohyoid membrane to enter the pharynx just cephalic to the superior laryngeal nerve. Although complete fourth-arch fistulae have yet to be described, there is an established clinical pattern for the internal sinuses, which are almost always left sided and present as suppurative thyroiditis. They typically manifest under the

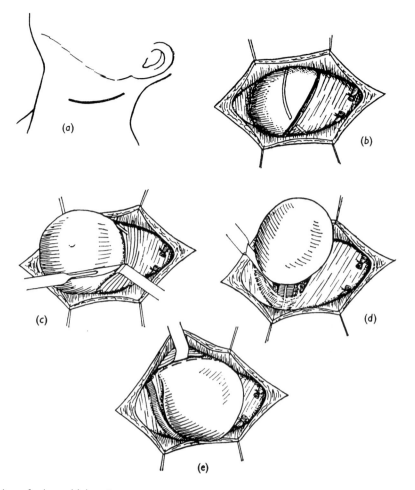

Figure 11.3 Excision of a branchial cyst.

age of 10 years, although adult presentation has been recorded. Barium swallow radiology and Valsalva manoeuvre may aid diagnosis. Treatment involves thyroid lobectomy with excision of the tract.

A branchial sinus should be excised in a stepladder fashion, removing the mouth of the pit in an ellipse. Follow the track upwards: the common second-arch variant takes a rather sharp bend upwards in most cases. The high exposure is best achieved by a vertical incision anterior to the ear, curving below the ear lobe and inferior to the jaw. The tract travels below the stylohyoid muscle and the posterior belly of the digastric, above the hypoglossal nerve and between the internal and external carotid arteries, usually below the postauricular and occipital branches of the external carotid. Thus, no arterial branches need to be tied, but the hypoglossal nerve must be identified. In other instances the track goes up towards the ear, and in this condition it is necessary to remove the superficial lobe of the parotid gland. Once this lobe is removed, finding the rest of the track is easy. It may be found to enter the junction of the cartilaginous and bony external auditory meatus. Some indication of this may be gained before operation if the patient also complains occasion-

ally of a discharging ear, for which no middle-ear cause can be found.

Complications of branchial sinus removal

- Damage to the hypoglossal nerve is most likely if one of the pharyngeal veins is cut and blind attempts are made to secure haemostasis as these veins disappear medial to the hypoglossal nerve.
- Carotid artery damage is unlikely if care is taken, and provided the operator realizes where the track goes
- The facial nerve can also be damaged, especially the mandibular branch, but this will be avoided if the previous steps described have been taken

---

Branchogenic carcinoma

This is a rare condition but a definite entity presenting as a single mass in the upper neck. It was at one time thought to be fairly common but it is now known that most previous reports have been of secondary malignancies.

> *Criteria for the diagnosis of branchogenic carcinoma*
>
> ◼ The carcinoma should be demonstrated as arising in the wall of a branchial cyst
> ◼ The tumour should occur in a line running from a point just anterior to the tragus along the anterior border of sternomastoid to the clavicle
> ◼ The histology should be compatible with a tissue origin from the branchial vestiges
> ◼ No other primary should become evident in a 5 year follow-up

The above criteria have been criticized for not allowing distinction from a cystic nodal secondary (e.g. from a tonsillar primary) and some authors continue to question its existence (Soh, 1998). Many series cite a fair proportion of later diagnosis of a tonsillar primary. A review of 67 reported cases indicated that at least 41 were not in fact branchiogenic carcinomas (Khafif *et al.*, 1989). Of the remaining 26 cases, 14 were felt to fulfill the required criteria, showing a branchial cyst with evidence of epithelial dysplasia progressing to carcinoma within the cyst wall. A therapeutic approach of wide local excision, radical neck dissection and radiotherapy has been recommended. Undoubtedly, where a cystic squamous lesion is diagnosed, tonsillectomy should accompany the essential panendoscopy.

Thymic cysts (Woodruff and Kennedy, 1997)

The thymus develops from the third pharyngeal pouch at 6 weeks' gestation and rests in the superior mediastinum at 12 weeks. Typically, a thymic cyst presents in boys aged 3–8 years as a painless swelling of 1–20 cm diameter. Half have a communication with the mediastinum.

Haemangiomas

Haemangiomas are the most common benign tumour of infancy and the head and neck is affected in 14–21%, most often within the masseter and trapezius muscles. They typically appear shortly after birth, proliferate for 6–12 months and up to 50% may then involute spontaneously. They are three times more common in females than in males.

Acquired neck masses

Ranulas

A ranula is a cystic mass in the floor of the mouth or tongue which arises as a result of obstruction of minor salivary glands or the sublingual gland. They are caused by trauma or ductal abnormality.

Simple ranulas are epithelial-lined cystic masses confined to the sublingual space, whereas plunging ranulas result from extravasation of mucus below the mylohyoid muscle and present as painless, non-mobile neck swellings.

There is a slight female predilection but no side dominance, and they present in the second to third decade.

Laryngoceles

Laryngoceles arise within the saccule of the laryngeal ventricle. If they extend through the thyrohyoid membrane, they tend to do so at the point of entry of the superior laryngeal vessels. Manual compression may result in the escape of fluid and gas into the airway (Bryce's sign).

> *Laryngocele*
>
> ◼ Rare: 1 per 2.5 million population per year
> ◼ Male:female 5:1
> ◼ Peak age: sixth decade
> ◼ 4/5 unilateral
> ◼ 30% external and expand through the thyrohyoid membrane
> ◼ 20% internal and present in the vallecula
> ◼ 50% combined
> ◼ 1% contain a carcinoma

Aetiology

There is no evidence to show that hobbies involving blowing, or jobs such as trumpet playing or glass blowing, cause laryngoceles. Lower animals have air sacs and it is considered that laryngoceles in humans represent atavistic remnants of these. Blowing hobbies increase the intralaryngeal air pressure and bring otherwise symptomless laryngoceles to light. Of more importance is the coexistence of a carcinoma of the larynx, which acts as a valve allowing air under pressure into the ventricle. External laryngoceles are said to be found in one in six laryngectomy specimens removed for laryngeal carcinoma, as opposed to one in 50 specimens removed for piriform sinus cancer. The difficulty in interpreting this statement is the absence of a definition of the level at which an enlarged saccule becomes a laryngocele.

> *Clinical features*
>
> ◼ Hoarseness
> ◼ Neck swelling
> ◼ Less common: stridor, sore throat, snoring, pain or cough
> ◼ 10% present with infected sacs (pyoceles)

On palpation the swelling over the thyrohyoid membrane can be easily emptied. Plain radiographs show the air-filled sac in all cases. The upper border of the thyroid cartilage may be taken as the dividing line between a large saccule and a laryngocele. Enlarged saccules can be found on a plain radiograph of the neck during the Valsalva manoeuvre in quite a large proportion of patients with hoarseness. Surgical therapy is probably unproductive.

Treatment

Laryngoceles are removed to prevent enlargement and eventual obstruction of the larynx (Fig. 11.4). Through a collar incision over the thyroid cartilage, the sac is located and followed downwards. To expose the neck of the sac, the perichondrium is elevated from the upper half of the thyroid cartilage on the same side. The upper half of the thyroid cartilage is removed, which allows the sac to be removed at its origin from the saccule. The sac is divided at its neck and stitched as in a hernia repair. The perichondrium is placed over the defect and the wound closed. A pyocele should be treated with antibiotics before surgery.

Pharyngeal pouches

Pathology

There are many types of pharyngeal diverticula but the most common type is the acquired pulsion diverticulum of the median posterior wall passing through Killian's dehiscence (Ellis, 1995). Pouch formation may relate to a restrictive defect of upper sphincter opening. This may result in an area of increased pressure in the hypopharynx and a herniation of mucosa above the cricopharyngeus through the dehiscence of Killian. Pathologically, biopsies of the cricopharyngeus in pharyngeal diverticulum patients show fibrotic changes, together with hypertrophy, necrosis and inflammation, some of which may be of autoimmune origin. There is a reduced ratio of muscle:connective tissue fibres in the cricopharyngeus muscle of diverticula patients (Zaninotto *et al.*, 1996). The effects of surgery on upper sphincter function are reported to include increased opening and reduced hypopharyngeal intrabolus pressure. Operation seems not to affect bolus flow rates and to have only minor effects on basal sphincter tone and the timing of swallow events (Shaw *et al.*, 1996). Hypopharyngeal intrabolus pressure is a useful indicator of sphincter compliance.

Clinical features of pharyngeal diverticula

- Male:female 2:1
- Peak age: seventh and eight decades
- Dysphagia most common symptom (98%)
- Halitosis
- Regurgitation of undigested food
- Weight loss (30%)
- Cough, recurrent chest infection due to aspiration (30%)
- Occasional hoarseness, neck mass

A barium swallow demonstrates the pouch in all cases. Pharyngo-oesophagoscopy is necessary in every patient. Firstly, to exclude a carcinoma, secondly, to look for a hiatus hernia, which often coexists and thirdly, to pass a feeding tube. Lastly, the technique is necessary to pack the pouch immediately before the operation. The pharyngoscope usually enters the pouch and it may be difficult to pass it over the bar of the cricopharyngeus muscle that separates the pouch from the mouth of the oesophagus.

Treatment

Unless the pouch is a tiny incidental radiological finding it will require treatment. Options are as follows.

Endoscopic. These are particularly appealing because of the mean age of patients and the high levels of comorbidity (von Doerstein and Byl, 1997).

Diathermy: Dohlman's procedure (Dohlman and Mattson, 1960). The original endoscopic method for treating a pharyngeal pouch was the application of insulated coagulation diathermy across both sides of the bar, followed by cutting diathermy applied to the central portion down to the level where it thins out inferiorly. The bar is demonstrated by the use of a slotted endoscope. Nasogastric

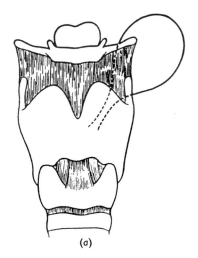
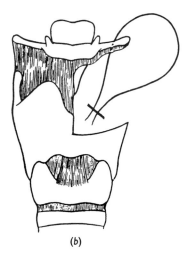

Figure 11.4 Removal of laryngocele: (a) laryngocele; (b) upper half of thyroid cartilage removed to expose the neck of the laryngocele.

feeding is common for 1–2 days postoperatively. At follow-up there is a residual pouch, but the height of the partition is reduced radiographically (Hadley *et al.*, 1997). If successful at a single sitting, which lasts for about 45 min, the procedure undoubtedly involves less morbidity than the open approaches and allows early hospital discharge at 48 h (von Doersten and Byl, 1997).

The complications of the procedure include a high recurrence rate of a symptomatic diverticulum, necessitating further procedures, and postoperative pyrexia, attributed to minor leakage at the apex of the coagulation site, which may occasionally progress to mediastinitis. More modern endoscopic procedures are therefore gaining popularity, although there is still some interest in coagulation, which has been successfully reported to have been applied without general anaesthesia using a flexible endoscope (Mulder *et al.*, 1995).

Endoscopic laser treatment (Bradwell et al., 1997). The bar is identified with a diverticuloscope and the operating microscope used (400 mm lens). The CO_2 laser is used on 15 W continuous power to divide the bar. Routine nasogastric intubation is not necessary and oral fluids are resumed at 24 h. The laser is claimed to have two advantages over endoscopic stapling, namely superior visualization (this being impeded by the presence of the gun) and the ability to treat small pouches, into which it can be almost impossible to insert the gun.

Endoscopic staple-assisted oesophagodiverticulostomy (Koay and Bates, 1996). This method also employs a distending diverticuloscope to display the common septum. The pouch is cleared and examined with a Hopkins' telescope to exclude a carcinoma. One of the commercially available stapling devices is then introduced such that its closure simultaneously cuts the bar and inserts bilateral double rows of sealing staples. Discharge is usually on the first postoperative day. With experience, the operative time is reduced to 10 to 15 min. In patients with residual or recurrent symptoms, the procedure can safely be repeated. In larger series, the cure rate is in excess of 90% (Scher and Richtsmeier, 1998), but with increasing use, the number of complications experienced has inevitably risen, including iatrogenic pharyngeal perforation, pyrexia and transient vocal-cord paralysis.

Open procedures

Diverticulectomy, pouch inversion or diverticulopexy; cricopharyngeal myotomy. To facilitate dissection and identification, the pouch is packed with acriflavine gauze before exploration. The pouch is approached through a collar incision (Fig. 11.5), at the level of the cricoid cartilage which marks the level of origin of the neck of the sac. The skin and platysma are divided, and the superior and inferior flaps elevated and retracted with Joll's clamp. The fascia is divided along the anterior border of the sternomastoid muscle and dissected down to the prevertebral fascia between the carotid sheath and the central structures of the neck, dividing the omohyoid muscle and the middle thyroid vein. The pouch should be found easily, lying posterior to the oesophagus. The pouch is dissected free of the surrounding tissues until its neck can be seen.

Cricopharyngeal myotomy. This procedure is also performed in isolation for certain highly selected patients with oropharyngeal dysphagia (Brouillette *et al.*, 1997). If a pharyngeal pouch is not present and the operation is performed for another indication, it may be helpful to inflate gently the balloon of an endotracheal tube to distend the cricopharyngeus muscle fibres and aid identification of the upper oesophageal sphincter. The approach is similar to that for a diverticulum. Where a pouch is present, the fibres are identified immediately inferior to the neck of the sac. Visualization is helped by retraction laterally of the carotid sheath and also of the thyroid contralaterally. The inferior thyroid artery is ligated as far laterally as possible, where it disappears under the carotid sheath. There is probably no need to dissect out the recurrent laryngeal nerve, but it may be palpated in the tracheo-oesophageal groove where it passes behind the inferior thyroid artery. At this point, the retraction of the thyroid and laryngopharynx is most gently achieved by the assistant's hand over a wet swab (Brouillette *et al.*, 1997). The division of the cricopharyngeal muscle in the posterior midline may be aided by inserting a right-angled clamp deep to the muscle. The division may be with a No. 11 blade or with low-intensity cutting diathermy. The myotomy should include 2 cm of the hypopharyngeal muscle and 2 cm of the upper cervical oesophageal muscle. With the 2 cm of the cricopharyngeus muscle, it thus measures 6 cm *in toto*. The hypopharyngeal portion may include some troublesome submucosal veins which may have to be ligated.

The neck of the sac is about 3 cm long. Excess traction on the pouch should be avoided as it can lead to overexcision and secondary narrowing of the oesophageal lumen. If the pouch can be inverted into the pharyngeal lumen without opening it, the site from which it arose can be oversewn using a polyglycol or non-absorbable suture. If the pouch is too large to invert (larger than 4 cm in length after dissection), it must be excised or suspended from the prevertebral fascia, i.e. diverticulopexy. Before removal of the sac, a stay suture is placed at its inferior and superior ends. Then the sac is excised, with scissors, about 5 mm from the oesophagus. The inner layer of the defect is closed with Connell's sutures, one beginning at the superior stay suture and proceeding about halfway down the defect, and the other beginning at the inferior end and proceeding superiorly to meet the point where the superior suture ended. Superior and inferior sutures are then tied to each other and cut and the end allowed to fall into the oesophageal lumen. A second layer of 3/0 catgut or 3/0 black silk in a continuous running suture is inserted to reinforce this first suture line. Alternatively, a short, straight stapler can be used to staple the neck of the pouch, while the residuum is excised and sent for histology. After excision and stapling, the patient can usually be discharged at 48 h. The wound is washed out and closed with a continuous suction drain.

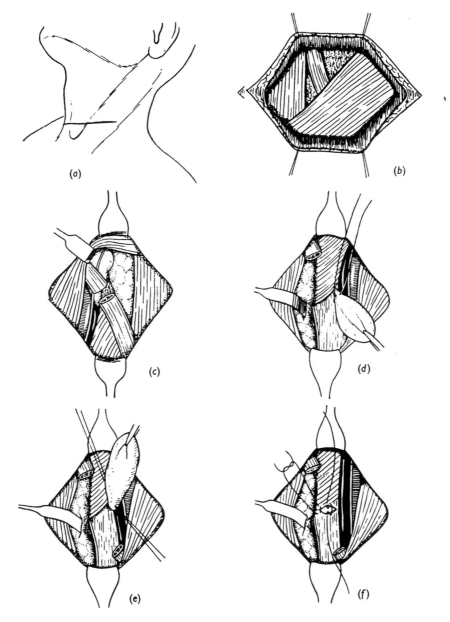

Figure 11.5 Removal of the pharyngeal pouch: (a) incision; (b) beginning of dissection medial to the sternomastoid; (c) retraction of the carotid sheath and sternmastoid muscle; (d) recurrent laryngeal nerve exposed: thyroid retracted medially and pouch exposed; (e) neck of pouch dissected out; (f) repair of the pharyngeal defect.

Complications

All large series show that primary healing after routine excision is far from usual. At least one-third of these patients still suffer major complications such as infection, fistulae, stenosis and vocal-cord paralysis. The incidence of major complications is dramatically reduced by inversion or suspension of the pouch. The incidence of recurrence is much reduced by the performance of a myotomy, without which up to one in five recurs. There is a poor correlation between symptoms postoperatively and objective radiographic signs of recurrence, which may be seen in up to 44% of subjects (Witterick *et al.*, 1995).

Carcinoma in a pharyngeal pouch

Carcinoma in a pharyngeal pouch

- Rare: incidence around 0.5% of pouches
- Male:female 5:1
- Affects long-standing diverticula (> 7 years)
- Due to chronic irritation from food retention
- Increased dysphagia
- Weight loss
- Occasionally blood in the regurgitated food
- Mass may be found in the neck

The usual lesion is an invasive squamous cell carcinoma, but a few cases of carcinoma *in situ* have been reported in the literature. Barium studies show a more constant filling defect than the variable defect of food debris. It is usually seen in the distal two-thirds of the pouch but can easily be missed. The diagnosis may be first made at operation. The unusual case with a tumour confined to the pouch should be treated by diverticulectomy. Most cases require total pharyngolaryngectomy as for a postcricoid carcinoma. The outlook is dismal.

Infective neck masses

Parapharyngeal abscess

Surgical anatomy of the parapharyngeal space

The parapharyngeal space extends from the skull base to the level of the hyoid bone, where it is bounded by the sheath of the submandibular gland. Laterally lie the lateral pterygoid muscles together with the sheath of the parotid gland, while medially the buccopharyngeal fascia overlies the pharyngeal constrictors. Posteriorly is the carotid sheath; anteriorly it tends to narrow like the prow of a ship towards the pterygomandibular raphe. The most pliable wall is the medial boundary with the pharynx, so that masses tend to displace the nasopharyngeal or oropharyngeal wall medially. The only truly pliable part of the lateral boundary is the retromandibular portion of the parotid (Som *et al.*, 1995a).

The roof of the parapharyngeal space is the junction of the medial pterygoid muscle and the superior constrictor. The space is divided by a tensor–vascular–styloid fascia with runs from the posteroinferior edge of the tensor palatini to the styloid apparatus, fusing anteriorly with the interpterygoid fascia and the buccopharyngeal fascia.

Surgical pathology

The most common neck swelling in children is an enlarged jugulodigastric lymph node secondary to tonsillitis. Although this can proceed to abscess formation the infection seldom extends to the parapharyngeal space. Parapharyngeal abscess is more common in adults and is a complication of tonsillectomy or tonsillitis in 60%, and of extraction of the lower third molar in a further 30%. The remaining 10% are due to extension of infection from the petrous apex or mastoid tip.

Clinical features of parapharyngeal abscess

- Elevated temperature
- Marked trismus
- Pain
- Tonsil is pushed medially but looks normal
- Neck swelling maximal at posterior mid-third of sternomastoid

---

Treatment

The patient is given antibiotics for at least 48 h. If there is not a good response, incision and drainage will be required, the space being opened from a point medial to the mandible down to the clavicle. The drain is left in for at least 72 h and antibiotics continued for 10 days.

Ludwig's angina

Surgical anatomy

The submandibular space lies below the floor of the mouth and tongue, and extends from the hyoid to the mandible. The space is divided into two by the mylohyoid muscle. The space above the muscle is called the sublingual space and contains the sublingual gland, the lingual and hypoglossal nerves and the submandibular duct. The space below the muscle is the submaxillary space, which contains the gland.

Surgical pathology

The source of the infection is dental in 80% of cases, especially from the lower molar and premolar teeth, the roots of which lie close to the lingual plate of the mandible; the roots of the second and third permanent molars lie below the mylohyoid line. If a dental root abscess drains into the space there will be little in the way of dental pain. The remaining 20% are due to soft-tissue and tonsillar infection. The microorganism usually implicated in simple dental infection is *Streptococcus viridans*.

Clinical features of Ludwig's angina

- Elevated temperature
- Pain
- Trismus
- Excessive salivation and brawny swelling of the submental and submandibular regions
- Floor of the mouth will become swollen and oedematous if in the sublingual space
- Tongue displacement may cause respiratory obstruction

Treatment

Incision and drainage should be postponed for as long as possible because pus is seldom found. The patient is treated with an antibiotic and analgesics. Tracheostomy is seldom necessary.

Tuberculous cervical adenitis

Pathology

In the Western world most of the morbidity and mortality from tuberculosis is caused by primary pulmonary tuberculosis. The majority of cases occurs in middle-aged and elderly subjects. Lymph-node tuberculosis remains a very common manifestation elsewhere in the world, especially in Asia. The enlargement of the node is usually painless. When the node caseates and liquefies, the swelling becomes fluctuant and sinus formation is common. The majority of infections are caused by *Mycobacterium tuberculosis* but *M. bovis*, endemic in cattle, can be spread to humans by milk. The primary infection of cervical tuberculosis is usually in the tonsil and in most people this and the associated lymph-node lesions heal and calcify. Where healing is incomplete, haematogenous lesions may develop in the lungs, bones or kidneys, sometimes after many months.

Clinical features of cervical tuberculosis
▪ Longstanding lymphadenopathy
▪ Pain (more recent onset)
▪ In Asia: 50% sinus formation, skin involvement or cold abscesses
▪ 90% single nodal group: usually the deep jugular chain, although the posterior triangle nodes are often affected

Diagnosis is by a positive skin test, demonstration of acid-fast bacilli in the lymph-node biopsy and growth of *M. tuberculosis* from the biopsy.

Treatment

If a patient presents with unconfirmed cervical tuberculosis, diagnosis may be possible on FNAC. Otherwise, a node is excised, and half sent for histology and half for culture. The patient with multiple infected nodes with sinus formation, in whom the diagnosis is already known, should be treated by antituberculous chemotherapy followed by excision of any residual disease. Short-course regimens lasting for 6 or 9 months are now the usual choice in the West; for example, a 6-month course of ethambutol or streptomycin plus isoniazid plus rifampicin plus pyrazinamide for 2 months, followed by a 4-month course of isoniazid plus rifampicin. Less expensive regimes are more appropriate in developing countries but need to be continued for 12 months; for example, a combination of isoniazid and thiacetazone which can be given by daily oral doses. Other important considerations in management are isolation of patients who are excreting tubercle bacilli, Ziehl–Neelsen stain examination of sputum smears and tuberculin testing of family contacts.

Aquired immunodeficiency syndrome (AIDS)

Head and neck manifestations of AIDS
▪ Multicentric simple parotid cysts
▪ Benign lymphoid follicular hyperplasia
▪ Cutaneous, oral or pharyngeal lesions of Kaposi's sarcoma
▪ Hairy leucoplakia
▪ Upper aerodigestive candidiasis

AIDS-related nodal inclusion cysts of the parotid

The differential diagnosis includes benign lymphoepithelial lesion, intraparotid branchial cysts and Warthin's tumour. The cysts of benign lymphoepithelial lesion, in contrast to AIDS-related cysts, arise not within nodes but from cystic dilatations of intranodal ductal inclusions,

similar to the probable origin of Warthin's tumour, but without the papillary hyperplasia (Som *et al.*, 1995b). The malignant diseases which are related to AIDS are described in full in Chapter 25.

Miscellaneous causes of lymphadenopathy

Toxoplasmosis

Toxoplasmosis is a world-wide infection caused by *Toxoplasma gondii*, a protozoon transmitted by the ingestion of cysts excreted in the faeces of infected cats, or from eating undercooked beef or lamb. Congenital infection causes hydrocephalus or microcephaly.

Acute acquired toxoplasmosis symptoms include
▪ Generalized aches and pains
▪ Fever
▪ Cough
▪ Malaise
▪ Maculopapular rash

Chronic toxoplasmosis may be asymptomatic or present as isolated lymphadenopathy. The peripheral blood picture shows lymphocytosis with some atypical mononuclear cells similar to Epstein–Barr virus (EBV) infection. Reactivation of latent toxoplasmosis may cause encephalitis in immunocompromised patients. Toxoplasmic encephalitis is estimated to develop in 25% of AIDS patients in much of Western Europe. Serological tests are usually negative. Diagnosis is confirmed by:

▪ serum antibodies,
▪ lymph node biopsy
▪ cerebrospinal fluid analysis.

Where treatment is indicated (in infants, immunosuppression or ocular involvement) a combination of sulphadimidine, pyrimethamine and folic acid is used and the blood count is monitored weekly.

Actinomycosis

Actinomycosis israelii is an anaerobic organism which is a commensal in the healthy oral cavity. The organism may become pathogenic when the mucous membrane is injured. Infection usually affects the cervicofacial region.

Clinical features of actinomycosis
▪ Severe dental caries and periodontitis
▪ Occasionally suppurative pneumonia and empyema develop
▪ Firm indurated mass with indefinite edges usually lateral to the mandible
▪ Untreated, invades adjacent tissue and becomes bony hard
▪ Multiple sinuses which discharge pus and watery fluid containing sulphur grains
▪ Give intravenous benzylpenicillin for up to several weeks

Cat-scratch disease

The illness is caused by small, pleomorphic, Gram-negative bacilli within the walls of capillaries and in lymph-node macrophages, but both the bacillus and its associated antibody are hard to identify.

Clinical features of cat-scratch disease

- acutely tender lymphadenopathy
- 30% pyrexial
- 90% give a history of contact with cats, most commonly kittens
- primary papule or vesicle develops at the site of a scratch after 1–2 weeks
- papule subsides after a few weeks and may be helpful in diagnosis
- slowly progressive chronic regional lymphadenopathy ensues 1–2 weeks later

---

Brucellosis

This is primarily a disease of domesticated animals and causes contagious abortion or other reproductive problems in cattle (*Brucella abortus*), pigs (*B. suis*), goats (*B. melitensis*), dogs (*B. canis*) and sheep (*B. ovis*). Human spread occurs by direct contact of infected tissue with conjunctiva or broken skin, by ingestion of contaminated meat or dairy products and by inhalation of infectious aerosols. Pasteurization of milk and other measures have greatly reduced the incidence in the Western countries, but stock producers, abattoir employees and veterinary surgeons remain at risk. The symptoms in humans are so variable that there is no characteristic clinical picture. The average incubation is 2–3 weeks and some infections are subclinical. In clinical cases most patients have drenching sweats, chills, fever and malaise. Although classically associated with undulating fever, the most common pyrexia pattern is a slight elevation in the morning with an increase in the afternoon. About 20% of patients have cervical and inguinal lymphadenopathy and a similar percentage have splenomegaly. Relapses occur in 5% of patients but are uncommon in appropriately treated individuals. Complications include arthritis, meningitis, depression, genitourinary symptoms, abnormal liver function tests, pulmonary symptoms and blood dyscrasias. A definitive diagnosis is made by recovering the organism from blood, fluid or tissue specimens. Blood cultures should be processed using the Castaneda biphasic medium bottle. The diagnosis can also be made serologically.

Treatment is probably best effected by combination therapy as most single agents are associated with a 30% chance of relapse. The presently favoured World Health Organization recommendation is a combination of doxycycline 200 mg and rifampacin up to 900 mg daily for 6 weeks. Prevention is by reducing the incidence of brucellosis in animal populations, e.g. the vaccination of cattle with *B. abortus* strain 19 vaccine.

Infectious mononucleosis

EBV is a member of the human herpes virus group which is found world-wide.

Clinical forms of EBV infection

- frequent subclinical infection in early childhood, e.g. UK and USA: 50% seroconversion <5 years of age.
- second wave of seroconversion associated infectious mononucleosis
- nasopharyngeal carcinoma
- African Burkitt's lymphoma, in which Epstein's group originally described the viral particles.

The C3d receptor for EBV is found on B-lymphocytes and nasopharyngeal epithelial cells of humans and certain primates. After attachment to the receptor (which is the receptor for the D-region of the third component of complement), the virus gains entry to susceptible B-lymphocytes. The virus persists in the oropharynx of patients for up to 18 months after clinical recovery and can be cultured from throat washings of 15% of normal healthy adults and 50% of renal transplant recipients. The virus may be spread by transfer of saliva with kissing. The virus infects susceptible B-lymphocytes within the pharynx and disseminates during the 1–2 month incubation period. The virus causes synthesis of antibodies directed against viral antigens and also antigens found on sheep, horse and bovine red cells (heterophile antibodies). During the first few weeks of clinical illness a mononuclear lymphocytosis is present. The white cell count comprises more than 50% mononuclear cells and more than 10% atypical lymphocytes.

Clinical features of infectious mononucleosis

- Fever
- Sore throat
- lymphadenopathy
- 5% have a rash; 100% if ampicillin is inadvertently administered
- Up to 50% have palatal petechiae or splenomegaly
- Elevated liver enzymes
- Complications
  - autoimmune haemolytic anaemia
  - thrombocytopenia
  - splenic rupture
  - encephalitis
  - cranial nerve palsies
  - acute upper airway obstruction

The vast majority of cases subside over 2–3 weeks. Treatment is largely supportive. Contact sports or heavy lifting should be avoided during the first 2–3 weeks of illness, and alcohol for a few months. Corticosteroids have a part to play in impending airway obstruction, in severe thrombocytopenia or haemolytic anaemia, and sometimes in the presence of other complications. The role of antiviral chemotherapy in the management of EBV infections is likely to broaden as new agents are developed. Given the potential oncogenicity of EBV, the risk of administration of inactivated EBV as a vaccination has not yet been fully evaluated and immunization against EBV has not been established.

Tumours of the parapharyngeal space

Almost all tumours which occur in the parapharyngeal space (see Surgical anatomy, above) arise from the deep portion of the parotid gland, anterior to the tensor–vascular–styloid fascia or from the cranial nerves travelling with the carotid sheath, which are posterior to this fascia. The medial wall of the space is pliable, but the only pliable area laterally is the retromandibular portion of the parotid gland, which thus tends to be displaced laterally irrespective of whether the lesion is intraparotid or extraparotid in origin. Masses may grow silently to a diameter of 4–5 cm.

Presenting symptoms of parapharyngeal mass

- Painless mass
- Sore throat
- Dysphonia
- Dysphagia
- Trismus
- Nasal obstruction
- Oral fullness

The most common non-neoplastic lesions are reactive nodes. Rarer causes include

- thrombosis of the internal jugular vein
- carotid artery aneurysm.

Open biopsy is usually best avoided. In some conditions it may be dangerous (e.g. paragangliomas) or have an adverse effect on outcome (e.g. salivary tumours). A combination of clinical and radiographic features, with FNAC as needed, will usually provide all of the necessary information.

Parapharyngeal tumours (in descending frequency of occurrence)

- Secondary node, e.g. lymphoma, nasopharyngeal
- Salivary (45%)
  parotid gland
  prestyloid salivary rests
  minor salivary glands
- Neurogenic (25%)
  schwannoma
  neurofibroma
  neurosarcoma
- Paragangliomas (chemodectomas) (15%)
  glomus vagale
  carotid body*
  glomus jugulare
- Miscellaneous: lipoma, liposarcoma

*10% are large enough to present in the parapharyngeal space

Salivary gland tumours are the most common primary lesions (45% of all primary parapharyngeal space masses). Up to 90% are pleomorphic adenomas of the parotid gland. Other parotid lesions (mucoepidermoid carcinomas, adenoid cystic carcinomas and acinar cell carcinomas) are uncommon and mostly arise from the minor pharyngeal submucosal salivary glands. These are a much less common source of extraparotid salivary gland tumours than the prestyloid salivary rests. On CT, extraparotid lesions are seen to be separated from the gland by a fat plane.

Deep lobe parotid tumours escape into the parapharyngeal space via the stylomandibular tunnel, i.e. between the ascending ramus of the mandible and the stylomandibular ligament/styloid process. The passage through this narrow constriction gives rise to the 'dumb-bell' appearance. If the lesion is an adenoid cystic rather than a mixed tumour, upward extension culminates in involvement of the skull base and eustachian tube.

Neurogenous tumours

Neural tumours are derived from neural crest cells. They can be divided into two main groups: the nerve sheath tumours and tumours derived from the sympathoblast. The normal nerve fibre is ensheathed by Schwann cells and by loosely distributed endoneural fibroblasts. The Schwann cell is the parent cell of both common clinical tumours, the schwannoma (neurilemmoma) and the neurofibroma, but the neurofibroma also has an origin from the perineurium and is thus linked inseparably from the nerve of origin.

Most parapharyngeal neurogenic tumours are vagal schwannomas (less commonly arising from the sympathetic chain or one of the other local nerves). Even vagal nerve tumours comprise only 1% of head and neck neoplasms. Typically they are associated with neurofibromatosis. They may have a deceptive postcontrast enhancement on MRI, apparently due to extravascular accumulation of contrast material. The tumour is solitary and encapsulated, being attached to or surrounded by the nerve. Paralysis of the associated nerve is thus unusual. Malignant change is also very unusual and may not occur at all.

Neurofibromas

These may form part of von Recklinghausen's syndrome [neurofibromatosis type 1 (NF1)] or rarely may be single. NF1 is an autosomal dominant hereditary disease, often present at birth. *Cafe-au-lait* spots associated with this disease are patches of skin which are hyperpigmented; hence, in white skins they appear like milky coffee, whereas in darker skinned individuals they appear almost black. More important in NF1 are other neurological lesions such as gliomas, meningiomas, and the neuropolyendocrine syndrome of mucosal neuromas and medullary thyroid carcinomas. Neurofibromatosis type 2 is less common and is associated with bilateral acoustic neuromas and phaeochromocytoma. Neurofibromas tend to undergo fatty degeneration and may thus have no identifiable capsule on imaging. Malignant change in some tumours, so that the disease may be fatal. These tumours incorporate nerve fibres and generally cause paralysis of their nerve of origin.

Clinical features

Slowly enlarging painless neck mass develops over a period of years. Angiography is needed to differentiate these tumours from paragangliomas, but the final diagnosis must usually wait until excision.

Treatment

The nerve from which the tumour arises is only evident in one in three operations. It may be stretched over the capsule of the tumour, or the tumour can be in the central core of the nerve with the fibres spread around it. All simple tumours should be excised and an attempt made to rejoin or graft the nerve. Entry into the parapharyngeal space can be posterior to the submandibular gland, beneath the parotid, i.e. a cervical rather than a trans-parotid approach. Although some neurogenous tumours can be removed from the surface of the nerve it is inevitable that others are so closely integrated to the vagal trunk that a section of the cranial nerve has to be resected with secondary rehabilitation of the larynx.

Malignant neurogenic tumours

Most malignant tumours of peripheral nerve origin arise, malignant *ab initio*, from the Schwann cell. Neuroblastomas are tumours of childhood, and in the head and neck may be secondary from an abdominal tumour or may arise primarily from the cervical sympathetic chain.

Paragangliomas (chemodectomas)

The paragangliomas arise from chemoreceptor bodies. At imaging, the three sites of origin may be distinguished. Glomus vagale and jugulare tumours tend to displace the internal carotid artery anteriorly. Carotid body tumours show a greater tendency to splay the internal and external carotids. Glomus vagale tumours have smaller intracranial extensions and better developed capsules than glomus jugulare tumours.

Glomus vagale tumours

Vagal paragangliomas arise from nests of paraganglionic tissue within the perineurium of the vagus nerve at its ganglion nodosum, i.e. just below the skull base. In large tumours there may be a small extension through the foramen jugulare. Intravagal tumours, however, are not restricted to this site and may be found at various sites along the nerve and down to the level of the carotid artery bifurcation.

> ### Clinical features of glomus vagale
>
> - Most commonly present as slowly growing and painless masses
> - Pulsating tinnitus
> - Deafness
> - Syncope
> - Vertigo
> - 50% > 3 year history
> - Pharyngeal pain: late sign indicating irritation of the pharyngeal plexus, often preceding the onset of cranial nerve palsies

The mass is high in the anterolateral aspect of the neck, often noted near the origin of the sternomastoid muscle with medial displacement of peritonsillar structures. The diagnosis is confirmed by arteriography. which tends to overestimate size owing to a surrounding pharyngeal plexus of veins.

Surgery is indicated for vagal paragangliomas because of their tendency to spread into the cranial cavity. The approach used is that described below for parapharyngeal tumours. The numerous thin-walled veins should be dealt with in the same way as for carotid body tumours. The most dangerous part of the dissection is superiorly where the internal carotid artery loops over the tumour and then immediately enters the skull. Injury is frequent at this site and therefore the help of a vascular surgeon is advisable.

Carotid body tumour

The carotid body tumour has a much more prominent surface vasculature than the glomus vagale and can be deeply embedded in the vessel wall, making resection extremely painstaking.

> ### Pathology
>
> - High incidence in Peru, Colorado and Mexico City, i.e. at high altitudes chronic hypoxia leads to carotid body hyperplasia
> - Average presentation in the fifth decade
> - Male:female 1:1
> - 10% positive family history:
>   - autosomal dominant
>   - 30% with bilateral tumours
>   - may have phaeochromocytoma
> - Arises from the chemoreceptor cells on the medial side of the carotid bulb
> - Cells histologically similar to normal carotid body cells: large, uniform epithelioid cells surrounded by a vascular stroma
> - Hormonally inactive
> - Proven metastases are rare

Clinical features

Patients present with a long history (5–7 years) of a slowly enlarging painless lump in the region of the carotid bulb. About 30% present with a pharyngeal mass pushing the tonsil medially and anteriorly. Thus, biopsy of a pharyngeal swelling must never be taken from within the mouth. On palpation the mass is firm, rubbery ('potato tumour') and pulsatile, and refills in steps synchronous with the pulse after compression. A bruit may be present and the mass may decrease in size with carotid compression. It is said that it can be moved from side to side but not up and down; this is also true of most other lumps in the neck. Nerve involvement is rare.

Investigation

Whenever a carotid body tumour is suspected biopsy is contraindicated, but careful FNAC with a very narrow-gauge needle has been described. Carotid angiography will demonstrate a tumour circulation, and determine the extent of the tumour and whether there is a cross-circulation. CT or MRI is also useful to determine its extent. Some paragangliomas are demonstrated by metaIodo-Benzyl Guanidine (^{125}I-MIBG) mIBG scintigraphy.

Treatment

Metastases are exceptionally rare and the disease is rarely fatal. Thus, the mere presence of a carotid body tumour does not justify an attempt at removal.

Indications for removal of carotid body tumours

- Good general health
- Age < 50 years
- Small or medium-sized tumour
- Tumours extending into the palate or pharynx interfering with swallowing, speaking or breathing
- Tumours with an aggressive growth pattern

Although these tumours were originally thought to be radioresistant, cures have been reported in recent publications. Radiotherapy should be used in patients who refuse surgery, in high-risk cases or in metastatic disease. [131I]MIBG therapy can be of value in patients with metastatic disease.

Removal of a carotid body tumour

An incision is made from the mastoid process to the clavicle down the anterior border of the sternomastoid muscle: this is one of the few occasions on which this long incision is justified. Dissection is continued down to the carotid sheath, and the common carotid artery, internal jugular vein and vagus nerve are located. The common carotid artery is freed on all sides, preserving the vagus nerve carefully. A tape is placed loosely around the common carotid artery and tagged with an artery forceps. The tape is placed at this stage to allow easy and rapid occlusion of the carotid artery if the internal carotid artery is damaged later in the operation.

The common carotid artery is followed upwards, dissecting along the adventitia and mobilizing the vagus nerve. On approaching the tumour one will encounter large numbers of thin-walled veins, more brown than red in colour. These veins bleed very easily and are a source

of difficulty in this procedure. This difficulty can be overcome by dissection with two non-toothed dissecting forceps with fine points. The tissue is grasped close to the adventitia of the artery with these forceps and pulled apart. Surprisingly, this produces much less bleeding than attempts at sharp dissection, which are slow, tedious and attended by steady bleeding. The surgeon continues in this fashion, freeing the tumour from the internal carotid artery in particular with great care. It should always be possible to preserve the vagus nerve but the hypoglossal nerve is often stretched and may need to be divided.

Glomus jugulare

The glomus jugulare arises from the non-chromaffin para-ganglionic cells around the jugular ganglion in the jugular bulb. There is usually a similar disease bulk above and below the skull base, in contrast to the glomus vagale. Advanced lesions erode the skull base and extend laterally to the middle ear cleft.

Surgical approaches to the parapharyngeal space

- Transparotid
- Anterior transantral – inferior
- Midline transmandibular oropharyngeal

Transparotid

Total conservative parotidectomy is suitable for deep lobe parotid tumours extending through the stylomandibular tunnel. The superficial lobe is ideally pedicled inferior to the mandibular branch, above the cervical branch of the facial nerve. Conservative and radical lateral approaches may also be used, which allow access to the infratemporal fossa as described in Chapter 17.

Anterior inferior approach

A horizontal incision is made at the level of the hyoid, from the midline to cross the anterior border of sternomastoid. The submandibular gland is excised. The approach then is essentially blind, at least in the upper part of the dissection. Blunt dissection opens the plane between the medial pterygoid and deep surface of the parotid laterally and the lesion medially. It may be possible to gain adequate access simply by forward dislocation of the mandible. Otherwise, it is divided close to the angle, to improve access to the upper part of the tumour. This approach is particularly good for extraparotid lesions such as lipomas.

Midline transmandibular oropharyngeal

This approach may be necessary for very large primary parapharyngeal pleomorphic adenomas, for certain malignancies or if the lesion is very vascular, when excision under direct vision is required. Following a mandibular swing approach, the medial pterygoid is divided, allowing removal of the lesion by a combination of sharp and blunt dissection under direct vision.

References and further reading

Bardales R. H., Sutherland M. J., Korourian S., *et al.* (1996) Cytologic findings in thyroglossal duct carcinoma, *Am J Clin Pathol* **106**: 615–19.

Benjamin B. and Innocenti M. (1991) Laser treatment of pharyngeal pouch, *Aust NZ J Surg* **61**: 909–13.

Bradwell R. A., Bieger A. K., Strachan D. R. and Homer J. J. (1997) Endoscopic laser myotomy in the treatment of pharyngeal diverticula, *J Laryngol Otol* **111**: 627–30.

Brouillette D., Martel E., Chen L.-Q. and Duranceau A. (1997) Pitfalls and complications of cricopharyngeal myotomy, *Chest Clin North Am* **7**: 457–75.

Choe S. S. and Zalzal G. H. (1995) Branchial anomalies: A review of 52 cases, *Laryngoscope* **105**: 909–13.

Civantos F. J. and Holinger L. D. (1992) Laryngoceles and saccular cysts in infants and children, *Arch Otolaryngol Head Neck Surg* **118**: 296–300.

Cohen S. R. and Thompson, J. W. (1986) Lymphangiomas of the larynx in infants and children: a survey of pediatric lymphangioma, *Ann Otol Rhinol Laryngol* **127** (Suppl): 1–20.

Deitel M., Bendago M., Krajden S. *et al.* (1989) Modern management of cervical scrofula, *Head Neck* **11**: 60–66.

Doersten von P. G. and Byl F. M. (1997) Endoscopic Zenker's diverticulotomy (Dohlman procedure), *Otol Head Neck Surg* **116**: 209–12.

Dohlman G. and Mattson O. (1960) The endoscopic operation for hypopharyngeal diverticula, *Arch Otolaryngol* **71**: 744–52.

Ellis F. H. (1995) Pharyngoesophageal (Zenker's) diverticulum, *Adv Surg* **28**: 171–189.

Ferreiro J. A. and Weiland L. H. (1994) Pediatric surgical pathology of the head and neck, *Semin Pediatr Surg* **3**: 169–81.

Fishman S. J. and Mulliken J. B. (1993) Hemangiomas and vascular malformations of infancy and childhood, *Pediatr Clin North Am* **40**: 1177–200.

Friedberg J. (1989) Pharyngeal cleft sinuses and cysts, and other benign neck lesions, *Pediatr Clin North Am* **36**: 1451 69.

Fritsch M. H. (1992) Branchial cleft cyst with fistula, *Otolaryngol Head Neck Surg* **107**: 133–4.

Greinwald J. H., Leichtman L. G. and Simko E. J. (1996) Hereditary thyroglossal duct cysts, *Arch Otol Head Neck Surg* **122**: 1094–6.

Hadley J. M., Ridley N., Djazaeri B. and Glover G. (1997) The radiological appearances after the endoscopic crico-pharyngeal myotomy: Dohlman's procedure, *Clin Radiol* **52**: 613–15.

Howard D. J. and Lund V. J. (1986) Thyroglossal ducts, cysts and sinuses: a recurrent problem, *Ann R Coll Surg* **68**: 137–8.

Jackson C. G., Harris P. F., Glasscock M. E. *et al.* (1990) Diagnostic and management of paragangliomas of the skull base, *Am J Surg* **159**: 389–93.

Khafif R. A., Prichep R. and Minkowitz S. (1989) Primary branchiogenic carcinoma, *Head Neck* **11**: 153–63.

Koay C. B. and Bates G. J. (1996) Endoscopic stapling diverticulotomy for pharyngeal pouch, *Clin Otol* **21**: 371–6.

Kraus D. H., Rehm S. J., Orlowski J. P., Tubbs R. R. and Levine H. L. (1990) Upper airway obstruction due to tonsillar lymphadenopathy in human immunodeficiency virus infection, *Arch Otolaryngol Head Neck Surg* **116**: 738–40.

Langlois N. E. I. and Kolhe P. (1992) Plunging ranula: a case report and literature review, *Hum Pathol* **23**: 1306–8.

McCaffrey T. V., Meyer F. B., Michels V. V. *et al.* (1993) High resolution computed tomography of palpable masses of the neck and face, *Radiol Graphs* **3**: 645–78.

Micheau C., Klijanienko J., Luboinski B. and Richard J. (1990) So-called branchiogenic carcinoma is actually cystic metastases in the neck from a tonsillar primary, *Laryngoscope* **100**: 878–83.

Mikaelian A. J., Varkey B., Grossman T. W. and Blatnik D. S. (1989) Blastomycosis of the head and neck, *Otolaryngol Head Neck Surg* **101**: 489–95.

Mitchell O. B., Irwin C., Bailey O. M. and Evans J. N. G. (1987) Cysts of the infant larynx, *J Laryngol Otol* **101**: 833–7.

Mulder C. J. J., Hartog G., Robijn R. J. and Thies J. E. (1995) Flexible endoscopic treatment of Zenker's diverticulum: a new approach, *Endoscopy* **27**: 438–42.

Radkowski D., Arnold J., Healy G. B. *et al.* (1991) Thyroglossal duct remnants: preoperative evaluation and management, *Arch Otolaryngol Head Neck Surg* **117**: 1378–81.

Ricciardelli E. J. and Richardson M. A. (1991) Cervicofacial cystic hygroma: patterns of recurrence and management of the difficult case, *Arch Otolaryngol Head Neck Surg* **117**: 546–53.

Roback S. W. and Telander R. L. (1994) Thyroglossal duct cysts and branchial cleft anomalies, *Semin Pediatr Surg* **3**: 142–6.

Rothstein S. G., Persky M. S., Edelman B. A., Gittleman P. E. and Stroschein M. (1989) Epiglottitis in AIDS patients, *Laryngoscope* **99**: 389–92.

Scher R. L. and Richtsmeier W. J. (1998) Long-term experience with endoscopic staple-assisted esophagodiverticulostomy for Zenker's diverticulum, *Laryngoscope* **108**: 200 5.

Shaheen O. H. (1997) Tumours of the infratemporal fossa and parapharyngeal space, in *Scott brown's Otolaryngology*, 6th edn, Vol. 5, *Laryngology Head and Neck Surgery* (A. G. Kerr, ed.), Butterworth, Oxford, pp. 22/1–19.

Shaw D. W., Cook I. J., Jamieson G. G. *et al.* (1996) Influence of surgery on deglutitive upper oesophageal sphincter mechanics in Zenker's diverticulum, *Gut* **38**: 806–11.

Soh K. B. K. (1998) Branchiogenic carcinomas: do they exist?, *J R Coll Surg Edin* **43**: 1–5.

Som P. M. and Curtin H. D. (1995a) Lesions of the parapharyngeal space role of MR imaging, *Otolaryngol Clin North Am* **28**: 515–542.

Som P. M., Brandwein M. S. and Silvers A. (1995b) Nodal inclusion cysts of the parotid gland and paraphyngeal space, *Laryngoscope* **105**: 1122–8.

Stern J. C., Lin P.-T. and Lucente F. E. (1990) Benign nasopharyngeal masses and human immunodeficiency virus infection, *Arch Otolaryngol Head Neck Surg* **116**: 206–8.

Todd N. W. (1993) Common congenital anomalies of the neck, *Surg Clin North Am* **73**: 599–610.

Witterick I., Gullane P. J. and Yeung E. (1995) Outcome analysis of Zenker's diverticulectomy and cricopharyngeal myotomy, *Head Neck* **17**: 382–8.

Woodruff W. W. and Kennedy T. L. (1997) Non-nodal neck masses, *Semin Ultrasound CT MRI* **18**: 182–204.

Zaninotto G., Costantini M., Boccu C. *et al.* (1996) Functional and morphological study of the cricopharyngeal muscle in patients with Zenker's diverticulum, *Br J Surg* **83**: 1263–7.

12 Metastatic neck disease

'Subclinical disease is not early cancer'
Helmuth Goepfert, 1988

Introduction

One of the most important prognostic factors in head and neck cancer is the presence or absence, level and size of metastatic neck disease. Many carcinomas within the head or neck will sooner or later metastasize to lymph nodes and various factors control the natural history of this event. Once a neck-node metastasis has occurred, further spread of the disease may not happen for many months or indeed years in conditions such as papillary carcinoma of the thyroid.

The assessment of any head and neck tumour should include careful attention to both sides of the neck for consideration of neck node metastases and treatment as appropriate. The subsequent discussion in this chapter relates principally to squamous cell carcinoma.

Surgical anatomy

*'Anatomy is a language,
As dead as dead can be,
It killed the ancient medics,
And now it's killing me'.*

It is impossible to understand the diagnosis, assessment or detailed surgical treatment of any procedure within the neck without understanding the underlying anatomy.

Anatomical divisions

The neck is divided into triangles which, by convention, are known as the anterior and posterior triangles of the neck (Fig. 12.1). These triangles are three-dimensional in shape and change with the position of the neck.

The posterior triangle is bounded by the trapezius muscle, the middle third of the clavicle and the posterior border of the sternomastoid muscle. It can be divided further by the omohyoid muscle into the occipital triangle above and the subclavian triangle below. Although this is an anatomical division, a more important division is that

made by the accessory nerve which travels in the roof of the triangle from 1 cm above Erb's point (where the greater auricular nerve curves around the sternomastoid muscle) down to entering trapezius in its lower third. Everything that is important in the posterior triangle lies below and inferior to this nerve.

The anterior triangle is bounded by the anterior border of the sternomastoid, the mandible and by the midline of the neck anteriorly. It may be further divided into the submandibular, submental and carotid triangles which together make up the supraomohyoidtriangle. From this it will be noted that the sternomastoid muscle and the structures beneath it, by definition, are excluded from either triangle, but most surgeons teach that these structures lie in the posterior triangle. It would be easier if the posterior limit of the anterior triangle were defined as the posterior border of the sternomastoid so that the muscle and associated structures be included in the anterior triangle where they more rightly belong.

Each triangle in the neck has a floor, a roof, important boundaries and a number of important contents. This facilitates easy learning of surgical procedures.

Fascial neck spaces

An understanding of the fascial spaces of the neck is crucial since operative procedures appear easier, more avascular and are better controlled if they proceed along fascial spaces rather than through them. Removal of the fascia is a crucial part of neck dissection technique since it surrounds those tissues which need to be surgically removed and by dissecting along the fascia, important structures within the head and neck can be preserved.

The superficial fascia of the neck is a single layer of fibrofatty tissue which lies superficial to the platysma muscle. The deep cervical fascia is more extensive and a much more important layer than the superficial fascia, and lies deep to platysma and occupies important spaces between muscles, blood vessels, lymph nodes and the

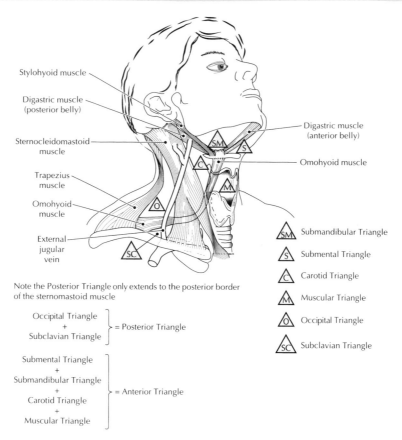

Stylohyoid muscle

Digastric muscle
(posterior belly)

Sternocleidomastoid
muscle

Trapezius
muscle

Omohyoid
muscle

External
jugular
vein

Digastric muscle
(anterior belly)

Omohyoid muscle

Submandibular Triangle

Submental Triangle

Carotid Triangle

Muscular Triangle

Occipital Triangle

Subclavian Triangle

Note the Posterior Triangle only extends to the posterior border
of the sternomastoid muscle

Occipital Triangle
+
Subclavian Triangle
} = Posterior Triangle

Submental Triangle
+
Submandibular Triangle
+
Carotid Triangle
+
Muscular Triangle
} = Anterior Triangle

Figure 12.1   Triangles of the neck.

viscera in the neck. In areas it may be very thin whilst in others it can be rather thick.

> ### Three layers of deep cervical fascia
>
> ■ The investing or outer layer
> ■ The visceral or middle layer
> ■ The internal layer

The investing layer of fascia invests the whole of the neck and splits to surround the trapezius muscle posteriorly and the sternomastoid muscle laterally (Fig. 12.2). Above it is attached to the superior nuchal line, the mastoid process and the mandible, and below this to the spine of the seventh cervical vertebra, the spine of the acromion, the clavicle and the manubrium. It forms the roof of the posterior and anterior triangles. It also splits to provide fascial sheaths for the parotid and submandibular glands and forms the carotid sheath which surrounds both the internal and external carotid arteries and the common carotid artery, along with the internal jugular vein and vagus nerve. Such a fascial envelope allows movement of these structures upon each other and hence dissection both around and between them. Other cranial nerves are also surrounded by this fascia and these include the glossopharyngeal, the accessory and the hypoglossal nerves, along with the ansa hypoglossi.

The visceral or middle layer of fascia surrounds the middle compartment of the neck to include the pharynx, larynx, oesophagus and trachea, and allows these structures to move upon each other. Included here is the pretracheal fascia which surrounds and envelops the thyroid gland and the parathyroid glands, by convention, lie outside this layer although sometimes it may contain them.

The internal layer of the deep fascia is known as the prevertebral fascia. This surrounds the deep muscles of the neck, i.e. the erector spinae, the levator scapula, the three scalenus muscles, the longus capitus and longus colli. It is crucial to understanding the surgical anatomy of the neck because it provides the floor to the posterior triangle, and has important relations with some important nerves in the neck. The cervical sympathetic trunk lies superficial to the prevertebral fascia under the carotid sheath, the branches of the cervical plexus lie deep to the fascia but pierce it as they become more superficial to enter the posterior triangle, and both the phrenic nerve and the brachial plexus lie deep to this layer.

Head and neck lymphatics

The lymphatic drainage of the head and neck is conventionally divided into three systems. These are discussed in turn.

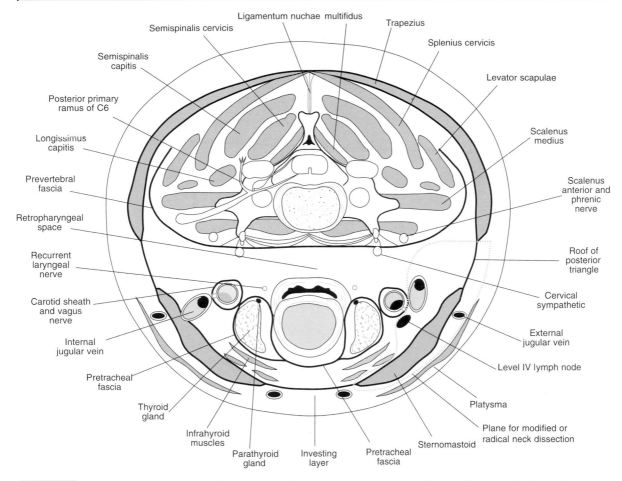

Figure 12.2 Three layers of deep cervical fascia. Dotted line marks resection margins for modified or radical neck dissection.

Waldeyer's internal ring

Within the pharynx at the skull base, there is a circular collection of lymphoid tissue aggregates which plays an important part in early immunological development. They consist of a collection of lymphoid tissue and were described by Waldeyer (who was Professor of Anatomy in Berlin) in 1884, 4 years before he introduced the word 'chromosome'. The ring includes the adenoid, the tubal and lingual tonsils, the palatine tonsil and aggregates of lymphoid tissue on the posterior pharyngeal wall. Tumours arising in this area have a high propensity for lymphatic spread.

Superficial lymph-node system (Waldeyer's external ring)

The lymphatic drainage of head and neck tissue is divided into a superficial and a deep system and usually, but not always, the passage of lymph is lateralized and sequential and follows a predefined route from superficial to deep. The superficial nodal system, which drains the superficial tissues of the head and neck, consists of two circles of nodes, one in the head and the other in the neck. In the head, the nodes are situated around the skull base and are known as the occipital, postauricular, parotid or preauricular and then buccal or facial nodes. They are in

continuity with the superficial nodes in the upper neck consisting of the superficial cervical, submandibular and submental nodes, along with the anterior cervical nodes. These latter nodes are situated along the external jugular vein and the anterior jugular veins, respectively.

This superficial system receives drainage from the skin and underlying tissues of the scalp, eyelids and face, along with Waldeyer's internal ring, nasal sinuses and oral cavity.

Deep system (cervical lymph nodes proper)

The deeper fascial structures of the head and neck drain either directly into the deep cervical lymph nodes or through the superficial system first and then into the deep system. These superficial nodes have already been described. The deep cervical lymph nodes proper (Fig. 12.3) consist of the junctional nodes, the upper, middle and lower cervical nodal groups which are situated along the internal jugular vein, the spinal accessory group which accompanies the accessory nerve in the posterior triangle, the nuchal nodes, the visceral nodes in the midline of the neck and nodes in the upper mediastinum. The junctional nodes represent the confluence of nodes at the junction of the posterior part of the submandibular

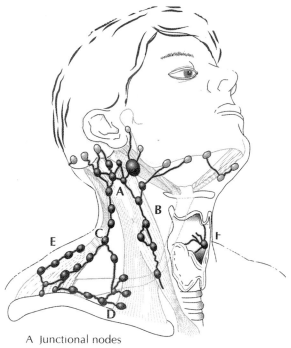

A Junctional nodes
B Internal jugular nodes
C Spinal accessory nodes
D Supraclavicular nodes
E Nuchal nodes
F Deep medial visceral nodes

Figure 12.3 Deep cervical lymph nodes.

triangle with the retropharyngeal nodes where they meet at the junction of the upper and middle deep cervical nodes.

In general, the passage of lymph within these systems has been well documented using lymphography and it follows a sequential pattern from superficial to deep, and from the upper to lower parts of the neck. These lower confluent vessels form into a jugular trunk which on the right side ends at the junction of the jugular vein and the brachiocephalic vein or joins the right lymphatic duct.

On the left side the trunk will usually join the thoracic duct as it arches behind the lower part of the carotid sheath and in front of the subclavian artery to enter the junction of the internal jugular vein with the brachiocephalic vein.

Natural history and evolution of malignant disease in the neck

It is possible to predict the site of a primary tumour based on the distribution of cervical metastases, and this was done by Lindberg in a classic study in 1972 whereby he was able to identify likely sites of metastases related to the site of the primary tumour (Fig. 12.4). It is the accepted rule that patterns of subclinical microscopic metastases follow a similar distribution. Following Lindberg's work, the Memorial Sloan-Kettering Hospital published in 1981 a number of levels or regions within the neck which contain groups of lymph nodes that represent the first echelon sites for metastases from head and neck primary sites. These are described below (Fig. 12.5).

Level I: submental and submandibular groups

This consists of the submental group of lymph nodes within the triangle bounded by the anterior belly of digastric and the hyoid bone, and the submandibular group of nodes bounded by the posterior belly of digastric and the body of the mandible.

Level II: upper jugular group

This consists of the lymph nodes located around the upper third of the internal jugular vein and adjacent spinal accessory nodes extending from the skull base down to the level of the carotid bifurcation where the digastric muscle crosses the internal jugular vein. This point relates to level of the hyoid bone on a computed tomographic (CT) scan. It contains the junctional and sometimes the jugulodigastric nodes.

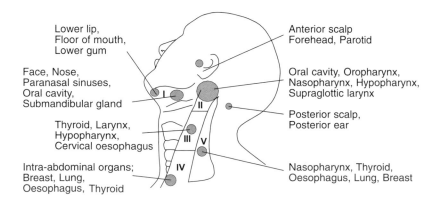

Figure 12.4 Likely primary tumour sites based on the distribution of cervical metastases

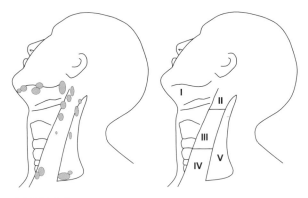

Figure 12.5 Lymph-node levels in the neck. (After Memorial Sloan Kettering Hospital, New York.)

The factors which affect the pattern of spread of malignant disease to the neck depend on both tumour and patient factors. The site of the primary tumour is important, with some sites having a high incidence of metastases, both palpable and otherwise, at presentation (Table 12.1).

It is important to note that the above drainage patterns apply in the non-violated neck. Once the natural history of the disease is changed, lymph-node metastases can occur anywhere. This explains why the operation of selective neck dissection is usually only suitable in the previously untreated neck.

An incision in the neck for a neck-node biopsy can alter patterns of lymphatic drainage for up to 1 year following surgery. Further shunting of lymph with opening up

Level III: middle jugular group

This consists of lymph nodes located around the middle third of the internal jugular vein extending from the carotid bifurcation superiorly (bottom of level II) down to the upper part of the cricoid cartilage (seen on a CT scan) and represents the level where the omohyoid muscle crosses the internal jugular vein. It usually contains the jugulo-omohyoid nodes and may contain the jugulo-digastric node.

Level IV: lower jugular group

This consists of lymph nodes located around the lower third of the internal jugular vein extending from the cricoid cartilage down to the clavicle inferiorly. It may contain some jugulo-omohyoid nodes.

Level V: posterior triangle group

These nodes are located along the lower half of the spinal accessory nerve and the transverse cervical artery. Supraclavicular nodes are also included in this group. The posterior border is the anterior border of the trapezius and the anterior boundary is the posterior border of the sternomastoid muscle.

Level VI: anterior compartment group (visceral group)

This consists of lymph nodes surrounding the midline visceral structures of the neck extending from the hyoid bone superiorly to the suprasternal notch inferiorly. The lateral border on each side is the medial border of the sternomastoid muscle. It contains the parathyroid, the paratracheal and pretracheal, the perilaryngeal and precricoid lymph nodes.

Level VII

These are the lymph nodes in the upper anterior mediastinum.

Table 12.1 The probability of cervical metastases (N) related to primary (T) staging in patients with head and neck squamous carcinoma

Primary site	T-Stage	N_0 (%)	N_1 (%)	N_2–N_3 (%)
Floor of mouth	T_1	89	9	2
	T_2	71	18	10
	T_3	56	20	24
	T_4	46	10	43
Oral tongue	T_1	86	10	4
	T_2	70	19	11
	T_3	52	20	31
	T_4	24	10	66
Retromolar trigone anterior faucial pillar	T_1	88	2	9
	T_2	62	18	20
	T_3	46	21	33
	T_4	32	18	50
Nasopharynx	T_1	8	11	82
	T_2	16	12	72
	T_3	12	9	80
	T_4	17	6	78
Soft palate	T_1	92	0	8
	T_2	64	12	24
	T_3	35	26	39
	T_4	33	11	56
Base of tongue	T_1	30	15	55
	T_2	29	14	56
	T_3	26	23	52
	T_4	16	8	76
Tonsillar fossa	T_1	30	41	30
	T_2	32	14	54
	T_3	30	18	52
	T_4	10	13	76
Supraglottic larynx	T_1	61	10	29
	T_2	58	16	26
	T_3	36	25	40
	T_4	41	18	41
Hypopharynx	T_1	37	21	42
	T_2	30	20	49
	T_3	21	26	54
	T_4	26	15	58

Lindberg (1972); Sessions *et al*. (1986).

of abnormal channels occurs when more extensive surgery and radiotherapy is undertaken, and once a lymph node is palpable and contains tumour there may be early shunting of cells to the contralateral neck. All of these factors play a part in the management of neck disease.

Organ-specific drainage

The nasopharynx, nasal cavities and sinuses drain via the junctional nodes into the upper deep cervical nodes (levels II and III) having passed through retropharyngeal or submandibular lymph nodes.

The oropharynx similarly drains into the upper and middle deep cervical nodes, again either directly or via the retropharyngeal or submandibular nodes. Within these areas of deep lymph-node collections in the neck, certain nodes can reach quite large proportions and some are named. There are 500 lymph nodes in the body and of these 200 are in the head and neck. They normally range in size from 3 mm to 3 cm but most nodes are less than 1 cm. Within the upper deep cervical nodes in low level II or high level III, the largest node is often called the jugulodigastric node and is usually situated within the triangle formed by the internal jugular vein, the facial vein and the posterior belly of the digastric muscle. It is important because it receives lymphatic tissue from a wide area to include the submandibular region, along with the oropharynx and oral cavity. The jugulo-omohyoid nodes are situated at the junction between the middle and lower cervical group (low level III/high level IV) where the omohyoid muscle crosses the internal jugular vein and again receives lymphatic vessels from a wide area to include anterior floor of mouth, oropharynx and larynx.

The oral cavity has a wide area of drainage and this is important because there is often free communication between the two sides of the tongue. This means that the normal acts of mastication and swallowing facilitate tongue massage and can promote early and rapid lymphatic spread directly to low in the neck. The posterior parts of the oral cavity drain either directly into the upper deep cervical nodes (level II/III) or indirectly via the submandibular nodes in level I. More anterior parts of the oral cavity and tongue also drain to these nodes but, in addition, may drain to the submental nodes (level I) or directly to the jugulo-omohyoid nodes (levels III/IV) low in the neck. Given the previous anatomical considerations, it is important to realize that contralateral neck spread may occur early in those tumours situated in or near the midline.

The larynx drainage is separated into upper and lower systems with embryological connotations and a division that occurs at the level of the true vocal cord. The supraglottis drains through vessels which accompany the superior laryngeal pedicle through the thyrohyoid membrane to reach the upper deep cervical nodes (levels II/III). The lower system drains directly into the deep cervical nodes (levels III/IV) through vessels which pass through or behind the cricothyroid membrane or drain into the

prelaryngeal, pretracheal or paratracheal nodes (level VI) before reaching the deep cervical nodes. Because the vocal cords are relatively avascular, they have an extremely sparse lymphatic drainage and, as such, lymph-node metastases from carcinomas of this site are uncommon in early stages.

The hypopharynx is similar to the larynx and both may have contralateral spread, particularly in those areas that are either close to the midline or have significant communication across the midline such as the epiglottis, the posterior pharyngeal wall and the postcricoid region. Drainage is to levels IV, VI and VII.

Tumours in the oral cavity and pharynx have a higher incidence of metastatic disease at presentation than those in the larynx and it is important to take this into account when treating these sites. The high incidence of occult metastases in tumours of the oral cavity, pharynx and, to a lesser extent, the supraglottic larynx forms the basis for selective neck dissection and, assuming that the patterns of spread from tumour sites is applicable to subclinical microscopic metastases, the following rules apply.

The first echelon lymph nodes for the oral cavity lie in levels I, II and III. The first echelon lymph-node levels for the larynx and pharynx lie in levels II, III and IV. The first echelon lymph nodes for the thyroid lie in the tracheo-oesophageal groove in level VI, the superior mediastinum (level VII) and in level IV. For the parotid gland, the first echelon lymph nodes, are the preauricular, periparotid and intraparotid lymph nodes along with those in levels II, III and the upper accessory chain (level V). For the submandibular and sublingual gland, the first echelon lymph nodes lie in level I, II and III.

Other factors that affect the natural history of neck disease are the size and thickness of the primary tumour, the laterality of the tumour and whether or not there has been any previous treatment to affect patterns of spread. Perineural and perivascular invasion, the degree of differentiation of the tumour and whether or not there is any recurrence at the primary site are all important. It has also been shown that those tumours with an infiltrating margin are much more likely to metastasize.

With regard to host factors, few would argue that the immulogical response of the host to the tumour is crucial in determining spread and ultimately prognosis in head and neck cancer, but there is little quantitative evidence to support this statement.

Clinical staging

There is now a joint International Union Against Cancer (UICC)/American Journal of Cancer (AJC) joint classification for regional cervical lymphadenopathy (Table 12.2).

This is based not only on the presence or absence of cervical lymphadenopathy but also on the size of the lymph node and the number of lymph nodes but, as yet, not the level. It applies to all head and neck tumours (Fig. 12.6) apart from the nasopharynx and thyroid, which are discussed separately in Chapters 20 and 23.

Table 12.2	TNM classification of regional nodes
Node	**Description**
N_x	Regional lymph-nodes cannot be assessed
N_0	No regional lymph node metastasis
N_1	Metastasis in a single ipsilateral lymph node 3 cm or less in greatest dimension
N_2	Metastasis in a single ipsilateral lymph node, more than 3 cm but no more than 6 cm in greatest dimension, or in multiple ipsilateral lymph nodes no more than 6 cm in greatest dimension, or in bilateral or contralateral lymph nodes, no more than 6 cm in greatest dimension
N_{2a}	Metastasis in a single ipsilateral lymph node, more than 3 cm but no more than 6 cm in greatest dimension
N_{2b}	Metastasis in multiple ipsilateral lymph nodes, no more than 6 cm in greatest dimension
N_{2c}	Metastasis in bilateral or contralateral lymph nodes, no more than 6 cm in greatest dimension
N_3	Metastasis in a lymph node more than 6 cm in greatest dimension

UICC (1997).

Behaviour of disease within cervical lymph nodes

The spread of disease from the primary tumour to the regional lymph nodes occurs by passive transport within lymph. Metastatic involvement of various lymph-node regions usually progresses from superior to inferior in an orderly fashion but it has been shown that in some situations lymph-node groups can be bypassed even in the normal lymphogram. Once tumour cells arrive at a draining lymph node, they can proliferate, die, remain dormant or enter the blood circulation through blood vessels in the node. The process of metastasis is not a random phenomenon, although random events may be important. Paget's seed and soil hypothesis was an attractive one and, although largely disproved, a number of important properties have recently been assigned to tumour cells or metastatic seeds and these include cell growth, chemotaxis, and immunological, metabolic and hormonal factors. Similar host environmental (soil) factors include the tissue and stromal environment, hormones, inflammatory and immunological responses and the presence or absence of vital nutrients.

There are several stages of metastasis via lymphatic pathways. Premetastatic invasion of the epithelial basal lamina of the primary tumour is followed by subsequent encroachment, penetration and translocation of cells through a lymphatic. This is followed by intranodal settling, proliferation and destruction of the lymph node. Secondary metastases to other lymph nodes soon develop, although their occurrence is not always accompanied by the destruction by the primary echelon node. Metastatic squamous

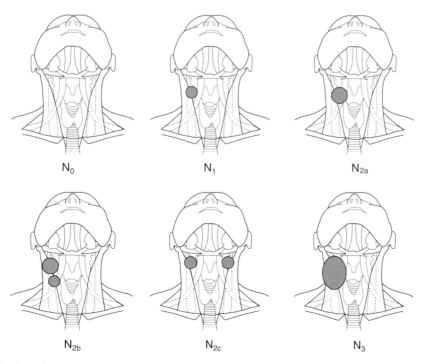

Figure 12.6 Clinical staging of malignant cervical lymphadenopathy.

cell carcinoma within a cervical lymph node can stimulate the stroma in a variety of ways and a number of histological and immunological patterns have been described.

There are four distinct growth patterns of squamous cell carcinoma within cervical lymph nodes.

1. Following original cancerous deposits in the subcapsular sinus, growth within the affected node proceeds to a considerable extent before extranodal spread occurs. Ultimately, extranodal extension occurs by the direct penetration and destruction of the capsule, or by the arrest of further underlying capsular or juxtacapsular lymphatics.
2. Extranodal spread occurs at an early stage in the genesis of the tumour growth within the node.
3. A less common pattern involves the deposition of a malignant embolus within the subcapsular sinus together with the simultaneous arrest of tumour within capsular or juxtacapsular lymphatics. This results in the coincident and equivalent proliferation of cancer both within and outside the node.
4. The least common growth pattern shows capsular or juxtacapsular emboli with no intranodal cancer. This is important to realize since, in some instances, extranodal spread can occur much earlier in the natural history of the disease process and, as such, may be important when undertaking conservation neck surgery.

Distant metastases from head and neck cancer may occur from haematological spread by direct invasion into blood vessels or by spread to regional lymphatic nodes and subsequent entry into the circulation through blood vessels or lymphaticovenous communications. Vascularization of tumours usually occurs when growths are greater than 0.1–1 mm in size and, following this, rapid rates of neoplastic growth and increased rates of vessel invasion can occur. Animal studies have shown that tumours in the range 2–4 g release up to 4×10^6 cells per gram of tumour tissue per day. These may be released as single cells, more often as cell clumps, and more often still, as a thrombus fragment containing tumour cells. It is now generally accepted that considerable fragments of tumour are required to cause bloodborne metastases and the success of their implantation is determined by both tumour and host factors.

Assessment of cervical lymphadenopathy

Any patient with a head and neck primary tumour requires assessment of the neck. This begins with a history and full clinical examination which may be supplemented by an examination under anaesthetic. Further assessment with radiology may be appropriate and fine-needle aspiration cytology (FNAC) can help to confirm or refute the diagnosis. If surgery is undertaken then a full pathological examination will allow final staging in relation to the presence or absence, size and number of lymph nodes, along with pathological grading, the presence or absence of extracapsular spread and also whether there is any vascular and lymphatic permeation.

Criticisms of the current staging system

Careful pathological studies now cast grave doubts on the significance of clinical staging. The most important prognostic factors are the number of nodes involved and, in particular, the presence of any extracapsular spread. Neither of these parameters can be measured clinically. In addition, no account has been taken in clinical series of the level of lymph node with regard to prognosis.

Furthermore, clinical staging gives great weight to laterality, whereas pathological studies have shown that bilateral nodes, particularly if they are N_1, do not carry a worse prognosis than unilateral N_1 nodes at certain sites, e.g. supraglottis. For other sites, contralateral and bilateral nodes carry a dismal prognosis and, as such, probably deserve an N_3 grouping. Finally, this scheme does not allow independent classification of massive nodes on both sides of the neck, which are usually fixed and almost universally fatal.

Assessment of cervical lymph nodes

Despite the above reservations, clinical examination remains an important method of assessing the regional lymph nodes. Great care should be taken in the neck examination, and this has been discussed in detail in Chapter 2. It must be remembered that not only are some necks more difficult to examine than others, but some regions are inaccessible, e.g. the retropharyngeal area. Nodes in these areas are impossible to palpate until they reach a considerable size. Clinical examination of the neck has a variable reliability with an inevitable false-positive and false-negative rate of around 20–30%.

The addition of radiological imaging represents the limit of clinical staging and further examination of surgical specimens by the histopathologist will supply the information described above to allow further sophisticated staging in relation to prognosis.

Computed tomography

There is no doubt that CT scanning can detect cervical lymphadenopathy within the neck. Its sensitivity and specificity compared with clinical examination vary from series to series but in essence it is more accurate than clinical examination, particularly in necks that are difficult to examine, for restaging and for the inaccessible areas such as the retropharynx. The detection of malignant disease is based on the fact that as the cancer invades the lymph node, its size, shape and characteristics change so that it becomes larger, has a thin rim of inflammation around its edge which shows up on the scan as an area of enhancement and, as the centre of the cancer dies, it appears as a necrotic centre. The range of normal cervical lymphadenopathy is 3 mm to 3 cm but most workers realize that nodes greater than 1 cm in size on CT scanning may contain metastatic disease. At present, the literature suggests that approximately an 80% overall accuracy rate can be achieved on CT by considering all nodes greater than

1 cm in size as containing malignant disease, except for those in the low level II, high level III (jugulodigastric) region, where a 1.5 cm size criterion is applied.

Suspicious nodes on cross-sectional imaging

- Size greater than 1 cm
- Rim enhancement following IV contrast
- Central necrosis
- Spherical shape

It is important to realize that the two difficult areas in imaging head and neck cancer are the detection of low-volume disease in the neck and residual and recurrent disease following surgery and irradiation. With regard to the former, it is possible on current criteria to miss cancer in an 8 mm cervical lymph node. This can be disastrous since such cancer is not early disease. Such a lymph node would contains 10^8 malignant cells, with 10^{13} cells representing an incurable growth. Therefore, it is important not to rely solely on CT scans and to treat the patient rather than the scan, and base management decisions on the natural history of the disease in question.

At present in the UK routine scanning of the neck in a patient with a head and neck cancer is probably not justified in terms of either time or cost but, with advances in current CT scanning and increased availability, this is likely to change so that routine evaluation of most head and neck squamous carcinomas (excluding T_1 larynx) will include a skull base to diaphragm CT.

At present, a CT scan of the neck should be considered in the following situations:

- if the neck is being scanned as part of the assessment of a primary tumour
- if there is a high chance of occult disease (>20%) as an alternative to elective treatment
- in the presence of significant ipsilateral disease when the presence of deep fixation or contralateral spread may change management from surgery to no treatment at all
- to assess the difficult neck
- for restaging.

Magnetic resonance imaging

Magnetic resonance imaging (MRI) can undoubtedly detect cervical lymphadenopathy and has similar accuracy rates to CT. Similar criteria for malignancy are used in both techniques. The various indications where MRI might be more suitable than CT are discussed in Chapter 3 but, in principle, the indications for performing a scan are similar to those for CT.

Ultrasound

There is no doubt that enlarged metastatic cervical lymphadenopathy can be demonstrated on an ultrasound scan, but that the absolute criterion for differentiating benign from malignant disease is notable by its absence. There are some workers at present who are using ultrasound-guided FNAC in the assessment of the neck to try to detect occult malignant disease, but this technique is labour intensive and operator dependent, and may miss disease which might condemn patients to a policy of 'wait and see' rather than elective treatment. In such necks, a policy of elective neck treatment is usually better than elective neck investigation.

Radionuclide scanning

- Pentavalent DMSA
- SPECT
- PET

Since the 1960s, various workers have used a number of radionuclides to detect metastatic cervical lymphadenopathy. Gallium citrate, cobalt bleomycin and more recently technetium-99m dimercaptosuccinic acid (pentavalent DMSA) have all been used, but all suffer from a low sensitivity and specificity and an inability to detect nodes less than 2 cm in size, by which time they are usually clinically palpable. The application of Erhlich's magic bullet theory and the use of radiolabelled monoclonal antibodies were attractive propositions but the *in vivo* problems of increased vascularity in the neck associated with a low sensitivity and specificity meant that these techniques using labelled antibodies to, for example, the epidermal growth factor receptor have not been introduced into routine clinical practice and further research is awaited.

A planar isotope image creates a two-dimensional picture but sensitivity and specificity can be increased using three-dimensional techniques in the form of single photon emission computed tomography (SPECT). Although this can increase the sensitivity and specificity of pentavalent DMSA scanning, the technique is still inferior to clinical examination.

These techniques rely on both anatomy and physiology to demonstrate the presence of pathological disease, and the uptake of a radionuclide into a tumour is often related to high blood flow, which explains overlap in the detection of inflammatory disease. The introduction of positron emission tomography (PET) means that the metabolic activity of cervical lymph nodes can now be assessed using 18-fluorodeoxyglucose (^{18}FDG). Although in theory this has certain attractions, problems inherent in the technique mean that there is a poor sensitivity and specificity for low-volume disease. The role of PET will almost certainly be confined for the foreseeable future to the detection of the occult primary and in the assessment of residual and recurrent disease following surgery and irradiation.

Fine-needle aspiration cytology

Not every lymph node in the neck requires FNAC investigation. In the presence of palpable disease and a proven primary then treatment will usually be directed towards the assessment of the neck disease rather than confirming that a metastasis is present. However, it is in many cases beneficial to perform FNAC on palpable nodes since the result showing squamous cell carcinoma is usually returned before the examination under anaesthesia is performed.

Few surgeons would ignore a clinically palpable node in the presence of proven primary disease, particularly as the aspiration cytology test may not be sufficiently reliable. The technique is particularly useful in the assessment of a palpable node when searching for an unknown primary, when the nature of the histology may help in the search for the primary tumour. The possibility of anaplastic carcinoma or lymphoma makes an open biopsy mandatory.

Pathology

The head and neck pathologist has the ultimate say in the assessment of cervical lymphadenopathy. Following neck dissection, the specimen should be pinned out on a board and presented to the pathologist. It will then be examined in a conventional manner to assess the total number of lymph nodes in the specimen, the number that are positive and the levels that are involved, along with the presence or absence of extracapsular spread, vascular and lymphatic permeation. This information is recorded on a diagram within the pathological report and stored in the notes. Within the current UICC classification, histological examination of a selective neck dissection will ordinarily include six or more lymph nodes and examination of a radical neck dissection will include 10 or more lymph nodes.

Histology reporting

- Prepare specimen on board
- Report number of nodes
- Report nodal levels
- Is there any extracapsular spread?
- Draw a diagram of results

Treatment of metastatic neck disease

The presence of metastatic cervical lymphadenopathy has an adverse effect on survival. At the same time, careful and effective treatment can provide a cure in a significant proportion of node-positive patients. The treatment of a patient with disease in the neck is clouded with controversial areas.

Treatment controversies

- Treatment of the N_0 neck
- Role of selective neck dissection in the management of N_1 disease
- Role of radiotherapy in the management of neck disease
- Role of modified radical neck dissection, radical neck dissection and extended radical neck dissection
- Treatment of neck disease in a patient who has an occult primary
- Treatment of suspected or established bilateral neck disease
- Management of the difficult, untreatable or inoperable neck
- Role of salvage surgery in the management of recurrent neck disease
- Role of chemotherapy

Whatever one's approach to the management of metastatic neck disease, it is important to remember a number of general principles. In the untreated neck, patterns of spread are often predictable and in the N_0 neck occult metastatic disease is usually found in the first echelon lymphnode drainage areas. This permits the principle of selective neck dissection. Once the patient has had previous radiotherapy or surgery, drainage patterns are often altered so, although the neck may be clinically N_0, all five levels in the neck should be treated by surgery or radiotherapy. In those patients with palpable neck disease, non-palpable spread may be present anywhere in the neck and, as such, the correct approach is to completely encompass the disease. This usually involves surgery, although radiotherapy may have a place for 'small' N_1 (less than 2 cm) necks. Postoperative radiotherapy is given in certain situations (see later).

Patients with no palpable nodes (N_0)

The evaluation and treatment of the N_0 neck has been one of the greatest problems in head and neck surgery and treatment remains controversial. The problem that faces the head and neck oncologist is whether or not to treat electively. Elective treatment to the N_0 neck has been proposed because on retrospective evidence from elective radical neck dissection specimens, there is a high incidence of subclinical disease in the neck, particularly for squamous carcinomas affecting the oral cavity, pharynx and supraglottic larynx. However, the likelihood of there being involved nodes depends not only on the site of the primary tumour but also its size and histological differentiation. The controversy extends into when, and how, the N_0 neck should be treated.

Treatment options for the N_0 neck

- Elective surgery
- Elective radiotherapy
- Elective neck investigation (CT or MRI)
- Adopt a policy of 'wait and see'

In the past there have been several proponents for elective neck dissection, and a case for and against elective surgery to the neck rests on the following key points.

Arguments for elective neck surgery:

- High incidence of occult metastatic disease
- If limited, neck dissection has a low morbidity and mortality
- If the neck has to be entered to remove the primary lesion, it is better to perform an incontinuity resection at that time
- It is impossible to provide the clinical follow-up necessary to detect the earliest conversion of the neck from N_0 to N_1
- Allowing neck metastases to develop increases the incidence of distant metastases
- Cure rate for neck dissection is decreased if gland enlargement occurs or multiple nodes appear

---

Until 1980, all of the evidence for and against elective surgery was retrospective. A consensus of opinion was that there was no place for elective surgery and to date there have been two controlled prospective trials which offered no benefit from elective surgery to the clinically N_0 neck (Vandenbrouck *et al.*, 1980; Fakih, 1989). It also became apparent that elective neck irradiation could irradicate more than 90% of subclinical disease in the neck.

There have been no published controlled prospective trials evaluating elective neck irradiation, although meta-analysis of the results of two retrospective series evaluating its role in the treatment of patients with squamous cell carcinoma of the oral cavity and tongue (Pointon *et al.*, 1990; Dearnaley *et al.*, 1991) showed that elective neck irradiation may prolong survival by reducing subsequent local recurrent metastatic disease.

Current data suggest that the principal value of prophylactic neck treatment, whether by surgery or irradiation, is to reduce significantly the chance of relapse in the neck, which may in some situations translate into improved outcome.

On the basis of these retrospective and prospective studies it seems reasonable to suggest that in those patients with a greater than 20–25% chance of subclinical neck disease, where vigilant follow-up is not possible, where clinical evaluation of the neck has proven difficult, where the neck is being entered for access for reconstruction or where imaging of the neck suggests possible occult nodal spread, then elective treatment with surgery or external beam radiotherapy should be considered.

When the primary tumour is being treated with radiotherapy (e.g. T_1 lateral tongue border or floor of the mouth), then the elective treatment to the neck should be with radiotherapy to the first echelon lymph nodes or the whole neck, and where midline extension occurs treatment should be bilateral.

Where the primary tumour is being treated with surgery (e.g. larger T_2/T_3 squamous cell carcinoma of the lateral tongue border), elective neck surgery should be carried out on the basis that it provides further information for clinical staging, lymph nodes in the area are cleared to give access to vessels for reconstruction purposes, local recurrence rates may be reduced and survival enhanced. The choice of selective neck resection to perform is based on the site of the primary tumour and this is discussed in Chapter 13.

A further option in the N_0 neck is to consider elective neck investigation. In other words, although no nodes are clinically palpable, can a radiological investigation such as CT or MRI demonstrate nodes and, if so, can a treatment plan be adopted on the basis of such scans?

In view of this, it would seem that many of the arguments levelled against neck dissection could be levelled against elective neck imaging. For example, in one series only 5% of clinically N_0 necks were correctly upstaged by CT (Watkinson, 1991) and, if false-positive results are inevitable in the presence of inflammatory neck nodes and false negatives do occur, then surely CT should play no role in the routine evaluation of the N_0 neck. Treatment should be based on the understanding of the natural history in question, and at present it is probably cheaper and as effective to offer elective treatment to those high-risk patients who need it and 'wait and see' in the others. This will avoid large numbers of unnecessary CT scans and subsequent inevitable inappropriate surgery since, as already explained, false positives are inevitable and the natural history of the tomographically positive node is not known. In addition, some patients in high-risk groups with negative scans may be offered a policy of 'wait and see' with possible disastrous results.

A recent study evaluated the outcome of observing the clinically N_0 neck in high-risk patients (mainly oral carcinoma) using ultrasonographic-guided (US)-FNAC for follow-up after transoral excision. Patients were followed up for between 1–4 years using palpation and US-FNAC. Fourteen patients (18%) had occult lymph node metastases and subsequent neck failure. Of the 14 neck failures, nine were detected within 7 months and, of these, six were not palpable. Ten out of 14 patients were successfully salvaged but four died of uncontrolled disease. The authors concluded that the high salvage rate (71%) indicated that a strict follow-up policy using US-FNAC enables early detection of recurrence in the high-risk N_0 neck and justifies a policy of wait and see.

However, although the authors do not identify the T staging of the primary tumour, some neck failures (and indeed subsequent death) might have been prevented by elective treatment rather that elective investigation.

Because of this, most surgeons would recommend elective treatment rather than elective neck investigation. It is perfectly reasonable to adopt a policy of wait and see in patients with low-risk necks, e.g. carcinoma of the glottis or soft palate, but for those that are high risk, the evidence that waiting for the neck to develop from N_0 to N_1 can have a detrimental effect on the patient is quite strong (Shah, 1996; van den Brekel *et al.*, 1999), and does not justify its routine use in current clinical practice.

Single palpable metastasis in one side of the neck less than 3 cm in diameter (N_1)

The majority of these patients will have metastatic lymphadenopathy and even if FNAC is negative or inconclusive, it is a brave person who ignores a palpable node in the neck. In general, the treatment of such nodes is surgery and as extranodal spread may be uncommon in this group, it is possible to consider conservation neck surgery.

It is important to remember that in palpable neck disease, all five levels may be involved and should be dissected. Therefore, the minimum operation that should be performed is a modified radical neck dissection. In these cases it is usually possible to preserve the accessory nerve but, in general, unless a second side neck resection is being performed or the internal jugular vein is required for reconstructive anastomotic purposes, the sternomastoid muscle and the internal jugular vein should be sacrificed. This is because the spread of disease is often between these two structures in an orderly progressive manner down the neck and in order to get it right first time, it is important to encompass the area involved in question rather than violate it and risk the possibility of spreading malignant cells, which can lead to less efficient surgery and local recurrence.

There are proponents of a 'less than five level' neck dissection for N_1 disease, on the basis that in the untreated neck, the arguments for the distribution of metastases in first echelon lymph nodes in non-palpable disease can be applied to early palpable disease. However, this sort of surgery requires considerable expertise, it is fraught with danger and many of these cases are also treated with subsequent postoperative radiotherapy to all five levels. The results of prospective trials are awaited but, at present, caution should be adopted in performing such limited surgery for clinically evident disease.

The role of radiotherapy in the treatment of N_1 disease is controversial. The current consensus is that it is less efficient than surgery and, in general, represents a less preferred option unless the primary site is also being treated with radiotherapy. The classic example of this is carcinoma of the nasopharynx with unilateral or bilateral cervical lymphadenopathy, where the conventional approach is radical radiotherapy and subsequent surgery for salvage.

Large (greater than 3 cm less than 6 cm) nodes (N_{2a}) or multiple unilateral nodes (N_{2b})

This group represents advanced neck disease and once deemed operable should be treated with radical surgery. In many cases the accessory nerve can be preserved, so the operation of choice is either a modified radical neck dissection (type I) or a radical neck dissection. Depending on the pathological findings, postoperative radiotherapy may be administered.

Bilateral and contralateral nodes (N_{2c})

Cases with bilateral neck nodes are uncommon and occur in about 5% of head and neck cancers overall. The common primary sites involved are usually the tongue base, the supraglottic larynx and the hypopharynx. Conventionally, it used to be thought that the presence of bilateral neck disease was a grave prognostic sign and this was indicated in the staging that such disease received in the past. However, subsequent careful pathological studies have shown that, in certain instances, this is not so. The prognosis is determined more by the size, number of nodes and by the presence or absence of extracapsular spread within the neck rather than by pure laterality. This is particularly true for the supraglottic larynx, and in those patients where the bilateral nodes are either N_1 or N_{2a} treatment is often worthwhile and is in the conventional manner described above. Postoperative radiotherapy will usually be administered. The decision to treat will often be helped by the location and size of the primary site. Supraglottic tumours with bilateral nodes are often eminently treatable with a laryngectomy and the appropriate neck dissections, but patients with an extensive tongue-base tumour and bilateral cervical lymphadenopathy will usually be inoperable at presentation. Patients with bilateral nodes where one side is fixed are usually incurable.

Interval contralateral lymphadenopathy

A proportion of patients in whom a node appears on the contralateral side of the neck some time after a dissection on one side will be salvaged, provided that recurrence at the primary site has not occurred. In this situation, a modified radical or radical neck dissection will produce a 5 year survival of approximately 30%. The incidence of such second side modified radical or radical neck dissections may have been reduced by the administration of postoperative radiotherapy to both sides of the neck in high-risk patients.

Massive nodes (greater than 6 cm): (N_3)

The presence of massive nodes is again an uncommon event occurring in patients with head and neck cancer. Only 5% of all patients will present as N_3 swellings. In previous classification systems, such nodes were referred to as fixed but because of the difficulty in both defining and assessing what this meant, fixation has been removed from the current staging system. However, it is important to realize that many nodes that reach 6 cm in size are often fixed to skin and/or underlying structures.

Many of these patients will be incurable but surgery may be possible in certain instances. The decision on whether or not to operate depends on the staging of the disease, the presence or absence of fixation and the structure to which the node is fixed.

The incidence of true fixation of neck masses is often difficult to determine from the literature and varies from series to series, with figures ranging from 23% in Stell's series (Stell *et al.*, 1984) up to 30% in Snow's series (Snow *et al.*, 1982). Fixation to the mandible, sternomastoid muscle and prevertebral fascia or muscles in the midline may not represent as much of a problem as fixation to the brachial plexus or carotid artery.

Careful clinical assessment with mandatory radiological imaging will help to assess operability and some of these patients will be helped by extended radical neck dissection. Fixation to the skull base and the brachial plexus is almost certainly a contraindication to surgical treatment, but fixation to the skin may be treated by wide resection and flap repair.

Assessment of tumour invasion of the arterial tree requires careful consideration. In the past, replacement of the common or internal carotid arteries by a vein graft has been practised. This has a high operative morbidity (33% hemiplegia) and mortality (12%), but there are reports of some patients living for a number of years. If the carotid artery is involved, the disease should be assessed as to whether or not cure may be achieved by its resection. If this is the case, then the best option is to resect the carotid artery. This is particularly true in patients who have non-squamous carcinoma disease, e.g. young patients with a malignant glomus vagale tumour surrounding the internal carotid artery at the skull base. If the carotid artery is to be resected and not replaced, the patient needs to be assessed as to whether or not this can be done safely without a significant risk of hemiplegia. This may be done preoperatively by measuring the cross-cerebral flow and pressure in the carotid stump, which can be combined with psychometric testing during digital carotid pressure. Alternatively, the carotid stump pressure may be measured at surgery.

In either case, unless the carotid stump pressure exceeds 70 mmHg, resection alone carries a high risk of significant morbidity and inevitable mortality and replacement of the carotid should be carried out. This requires the help of a vascular surgeon. This technique is associated with inevitable morbidity and possibly mortality, the graft may become infected and a subsequent blowout can occur. However, in certain instances, particularly in young patients and in those with non-squamous disease, it may be worthwhile.

Contraindications to neck dissection

Patients with metastatic neck disease who should not undergo surgery

- Those patients whose primary tumours are untreatable
- Any patient who is unfit for major surgery because of a serious medical condition which would render anaesthesia and major surgery unsafe
- Patients with inoperable neck disease
- Patients with distant metastases

In those patients who are deemed inoperable, radical radiotherapy with or without adjuvant chemotherapy is seldom curative but may provide excellent palliation. Appropriate assessment is crucial in patients with advanced disease and for some, palliative care in the form of appropriate pain relief and supportive nursing is all that is required.

Recurrence and salvage surgery

Recurrence in the neck following neck dissection carries a gloomy prognosis. Careful evaluation and staging with imaging are essential. Many of these masses will be fixed to vital structures which will negate extensive surgery. If surgery is possible, wide resections should be undertaken and postoperative radiotherapy given. If the patient has already received postoperative radiotherapy, then further radiotherapy may be given when margins are close or when complete resection is not possible in the form of local brachytherapy (see Chapter 5).

Non-squamous carcinoma neck disease

Some benign conditions in the neck, e.g. an infected branchial cyst, because of their location and immediate association with surrounding structures, to include the internal jugular vein, are best dealt with using the technique of conservative neck dissection to facilitate their removal.

The occult primary

This section will discuss the all too common clinical situation of a patient over the age of 45 years (often a smoker) who presents with a single lump in the upper lateral neck which is thought to be a metastatic malignancy from an occult primary. These patients should be approached in a logical manner and it is important to remember that in 90% of cases the cause of a neck lump will be in the head and neck, and a vigilant search above the clavicles will provide the primary tumour site in approximately 50% of cases.

Most carcinomas of the central head and neck metastasize to the lymph nodes in the deep cervical chain. A lymph node in the posterior triangle, particularly in young people, may represent a metastasis from the postnasal space. A secondary malignant node in the neck may also be due to a tumour below the clavicle; the lung, stomach and breast are common sites, although on occasions others can arise from a primary elsewhere in the body such as the ovary or testis. These nodes are often low, in the supraclavicular fossae, and with a lower limit which cannot be reached – the 'rising sun' appearance. These nodes usually herald occult malignancy in the chest or gastrointestinal tract and are known as Virchow's node or Troisier's sign. A cancer presenting with a node in the neck is four times more common in men than in women, with a mean age of 65 years in men and 55 years in women.

The histology of the occult nodal carcinoma of unknown primary varies from case to case but between one-third and one-half of all such nodes are infiltrated by squamous carcinoma, with about one-quarter reported as undifferentiated or anaplastic carcinoma and a similar number as adenocarcinoma if the supraclavicular nodes are involved.

A small number of nodes are involved by miscellaneous tumours, including malignant melanomas and thyroid tumours. In about one-third of patients, the primary tumour can be found by careful investigation at the time of presentation. The primary sites in order of frequency are the nasopharynx and tonsil, along with the retromolar trigone, tongue base and piriform sinus, followed by other miscellaneous head and neck sites and then the bronchus, breast and stomach. Careful follow-up will later show the primary site in a further third of patients, although this figure may be reduced if the so-called 'coffin corner' primary sites are irradiated following definitive surgery to the neck. The primary site is more commonly found in the head and neck than anywhere else and there are times when a carcinoma of the tonsil may not be apparent for several years after the gland appeared in the neck.

Finally, a branchogenic carcinoma should not be forgotten. This usually occurs at a younger age but any age group can be affected. It usually feels clinically exactly like a malignant lymph node, from which it should be differentiated as the latter is much more common.

Investigation

Patients with an occult head and neck primary (if treated properly) have a 50% chance of living for 5 years. However, it is important to follow the correct sequence of investigations, which include history, examination, radiology, laboratory tests and finally endoscopy, before embarking on treatment (Fig. 12.7).

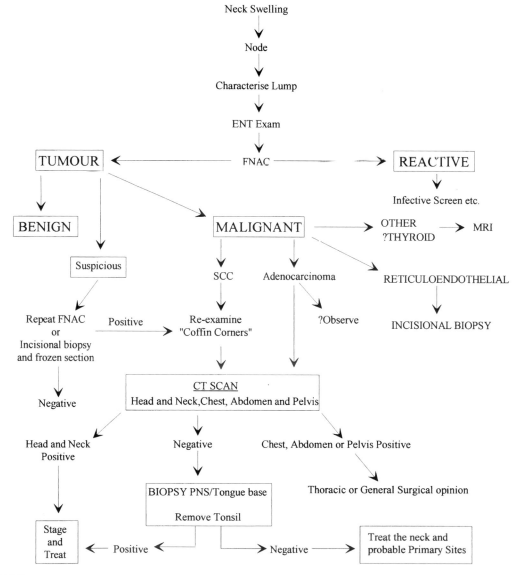

Figure 12.7 Diagnostic approach to the patient with carcinoma in the neck from an unknown primary.

History. Often the history does not help very much in arriving at a diagnosis. The mass in the neck has usually been present for several weeks and has increased quickly in size but is often painless. It is important to ask about other symptoms of disease within the head and neck, particularly, dysphagia, hoarseness, sore throat and nasal obstruction, and for pulmonary and gastric symptoms such as cough, haemoptysis, indigestion and loss of weight. The rare laryngocoele fluctuates in size and a tumour arising from the vagus nerve may cause hoarseness due to paralysis of the nerve. Finally, patients who are Cantonese with a node in the neck will have a nasopharyngeal cancer until proven otherwise. Apart from these points the history is of little help in making the diagnosis.

Examination. The lump should be examined for size, mobility and possible fixation to deep tissues. It is often said that a carotid body tumour is mobile from side to side and not up and down, but this is also true of virtually every other lump in this area. Do not forget that a neck lump in a patient with a tumour of the piriform sinus or tonsil may not be a secondary in a lymph gland, but a direct extension of the tumour through either the thyrohyoid membrane or the pharynx. This should be assessed by asking the patient to swallow, upon which a lump due to direct extension will move up and down. In addition, such lumps are often painful. A carotid body tumour can be compressed and made smaller by gentle pressure and the lump slowly refills upon removal of the finger.

A full clinical examination of the head and neck is carried out, paying particular attention to the classic sites for occult primaries listed above. Other lymphatic sites in the axillae, groins, liver and the spleen are also examined and the abdomen palpated for enlargement of the stomach, liver and spleen. In men, testicular examination is mandatory. Tumours arising in these sites may all present with a gland in the neck and many are eminently treatable with good 5 year survival figures. It is important to realize that an incisional biopsy of the neck node should not be performed, as this may have deleterious effects on the ultimate outcome for squamous carcinoma.

Fine needle aspiration cytology. FNAC is performed at the first visit. This may confirm the diagnosis of squamous cell carcinoma and can direct one with further investigations to include imaging if an adenocarcinoma is suspected, for example, of the thyroid gland. If there is any suggestion of a lymphoma, then an open neck node biopsy should be performed.

Radiology. The majority of patients will have an occult primary within the head and neck. However, all patients should have a CT scan of the neck, chest, abdomen and pelvis. This may identify the primary tumour site and visceral metastases. The chest views either show a second primary or reveal a primary site within the lung. If this mode of investigation fails to identify the primary site, further investigations may be indicated. If a primary dif-

ferentiated thyroid tumour is suspected and an image required, it is better to perform coronal MRI than CT since better images can be obtained and iodine contrast is required with the latter, which may negate the use of postoperative radioiodine for up to 6 months following the scan.

Endoscopy. Following the history and examination and more importantly radiology, the patient should be examined under a general anaesthetic which will allow the entire upper respiratory tract to be palpated; some small tumours, particularly in the tongue base and tonsil, can often be better felt and seen and the nasopharynx can be carefully examined. If the tumour is discovered, a biopsy is taken and the examination completed. Often no tumour will be found and in this situation blind biopsies are taken of both sides of the nasopharynx and the tongue base, and tonsillectomy performed on the side of the node. It is important to remember at the time of performing the tonsillectomy that the tonsil may contain cancer and as such the tonsil should be assessed, the ease of tonsillectomy should be noted and a wide resection should be carried out.

Treatment

Approaching these patients correctly will produce a diagnosis in many, but there will remain some where the primary site cannot be identified. In those where the primary site is known, the tumour will be small and submucosal, e.g. the nasopharynx or tongue base, and surgery to the primary site would be inappropriate. If the tumour is in the tonsil, is well localized (T_1 and T_2) and has been widely resected, then no further pharyngeal surgery is appropriate. All patients should undergo modified radical or radical neck dissection and then postoperative radiotherapy to the neck and the primary site.

If the disease is in the midline, such as the nasopharynx, then both sides of the neck should be irradiated. If the primary site is not identified and the FNAC shows squamous cell carcinoma, then a similar treatment plan with radical or modified radical neck dissection and postoperative radiotherapy should be adopted. If the histological diagnosis is not clear, then the patient's permission should be obtained for carrying out modified radical or radical neck dissection. Under anaesthetic, an incision is marked out for neck dissection and an incision made over the lump to facilitate an on-table incisional biopsy, which is then sent for frozen section analysis. If this confirms squamous cell carcinoma and the disease is operable, then the treatment plan continues as described previously with radical surgery to the neck and postoperative radiotherapy to the presumed primary site. This is because it is highly likely that the primary tumour site is within the head and neck. Following surgery, the patient should be followed up for at least 5 years, during which time the primary site will be revealed in up to 33% of cases and, if appropriate, can be further treated. Adopting such a policy will cure between 30 and 50% of patients.

However, if the neck-node disease is extensive with extra-nodal spread (or if the histologist is uncertain about the nature of the tumour), then the neck should be closed at this point and the patient referred back to the combined head and neck clinic to see the clinical oncologist again. If the frozen section shows an adenocarcinoma arising from the thyroid gland then this should be treated on its merits. Anaplastic carcinoma or squamous carcinoma of the supraclavicular nodes should not be treated radically because the primary site is presumably below the clavicles, and the patient should again see the clinical oncologist.

Branchogenic carcinoma

This is a very rare condition but a definite entity presenting as a single mass in the upper neck. It was at one time thought to be fairly common, but it is now known that the majority of these represent secondary malignancies in cervical lymph nodes, as described above. A diagnosis of branchogenic carcinoma arising within the branchial system can only be made if the following criteria are fulfilled.

Criteria for the diagnosis of branchogenic carcinoma

- Carcinoma should be demonstrated as arising in the wall of a branchial cyst
- Tumour should occur in a line running from a point just anterior to the tragus along the anterior border of sternomastoid muscle to the clavicle
- Histology should be compatible with an origin from tissue found in branchial vestiges
- No other primary should become evident within a 5 year follow-up

---

Treatment is with radical surgery to the neck with postoperative radiotherapy.

Thyroglossal duct carcinoma

This is a rare tumour: only approximately 100 cases have been described. It is nearly always a papillary thyroid carcinoma and few are diagnosed preoperatively. Many present as presumed benign thyroglosal cysts and are usually treated with Sistrunk's operation, and the diagnosis is made histologically following surgery. There is no sex predominance and the peak incidence in women is the fourth decade and in men the sixth decade. Only 10% have evidence of metastatic disease, compared with 50% with carcinomas arising in an ectopic thyroid.

If the disease is localized within the thyroglossal duct-cyst and has been completely excised with a Sistrunk procedure, and as long as the thyroid gland is normal on palpation and on scanning with either ultrasound or radionuclide imaging, then no further surgical treatment is necessary. Further follow-up involves suppressive doses of thyroxine and annual thyroglobulin measurements. If there is any suggestion that the thyroid is abnormal, the patient should have a total thyroidectomy (see Chapter 23).

Carcinoma in the pharyngeal pouch

This is a rare disease, with only about 30 cases having been reported in the English literature. The incidence of malignancy is probably between 0.5 and 1%. It affects men predominantly in a ratio of about 5:1, and usually occurs in a long-standing diverticulum with the average duration of symptoms being greater than 7 years. The age at diagnosis is usually over 50 years. The main predisposing factor is thought to be chronic irritation and inflammation of the diverticulum lining from food retention. Symptoms indicating carcinomatous change are increasing dysphagia, weight loss and occasionally blood in the regurgitated food. A mass may be found in the neck. The usual lesion is an invasive squamous cell carcinoma, but a few cases of carcinoma *in situ* have been reported in the literature.

Barium studies show a constant filling defect, unlike food debris which changes between films or repeat swallows. It is usually seen in the distal two-thirds of the pouch but can easily be missed. The diagnosis may be first made at operation.

The unusual case with a tumour confined to the pouch should be treated by diverticulectomy. Most cases require total pharyngolaryngectomy as for a postcricoid carcinoma. The outlook is dismal.

Radiotherapy in the management of metastatic neck disease

Radiotherapy may be used to treat the neck in the following clinical situations:

- the clinically negative neck (N_0 neck)
- the clinically positive neck
- electively after surgery
- neck disease developing or recurring after initial treatment: (i) nodal metastases developing in the untreated neck after initial treatment of the primary tumour alone; (ii) recurrence after previous surgery to the neck; or (iii) nodal recurrence after combined treatment.

The clinically N_0 neck

No survival advantage from elective treatment of the N_0 neck in squamous cell carcinoma has so far been demonstrated by controlled trials, although there is some evidence from multivariate analysis of retrospective data to suggest a significant benefit in locoregional control. There is now a consensus view that the neck should be treated in cases with a high probability (> 25%) of cervical micrometastases. The choice between elective neck dissection and radiotherapy will depend on the method of treatment of the primary tumour but Fletcher (1972) has shown that elective neck irradiation can eliminate at least 95% of nodal micrometastases and has less morbidity than surgery. It is therefore preferable when the primary tumour site is being treated by radiotherapeutic means.

The clinically positive neck

Generally speaking, involved nodes are best managed with surgery and postoperative radiotherapy when indicated, although there is no prospective trial to confirm this. This is especially true if there are large lymph-nodes masses. This is not just because large lymph-node metastases are resistant to radiotherapy, but because of the greater difficulty in diagnosing and surgically salvaging recurrences in the neck compared with those of the primary site. This does not apply to very radiosensitive tumours such as lymphoma or undifferentiated nasopharyngeal carcinoma, which can often be controlled locally with radiotherapy. Radical radiotherapy may be used as an alternative to surgery in patients unfit for surgery or with unresectable disease. Cure rates depend on both the size of the nodes and the dose of radiotherapy. Two year local control rates as high as 81% for nodes not exceeding 3 cm in diameter have been published, but such figures are probably higher than expected owing to the exclusion from the data analysis of those patients who had recurrence at the primary site. The results of irradiating large, unresectable neck masses are usually disappointing.

Electively after surgery

Postoperative radiotherapy is usually indicated in those cases with risk factors for local recurrence. These include node-positive disease (with or without extracapsular spread). To date, there have been no controlled trials of postoperative radiotherapy, but analysis of retrospective data has strongly suggested that it is of significant value in reducing the possibility of neck recurrence. Although planned preoperative radiotherapy has been used in the past, at present it is rarely indicated apart from in cases of doubtful operability.

Neck disease developing or recurring after initial treatment

Nodal metastases developing in the untreated neck after initial treatment of the primary tumour alone. In this situation, neck dissection is usually the preferred treatment, with or without postoperative radiotherapy. Alternatively, initial radical radiotherapy may be used.

Recurrence after previous surgery to the neck. Radical radiotherapy can be used if there is recurrent disease in the neck developing after an earlier elective or therapeutic neck dissection which was not followed by elective postoperative radiotherapy.

Nodal recurrence after combined treatment. The prognosis is extremely poor in those patients who suffer a neck recurrence following surgery and radiotherapy. This clinical situation is often associated with distant metastases. However, the presence of such disease in the neck causes distressing symptoms such as pain, bleeding and offensive fungation and, in selected cases, further treatment may be appropriate to include wide excision of the tumour and the overlying skin, myocutaneous flap reconstruction and concominant brachytherapy.

References

Ali S., Tiwari R. M. and Snow G. B. (1985) False-positive and false-negative neck nodes, *Head Neck Surg* 8: 78–82.

Baatenburg de Jong R. J., Rongen R. J., De Jong P. C., Lameris J. S. and Knegt P. (1988) Screening for lymph nodes in the neck with ultrasound, *Clin Otolaryngol* 13: 5–9.

Carter R. L., Barr L. C., O'Brien C. J., Ko K. C. and Shaw H. J. (1985) Transcapsular spread of metastatic squamous cell carcinoma from cervical lymph nodes, *Am J Surg* 150: 495–9.

Cornes P., Cox H. J., Rhys-Evans P. R., Breach N.M. and Henk J. M. (1996) Salvage treatment for inoperable neck nodes in head and neck cancer using combined iridium-192 brachytherapy and surgical reconstruction, *Br J Surg* 83(11): 1620–2.

Dearnaley D. P., Dardoutas C., A'Hearn R. P. and Henk J. M. (1991) Interstitial irradiation for carcinoma of the tongue and floor of the mouth. Royal Marsden Hospital Experience 1970–1986, *Radiother Oncol* 21: 183–92.

Fakih A. R. (1989) Elective versus therapeutic neck dissection in early carcinoma of the oral tongue, *Am J Surg* 158: 309–13.

Fisch U. P. and Sigel M. E. (1964) Cervical lymphatic systems as visualised by lymphography, *Ann Otol* 73: 869–83.

Fletcher G. (1972) Elective irradiation of subclinical disease in cancers of the head and neck, *Cancer* 29: 1450–1454.

Goepfert H. (1988) Subclinical cancer (Editorial), *Head Neck Surg* 10: 217–18.

Hibbert J. (1997) Metastatic neck disease, in *Scott-Brown's Otolaryngology*, 6th edn, Vol. 5, *Laryngology and Head and Neck Surgery*, Butterworth Heinemann, Oxford, Chap. 17, pp. 1–18.

Johns M. E., Neal D. A. and Cantrell R. W. (1984) Staging of cervical lymph node metastasis: Comparison of two systems, *Ann Otol Rhinol Laryngol* 93: 330–?

Larson D. L., Ballantyne A. J. and Guillamondegui O. M., eds (1986) Pathological evaluation of neck dissection lymph nodes: a status report, in *Cancer in the Neck: Evaluation and Treatment*. MacMillan, New York, pp. 33–9.

Lindberg R. (1972) Distribution of cervical lymph nodes metastases from squamous cell carcinoma of the upper respiratory and digestive tracts, *Cancer* 29: 1146–9.

Pointon R. C., Gleave E. N., Sikora K. and Halnan K. E., eds (1990) *Lymphatic Spread in Treatment of Cancer*, Chapman and Hall, London, pp. 323–7.

Sessions R. B. and Picker C. A. (1986) Malignant cervical adenopathy, in *Otolaryngology – Head and Neck Surgery* (Cummings C. W., Fredrickson J. M., Harker L. A., Krause C. J., Richardson M. A. and Schuller D. E., eds), Vol. 3, C.V. Mosby Co., St Louis, MO, pp. 1737–57.

Shah J. (1996) *Cervical Lymph Nodes in Head and Neck Surgery*, 2nd edn, Mosby-Wolfe, London, pp. 355–92.

Shah J. P. (1990) Cervical lymph node metastasis, its diagnostic, therapeutic and prognostic implications, *Oncology* 4: 61–9.

Shah J. P., Strong E., Spiro R. H. and Vikram B. (1981) Neck dissection: current status and future possibilities, *Clin Bull* 11: 25–33.

Snow G. B., Annyas A. A., Van Slooten E. A., Bartelink H. and Hart A. A. M. (1982) Prognostic factors of neck node metastasis, *Clin Otolaryngol* 7: 185–92.

Soo K. C., Ward M., Roberts K. R., Keeling F., Carter R. L., McCready V. R. *et al.* (1987) Radioimmunoscintigraphy of squamous carcinomas of the head and neck, *Head Neck Surg* 9: 349–52.

Spiro R. H., Huvos A. G., Wong G. Y., Spiro J. D., Gnecco C. A. and Strong E. W. (1986) Predictive value of tumour thickness in squamous carcinoma confined to the tongue and floor of the mouth, *Am J Surg* 152: 345–50.

Stell P. M. (1983) Fixed bilateral cervical nodes, *J Laryngol Otol* 97: 851–6.

Stell P. M., Morton R. P. and Singh S. D. (1983) Cervical lymph node metastases: the significance of the level of the lymph node, *Clin Oncol* 9: 101–7.

Stell P. M., Dalby J. E., Singh S. D. and Taylor W. (1984) The fixed cervical lymph node. *Cancer* 53: 336–41.

Traynor S. J., Cohen J. I., Gray J., Anderson P. E. and Everts E. C. (1996) Results of selective neck dissection in the clinically positive neck (Abstract), *Am. J. Surg.* 172: 654–657.

UICC (International Union Against Cancer) (1997) *TNM Classification of Malignant Tumours*, 5th edn, Wiley-Liss, New York.

Vandenbrouck C., Sancho-Garnier H., Chassagne D., Saravene D., Cachin Y. and Michear C. (1980) Elective versus therapeutic radical neck dissection, in Epidermoid carcinoma of the oral cavity – results of a randomised clinical trial, *Cancer* 46: 386–90.

Van den Brekel M. W. M., Stell H. V., Castelijns J. A., Nauta, J. J. P., Waal, I. V. D. and Valk J. (1990) Cervical lymph node metastasis: assessment of radiologic criteria, *Radiology* 177: 379–84.

Van den Brekel M. W. M., Castelijns J. A., Reitsma L. C., Leemans C. R. and van der Waal I. (1999) Outcome of observing the N0 neck using ultrasonic-guided cytology for follow-up. *Arch Otolaryngol Head Neck Surg* 125: 153–6.

Vikram B., Strong E. W., Shah J. P. and Spiro R. (1984) Failure in the neck following multimodality treatment for head and neck cancer, *Head Neck Surg* 6: 720–3.

Watkinson J. C. (1991) Some aspects of imaging squamous cell carcinoma using technetium 99m(V) dimercaptosiccinic acid, MS Thesis, University of London.

Watkinson J. C. (1993) The clinically N0 neck: investigation and treatment (Editorial), *Clin Otolaryngol* 18: 443–5.

Watkinson J. C., Johnston D., Coady M. *et al.* (1990) The reliability of palpation in the assessment of tumours, *Clin Otolaryngol* 15: 405–10.

Watkinson J. C., Todd C. E. C., Paskin L. *et al.* (1991) Metastatic carcinoma in the neck: a clinical, radiological, scintigraphic and pathological study, *Clin Otolaryngol* 16: 187–92.

Wong W. L., Chevretton E. B., McGurk M., Hussain K., Davis J., Beaney R. *et al.* (1997) A prospective study of PET–FDG imaging for the assessment of head and neck squamous cell carcinoma, *Clin Otolaryngol* 22: 209–14.

13 Neck dissection

'Pay attention to the corners of consternation'

Introduction

The operation of neck dissection dates back to 1906 when Crile described the classic radical neck dissection. This was subsequently popularized by Hayes Martin and still remains the gold standard by which other operations are judged. This operation removes the lymph-node-bearing areas of the neck along with the sternomastoid muscle, the internal jugular vein and the accessory nerve. The inevitable morbidity to which this led fuelled an interest in more conservative approaches and during the 1980s and 1990s, a number of less radical procedures has been popularized based on the staging of the disease at presentation. The following neck dissections can be performed.

- Classic radical neck dissection
- Extended radical neck dissection
- Modified radical neck dissection (types 1–3)
- Selective neck dissection

Preoperative preparation

The patient is advised preoperatively about the risks and possible complications of the appropriate neck dissection in question. A patient undergoing a unilateral neck dissection does not usually require a tracheostomy unless the operation is combined with the incontinuity removal of the primary tumour. It may be advisable to perform an elective tracheostomy for a patient who is undergoing a bilateral or a second neck dissection and one should also consider a tracheostomy in patients who are having neck dissections (particularly bilateral or second side procedures) following previous radiotherapy.

Position

The patient is intubated and laid supine on the operating table with the head extended on a head ring, a sandbag is placed under the shoulders and the head turned to the opposite side. By placing the sandbag more on the ipsilateral side, the dissection of the posterior triangle is made easier.

Incision

A neck dissection can be performed through a number of incisions and these are shown in Fig. 13.1. The decision to use a certain incision will be based on a number of factors which will include personal preference, previous radiotherapy, the number of levels required for access purposes, any previous surgical incisions and the site of the primary tumour if that is being resected as well. If the patient has not been irradiated, probably the most common used incision is the Y type (or Crile) or the Schobinger incision with a lazy S on the vertical limb to reduce scar tissue contracture (Fig 13.1a). If the patient had been irradiated, it was popular in the past to use two separate incisions as described by McFee (Fig. 13.1c), but the rationale for this was based on the radiotherapy of the 1970s and nowadays there is little evidence to suggest that wound breakdown rates are any greater in irradiated than in non-irradiated patients, and there are problems with the McFee incision. It makes the dissection more difficult through limited access, there may be troublesome bleeding from the undersurface of the bridge flap and consequently it has now been abandoned by many surgeons. Other popular incisions are the horizontal-T (Hetter) and the utility incision. The vertical limb should not cross the clavicle since this may compromise any future chest flaps. The McFee incision consists of two horizontal limbs and is the one incision in the head and neck where anatomical landmarks are given, although they are rarely used nowadays. The first limb begins over the mastoid process, descends to the hyoid bone and then ascends to the point of the chin. The second limb lies about 2 cm above the clavicle. It starts laterally at the anterior border of the trapezius and ends medially at the midline. The lateral end of this lower incision can be turned up if necessary to improve access.

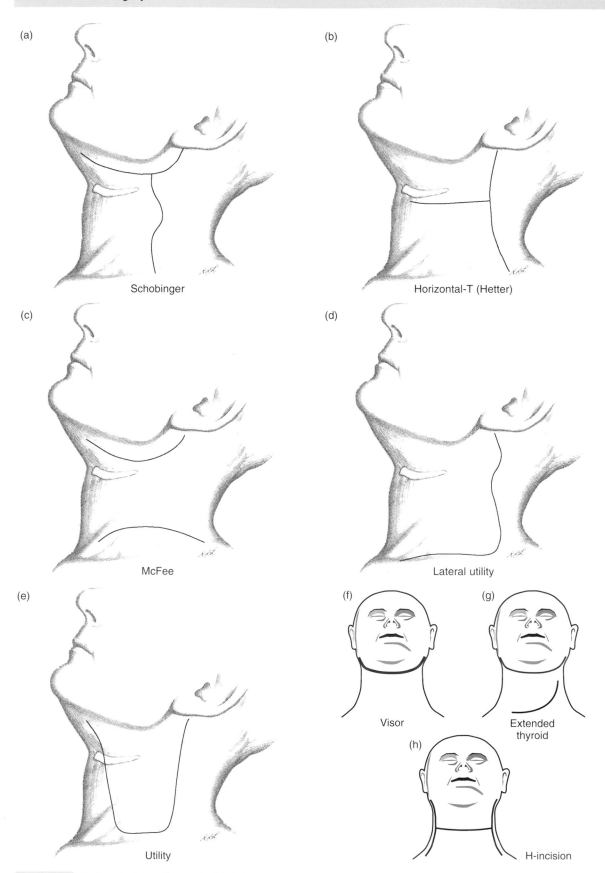

(a)

Schobinger

(b)

Horizontal-T (Hetter)

(c)

McFee

(d)

Lateral utility

(e)

Utility

(f)

Visor

(g)

Extended thyroid

(h)

H-incision

Figure 13.1 Various incisions for neck dissection.

Radical neck dissection

Definition

This operation removes the lymph-node-containing levels in the neck (I–V) and all three non-lymphatic structures (spinal accessory nerve, sternomastoid muscle and internal jugular vein).

Indications

The indications and contraindications for performing a radical and modified radical neck dissection are controversial but the following view represents a majority opinion.

First, for significant operable palpable neck disease in the presence of a primary tumour (or an occult primary) in the upper aerodigestive tract, an incontinuity resection with the primary site represents the best chance of a cure. Second, when significant operable palpable disease is present in the neck and the primary tumour has been previously well controlled, a neck dissection is indicated for salvage. Previously, the indications for a radical neck dissection rested on the size and site of the disease in relation to the accessory nerve but it is now usually possible to perform less than radical procedures for the above indications.

Indications for radical neck dissection

- Significant operable neck disease (N_{2a}; N_{2b}, N_3)
- Access prior to pedicled flap reconstruction

Other more controversial indications include a patient with an extensive primary lesion which is being treated

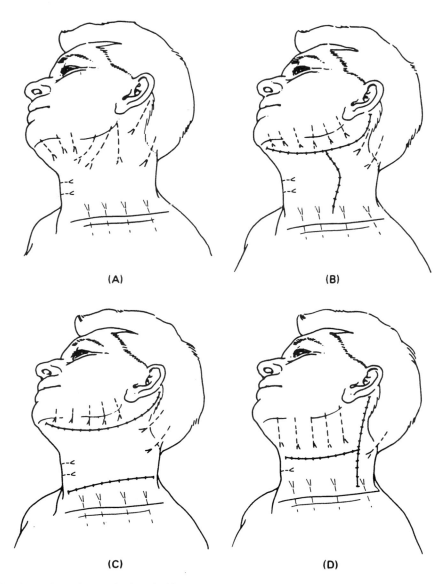

(A)　　　　　　　　　　(B)

(C)　　　　　　　　　　(D)

Figure 13.2　Blood supply to the cervical neck skin.

surgically and who has an N_0 neck but where a flap is required, e.g. pectoralis major or latissimus dorsi, and a modified radical or radical neck resection is appropriate for both access and staging purposes, as well as electively treating the N_0 neck. In the presence of a large primary tumour which by its size, site and nature carries a high risk of occult metastases, elective neck surgery may be indicated, but it is now usual in this instance to adopt more conservative approaches. This has been discussed in Chapter 12 relating to arguments for and against elective neck dissection. Lastly, a radical or modified radical neck dissection is indicated in the presence of an occult primary.

The blood supply to the cervical neck skin is shown in Fig. 13.2. Blood enters from above, below and either side with a resultant watershed in the middle of the neck. Incisions can be planned to utilize this (Fig. 13.1) so as to maximize blood supply to each of the neck flaps when raised.

The contraindications for radical and modified radical neck resection should include those patients whose primary tumours are untreatable, those who are unfit for major surgery and those with distant metastases apart from those with thyroid cancer, where radical surgery is sometimes carried out prior to systemic treatment with radioiodine therapy, although this is rarely a traditional radical neck dissection. Finally, it is generally accepted that a patient with significant bilateral neck disease is regarded as incurable and, in this situation, extensive surgery offers little or no chance of cure and indeed may make the patient's plight worse. There are times when it may be worth operating on bilateral neck disease, for example, supraglottic laryngeal tumours, and the final decision based on bilaterality of disease must rest with both the surgeon and the patient.

Contraindications to radical neck dissection

- Untreatable primary tumour
- Patients unfit for major surgery
- Distant metastases
- Significant bilateral neck disease
- Inoperable neck disease

A radical neck dissection or modified radical is also contraindicated for what is regarded as inoperable, i.e. unresectable, disease in the neck. Again, this is controversial but most would agree that as a general rule, involvement of the common carotid or internal carotid arterial tree, invasion of the prevertebral fascia and muscles along with the brachial plexus and extension onto and into the skull base all make surgery rather futile, but again any final decision must rest both with the surgeon and the patient.

Raising the flaps

The skin is prepared in the standard manner and the skin incision marked out using a marking pen. The incision, as described previously, is based on personal preference but should provide suitable access to the four corners of consternation, which define the limits of the dissection and can make all the difference between success and failure.

Corners of consternation

- Lower end of internal jugular vein
- Junction of lateral border of clavicle with the lower edge of trapezius
- Upper end of internal jugular vein
- Submandibular triangle

This is important because this operation aims not only to remove the palpable disease but also to understand where any other further occult disease may lurk. Any three-point junctions should be placed away from the carotid artery. Once the incision is made, the tip of an intramuscular green needle (2I FG) can be dipped in the appropriate ink and dots made on the skin in three or four places to facilitate placement of critical sutures. Appropriate access will usually mean that the ear is left uncovered, and a suture may be placed in the earlobe to retract it backwards to facilitate access to the parotid and skull base.

With traction and countertraction, the skin is incised in one movement with a no. 10 blade down to and through the platysma muscle, the fibres of which spring apart if strong tension is applied. In the posterior part of the neck, the fibres of the sternomastoid muscle are inserted directly into the skin, which makes the dissection and identification of the appropriate plane more difficult and results in more bleeding. It is important to keep the platysma on the skin flaps as it not only increases the strength of the wound in the postoperative period, but also provides important blood supply to the flaps. In certain instances in isolated situations, the platysma may have to be removed because disease extends onto, into or even through it. In this situation, the overlying skin may have to be removed as well. In the past the platysma was removed as part of the routine operation because there are lymphatics within in, but if these lymphatics are invaded by cancer then the patient is incurable by surgery.

The assistant places double skin hooks or a rake retractor under the platysma and applies traction in an upward direction. Similar countertraction to the specimen identifies the subplatysmal plane and the dissection con-

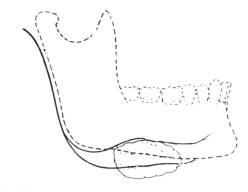

Figure 13.3 Cervical and marginal mandibular branches of the facial nerve.

tinues using a knife so that the flaps are quickly raised. Dissection here causes very little bleeding, provided the branches of the external and anterior jugular veins are tied. Any significant bleeding usually means that the operator is in the wrong place.

In a double horizontal incision (McFee), the lower flap and the lower half of the middle flap are raised from below, and the upper flap from the upper half of the middle flap from above. Access is gained by retracting the middle bridging flap with tapes. Bleeding from the inner surface of the bridge flap can be cumbersome and this should be stopped at this point.

During the dissection in the upper part of the neck when the upper flap is being raised, there are two branches of the facial nerve which should be preserved if possible. The most important of these is the marginal mandibular nerve and, of somewhat less importance, is its cervical branch (Fig. 13.3). The former supplies the muscles around the mouth and the latter supplies the part of the platysma that crosses the mandible and is inserted into the corner of the mouth, so that division of either nerve will lead to a weakness of the lower lip. Both nerves curve downwards below and in front of the angle of the mandible across the facial vessels about one finger's breadth below the mandible. The marginal mandibular nerve then runs immediately superior to the submandibular gland, while the cervical branch runs lateral to this gland. Both of the nerves then curve upwards again to reach their destination (Fig. 13.3).

There are a number of ways to protect these nerves. The easiest way to preserve the branches of the facial nerve is to cut through the deep investing layer of fascia at the level of the hyoid bone and to expose the capsule of the lower part of the submandibular gland. The fascia can then be elevated as a flap over the mandible, taking the nerve with it, and then is sutured superiorly. Care should be taken not to transfix the nerve and to use bipolar diathermy on the upper flap. A less reliable method of protecting these nerves is to ligate and divide the facial vessels on the submandibular gland and lift them over the mandible. However, this technique fails when the nerve's course is lower than usual and it can also compromise the removal of prefacial and postfacial nodes, which can be affected in tumours of the oral cavity. At times it is difficult to preserve the nerve when disease extends through the deep fascia and approaches the platysma, but this is an oncological operation and, for the sake of cancer cure, the nerve must sometimes be sacrificed.

In summary, if there are metastatic glands in close relationship to the nerve, the cancer operation must not be compromised.

The flaps are elevated, the neck is exposed with access to the corners of consternation and the resulting skin flaps are sutured back to the towels using strong silk sutures (Fig. 13.4).

Lower end of the internal jugular vein

There is some predefined order in the operation of rad-

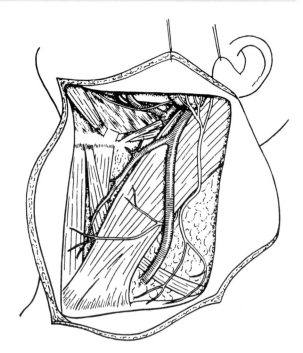

Figure 13.4 Flaps raised showing the four corners of consternation.

ical and modified radical neck dissection. It is, by convention, usual to begin at the lower end in the first corner of consternation (lower end of the internal jugular vein) or corner 2 (junction of the lateral border of the clavicle with the lower edge of the trapezius) but occasionally some surgeons like to find the accessory nerve early and then proceed to the lower end.

It is a basic principle of cancer surgery that the main vein draining the primary tumour that is being removed should be divided first. This step reduces the number of systemic metastases because small tumour emboli released by manipulating the tumour are unable to find their way into the general circulation. Whether this is important in head and neck cancer surgery is uncertain and some have argued that ligation of the internal jugular vein should be left as late as possible since this may reduce bleeding. However, the lower end of the internal jugular vein is usually approached early in the operation and this is done by dividing the sternomastoid muscle (Fig. 13.5). The assistant applies traction in an upwards direction while the surgeon applies traction to the lower end of the muscle and cuts it with a no. 10 blade. The muscle fibres separate easily, which allows the blueness of the internal jugular vein to be identified. One or two smaller arteries usually need to be diathermied in the sternomastoid muscle during this procedure.

The carotid sheath is opened to expose the internal jugular vein and it is important to identify a length of at least 2 cm to facilitate ligation with adequate control. Ligatures of either silk or vicryl are placed around the vein, making sure to check that the vagus is not included. Three ligatures are used, two at the lower end and one at the

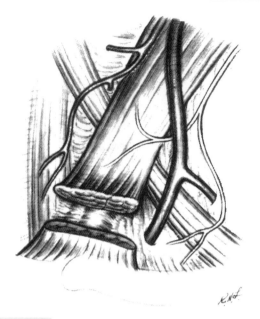

Figure 13.5 Division of the lower end of the sternomastoid.

upper end, and both ends are transfixed (Fig. 13.6). The transfixion stitch on the lower end is known as the 'houseman's suture' since, if it fails in the early hours of the morning following surgery, it is the houseman who knows about it first! This is one area of the operation where it is worth spending some time ensuring proper placement of all the sutures.

The internal jugular vein can be easily torn by injudicious passage of artery forceps beneath the sternomastoid muscle to mobilize it prior to its division or by opening scissors longitudinally next to the vein. This manoeuvre tears small tributaries and can contribute to alarming bleeding.

If bleeding occurs, the assistant must not be allowed to grab a large bleeding vessel with artery forceps or attempt diathermy as this will only convert a small hole into a large one. The bleeding injured vessel should be identified and occluded temporarily with pressure or arterial clamps and the defect repaired using 6.0 Ethilon.

The danger of tearing the lower end of the vein is not blood loss, but air embolism. If the vein is torn before it is divided, a finger should be placed over the hole and the anaesthetist asked to tilt the patient's head downwards. The area of the vein above and below the hole is tied and ligatures passed above and below the tear. When these are tied, the finger may be lifted off the vein.

If sutures slip off the lower end of the vein after it has been divided, again a finger is placed on the hole, the patient tilted feet down and, when the sucker is turned up to full power, the finger is gradually slid off the hole, arterial clamps are applied and the hole is stitched with a non-absorbable suture. When dealing with extensive disease low in the neck, it may be necessary to gain access to the junction of the internal jugular vein with the subclavian vein. If this is anticipated, it may be prudent for both oncological and safety reasons to gain appropriate control in the upper mediastinum and for this reason the upper part of the sternum and medial end of the clavicle

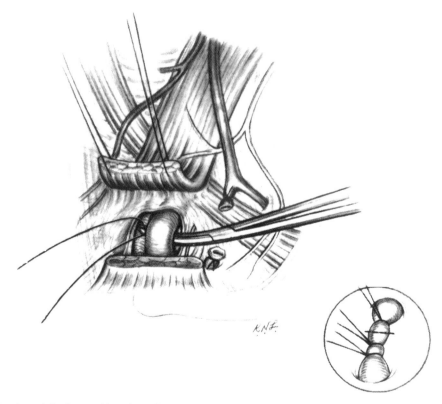

Figure 13.6 Ligation of the internal jugular vein.

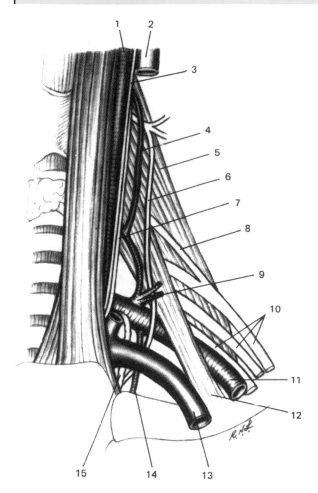

Figure 13.7 Anatomy of the root of the neck. 1= Common carotid artery; 2 = internal jugular vein; 3 = vagus nerve; 4 = ascending cervical artery; 5 = scalenus medius muscle; 6 = phrenic nerve; 7 = interior thyroid artery; 8 = C5 nerve; 9 = thyrocervical trunk; 10 = brachial plexus; 11 = subclavian artery; 12 = scalenus anterior muscle; 13 = subclavian vein; 14 = internal thoracic artery; 15 = thoracic duct.

sionally one will find a whole leash of lymphatic vessels terminating in this area and no one large duct can be identified. In this situation, the whole area should be oversewn taking large bites with a non-absorbable silk suture since this incites a vigorous inflammatory reaction.

> **Critical steps in radical neck dissection: lower neck**
>
> ■ Divide the lower end of sternomastoid in corner 1
> ■ Isolate and ligate the internal jugular vein
> ■ Look for and avoid the thoracic duct and/or branches of the jugular lymph duct in Chaissaignac's triangle
> ■ Remove any Scalene nodes
> ■ Divide and retract the omohyoid muscle upwards
> ■ Mobilize the fat pad overlying the prevertebral fascia
> ■ Identify and preserve the brachial plexus and phrenic nerve
> ■ Deal with corner 2

Supraclavicular dissection

Once the first corner of consternation has been dealt with (Fig. 13.8) the dissection proceeds towards corner 2 at the lateral end of the clavicle and this is done by supraclavicular dissection (Fig. 13.9). This area of the operation may be approached by dissecting area 2 and approaching area 1 or, as previously described, one may deal with area 1 and approach area 2. One trick is to tie off the internal jugular vein, then move straight to the

may be removed to facilitate this. On the left side, the thoracic duct passes medial to the jugular vein, then posterior to it and finally curves around to enter the junction of the internal jugular vein and the subclavian vein (Fig. 13.7). Once the internal jugular vein has been tied, the dissection extends laterally to approach Chaissaignac's triangle, which is defined as a triangle between where the longus colli and scalenus anterior attach to the tubercle of C_6 (Chaissaignac's or carotid tubercle) with the subclavian artery as the base (Fig. 13.7). Here are found the Scalene node(s) (which should be removed) and also the main jugular lymph duct that terminates here on the left with the thoracic duct, which is at risk and if it is seen it should be tied off and any chylous leak (recognized as milky fluid) should be dealt with immediately. The duct should be isolated and oversewn with fine silk. At the end of the operation it is important to return and check that there are no further leaks. Occa-

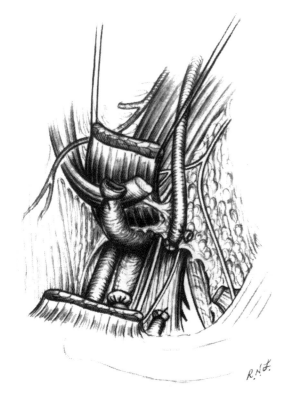

Figure 13.8 Ligation and division of the lower end of the internal juglar vein and dissection from the carotid sheath.

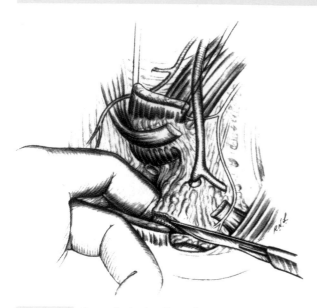

Figure 13.9 Supraclavicular dissection.

bottom end of the trapezius muscle and begin the dissection there, behind the omohyoid muscle, and then approach the ligated internal jugular vein from lateral to medial. Either way, the omohyoid muscle is divided without any clamping and is retracted in a upwards direction. It should not bleed if cut through the tendon, and at this point the transverse cervical artery and vein may be encountered and should be ligated. Medial to the omohyoid muscle, the fascia over the fat pad lateral to the internal jugular vein should be incised and then the prevertebral fascia may be exposed by sharp or blunt dissection with a swab in an upward direction. Here, the phrenic nerve is identified as it runs over scalenus anterior from lateral to medial. It lies behind the prevertebral fascia and is safe as long as this fascia is not breached, since the fascia protects not only this nerve but also the brachial plexus, which is the next structure to be encountered in the dissection. Bipolar diathermy should be used in this region since conventional diathermy can damage the nerves. It is crucial at this point to clear Chassaignac's triangle, which lies between the scalenus anterior and the vagus nerve and common carotid artery overlying the longus colli, and which occupies territory that has, in part, been vacated by the internal jugular vein. This triangle contains branches of the thyrocervical trunk, the vertebral vein and the thoracic duct and it is here that the cervical lymphatics terminate and occult disease may lurk in the Scalene nodes. This area should be cleared as part of dissection in the first corner of the consternation.

Once the supraclavicular dissection has been completed towards the anterior border of trapezius, the operation continues in an upward direction to dissect the posterior triangle. The completion of the supraclavicular dissection means that the transverse cervical artery and vein can be encountered anywhere in the lateral half of this manoeuvre and can be met again distally as dissection of the posterior triangle begins. The external jugular vein also needs to be divided in this area and the fat in the supraclavicular fossa can be divided with minimal bleeding, but one should avoid excessive traction in this area since the subclavian vein can be pulled out of the upper chest, with obvious consequences.

Dissection of the posterior triangle (Fig. 13.10)

This dissection continues up the anterior border of trapezius to the mastoid tip. It should be remembered that everything that is important in the posterior triangle lies below, i.e. caudal to, the accessory nerve. This nerve runs in the roof and not the floor of the posterior triangle and can therefore be damaged early in the dissection, either in the elevation of the flaps or in this part of the dissection.

It is important that the accessory nerve is identified before dissecting the posterior triangle. This should be done as a matter of routine and in some cases, the nerve may be preserved based on the operative findings. The technique of preserving the nerve is discussed later (modified radical neck dissection). There is a number of ways to identify the nerve. The nerve exits the lateral border of the sternomastoid muscle at the junction of its upper third with the lower two-thirds and then has a sinuous course before arriving at the lower anterior border of trapezius to supply this muscle. In view of its unpredictable position within the posterior triangle, one of the best ways to identify the nerve is at its exit from the sternomastoid muscle. This is known as Erb's point and can be identified in the operating room as being 1 cm above the point above where the great auricular nerve winds around the sternomastoid muscle on its way to supply the parotid gland. Once identified, the nerve may be mobilized and preserved. Another way to identify it is to dissect up the anterior border of trapezius in the posterior triangle until the nerve is encountered, when it may be confirmed by stimulation. This is a more difficult technique because the nerve may be confused with branches of the cervical plexus, which can be quite large, although the use of the stimulator helps. Another way of finding the nerve is to draw a line laterally from the laryngeal prominence through the posterior triangle. The nerve will usually cross this line as it runs from Erb's point to the lower posterior corner of the posterior triangle.

During the dissection, which is performed using both scissors and the knife, ascending branches of the transverse cervical artery and vein run up the anterior border of the trapezius and make a bloodless dissection along this part of the muscle difficult. This is to be expected and there is no substitute at this point for careful dissection, appropriate diathermy and vessel ligation. This is the only way to prevent damage to the accessory nerve. At this point, every attempt should be made to preserve shoulder function and even if the accessory nerve has to be divided, it is wise to preserve the branches to the trapezius muscle from the third and fourth cervical nerves. These lateral branches arise from the cervical plexus, being ultimately derived from C_3 and C_4 (Fig. 13.11). They arise deep within the sternomastoid muscle, pass

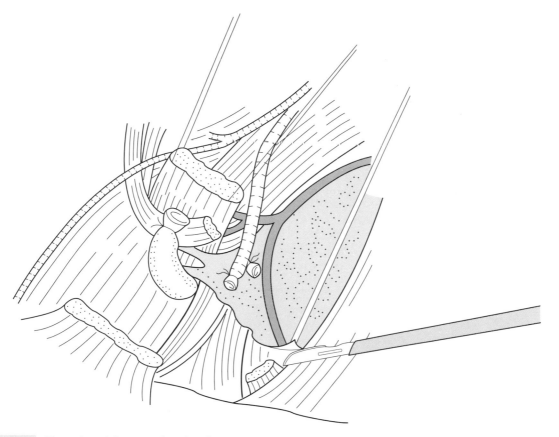

Figure 13.10   Dissection of the posterior triangle.

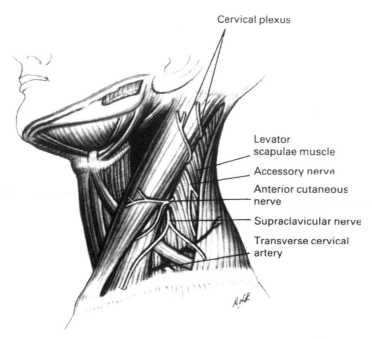

Cervical plexus

Levator
scapulae muscle

Accessory nerve

Anterior cutaneous
nerve

Supraclavicular nerve

Transverse cervical
artery

Figure 13.11   Anatomy of the cervical plexus and its cutaneous branches.

laterally beneath the fascia covering the floor of the posterior triangle to supply the trapezius muscle and also to give off a communicating branch to the accessory nerve. In order to preserve these nerves, it is essential that the fascia is preserved on the floor of the posterior triangle.

The dissection continues quickly, dividing the fascia from the anterior border of trapezius up to the mastoid tip where the sternomastoid joins the trapezius. If there are nodes involved in the upper spinal accessory chain, then it is wise not to preserve the nerve. Otherwise, the nerve may be followed through the sternomastoid and this is one way to identify the upper end of the internal jugular vein. Clips are placed on the sternomastoid muscle and a tunnel is formed so that the nerve can be followed and dissected free of the muscle up to level II, to the point where it lies on top of the internal jugular vein. At this point, it is prudent to divide the upper end of the sternomastoid muscle to facilitate further identification of the upper end of the internal jugular muscle prior to its ligation. Firm traction is applied to the upper end of sternomastoid and, with the surgeon pulling down on the body of the muscle, the upper end of the muscle is cut under tension and haemostasis secured. The level of transection is at the angle of the jaw and would normally include the lower pole of the parotid gland. With an assistant placing a Langenbeck retractor under the digastric muscle, the upper end of the internal jugular vein is identified, the accessory nerve may be transposed laterally, and the upper end of the transected sternomastoid muscle passed under the nerve and its division completed to facilitate ligation of the upper end of the internal jugular vein.

Division of the upper end of the internal jugular vein

This is the third corner of consternation. Access is crucial in a cephalic direction to allow access above the disease and to obtain control of the upper end of the internal jugular vein. The upper end of the internal jugular vein is identified by the division of the sternomastoid muscle as described previously (Fig. 13.12). Its position may be located by palpating the transverse process of C_2 over which it lies, but with the neck extended to the contralateral side, this landmark is usually just in front of the vein. The vein is mobilized, and using right-angled Lahey forceps, non-absorbable sutures are placed to facilitate its ligation; two sutures above and one below the point of division, along with transfixing sutures, will usually suffice.

It is not usually necessary to remove the posterior belly of digastric muscle, unless to facilitate access into level II (Fig. 13.13). This muscle may be retracted upwards but if there is any problem with regard to disease extension, the muscle may be removed with the specimen. Before tying any ligatures, **the vagus and hypoglossal nerves should be identified and preserved**. If any venous tributaries of the venae nervi hypoglossi comitantes are seen, these should be ligated carefully as they can cause troublesome bleeding (Fig. 13.14).

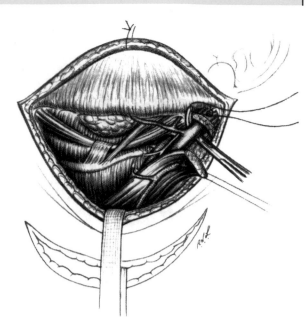

Figure 13.12 Division of the upper end of the internal jugular vein.

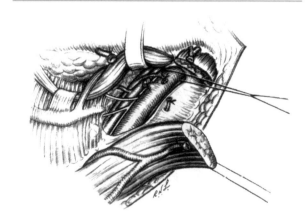

Figure 13.13 Retraction of the posterior belly of the digastric to show the upper end of the internal jugular vein in level II (third corner of consternation).

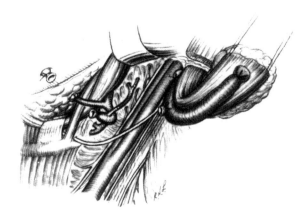

Figure 13.14 Division of the veins related to the hypoglossal nerve.

The hypoglossal nerve runs across the external carotid, lingual and occipital arteries and may form, like the digastric, a convenient tunnel which can be followed anteriorly. The hypoglossal tunnel is a particularly useful landmark when tumour is stuck near the carotid bifurcation.

The occipital artery crosses the posterior part of the internal jugular vein and this should also be ligated now to prevent further troublesome bleeding. If a tie comes off the jugular stump, the pressure inside is only about 4 cmH$_2$O so the bleeding can easily be controlled by packing, and then ligation and oversewing as appropriate. If control cannot be achieved, then the area can be packed off and the pack removed a couple of weeks later.

The specimen is now mobilized both top and bottom, and the top section is completed by finding the posterior branch of the posterior facial vein 12 mm (0.5 inch) anterior to the interior jugular vein. This is ligated and divided. The division of the lower portion of the parotid gland is completed and the hypoglossal nerve preserved as it turns sharply to cross the branches of the external carotid artery on its way to the submandibular triangle.

Critical steps in radical neck dissection: upper neck

- Divide the upper end of sternomastoid in corner 3
- Retract the posterior belly of the digastric upwards
- Identify and ligate the internal jugular vein
- Identify and preserve the hypoglossal nerve

The dissection of the posterior triangle may now be completed by lifting the specimen upwards and taking a scalpel to dissect between the contents of the posterior triangle and the prevertebral fascia. The branches of the cervical plexus can be clearly identified running upwards and these are cut and the accompanying arteries and veins diathermized. The common carotid artery and the vagus nerve can be identified clearly, along with the stump of the internal jugular vein, and the operation continues with sharp dissection between the internal jugular vein above the common carotid artery and the vagus nerve below (Fig. 13.15). This facilitates removal of the carotid sheath and lymphatics that are contained within it.

Anteriorly low down, dissection is completed taking the specimen with omohyoid up to the junction with the hyoid bone (omohyoid tunnel) so that the submandibular triangle can be dissected.

Dissection of the submandibular triangle

This dissection represents the fourth corner of consternation (Fig. 13.16). The fat is divided in the submental area and this displays the anterior belly of the diagastric muscle. The anterior part of the submandibular gland is then identified and this is dissected to the posterior border of the mylohyoid muscle. The upper border of the submandibular gland is freed by dividing and tying the vessels, including the facial artery, that cross the lower border of the mandible.

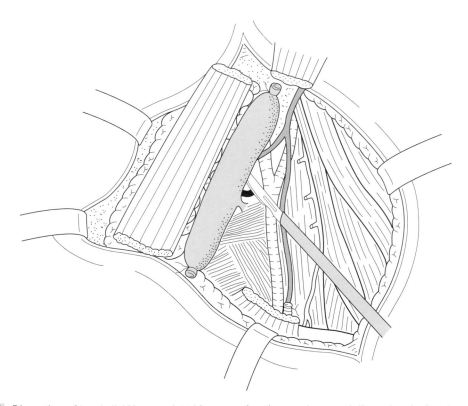

Figure 13.15 Dissection of levels II–V is completed by removing the specimen and dissecting the jugular vein free from the carotid artery and vagus nerve.

The mylohyoid muscle is retracted in a forward direction to reveal the submandibular duct and, at this point, the lingual nerve is pulled down in a curve. The latter is freed by dividing the fascia around the submandibular ganglion with a knife. The lingual nerve gives off a small but constant branch to the submandibular ganglion and this branch is usually accompanied by a vessel that can cause troublesome bleeding if it is not ligated properly. The lingual nerve is identified and two artery forceps are placed below it to divide the branch to the submandibular gland. This allows the lingual nerve to spring back upwards behind the body of the mandible. The submandibular duct is then tied and divided. During both of these manoeuvres, the hypoglossal nerve is kept under constant direct vision to avoid any damage. The specimen is then removed following transfixion and division of the facial artery as it winds over the posterior border of digastric muscle at the posterior inferior border of the submandibular gland.

Once the dissection is completed, a warm pack is placed in the wound and, following a Valsalva manoeuvre, haemostasis is completed. The wound is then irrigated with first saline and then sterile water, and any further bleeding points are secured.

Closure

Following the washing of the wound, dirty instruments should be discarded and new gloves may be worn to close the wound. Two large drains (12 Fr) are placed through the posterior flap and securely tied. Drains should never cross the carotid sheath, they should be cut to the correct length and should be kept well away from any microvascular anastomosis.

Finally, a check is made for any chylous leak, any bleeding from the veins accompanying the hypoglossal nerve (the venae nervi hypoglossi comitantes) and any bleeding on the undersurface of the middle flap if a McFee incision has been used. The wound is closed in two layers with an absorbable Vicryl or catgut stitch to the platysmal layer and the skin closed using either interrupted or continuous sutures of ethilon or staples. If staples are used, the three-point junction should be closed accurately with ethilon.

The wound may be left uncovered or gauze dressing may be applied to the suture line prior to release of the drains. It is important at this stage to check for an air leak as a subsequent collection can have disastrous results.

Radical neck dissection as part of a combined procedure

When a primary tumour is removed in continuity with a neck dissection, a band of continuity should be kept between the neck dissection and the primary growth. This is not, however, always essential oncologically as has been taught in the past.

Laryngeal cancer

In a total laryngectomy, the neck dissection should be left attached along the whole length of the larynx to include the superior and inferior lymphatic pedicles. A neck dissection is never performed with a hemilaryngectomy, but when carried out with a supraglottic laryngectomy it is pedicled on the thyrohyoid membrane.

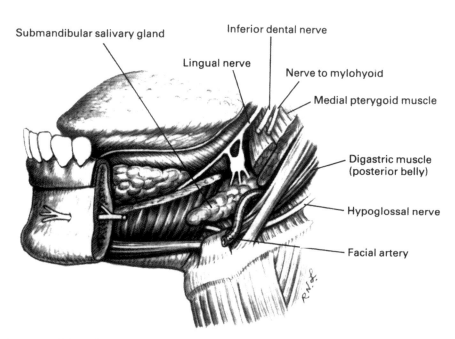

Figure 13.16 Anatomy of the submandibular triangle.

Pharyngeal cancer

When a pharyngectomy is performed, the pedicle must be as broad as possible and it is best if it is left along the whole length of the pharynx.

Oral cancer

Oral cancers drain to the submandibular, submental and upper deep cervical lymph nodes in levels I, II and III. Therefore, the specimen remains attached along the lower border of the mandible and the inner layer of periosteum is included to preserve continuity.

Oropharyngeal cancer

Tumours of the oropharynx drain by a pedicle to the upper deep cervical nodes in levels II, III and IV. Therefore, the specimen should remain attached near to the tail of the parotid gland whenever possible.

Post-operative care

No specific postoperative care is needed other than that already outlined in Chapter 4.

Complications

Most of the complications of radical neck dissection have already been discussed in Chapter 6. The most crippling long-term complication is the 'shoulder syndrome'. The main effects of this syndrome are long-standing pain in the shoulder and the inability to perform certain manocuvres such as putting on a jacket. Two important movements at the shoulder joint must be considered. abduction and flexion. Denervation of the trapezius muscle allows the shoulder girdle to rotate through 30° anteriorly. Abduction in these patients then becomes the equivalent of extension in the normal subject. The normal subject is unable to extend the arm beyond 45° because of locking of the glenohumeral joint. Abduction of the shoulder beyond 45° is therefore physically impossible in the patient with a denervated trapezius muscle. Flexion at the shoulder joint in the patient with a denervated trapezius is the equivalent of abduction in the normal subject. Abduction of the arm is a combination of two movements: firstly, elevation and rotation of the scapula on the trunk achieved by the trapezius muscle, and secondly, abduction of the humerus on the scapula mainly achieved by the deltoid muscle, assisted by the supraspinatus muscle, which helps to prevent displacement of the head of the humerus during strong deltoid action. The first 90° of the movement takes place at the shoulder joint under the control of the deltoid muscle and remains possible in the patient with a denervated trapezius. However, this 90° of movement only brings the arm to about 75° from the trunk because the shoulder girdle is tilted downwards. Furthermore, the remaining 90° of movement due to movement of the shoulder girdle on the trunk by the trapezius muscle is no longer possible. In summary, therefore, a patient with a denervated trapezius muscle can only abduct the arm from the trunk to an angle of 75° and abduction beyond that

point is prevented by locking of the glenohumeral joint. He or she can flex the arm from the trunk to an angle of about 45° by the action of the deltoid muscle, but further flexion is prevented by a downward tilt of the shoulder girdle and the loss of the rotation of the shoulder girdle on the trunk by the trapezius.

The best way to prevent this syndrome is to preserve both the accessory nerve and the separate branches from the cervical plexus (C_3 and C_4) to the trapezius muscle. If the spinal accessory nerve cannot be preserved, then the branch from the cervical plexus should be preserved if possible. If both nerves are divided, it is then important to refer the patient postoperatively to a physiotherapist for early mobilization and treatment.

Carotid artery protection

It is no longer routine practice to protect the carotid artery in a radical neck dissection, but if this is required it may be done at the time of surgery using a Levator scapulae muscular flap (Fig. 13.17). This may be swung forwards pedicled on its anterior border like the page of a book. It is important to avoid any damage to the brachial plexus during the division of the lower end of the muscle. The muscle can then be sewn over the carotid artery using an absorbable stitch such as chromic catgut or vicryl and suturing is usually performed to the sternohyoid muscle (Fig. 13.18). When suturing the lower end, the phrenic nerve must not be included in the stitch. This technique is usually unsuitable if the cervical nerves arising from C_3 and C_4 have been preserved, as they will inevitably be cut in the process of lifting the muscle but, as previously stated, it is very rare nowadays to have to carry out this manoeuvre for carotid artery protection.

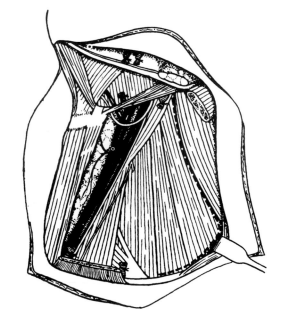

Figure 13.17 Levator scapulae flap marked out.

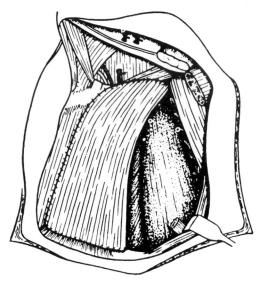

Figure 13.18 Levator scapulae flap rotated and stitched into place.

Extended radical neck dissection

This operation consists of removal of all of the structures resected in a radical neck dissection, along with one or more additional lymph-node groups or non-lymphatic structures or both. The additional lymph-node groups include the retropharyngeal lymph nodes, the parotid nodes, or lymph nodes in level VI or VII. The non-lymphatic structures that may be removed include part or all of the mandible, the parotid gland, part of the mastoid tip, prevertebral fascia and musculature, the digastric muscle, the hypoglossal nerve, and the external carotid artery and skin.

The operation is indicated when neck disease invades any of the previously non-lymphatic structures, which then have to be excised in continuity with the neck dissection to facilitate clearance. It is also indicated when the primary tumour arises in the parotid gland or the pharynx when a retropharyngeal node dissection is required. Finally, it is indicated for transglottic and subglottic carcinomas, along with carcinomas of the cervical oesophagus and thyroid, when it is necessary to remove the paratracheal, pretracheal and anterior compartment nodes with an associated neck dissection.

The operation is carried out as described previously to include the whole of the parotid as required or extension into the retropharyngeal area to dissect any nodes there. Level VI dissection may be carried out as described later and the appropriate non-lymphatic structures are excised in a conventional manner.

Modified radical neck dissection

This operation consists of the removal of all lymph-node groups (levels I–V) with preservation of one or more non-lymphatic structures (Table 13.1). A type 1 modified radical neck dissection preserves the spinal accessory nerve, a type 2 preserves not only the spinal accessory nerve but also the internal jugular vein, and a type 3 is when the spinal accessory nerve, the internal jugular vein and the sternocleidomastoid muscle are all preserved (Fig. 13.19). Type 3 modified radical neck dissection is also known as a comprehensive functional or selective neck dissection.

Indications

Type 1

This operation is indicated for patients with cervical metastases where the spinal accessory nerve is not involved by tumour and its preservation will not involve encountering tumour, thereby compromising the results of the resection. It may be used for elective treatment of the N_0 neck but, as previously described, more conservative procedures are currently available to treat this condition.

Type 2

Preservation of the internal jugular vein in squamous cell carcinoma is not usually carried out when operating for

Table 13.1 Modified radical neck dissection

Type	Indications
Type 1: removal of all lymph-node groups (levels I–V) with preservation of the spinal accessory nerve	Operable palpable neck disease (usually N_1, N_{2a}, N_{2b}) not involving the accessory nerve Occasionally can be performed for the N_0 neck
Type 2: removal of all lymph-node groups (levels I–V) with preservation of the spinal accessory nerve and the internal jugular vein	Occasionally performed for the same indications as for a type 1 procedure, particularly for a second side operation, when there is a need for microvascular anastomosis or when histology dictates that the internal jugular vein need not be resected, e.g. differentiated thyroid cancer
Type 3: removal of all lymph-node groups (levels I–V) with preservation of the spinal accessory nerve, internal jugular vein and the sternomastoid muscle	• Treatment of the N_0 neck • Treatment of differentiated thyroid cancer • Skin tumours such as melanoma, squamous cell carcinoma and Merkel cell carcinoma in the narrow band of scalp between the ears

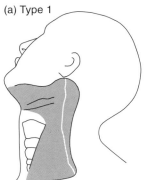

(a) Type 1

- Lymph Node levels dissected I-V
- *Also excised*
  Sternomastoid muscle
  Internal jugular vein
  Submandibular gland
- Accessory nerve is preserved

(b) Type 2

- Lymph Node levels dissected I-V
- *Also excised*
  Sternomastoid vein
  Submandibular gland
- Accessory nerve and internal jugular vein are preserved

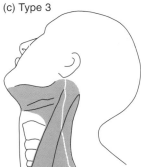

(c) Type 3

- Lymph Node levels dissected I-V
- *Also excised*
  Submandibular gland
- Sternomastoid muscle, internal jugular vein and accessory nerve are preserved

Figure 13.19 Types of modified radical neck dissection.

palpable disease but, in addition to the indications described above for a type 1 dissection, a type 2 dissection may be carried out where preservation of the internal jugular vein is important either for a second side operation or for microvascular anastomosis, and where histology dictates that the vein need not be resected, e.g. differentiated thyroid cancer.

Type 3

This operation, otherwise known as a comprehensive or functional selective neck dissection, has been used for elective treatment for the N_0 neck in patients with squamous cell carcinoma of the upper aerodigestive tract. This is appropriate treatment if the patient has had previous radiotherapy but, if not, it is questionable whether all five levels need to be dissected or whether a more selective neck dissection (see below) will suffice. Some surgeons advocate its use for the treatment of carcinoma of the thyroid gland with palpable lymph nodes in the lateral compartment of the neck but, as previously stated, level I does not usually have to be dissected in the treatment of previously untreated differentiated thyroid cancer. It is also indicated for patients with skin tumours such as melanoma, squamous cell carcinoma and Merkel cell carcinoma that originate in the narrow band of the scalp within the confines of the anterior and posterior aspects of the auricle.

Operative technique

The incisions and exposure for a modified radical neck dissection are the same as for radical neck dissection. The nerve is identified as described previously. It is isolated using a nerve hook or sloop and followed to Erb's point. Clips are placed on the sternomastoid muscle on either side of the nerve and lifted up, a tunnel is made following the nerve and the overlying muscle divided. At this point, the branch to sternomastoid is divided. The nerve can then be followed up to the skull base, where it runs on the anterior surface of the internal jugular vein and forms one method of identifying the vein. Its preservation does not guarantee function postoperatively since preserving the nerve involves its devascularization with associated, unpredictable loss of function in some cases.

Preservation of the sternomastoid muscle makes the operation more difficult. If the operation is for palpable disease, the surgeon should consider whether preserving the muscle adds anything to the procedure, particularly in the elderly patient for whom the length of time and the difficult dissection may compromise the ultimate outcome.

The deep investing layer of fascia is mobilized from the anterior part of the sternomastoid muscle and dissection of the muscle from the fascia below allows the muscle to be retracted up using sloops. The neck dissection proceeds under the muscle in the same manner as described previously for radical neck dissection. Another technique is to divide the muscle at the lower end, fold it upwards, complete the dissection and then return the muscle after the operation and resuture it. This is particularly useful in young patients with thyroid carcinoma where preservation of the muscle is possible since its removal can cause significant cosmetic deformity.

Preservation of the internal jugular vein involves dissection of the carotid sheath along with the deep investing layer of fascia and the contents of the posterior triangle. It proceeds in a plane above, not below, the internal jugular vein leaving the latter structure behind. The relevant branches of the vein are encountered in their usual position and ligated as appropriate.

Selective neck dissection

A selective neck dissection consists of preservation of one or more lymph nodes groups and all three non-lymphatic structures. They are named accordingly, depending on the lymph-node groups removed and are shown in Table 13.2 and diagrammatically in Fig 13.20.

Indications

Supraomohyoid and extended supraomohyoid (anterolateral)

This operation is indicated in squamous cell carcinoma of the oral cavity (T_1–T_4, with no palpable lymph nodes). A controversial indication is a single palpable mobile node in level I or II associated with squamous cell carcinoma of the oral cavity, lip or skin of the middle third of the face. It may also be used in conjunction with an elective superficial parotidectomy in patients who have intermediate thickness melanoma and T_4 squamous cell carcinoma in the facial region in a line anterior to the tragus.

Lateral

This operation is indicated in carcinomas of the larynx, oropharynx and hypopharynx that are staged T_2–T_4N_0 where the primary tumour is being treated surgically. Some proponents suggest that it may be indicated for carcinoma of the larynx, oropharynx and hypopharynx staged $T_{1-2}N_1$, when palpable lymphadenopathy is confined to levels II–IV. In both of the indications, these operations are usually carried out bilaterally as the natural history of the disease is associated with a high incidence of bilateral metastases.

Posterolateral

This operation is indicated for skin tumours such as melanoma, squamous cell carcinoma and Merkel cell carcinoma that originate in a line behind the posterior margin of the ear and arise in the posterior and posterolateral aspect of the neck and the occipital part of the scalp.

Anterior compartment (level VI)

This operation is indicated for differentiated and medullary thyroid cancer and is carried out in conjunction with a total thyroidectomy. It is also performed in conjunction with a lateral selective neck dissection for tumours of the hypopharynx and subglottis.

Level VII

During a level VI anterior compartment neck dissection for differentiated and medullary thyroid cancer, level VII can be palpated and lymphatic tissue cleared as part of the procedure. True lymph-node involvement demonstrated on computed tomography (CT) or magnetic resonance imaging (MRI) scanning requires a upper sternotomy and access to the area which clears the lymphatic tissue, including the thymus, on the medial aspects of both common carotid arteries overlying the trachea down to the brachiocephalic vein. It is indicated for suspected disease in differentiated thyroid cancer, medullary thyroid cancer, subglottic laryngeal cancer, hypopharyngeal and cervical oesophageal cancer. In the latter case, the dissection should only take place if the disease is completely resectable.

Operative technique

Access to the appropriate lymph-node areas required for selective neck dissection will be governed by the personal preference of the surgeon, the numbers and location of levels to be accessed and dissected, as well as the site of any primary tumour resection and the mode of reconstruction. Examples of incisions are shown in Fig. 13.1.

Table 13.2 Selective neck dissection (for the previously untreated N_0 neck)

Type	Levels dissected	Main indications
Supraomohyoid	I–III	T_1–T_4N_0 SCC oral cavity
Extended supraomohyoid (anterolateral)	I–IV	Skin cancer (SCC and melanoma) anterior to the line of the tragus. Performed in conjunction with a superficial parotidectomy
Lateral	II–IV	T_2–T_4: N_0 SCC larynx, oropharynx and hypopharynx
Posterolateral	II–V (plus postauricular and suboccipital nodes)	Skin cancer (SCC and melanoma) posterior to the the line of the tragus
Anterior or central	VI	Differentiated thyroid carcinoma Subglottic and hypopharyngeal SCC
Superior mediastinum	VII	Differentiated and medullary thyroid carcinoma Subglottic laryngeal and hypopharyngeal SCC Cervical oesophageal carcinoma

SCC: squamous cell carcinoma.

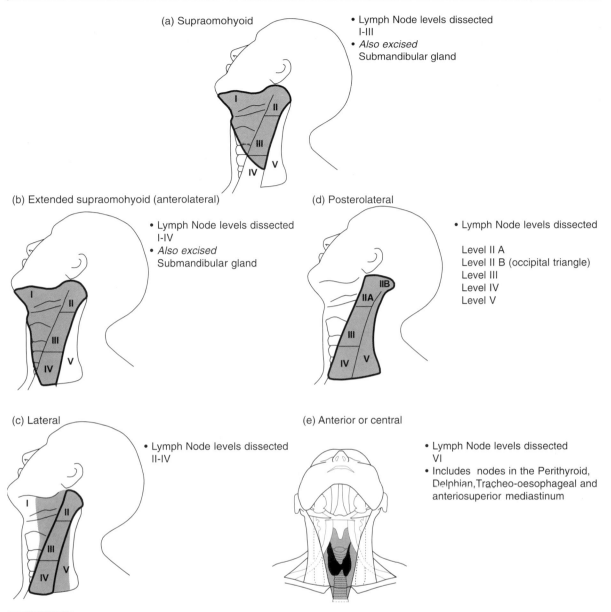

Figure 13.20 Types of selective neck dissection.

Supraomohyoid neck dissection levels I–III

For a selective supraomohyoid neck dissection (and extended supraomohyoid), the fascia overlying the sternomastoid muscle is mobilized anteriorly and the muscle retracted laterally. The fascia is dissected down to the posterior limit of the muscle, where the fascia is incised to expose the prevertebral fascia and the floor of the posterior triangle. This commences inferiorly and proceeds superiorly, dividing branches of the cervical plexus, and is taken up to the level of the digastric muscle. From this point, the dissection proceeds in a forward direction both superiorly and inferiorly to identify where the fascia approaches the internal jugular vein. This tissue, which includes the appropriate lymph nodes, is then folded over and dissected off the internal jugular vein,

the appropriate tributaries are tied and the dissection continues anteriorly, leaving the omohyoid muscle behind. As the dissection approaches the submandibular triangle, the hypoglossal nerve is identified and preserved and the submandibular gland excised in the same manner as described previously.

In this dissection, care must be taken to identify and preserve the accessory nerve in the upper posterior limit of the dissection where it enters the undersurface of the sternomastoid muscle.

Lateral

This operation is carried out in conjunction with excision of the primary tumour as described above, except that level 1 is not dissected.

Posterolateral

In this operation, access is obtained to the posterior triangle. The flaps are elevated, the fascia is mobilized off the sternomastoid from medial to lateral, the sternomastoid is retracted medially in the opposite direction as described for the previous selective neck dissections and levels II, III and IV are cleared from medial to lateral in the manner described above. The dissection extends laterally, preserving the accessory nerve, and clearance is completed by dissecting the postauricular nodes and the suboccipital triangle (level IIb).

Selective neck dissections are only indicated when the natural history of the disease in question is predictable and should not be done following previous surgery radiotherapy to the neck.

Level VI

This operation is carried out in conjunction with a total thyroidectomy. The lymph-node bearing areas in the prelaryngeal and pretracheal areas are dissected down to the level of the suprasternal notch and laterally, level VI nodes in the pretracheal area are dissected and removed. In particular, those nodes that lie medial and lateral to the recurrent laryngeal nerve in the paratracheal space are removed when present. It is important when this dissection is carried out that levels II, III, IV and VII are palpated and any disease suspected in these areas should be confirmed on frozen section and treated with an appropriate extended selective or comprehensive neck dissection.

Level VII

This is usually carried out in conjunction with an anterior central compartment neck dissection (level VI) and total thyroidectomy. An upper median sternotomy (with a lateral extension at the angle of Louis if required) is made to facilitate access to the upper mediastinum. However, if the operation is being performed with more radical surgery to the trachea, larynx and pharynx which involves the fashioning of a low end-tracheostome, the upper sternum should be removed to facilitate its exteriorization. Lymphatic tissue is cleared to the level of the clavicle medial to both carotid arteries and the area dissected, including the thymus gland, down to the level of the brachiocephic vein. Care must be taken to preserve the recurrent laryngeal nerves when appropriate; sometimes this operation facilitates their identification in the upper mediastinum well away from the disease which will be encountered later in the lower neck.

Postoperative management and complications

Postoperatively, all of these neck dissections are managed in the same way as for radical neck dissection. Prophylactic antibiotics are not indicated unless the length of the operation so dictates or the pharynx, oral cavity or upper airway is entered. Drains are removed separately in a conventional manner and closure of the skin is as per radical neck dissection. Complications are described in Chapter 6.

References and further reading

Crile G. W. (1906) Excision of cancer of the head and neck. With special reference to the plan of dissection based on one hundred and thirty-two operations, *JAMA* 47: 1780–6.

Martin H. (1941) The treatment of cervical metastatic cancer, *Ann Surg* 114: 972–86.

Martin H. (1961) Radical neck dissection, *CIBA Clin Symp* 13: 103–20.

Robbins K. T., Medina J. E., Wolfe G. T., Levine P. A., Sessions R. B. and Pruet C. W. (1991) Standardising neck dissection terminology. *Arch Otolaryngol Head Neck Surg* 117: 601–5.

Shah J. P. and Anderson P. E. (1994) The impact of patterns of neck metastasis on modifications of neck dissection, *Ann Surg Oncol* 1: 521–32.

Shah J. P. (1990) Cervical lymph node metastasis. Its diagnostic, therapeutic, and prognostic implications, *Oncology* 4: 1–69.

Shah J. P. (1996) Cervical lymph nodes, in *Head and Neck Surgery*, 2nd edn (J. P. Shah, ed.), Mosby-Wolfe, London, pp. 355–92.

The root of the neck, in *Last's Anatomy Regional and Applied*, ninth edn (R. M. H. McMinn, ed.), Churchill Livingstone, London, pp. 442–5.

Urquhart A. C. (1997) Radical and conservative neck dissections, in *Operative Otorhino-laryngology* (N. Bleach, C. Milford and A. Van Hasselt, eds), Blackwell Science, Oxford, pp. 444–53.

Tumours of the larynx

'In every age and clime we see, two of a kind can never agree'
Fables, 'The Rat Catcher and Cat', John Gay, 1927

Introduction

Carcinoma of the larynx, along with carcinoma of the oral cavity, is the most common primary head and neck malignancy (excluding skin). In the UK it represents approximately 1% of all malignancies in men but is less common in women. It often presents early when a high cure rate can be achieved. Treatment remains controversial but early cancers may be treated with either surgery or radiotherapy, depending upon size, site, and patient and doctor preference. Advanced disease is usually treated with radical surgery and postoperative radiotherapy. Alternatively, non-surgical treatment may be used for advanced disease with the aim of laryngeal conservation.

Surgical anatomy

The larynx is divided into three sites and each of these sites is divided into sub-sites. The current sites and subsites laid down by the International Union Against Cancer (UICC) are shown in Table 14.1.

The larynx also encompasses several spaces, or rather potential spaces, which are important in the spread of disease. These include the pre-epiglottic and paraglottic spaces, Reinke's space and the anterior subglottic wedge. The pre-epiglottic space is bound superiorly by the hyoepiglottic ligament, posteriorly by the epiglottis and anteriorly by the thyrohyoid ligament. Its apex inferiorly is limited by the attachment of the inferior end of the epiglottic cartilage by a strong fibrous band, the thyroepiglottic ligament, to the posterior surface of the thyroid cartilage below the median notch at the anterior commissure tendon. The epiglottic cartilage has numerous foramina through which carcinoma can pass from its posterior surface into the pre-epiglottic space (Fig. 14.1).

The paraglottic space, or rather potential space, lies lateral to the true and false cords. Medially, it is bounded by the vestibular fold and the quadrangular membrane and more inferiorly by the conus elasticus, which is covered by the mucosa of the subglottic space. Medially, the paraglottic space is continued through the pre-epig-

Table 14.1 Anatomical sites and subsites of the larynx

1. Supraglottis
(i) Suprahyoid epiglottis (including tip, lingual (anterior) and laryngeal surfaces)   — Epilarynx (including marginal zone)
(ii) Aryepiglottic fold, laryngeal aspect
(iii) Arytenoid
(iv) Infrahyoid epiglottis   — Supraglottis excluding epilarynx
(v) Ventricular bands (false cords)

2. Glottis
(i) Vocal cords
(ii) Anterior commissure
(iii) Posterior commissure

3. Subglottis

UICC (1997).

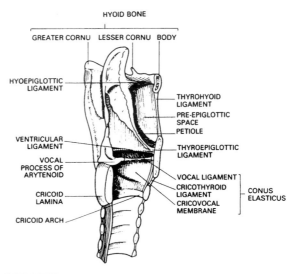

Figure 14.1 Pre-epiglottic space (sagittally bissected larynx).

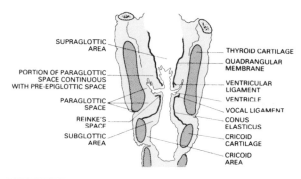

Figure 14.2 Paraglottic space.

lottic space, and superiorly it is bounded by the vallecula and the aryepiglottic fold. Its lateral relation is the mucosa of the medial wall of the piriform fossa posteriorly and the thyroid cartilage anteriorly. Inferolaterally, the space is bounded by the cricothyroid ligament (Fig. 14.2).

Reinke's space lies immediately beneath the laryngeal mucosa, i.e. superficial to the vocal ligament, and is bounded superiorly and inferiorly by the junction of the columnar squamous epithelium which represents the superior and inferior arcuate lines.

The anterior subglottic wedge is a triangular-shaped zone with an apex terminating just below the anterior commissure tendon and which is delineated inferiorly by the anterior arch of the cricoid (Fig. 14.1). Anterior commissure tumours commonly spread in a mushroom-like manner to involve this area and then penetrate the cricothyroid ligament.

The important tendons and ligaments of the larynx are the vocal ligament, the cricovocal membrane (conus elasticus), the vestibular ligament (the quadrangular membrane) and the anterior commissure tendon. The cricovocal membrane (conus elasticus) is attached below the entire border of the arch of the cricoid cartilage running round from one arytenoid facet to the other. Its median part, called the crico-thyroid ligament, is tense and strong and triangular in shape. Its apex is inserted into the prominence of the thyroid cartilage at the anterior commissure. The upper edge of the cricovocal membrane extends from this point backwards to be inserted into the inferior border of the vocal process of the arytenoid cartilage. This upper free border is thickened and forms the vocal ligament which is the supporting ligament of the vocal cord.

The quadrangular membranes have as their inferior margin the vestibular folds attached anteriorly to the depression between the two laminae of the thyroid cartilage above the vocal ligament and close to the attachment of the thyroepiglottic ligament. It extends backwards to be inserted into the tubercle on the anterolateral surface of the arytenoid cartilage. It is composed of elastic fibrous tissue and contains the cuneiform cartilages which attach to the anterolateral surface of the arytenoid cartilages and help to keep the glottis open when the laryngeal muscles are relaxed. Medially, the quadrangular membrane is loosely covered by mucosa and laterally it is bounded by the paraglottic space. Its upper free margin is the aryepiglottic fold. The anterior commissure tendon is formed by the fusion of the two vocal ligaments anteriorly to form a tendon inserted into the thyroid cartilage.

The supraglottic portion of the larynx is derived from the buccopharyngeal anlage (arches III and IV), whereas the glottic and subglottic portions derive from pulmonary anlage (arch VI). Thus, each major component has an independent lymphatic circulation, separated into an upper and a lower drainage system. They are collected together on the posterior wall of the cavity, but are separated laterally and anteriorly by the vocal folds. It is generally said that a vocal fold contains only a few capillary vessels, although some authorities disagree with this. It is this poverty of lymph drainage which is said to predispose Reinke's space to accumulation of oedema. The lymph vessels of the upper part pass alongside the superior laryngeal artery, pierce the thyrohyoid membrane and end in the upper deep cervical glands along with the lymph vessels of the pharynx (levels II and III). The efferent vessels from the anterior part of the lower segment of the larynx pierce the cricothyroid ligament and end in the prelaryngeal and pretracheal lymphatic nodal region (level VI) and the deep cervical chain (level IV). The efferents from the posterolateral region pierce the cricotracheal membrane and end in the paratracheal (level VI) and lower deep cervical nodes (level IV).

The free edge of the vocal cord is covered by squamous epithelium. Its superior and inferior surfaces are covered by respiratory epithelium and the junction between the respiratory and squamous epithelium above and below is marked by the superior and inferior arcuate lines, respectively. The subglottis can be divided into two parts. The anterior, fixed part is a triangle whose apex lies superiorly at the anterior commissure. Here, the mucosa is tightly bound to the cartilage, which has foramina through which tumour can pass. Laterally, the subglottic mucosa covers the conus elasticus and is mobile. The nerve supply of the larynx is best discussed under the heading of vocal-cord paralysis (see Chapter 18).

The TNM (tumour, node, metastasis) staging of laryngeal carcinoma is discussed later but there are a number of anatomical points that are important here that relate to the TNM classification.

A glottic tumour is described as being T_2 when the tumour extends to the supraglottis or to the subglottis. Unfortunately, the classification at present does not define where the glottis becomes the supraglottis above, and until recently did not define where the glottis became the subglottis below.

It is clear from the writings of many authors in the literature that there are many different definitions of these two boundaries, which has added to confusion with regards to staging in the past. Some regard the superior border of the glottis as being the superior arcuate line, whereas others include all of the superior surface of the vocal cord and the floor of the vestibule in the glottis. In the past, some authors have placed the lower border of the glottis at the inferior arcuate line, some at the level of the superior border of the cricoid cartilage and others at a point 1 cm inferior to the free edge of the vocal cord or 5 mm inferior to the free edge (at midcord level). In 1993, the UICC accepted the recommendation by Steiner and Amrosch that 'the inferior border of the glottis is a horizontal plane 1 cm inferior to the level of the upper surface of the vocal cord'.

The strict anatomical definition of the vocal cord is that part of the free edge of the cord, covered by squamous epithelium, which has a vertical height of about 5 mm, being bounded superiorly and inferiorly by the superior and inferior arcuate lines. The tissue above and below these lines is now included in the glottis. This means that a tumour may have already spread into this area of richer lymphatic drainage rather than the true vocal cords, so inevitably this change in anatomical classification may dramatically affect reported results.

The glottis is said to consist of the vocal cords, the space which lies in a horizontal plane 1 cm inferior to the level of the upper surface of the vocal cord, the anterior commissure and posterior commissure but, again, these latter two structures are not defined accurately. Strictly speaking, commissure means 'a point', so that the anterior commissure presumably means the point anteriorly where the vocal cords come together. It is clear, however, that many authors regard the anterior commissure as an area from which a tumour can arise. On passing along the vocal cords to the anterior end, the strip of squamous epithelium narrows, so that at the anterior end of the cord the strip of squamous epithelium is only about 1 mm high. Here, it may join its fellow of the opposite side, or there can be a narrow strip 1–2 mm wide covered with respiratory epithelium passing between the anterior end of the two vocal cords. Indeed, such an area is necessary on physiological grounds to allow mucus to pass up by ciliary action from the trachea to cross the vocal cords. At this point, the vocal cords are very narrow so that a tumour that crosses the anterior commissure spreads readily off the vocal cords, and in particular below the cord into the apex at the anterior part of the subglottic space (anterior subglottic wedge). At this point the mucosa is tightly bound to the thyroid cartilage, which has foramina for the passage of vessels, providing an easy route of escape for cancer into the prelaryngeal tissues.

The posterior commissure is not defined, but is taken to comprise the squamous epithelium lining the anterior surface of the arytenoid cartilage and that over the vocal processes of the arytenoid cartilage. The vocal cords form only a little over half of the glottis, the remaining part being formed by the mucosa over the vocal processes of the arytenoid cartilage and over the anterior surface of the arytenoid cartilage. Tumours seldom arise from this area.

Surgical pathology

Tumours of the larynx may be benign or malignant. True benign tumours constitute 5% or less of all laryngeal tumours and their relative incidence is shown in the box below.

Benign tumours of the larynx

■ Papilloma (85%)
■ Chondroma
■ Miscellaneous (granula cell myoblastomas, lipomas, haemangiomas, neurofibromas)

Benign tumours

Papillomas

True papillomas are by far the most common benign laryngeal tumour. They can be divided into two types: juvenile papilloma, which is multiple and usually regresses after puberty, and adult papilloma, which is usually single, does not undergo spontaneous resolution and comprises only about 25% of cases.

The juvenile papilloma arises mainly on the true and false cords and the anterior commissure, but often extends into the subglottic space, the trachea, bronchi and epiglottis. Human papilloma virus (HPV) types 6 and 11 are believed to be the causative agents. HPV-6, 11 and 16 have been demonstrated by, e.g. Southern blotting, *in situ* hybridization and immunocytochemistry. Viral DNA is found less consistently in adult papillomas. Fifty per cent of children with papillomas are born to mothers with active genital condylomata. Malignant change may occur in a juvenile papilloma but usually only if the patient has been irradiated. A hallmark of the juvenile papilloma is its multiple nature and notorious propensity to recur.

There are no histological differences between an adult and a juvenile papilloma, although the former do not usually recur after local removal.

The treatment of juvenile laryngeal papillomatosis is repeated and careful removal using a laser, e.g. CO_2 laser at 10 W power with 0.1 sec pulses and a small spot size. Theatre personnel should be protected from the laser fume, which may be contaminated with viral particles. Tracheostomy should be avoided at all costs if at all possible. Every effort should be made to avoid recurrence in the trachea or bronchi and if laryngeal trauma can be minimized, subsequent dysphonia and respiratory difficulty is usually slight.

Haemangiomas

Small cavernous haemangiomas present in any part of the larynx but favour the supraglottis. They are usually seen in adults and can be dealt with endoscopically. The Nd:YAG laser may be helpful to limit bleeding. Capillary haemangiomas are usually congenital and are rare in adults. They usually present with dyspnoea between the 3rd and 16th week of life. Five per cent of patients will also have other congenital abnormalities and half have cutaneous haemangiomas. Some 80% of cavernous haemangiomas arise from the posterior wall of the larynx or trachea and involve one side of the subglottis. Many respond well to one or two CO_2 laser vaporizations. Excision via laryngofissure, or excision with laser or cryotherapy has been tried but where laser therapy is unavailable, probably the best treatment option is a tracheostomy and to await resolution along with growth of the trachea. Some regress slowly after the age of 12 years. Steroid therapy may be of benefit.

Combined lymphangiomas and haemangiomas may be present along with haemangiopericytomas.

Cartilaginous tumours

This term is used deliberately to emphasize the fact there is no clear-cut histological or clinical distinction between chondromas and chondrosarcomas. Of those reported in the literature, 20% have been considered to be malignant. This is distinctly a male disease (sex ratio of 5:1), occurring between the ages of 40 and 60 years. Seventy per cent of cartilaginous tumours arise from the cricoid cartilage and in this situation most often from the posterior cricoid plate. Twenty per cent arise from the thyroid cartilage and the rest usually from the arytenoid. Clinically, these tumours present with dysphonia, dyspnoea and dysphagia. They are smooth and encapsulated, covered by intact mucosa, and radiographs often show mottled calcification.

Patients may present with progressive inspiratory stridor. Irrespective of the histological appearance, these tumours grow and extend locally and require removal with a good margin. If more than 50% of the cricoid is involved, it needs to be reconstructed. Radiotherapy is of little value. Local and distant metastases have only been recorded very rarely.

Schwannoma

Schwannomas of the larynx are extremely uncommon. They arise from the aryepiglottic fold close to the apex of the arytenoid cartilage at the laryngeal ventricle, arising from the internal branch of the superior laryngeal nerve. They usually occur in the fourth and fifth decades of life and are more common in women. Symptoms tend to develop insidiously and the tumours are usually small and can be dealt with endoscopically, but occasionally a lateral pharyngotomy is required for access. The necessity for a total laryngectomy is extremely rare. Only one case of a malignant schwannoma has been described.

Neurofibroma

Most neurofibromas are part of a generalized von Recklinghausen's syndrome (neurofibromatosis type I). Most cases arise in children and in adolescents, and usually occur in the supraglottis but they can occur as far down as the subglottis. Typically, they present as pink or yellow submucosal masses along the aryepiglottic folds. They are not suitable for endoscopic resection because of indistinct borders and a lateral pharyngotomy or thyrotomy is necessary for access. In approximately 10% of cases, neurofibrosarcoma can occur, especially in fully developed von Recklinghausen's disease (see Chapter 25).

Adenoma

Benign tumours arising from the seromucinous glands of the larynx are also rare and most occur in the subglottis. Symptoms are unusual until the tumour obstructs the airway and the differential diagnosis is limited to those lesions with smooth overlying mucosa in this area to include a retention cyst, haemangioma, internal laryngocoele or an adenoid cystic carcinoma. The most common variant is the oncocytoma or oxyphil adenoma. Oncocytes are cells found with ageing, which have eosinophitic cytoplasm and are often associated with salivary gland disease. Oncocytic tumours therefore tend to arise in the ventricle and false cords where these are numerous minor salivary glands. Histologically, they are cystic with intracystic papillary projections, rather like Warthin's tumours. Treatment is by surgical excision and the approach depends on the size and site of the lesion.

Granular cell myoblastoma

This uncommon lesion was once thought not be a true tumour at all but a degenerative disease of mature striated muscle cells, hence the name. Evidence now suggests that they arise from neural tissue, most likely the Schwann cell, because of cytoplasmic granules which show positive S100 immmunohistochemical staining. Most arise in the tongue and probably less than 10% are laryngeal. The vast majority of laryngeal granular cell tumours arise within the substance of the vocal cord and cause hoarseness. They are reported at all ages from infancy upwards. The most important point about them is that the overlying epithelium may show the appearance of pseudoepitheliomatous hyperplasia, which the pathologist might report as squamous cell carcinoma. If the clinician and the pathologist are unaware of this, unnecessary radical surgery may be advised. Treatment is by endoscopic excision.

Paraganglioma

Glomus tumours of the larynx arise from laryngeal paraganglia. These are paired structures on the internal branch of the superior laryngeal nerve on the upper anterior third of the false cord and a second pair lies on the terminal branch of the posterior branch of the recurrent laryngeal nerve close to the inferior horn of the thyroid cartilage/cricoid ring. Most tumours arise from the supraglottic paraganglia and less frequently from the inferior ones. Patients are usually aged between 50 and 70 years and men are affected slightly more often than women. The paraganglia look like haemangiomas and cause non-specific symptoms but occasionally can cause pain. They grow slowly and destroy the laryngeal skeleton. As they increase in size they cause symptoms such as hoarseness and stridor and occasionally haemoptysis can occur. Angiography can provide information about the vascularity of the tumours but computed tomography (CT) or magnetic resonance imaging (MRI) is the best radiological method to determine their extent. Most are relatively radioresistant and the preferred treatment is either excision or supraglottic laryngectomy. Excision is usually external since there is a risk of haemorrhage and recurrence when an endoscopic approach is employed. Histological examination confirms the presence of neurosecretory granules (see Chapter 25).

Leiomyoma

The leiomyoma is one of the most common benign laryngeal tumours in humans. They have been reported in children but usually occur more often in adults of all ages and are most common in the supraglottic region. Treatment is by surgical excision, which is usually endoscopic, or an external approach, depending on the tumour site.

Rhabdomyoma

True adult rhabdomyomas are extremely rare. Around 80% of non-cardiac lesions occur in the head and neck, principally in the larynx. Most originate in the vocal cord region and appear as a polypoid mass and can extend above and below the cords. Treatment is surgical excision and the endoscopic route is usually sufficient, although the surgeon must be aware of their occasional multicentric origin and propensity to recur.

Fibromas and lipomas

Fibromas occur in the larynx as soft pedunculated masses, whereas lipomas arise from adipose tissue, especially in the false cords. They are similarly encapsulated and lobulated, and the treatment of both lesions is surgical removal.

Malignant tumours

Squamous carcinoma forms the vast majority of malignant laryngeal disease. Its incidence in the UK is approximately 1% of all malignancies in men although it is less common in women. This is rather surprising in an organ which is at birth lined by respiratory epithelium and reflects the fact that squamous metaplasia is a common occurrence within the larynx presumably due, in part, to the aetiological factors that will be discussed subsequently. Because prognosis for laryngeal cancer varies with the site as well as the stage of disease, it is crucial that great care and attention is placed on the accurate assessment and staging of these tumours. The relative incidence of malignant tumours within the larynx is shown in the box below.

Malignant tumours of the larynx
■ Squamous cell carcinoma (85%)
■ Carcinoma *in situ*
■ Verrucous carcinoma
■ Undifferentiated carcinoma
■ Adenocarcinoma
■ Miscellaneous carcinomas (adenoid cystic, spindle cell, etc.)
■ Sarcomas (including reticulosis)

Squamous carcinoma

Carcinoma *in situ* generally only occurs on the vocal cord and it is discussed below. Frankly invasive squamous cell carcinoma is usually moderately to well-differentiated and may arise from the supraglottic, glottic or subglottic areas.

Epidemiology. The incidence of laryngeal cancer within the UK is approximately four per 100 000. Approximately 70% of laryngeal carcinomas in the UK occur in men (3–4:1), with a peak incidence between 55 and 65 years of age. In Scotland, the male: female ratio is 2:1 and in France 9:1. There are areas in the world where the incidence is higher (greater than 10 per 10 000), including Brazil (São Paulo), the Afro-caribbean populations in parts of the USA, India, France, Italy, Poland, Spain and Switzerland. Areas of low incidence (less than two per 100 000) include Japan, Norway, and Sweden. There is also a marked social class difference, in that carcinoma of the larynx is twice as common in men in social class V than men in social class I. There is also an urban variation, in that it is more common in people residing in cities than in rural areas.

Risk factors
■ Geographic
■ Social class V
■ Urban
■ Smoking
■ Alcohol
■ Radiation

These social and racial differences probably reflect different habits and confirm the already recognized effects of tobacco and alcohol. What is interesting is the low rate of laryngeal cancer in the UK, compared with the high rates of smoking-related lung cancer.

Aetiology. The exact cause of laryngeal cancer is unknown. At present, there is no one proven aetiological factor but there are several often interrelated factors (usually environmental) which are clearly associated with the increased incidence of laryngeal cancer, notably cigarette smoking and consumption of alcohol (especially dark spirits). Exposure to asbestos, formaldehyde and therapeutic radiation (thyroid) have also been postulated as aetiological factors. Further studies are awaited to identify genetic factors that may be of aetiological interest. Laryngeal keratosis and leucoplakia are related to carcinoma of the larynx but metaplasia, although it is smoking related, has not yet received designation as a clear precursor of neoplasia.

Squamous intraepithelial neoplasia

Squamous intraepithelial neoplasia
■ Keratosis: keratin formation by superficial layer only
■ Parakeratosis: nucleus retained abnormality in the superficial layer of keratin-producing cells
■ Dyskeratosis: keratinization within the prickle cell layer
■ Dysplasia: nuclear variation, mitosis, loss of normal epithelial layering
■ Carcinoma *in situ*: cells of malignant cytology but confined superficially to the basement membrane

To date there is no recognized uniform terminology for epithelial lesions occurring within the larynx. Many conditions are characterized by their gross appearance, i.e. leucoplakia, erythroleucoplakia and hyperkeratosis. Modern terminology is as follows.

Grade I squamous cell hyperplasia with mild dysplasia and keratosis is usually benign but should be regarded a premalignant disorder.

Grade II lesions exhibit keratosis and squamous cell dysplasia with occasional nuclear atypia which, if pronounced enough, may be premalignant.

Grade III squamous cell hyperplasia or carcinoma *in situ* shows coarse abnormalities of differentiation and nuclear atypia in almost all areas of the epithelium, with basal cell proliferation and mitoses.

Microcarcinoma and microinvasive carcinoma: the vocal cord is one of the few parts in the body where small carcinomas can develop relatively often. A micro-carcinoma describes a superficial carcinoma of a maximum size of $10 \times 10 \times 3$ mm and a microinvasive carcinoma tumour that has not yet infiltrated the submucosa of the vocal cord. It is important to remember that not all squamous cell carcinomas on the vocal cords arise from a previously existing premalignant lesion and that some arise directly from the basal epithelial layers and infiltrate deeply and, as such, are menacing lesions.

Clinically, carcinoma *in situ* comes in three very distinct clinical types. The first is a small, white patch on the vocal cord which, when removed, may be reported as carcinoma *in situ*. These patients can often be safely reviewed and told to stop smoking. Any further recurrence can be treated by vocal-cord stripping or laser vaporization, which can be repeated. In the presence of continual reports of carcinoma *in situ*, the lesion seldom progresses to involve any more of the larynx.

The second type is a widespread, white–grey change in the laryngeal epithelium. The third type is the same change, only with a reddish tinge to it and looks to all intents and purposes like erythroleucoplakia. Carcinoma *in situ* in this situation tends to behave badly and has a worse prognosis than the small T_1 glottic carcinoma. Localized vocal-cord stripping or laser excision is probably a waste of time in these patients and given the widespread field change of the disease, they should be treated aggressively with external radiation. Carcinoma *in situ* usually occurs in smokers but when it occurs in the young non-smoker, it is probably of a different biological entity and again should be treated more aggressively with irradiation.

Supraglottic carcinoma

Supraglottic carcinomas comprise about 40% of all laryngeal cancers in the UK and 30% in North America. The incidence appears to be higher in continental Europe owing to synergistic carcinogenesis of alcohol and tobacco affecting the epilarynx (aryepiglottic folds and suprahyoid epiglottis).

The most common supraglottic carcinoma is that occurring in the centre of the infrahyoid epiglottis (Fig.

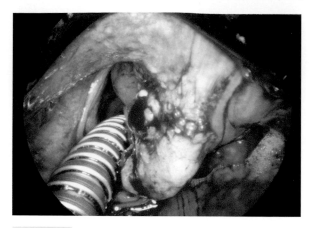

Figure 14.3 Extensive T_2N_0 squamous cell carcinoma of the right supraglottic larynx.

14.3). These tumours nearly always (90%) invade the fenestra in the epiglottic cartilage. About 50% invade the thyroid cartilage anteriorly or along its upper lateral edge. About half of these tumours also invade the pre-epiglottic space either by spreading through the fenestra or, more commonly, by destroying the thyroepiglottic ligament and passing through the resulting breach into the pre-epiglottic space. In contrast, tumours at the base of the epiglottis never invade the paraglottic space. It is thus safe in this instance, in the absence of previous radiotherapy, to carry out a horizontal supraglottic laryngectomy.

A small proportion, perhaps 5% or less, of the tumours extend inferiorly to invade the floor of the ventricle or the vocal cords. Carcinoma of the lateral supraglottic endolarynx (the ventricular bands) is much less common. These tumours tend to spread superficially on the mucosal surface to the laryngeal surface of the epiglottis and to the aryepiglottic fold. More important, however, is the spread into the paraglottic space. Involvement of this space is inferred from both clinical examination and radiological investigation which shows oedema and/or swelling increasing the distance between the piriform fossa and the false cord. Radiographic reversal of the subglottic contour is due to inferior paraglottic extension of disease. Extension into the paraglottic space can occur in tumours of the false cord or of the ventricle (the only mucosa embraced by this space), and in tumours of the glottis and of the medial wall of the piriform fossa. This is the cause of vocal-cord fixation seen in the latter tumours.

Supraglottic carcinomas may also extend cranially to the vallecula and the tongue base. Lastly, they may extend posteriorly to the arytenoid cartilage, the invasion of which seems only to occur when the arytenoids are grossly involved by tumour.

The UICC staging of supraglottic carcinoma is shown in Table 14.2. Note that involvement of the mucosa of the tongue base and medial wall of the piriform sinus represents T_2 disease while deep invasion is elevated from T_4 to T_3 status.

Table 14.2 Classification of supraglottic tumours

T	Primary tumour
T_{is}	Carcinoma *in situ*
T_1	Tumour limited to one subsite of supraglottis with normal vocal-cord mobility
T_2*	Tumour invades mucosa of more than one adjacent subsite of supraglottis or glottis or region outside the supraglottis (e.g. mucosa of base of tongue, vallecula, medial wall of piriform sinus) without fixation of the larynx
T_3*	Tumour limited to larynx with vocal-cord fixation and/or invades any of the following: postcricoid area, pre-epiglottic tissues, deep base of tongue
T_4*	Tumour invades through thyroid cartilage, and/or extends into soft tissues of the neck, thyroid and/or oesophagus.

*New inclusion.
UICC (1997).

Table 14.3 Classification of glottic tumours

T_{is}	Carcinoma *in situ*
T_1	Tumour limited to vocal cord(s) (may involve anterior or posterior commissures) with normal mobility
T_{1A}	Tumour limited to one vocal cord
T_{1B}	Tumour involves both vocal cords
T_2	Tumour extends to supraglottis and/or subglottis and/or with impaired vocal cord mobility
T_3	Tumour limited to the larynx with vocal cord fixation
T_4	Tumour invades through thyroid cartilage and/or extends to other tissues beyond the larynx, e.g. to oropharynx, soft tissues of the neck

UICC (1997).

Lymph-node metastases are classified as for head and neck squamous cell carcinoma (Chapter 12). The supraglottis is rich in lymphatics, which accounts for the high incidence of lymph-node metastases in supraglottic carcinoma. Even in early supraglottic cancers, the incidence of lymph-node metastases is not insignificant and because of the possibility of bilateral spread, both sides of the neck in levels II, III and IV should be considered at risk. Lymphatic spread occurs via the superior lymphatic pedicle which accompanies the superior laryngeal artery and nerve to levels II, III and IV in a previously untreated patient.

Supraglottic carcinoma: lymph-node metastases (UICC classification)

- N_0: 49%
- N_1: 18%
- N_2–N_3: 33%

Glottic carcinoma

The glottis is the site of the white lesion which has been called in the past either keratosis or leucoplakia. A neighbouring frank carcinoma should be carefully excluded if histology reporting carcinoma *in situ* is received. In North America, 60% of laryngeal neoplasms are glottic, whereas the figure is 50% for the UK. Glottic carcinoma may be divided into those small tumours that arise on one vocal cord and remain localized to it for long periods and those tumours, often called transglottic, that involve a large part of the laryngeal surface, cross the vocal cord and are extensive when first seen (Fig. 14.4). These tumours are not a later stage of a smaller tumour but probably represent a wide-field malignant degeneration.

Glottic carcinomas are classified according to the UICC as shown in Table 14.3.

It should be noted that tumours may also rise from the posterior third of the glottis, i.e. that part of the glottis which lies over the vocal process. For some reason, such tumours remain omitted from the current classification of laryngeal tumours within the UICC handbook. Glottic carcinomas arise on one or other of the vocal cords and spread along the cord in Reinke's space. These tumours may spread superficially into the neighbouring supraglottic or subglottic areas in about 10% of patients. Tumour may also spread across the anterior commissure to the opposite cord. Invasion of the intrinsic laryngeal muscles is common, especially the thyroarytenoid muscle. Small glottic tumours do not invade cartilage, but larger ones may involve the arytenoid cartilage or the thyroid cartilage at the anterior commissure. Once the carcinoma extends more than 1 cm inferior to the free edge of the vocal cord, it may invade the cricoid cartilage. Tumours that are limited to the glottis without fixation almost never transgress the conus elasticus.

If a glottic carcinoma arises from or reaches the anterior commissure, it can easily extend into the subglottis. The anterior midline is the most frequent location for invasion of the laryngeal framework. The tumour lies close to the cricothyroid membrane and can then escape early and easily by this route. This appears to be related to the close proximity of the mucosa to the thyroid ala at the anterior commissure and to the presence of the anterior commissure tendon. Tumour may spread along this route to invade the anterior supraglottis and subglottic larynx at the anterior subglottic wedge in the midsagittal plane.

Deep spread of glottic tumours. When the vocal cord muscles are invaded, the tumour may extend along the muscle bundles anteriorly or posteriorly and emerge lateral to the arytenoid cartilage, close to the mucosa of the piriform sinus, and invade the posterior cricoarytenoid muscle. Tumour extension lateral to the arytenoid cartilage is difficult to assess clinically but may be visualized on CT. Widening of the arytenoid space is

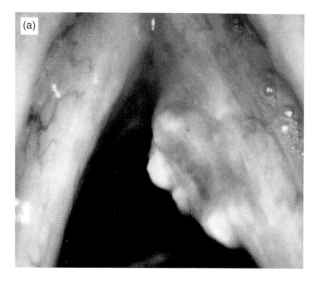

indicative of spread of disease and that the mucosa within the piriform sinus lateral to this point should be included in the resection.

Causes of vocal-cord fixation

- Vocal-cord fixation indicates deep invasion with involvement of at least the thyroarytenoid muscle
- When tumour involves the posterior part of the vocal cord, vocal fixation may be due to involvement of either the cricoarytenoid joint, the cricoid cartilage or the arytenoid, or a combination of these
- Perineural invasion may be another contributory factor but this is usually seen in larger tumours

Impaired mobility may indicate superficial invasion of the thyroarytenoid muscle and further assessment may suggest that conservation surgery is feasible, but fixation of a vocal cord usually means that the laryngeal framework is involved with tumour spread outside the larynx and that radical surgery is the only option.

Transglottic tumours. It is possible that some of these larger transglottic tumours originate in the ventricle. They invade the paraglottic space and are aggressive, almost always invading the laryngeal framework. They emerge from the cartilaginous part of the larynx between the thyroid and cricoid cartilages at the cricothryoid membrane. Up to 50% of transglottic tumours invade the ipsilateral lobe of the thyroid gland, which should be included in the resection if surgery is undertaken, and the strap muscles may also be involved. Transglottic tumours also extend posteriorly through the cricoarytenoid joint to invade the overlying pharyngeal mucosa, which must be included, as above, in the resection.

The lymphatics within the larynx can be divided into a supraglottic and subglottic network. These are separated by the free margins of the vocal cords, which under normal circumstances have minimal lymphatic drainage. This fact explains why there is an extremely low incidence of lymph-node metastases in those tumours that remain confined to the vocal cords. However, the incidence of lymph-node metastases in transglottic carcinoma increases in relation to the size of the primary tumour.

Incidence of lymph-node metastases in transglottic carcinoma

- N_0 70%
- N_1 20%
- N_2/N_3 7%

Figure 14.4 (a) Early squamous cell carcinoma of the right vocal cord ($T_{1a}N_0$ glottis); (b) extensive T_3N_0 transglottic squamous cell carcinoma.

Subglottic carcinoma

There are two types of subglottic tumour that should be distinguished from each other: first, a tumour which aris-

Table 14.4   Classification of subglottic tumours

T_{is} Carcinoma *in situ*

T_1 Tumour limited to the subglottis

T_2 Tumour extends to vocal cord(s) with normal or impaired mobility

T_3 Tumour limited to the larynx with vocal-cord fixation

T_4 Tumour invades through the cricoid or thyroid cartilage and/or extends to other tissues beyond the larynx, e.g. to oropharynx, soft tissues of the neck

UICC (1997).

Table 14.5   Overall staging grouping for laryngeal cancer (UICC 1997)

Stage 0	T_{is}	N_0	M_0
Stage I	T_1	N_0	M_0
Stage II	T_2	N_0	M_0
Stage III	T_1	N_1	M_0
	T_2	N_1	M_0
	T_3	$N0, N_1$	M_0
Stage IVA*	T_4	$N0, N_1$	M_0
	Any $T_{1,2,3}$	N_2	M_0
Stage IVB*	Any $T_{1,2,3}$	N_2	M_0
Stage IVC*	Any T	Any N	M_1

UICC (1997).
*New inclusion.

es primarily in the subglottic space and, secondly, a tumour which arises on or under the vocal cords and extends into the subglottic space, the latter being the more common. Subglottic carcinoma is uncommon in all published series, forming 5% or less of the total; indeed, subglottic extension of a glottic carcinoma is as common as, if not more common than a true subglottic carcinoma as previously described. The classification of these tumours is shown in Table 14.4.

True subglottic carcinoma is usually unilateral, virtually always ulcerative and fungating and not exophytic like many epiglottic carcinomas. It quickly invades the perichondrium of the thyroid and cricoid cartilages and always extends to and frequently through the cricothyroid membrane. These tumours almost always spread also through the conus elasticus to the glottic region, where the tumour margins tend to invade the intrinsic muscles of the true cord, producing the effect of a thickened and fixed cord, but not invading the free margin of the mucosa. True subglottic carcinoma usually presents with stridor, as distinct from subglottic spread of a glottic tumour which usually causes hoarseness. Vocal-cord fixation occurs in about 30% of both groups: 20% of true subglottic tumours have lymph-node metastases, compared with only 5% of the group with subglottic spread.

The overall group staging for laryngeal cancer shown in Table 14.5.

Histological confirmation of laryngeal cancer. At the time of direct endoscopy, a sample of the tumour is obtained for histological investigation. This is essential to confirm the diagnosis and thus to exclude non-malignant disease such as tuberculosis, chronic laryngitis and some benign tumours. In addition, the type of tumour can be identified, along with its degree of differentiation which may be of prognostic significance. A histopathological classification of squamous cell carcinoma can be performed based on Broder's method. Others (Jakobbson *et al.*, 1973) have applied a malignancy grading system to glottic carcinomas and identified nuclear poly-

morphism, mode of invasion and the total malignancy score as the most important factors in predicting patient outcome.

Prognostic factors. An adverse prognosis for laryngeal cancer relates to both the size of the primary tumour and the site, with a better prognosis being related to glottic disease. Prognosis is inversely related also to the N stage and the M stage and persistence of disease at the primary site. Biological prognostic factors can be assessed in DNA content and cell-cycle distribution. Aneuploid tumours have a worse disease-specific survival but further work has indicated that cell-cycle distribution has no prognostic importance other than G_0 nucleolar protein. Tissue eosinophilia may be helpful but oncogenic over-expression has not yet been established as important.

The administration of previous radiotherapy can have adverse effects for a number of reasons. First, a biopsy may be taken from an area of chronic inflammation and fibrosis which overlies or surrounds the current tumour, thus masking overt disease. Radiotherapy may cause chondronecrosis of the larynx, which may mimic recurrent disease and can coexist with recurrent disease. It may also affect and alter the normal patterns of spread of disease both within the larynx and to cervical lymph nodes on both sides of the neck, and following surgery can adversely affect healing and inversely increase complication rates such as fistula formation.

Distant metastases. It is uncommon for a patient with laryngeal cancer to present with a distant metastasis as their first symptom. Sometimes at the time of primary presentation, subsequent investigation elicits the presence of distant metastases and this has been reported to be in the region of 5%. In this setting the lung is the site most commonly involved.

It is becoming increasingly common for patients to survive their primary disease and succumb to distant metastases at some stage in the future. In one study of head and neck patients where death was studied with post mortem examination, 44% of patients with supraglottic and glottic laryngeal cancer had evidence of distant metastases (Kotwall *et al.*, 1987). It appears there is a relationship between the presence of distant metastases and T stage (Kotwall *et al.*, 1987), N stage, total stage, poorly differentiated tumours and the presence of recurrent disease. The N stage has a greater influence on the rate of distant metastases than T stage and the lungs and bones are the most common first sites of metastases.

Multiple primary tumours. Approximately 10% of patients with laryngeal cancer will have a second primary carcinoma within the respiratory tract and half of these are located distally in the lungs and have to be separated from distant metastases.

It is important to carry out panendoscopy at the time of primary presentation to exclude a second primary tumour, and in advanced laryngeal disease where radiological investigation is to be carried out, CT scan of the chest should be considered to exclude such pathology. This is discussed in Chapter 2.

Following treatment, there is a 3% cumulative rate per year of the development of synchronomous primary carcinomas. The value of prospective panendoscopy in such patients has been discussed already in Chapter 2.

Unusual tumours

Verrucous carcinoma

This tumour was first described by Ackerman in 1948 and usually occurs in the mouth but less commonly in the supraglottis and glottis. It is a relatively non-aggressive tumour which seldom metastasizes in the neck. The majority of patients are smokers and in a subgroup of patients previously reported (Olsen *et al.*, 1994) herpes virus DNA was detected in 85% of tissue samples by polymerase chain reaction, which suggests that herpes infection may also play an aetiological role. Hoarseness is the most common symptom and the lesion is often misdiagnosed as being benign.

The gross findings of verrucous carcinoma consist of a fungating, papillomatous, shaggy greyish white neoplasm. The characteristics of the tumour are shown in the box below.

Tumour characteristics

- It comprises unusually well-differentiated keratinizing squamous epithelium arranged in compressed invaginating folds
- It has a warty papillary surface
- The clefts between adjacent capillary folds can be traced to the depths of the tumour
- Infiltration is on a broad base with pushing margins against a stroma containing a prominent inflammatory reaction
- The usual cytological and infiltrating growth pattern of squamous carcinoma is absent

---

There are two principal controversies which relate to verrucous carcinoma. First, otolaryngologists and pathologists cannot agree about which cases should be included in this category and some respected authorities even deny that it is a true tumour. Secondly, there is argument about whether the apparent transition which is sometimes observed from a relatively benign to a highly malignant tumour is due to irradiation or is an independent phenomenon.

Verrucous carcinoma accounts for about 1% of cases of laryngeal carcinoma. The majority of cases occurs in the glottis (72% in one series; Olsen *et al.*, 1994) and the rest in the supraglottis. In Olsen's series there were no cases of subglottic disease. Its characteristic exophytic fungating microscopic appearance, likened to white fronds of seaweed, is distinct from that of typical squamous carcinoma. Many cases described as verrucous by the surgeon do not, however, fulfil the established criteria for a histopathological diagnosis of verrucous carcinoma. Because of its gross morphology, biopsies of verrucous carcinoma are often superficial, and the microscopic appearance is of mature squamous epithelium with hyperkeratosis and parakeratosis. However, 20% of cases of verrucous carcinoma have a hybrid nature with foci of poorly differentiated non-verrucous carcinoma. While it is true that some patients with verrucous carcinoma treated by radiotherapy have subsequently succumbed to metastatic anaplastic carcinoma, it is not proven that irradiation has caused malignant transformation in a benign tumour. It is equally possible that the treatment caused satisfactory regression of the well-differentiated component but a pre-existing focus of anaplastic carcinoma has escaped cure.

Certainly, this aggressive behaviour has been noted in patients treated by other modalities. It is now acceptable to regard verrucous carcinoma as a tumour with malignant potential from the start, and to treat it as one would any other squamous carcinoma. It is slow growing and locally invasive, and misdiagnosis can lead to a delay in both diagnosis and treatment. Patients with more advanced tumours appear to do worse. Small, early tumours should be treated by either an endoscopic approach, partial laryngectomy when appropriate or radiotherapy, but larger tumours which compromise the airway at presentation require radical surgery. Larynges, not lives, will be lost if radiotherapy is considered contraindicated and a policy of primary radical surgery is followed. In one series (Olsen *et al.*, 1994), the small number of patients who were treated by radiotherapy suffered no adverse effects and in that particular series, there were no cases of metastases or death from verrucous carcinoma alone. Hybrid cases carry a greater risk of recurrence.

Kaposi's sarcoma

This disease was rare in Europe and America until recently, when it has become more and more common in association with acquired immuno-deficiency syndrome (AIDS). A review of 13 cases of Kaposi's sarcoma in the larynx showed that all of these patients also had skin tumours. Involvement of the larynx is thus only to be expected in the late stages when the disease has already been diagnosed from the skin lesions.

Diagnosis of laryngeal cancer

The diagnosis of laryngeal cancer is based on a full history and examination together with clinical investigations, specialist radiology and subsequent endoscopy and biopsy.

History. It is important to take a full history and listen to what the patient says. Patients will present with a variety of symptoms as described above but the most common symptom is hoarseness and of the many patients presenting to an ear, nose and throat (ENT) clinic with this symptom, approximately 1% will have a laryngeal cancer. Because of this screening programmes for early diagnosis are not effective, although rapid access clinics to evaluate the hoarse voice do play a role (Hoare *et al.*, 1993). The presence of other symptoms will help alert the clinician to the possibility of a laryngeal cancer.

Symptoms and signs of laryngeal carcinoma

- Progressive continuous hoarseness
- Dyspnoea and stridor
- Pain
- Dysphagia
- Swelling in the neck

The common presentation of hoarseness occurs because the most common site for the disease is on the vocal cord and any alterations in the surface of this structure cause early symptoms. The hoarseness is progressive and unremitting, although in the very early stages it is not uncommon for these symptoms to fluctuate. It is also important to remember that some of these cancers develop on a background of chronic laryngitis in individuals who smoke and these people are particularly at risk of delayed diagnosis.

Dyspnoea and stridor are less common symptoms but may be the presenting feature of a supraglottic carcinoma. In glottic and transglottic disease they may occur sequentially to progressive neglected dysphonia, when their presence usually indicates advanced disease. Such symptoms may be the only presenting feature of subglottic carcinoma.

Pain occurs somewhat uncommonly in laryngeal cancer and is a late symptom. It is more typical of supraglottic and transglottic lesions and pain referred to the ear is an ominous sign and usually indicates extensive disease with cartilage invasion. One should beware of the elderly smoker with unexplained otalgia who may have a small carcinoma tucked out of sight in the ventricle.

Dysphagia is again a relatively rare presenting symptom of laryngeal cancer. It indicates advanced disease with involvement of the pharynx and may be the presenting feature of tranglottic disease with extension into the medial wall of the piriform sinus through the paraglottic space, or conversely a so-called marginal lesion which arises on the medial wall of the piriform sinus and extends medially. In this situation dysphagia and pain normally precede the stridor.

Swelling in the neck can occur as a result or either cervical lymphadenopathy, direct extension of the disease into the thyroid gland or direct extension of the disease through the thyroid cartilage into the lateral part of the neck. Its presence is uncommon in the absence of other presenting symptoms and signs. Occasionally, patients may present with cough and irritation in the throat. These are early non-specific symptoms but the irritation is often lateralized and may be picked up by the suspicious clinician. Rarely, patients present with haemoptysis when bleeding occurs from the epiglottis and in late cases symptoms of fetor and/or anorexia may be apparent.

Examination. All patients require a general ENT examination and particular attention is focused on examination of the larynx. This may be performed using indirect laryngoscopy with a mirror, but more commonly nowadays, nasopharyngoscopy allows rapid examination of almost every patient to provide vital information in the clinical setting. Any focal abnormality seen within the larynx should be drawn in the notes. The typical glottic lesion is a warty enlargement on one vocal cord, but there may be a variety of lesions from a nodule or thickening extending through hyperkeratosis to gross ulceration. Such lesions may extend into the supraglottis and the subglottis. Within the supraglottis there may be localized swelling, inflammation or ulceration, while within the subglottis a mass may be seen. Videostroboscopy may be particularly helpful in this situation.

A number of stroboscopic parameters are evaluated in the assessment of vocal cord function (see box) but in early glottic cancer the fifth, sixth and seventh parameters are particulary important. The videostroboscopic assessment of vocal-cord tumours has been studied and the following benefits have been identified. It can provide information on detailed vibratory behaviour in cases with hoarseness to obtain a reasonable diagnosis, the exact identification of surface lesions on the vocal fold mucosa can be shown during vibration, information can be provided in the out-patient clinical setting and the need for a biopsy and finally documentation can be obtained on the superficial extent and infiltrative depth of early malignant lesions on the vocal fold.

- Fundamental frequency
- Bilateral symmetry
- Periodicity of successive vibrations
- Glottal closure
- Amplitude of vibration
- Mucosal wave
- Non-vibrating portion

Advantages of videostroboscopy

- Information on detailed vibratory behaviour
- Exact identification of surface tensions
- Information provided in out-patient setting
- Histology and documentation can be obtained on superficial extent and infiltrative depth of early malignant lesions

The subglottis is difficult to examine in the clinical setting but it may be done using the following technique. Local anaesthetic (lignocaine) may be injected using an orange needle through the cricothyroid membrane in the midline (2–3 ml of anaesthetic will suffice). This initiates a cough which then vaporizes the anaesthetic back through the subglottis and into the larynx; 5 min later, the flexible scope may be passed through the vocal cords and the subglottis and trachea examined with ease down to the carina. Another difficult area to see in the clinic is the posterior surface of the epiglottis and similarly the laryngeal ventricle is also quite difficult to see where the only hint of a cancer may be a slight fullness in this area. If there is any suspicion of a carcinoma lurking in these areas and, in particular, if there are associated symptoms such as earache, the patient requires an urgent laryngoscopy under general anaesthetic.

It is important to assess the mobility of the larynx. Movements of the vocal cords, the arytenoid joints and the whole hemilarynx should be assessed. The mobility of the medial visceral compartment of the neck upon the prevertebral fascia should be assessed along with the presence of laryngeal crepitus. Invasion of glottic cancer into the muscle layers of the vocal cord changes staging and carries a sinister prognosis, but occasionally mobility may be impaired by the sheer size of a tumour and this must be distinguished from actual deep invasion. Lesions of the supraglottis and subglottis may affect mobility by direct muscular invasion, cricoarytenoid joint involvement or rarely perineural spread and carry a grave prognosis.

Examination of the neck. This has been discussed in Chapter 12. Each side of the neck should be examined for palpable lymphadenopathy and particular attention paid to the first-echelon nodal draining areas in levels II,

III and IV. In addition, direct extension of tumour should be felt for extending either through or posterior to the thyroid cartilage, or in the subglottic area into the thyroid gland.

General examination. Any patient with a suspected head and neck malignancy, and certainly any patient undergoing a general anaesthetic, should have a general physical examination and it is important to assess the chest and abdomen to exclude any obvious signs of distant metastases. This will not be detailed further here.

Radiology. All patients with a laryngeal cancer and any patient undergoing general anaesthesia require a chest X-ray.

In the evaluation of a known laryngeal tumour, the best radiological examination to assess the size and extent of the lesion is to perform either CT or MRI. Many patients with early laryngeal cancer will be treated by either radiotherapy or endoscopic excision. In this situation, the primary tumour volume is small and the incidence of neck metastases is extremely low, so that routine scanning for assessment of tumour size, stage or preradiotherapy planning is not usually required.

Pretreatment scanning may be required to assess patients for conservation surgery, to assess advanced disease (prior to definitive surgery or radiotherapy) where the extent of the primary tumour is required and when extensive or bilateral nodal disease may preclude radical surgery. It is also required for preradiotherapy planning in organ preservation, or the high-dose palliative setting and may be used to assess the chest and upper abdomen for a second primary or distant metastases. The techniques, advantages and disadvantages of CT versus MRI in this setting are discussed in Chapter 3. When assessing tumour spread within the larynx it is important to be aware of whether or not the patient has had previous radiotherapy and the radiologist should pay particular attention to the preglottic and paraglottic spaces, the anterior subglottic wedge, actual tumour volume, vocal cord and hemilaryngeal mobility, extension of the tumour outside the larynx to include thyroid and cartilage invasion, assessment of the thyroid and strap muscles and either side of the neck.

Clinical investigations. Patients undergoing a general anaesthetic for laryngeal staging may require a full blood count and urea and electrolytes. It addition, in the assessment of advanced disease liver function tests and a serum calcium are appropriate.

Endoscopy and biopsy. The biopsy of a laryngeal tumour is obtained at direct laryngoscopy under general anaesthetic. This in itself may pose problems because the airway may be compromised and it requires careful co-operation between the surgeon and anaesthetist to achieve the staging endoscopy, obtain the biopsy and control the airway. The difficult airway is discussed below. If the patient does not have respiratory obstruction, the most satisfactory method is to examine the larynx under general anaesthetic using a small microlaryngoscopy tube or through a stiff wired catheter (the insufflation technique). This ensures a good airway and allows the anaesthetist to oxygenate the patient but because the catheter does not occupy all the lumen of the larynx it is possible to examine it satisfactorily. If the laryngoscopy tube is used, it may be removed during the procedure and replaced with a wide catheter. Small lesions can be examined without a tube using spontaneous shallow ventilation in a similar manner to laser laryngeal surgery with an oxygen cannula in the pharynx. Alternatively, the examination can be continued using jet insufflation (Venturi technique), particularly if bronchoscopy is being performed. At this point, the subglottis may be examined, the investigation continued and bronchoscopy carried out.

A laryngoscopy should not be confined to confirming that there is a tumour present and taking the biopsy. It is vital to establish the limits of the tumour in three dimensions and to record these in the notes. The important points are as follows.

In supraglottic tumours, it is important to know the size of the tumour and its extent. In an upward direction, does it extend into the vallecula and the pre-epiglottic space and is the tongue base involved? Is there any extension laterally into the medial wall of the piriform sinus or on to the lateral pharyngeal wall and is there any loss of laryngeal mobility indicating paraglottic space involvement? It is most important to know how close the tumour comes to the true cords, and in particular the anterior commissure.

Laryngoscopy for supraglottic tumours

- The size, site and extent of the tumour are determined
- The tumour may extend into the vallecula or pre-epiglottic space
- Tongue base involvement is checked for
- The tumour may extend laterally on to the lateral pharyngeal wall or medial wall of the piriform sinus
- The vocal cords are checked (including mobility)
- The paraglottic space may be involved
- The hypopharynx is examined
- The neck is felt
- A drawing is made

In glottic tumours, it is important to assess whether the tumour is exophytic, or whether there is any evidence of deep ulceration and infiltration and what is the apparent size of the tumour. Does the tumour spread to the anterior commissure and on to the vocal cord or posteriorly does it involve the vocal process and, in particular, is there any evidence of subglottic or supraglottic spread? To assess this, it is important to retract the false cords with the beak of the laryngoscope and inspect the ventricle. The examination may be completed

by the use of Hopkin's rods with a 30° angle-viewing telescope to assess ventricular spread more accurately. The anterior commissure laryngoscope should be used to inspect the subglottic space and the examination completed by examining both piriform fossae, postcricoid region and cervical oesophagus. Drawings of the exact extent of the tumour with measurements should be recorded in the notes on the appropriate prepared diagram.

Laryngoscopy for glottic tumours

- The size, site and extent of the tumour are determined
- The tumour may be exophytic
- Deep infiltration may be present
- Vocal-cord mobility is checked
- The tumour may spread anteriorly towards the anterior commissure or posteriorly on to the vocal process
- There may be supraglottic or subglottic spread
- The ventricle is checked
- The paraglottic space may be involved
- The hypopharynx is examined
- A biopsy is taken
- The neck is felt
- A drawing is made

For subglottic tumours, the site, size and extent of the tumour are assessed. This may be difficult and the paediatric endoscope or Hopkin's rods are useful here. Vocal-cord movement and transglottic spread are assessed. Any involvement of the tracheal party wall is noted and the cervical oesophagus inspected. Then, a biopsy is taken, the neck and thyroid are felt and a picture is drawn.

Laryngoscopy for subglottic tumours

- The appropriate instruments must be used
- The size, site and extent of the tumour are assessed
- Vocal-cord mobility is checked
- The paraglottic space may be involved
- The posterior tracheal wall and cervical oesophagus are assessed
- The neck and thyroid are felt
- A biopsy is taken
- A drawing is made

In the future, contact microendoscopy and contact videoendoscopy using Methylene Blue may be used to delineate the extent of early lesions along with their margins. This may be particularly useful prior to conservation endolaryngeal surgery.

The neck is examined and the larynx assessed for laryngeal crepitus, visceral mobility on the prevertebral fascia and tracheal mobility within the suprasternal notch, all of which may indicate signs of inoperability. Next, a biopsy of the tumour is taken, using as large a pair of forceps as possible and care is taken not crush the specimen. It is not necessary and indeed may be misleading to take a biopsy specimen including an area of apparently normal epithelium, because this may show only pre-malignant changes and lead to an indefinite report. Therefore, several biopsies are taken from the growing edge of the tumour, since material at the centre is often necrotic.

All tumours should be examined using this technique. In addition, for the assessment of smaller tumours in the glottis and supraglottis, particularly where conservation endolaryngeal surgery may be required, i.e. the treatment of the T_{1a} midcord lesion, microlaryngoscopy should also be used since it provides a more accurate assessment and staging, facilitates subsequent treatment and allows photodocumentation.

Stridor and the difficult airway

Some laryngeal tumours, in particular the transglottic tumour, present with stridor. This may be dealt with in a number of ways depending on the degree of the problem. Any patient with a laryngeal cancer who presents with stridor should be assessed by the most experienced surgeon available at the time in conjunction with an experienced anaesthetist.

Mild stridor indicates a potential airway problem. Consideration should be given to admitting the patient to hospital for observation, treatment of the compromised airway to include steroids, appropriate assessment before proceeding to urgent examination under anaesthesia (EUA) and biopsy, and management as appropriate. If the stridor is severe, then this may be dealt with in a number of ways depending on the degree of stridor, the setting in which the patient presents, the time of day at which the presentation occurs, the level of experience of staff that are available and whether or not a definitive biopsy has already been obtained. The following is not meant to be a protocol cookbook but more a guide on which treatment can be based depending on a number of patient, tumour and physician factors.

The safest option is to perform a tracheostomy. This should be done under local anaesthetic to secure the airway. An experienced anaesthetist may offer a light inhalational (sleep-dose) anaesthetic. Muscle relaxants must never be used in patients with compromised airways. In an emergency setting, a cricothyrotomy may be necessary to establish the airway. A subsequent general anaesthetic facilitates assessment of the tumour, biopsy as appropriate and debulking may be performed if the patient is going to undergo radiotherapy. The tracheostomy is performed in the conventional manner but consideration should be given to the siting of the tracheostomy because this technique has been implicated in an increased risk of stomal recurrence, although there is little evidence that this occurs. The following policy is recommended.

If the patient has a long, slim neck and it is possible to perform a tracheostomy safely below the tumour, then this should be the technique of choice. The surgeon must not go too low, so that when subsequent surgery is carried out, the tracheostomy track can then be excised within a Gluck–Sorenson incision and a stoma fashioned using healthy trachea below. If the patient has a short, stocky neck and if the tracheostomy is difficult then it may be necessary to make the tracheostomy high. The theoretical risk is of going through tumour. Even in this situation, however, unless there is extensive subglottic and upper trachea extension, such a technique will usually pass below the tumour. Following this technique, definitive surgery includes excision of the tracheostomy as part of the surgical specimen, and the use of healthy trachea to fashion the stoma.

A problem arises when a tracheostomy has been fashioned through tumour and the intended definitive treatment is radiotherapy, since in this setting it is unlikely to be curative. Therefore, if definitive treatment is planned and one needs to perform a tracheostomy, then the best form of treatment is surgery.

The second alternative is following experienced assessment, the patient is anaesthetized and the airway controlled with a small microlaryngoscopy tube. If there is any difficulty with this intubation then the surgeon may intubate the airway with either a tube, or a bronchoscope prior to passing the tube, or proceed to tracheostomy. Once the airway is controlled, the tumour is assessed, biopsies are taken and then the airway is debulked using the CO_2 laser, the patient is extubated under controlled situations and appropriate definitive treatment is planned.

In the past, some authors have suggested the performance of an emergency laryngectomy. This is defined as a total laryngectomy which is carried out within 24 hours of presentation. It is doubtful whether the patient can give true and informed consent in such circumstances and, furthermore, experience has shown that the mortality from this procedure is roughly the same as that from stomal recurrence if a preoperative tracheostomy is performed. While emergency laryngectomy is not normally an option, there may rarely be situations when a patient with laryngeal cancer (in whom the diagnosis is known and confirmed histologically) presents with significant stridor. If the situation allows where theatre space is available in the 24 h following admission, the appropriate surgical and anaesthetic staff are also available and true informed consent is achieved, it is reasonable to proceed to definitive laryngectomy. However, this should be re-defined as urgent laryngectomy rather than emergency laryngectomy.

In certain situations where the age and condition of the patient and the extent of the tumour dictate that no definitive treatment is indicated, then the appropriate palliative care should be undertaken, and the treating physician or surgeon may make the decision to treat airway obstruction conservatively. This is discussed under treatment policy.

Controversies in staging

There are a number of problems with the current staging system relating to laryngeal cancer and some of these have been referred to earlier in the text. For staging criteria to be successful they should be reproducible from one individual and one institution to another, and they should be uniformly applied and constant over a longitudinal time scale so that results can be analysed and validated to assess their prognostic significance. The first problem with the current staging system of laryngeal cancer is one of arbitrariness. This means that there are different criteria for the assignment of the same T stage which carry markedly differing prognoses. Take, for example, T_3 supraglottic cancer. The criteria for such a designation include a fixed cord, invasion of the pre-epiglottic space, involvement of the medial wall of the piriform sinus or postcricoid invasion. These four categories certainly do not carry the same prognosis, and data from the University of Florida show that one of the important prognostic factors on outcome in this disease is the size of the tumour. T_3 lesions <6 cm have a much higher control rate with radiotherapy than those that exceed this measurement.

The next problem is subjectivity. There are parameters within the current classification system where a high observer subjectivity rate may lead to a lack of reproducibility and bias. A classic example of this is mobility. Experienced observers disagree as to whether the cord is moving normally or whether its mobility is impaired. Such problems with staging can lead to both apparent upstaging and improvement in survival.

The other problem to consider is that of stage migration or the Will Rogers' phenomenon. The development of better imaging means that systematic upstaging of tumours will occur when imaging data are added, so that tumours are upstaged and apparent cure rates improve.

Finally, in the staging of laryngeal cancer, conventionally assigned Roman numeral groupings provide ambiguous heterogeneous aggregates of patients, since a T_3N_0 tumour is certainly not the same as a T_1N_2, yet both are stage III.

The definition of the inferior border of the glottis as a horizontal plane 1 cm inferior to the level of the upper surface of the vocal cord is most welcome. In the past, radiotherapy has been equally successful in treating both 'T_1' and 'T_2' lesions of the glottis, so defined when an early mucosal lesion has spread just

inferior to the phonating surface and is limited to the mucosa and has been classified as T_2 in the past. In the future most of these will be classed as T_1 and quite rightly so.

Within the T_2 classification there is no mention of bilateral disease with an 'a' and 'b' subclassification as there is in the T_1 section. Bilateral disease represents an increase in tumour volume requiring more extensive surgery or proving more resistant to radiotherapy and might be better classified as T_{2b}.

Within the T_3 glottic classification, there are two different types of tumour with two different prognoses, yet both are staged similarly. The T_3 lesion arising from the vocal-cord surface with some underlying vocalis muscle involvement producing cord fixation is a T_3 lesion by definition. This may be considered a favourable tumour since it may be treated with a high success rate with either vertical partial laryngectomy or radiotherapy and salvage. In contrast, an advanced transglottic T_3 lesion involving the free cord margin with supragottic and subglottic spread can infiltrate through the conus elasticus and treatment of this lesion by anything other than a total laryngectomy would be ill-advised.

Clinical surveys supplemented by laryngeal serial sectioned studies have highlighted that glottic cancers tend to spread horizontally but the more advanced and aggressive lesions also spread vertically. Subglottic spread greater than 1 cm is often associated with erosion into the thyroid and cricoid cartilages. In view of these findings not only should bilateral T_3 lesions be classified as T_{3b}, and when a tumour is limited to the glottis with a fixed cord it is glottic T_3, but when there is subglottic spread beyond 1 cm from the cord surface, the tumour should be classified as glottic–subglottic T_3 rather than T_4. A final point merits mention: the anterior subglottic wedge. Certain glottic cancers affecting the anterior commissure can bridge the gap between the anterior subglottic wedge and the epiglottis without affecting vocal-cord fixation. In this situation, a fronto-lateral laryngectomy may be contraindicated and some have suggested that these tumours should be classified as T_3 regardless of vocal-cord movements (Smee and Bridger, 1994).

Treatment policy

Over 95% of patients with laryngeal carcinoma are treatable. The causes of untreatability include distant metastases (less than 5%), poor general health along with rare refusal by the patient and those patients with advanced tumours that involve all compartments of the larynx with a fixed cord and bilateral nodes of which one side is fixed. These patients do very badly, having a 5 year survival of less than 5% compared with an overall 5 year survival of 55–60% in the UK. Radical surgery for these patients is therefore unjustified.

Treatment planning may fall into the following categories:

- curative intent:
  - surgery
  - radiotherapy (organ preservation) with or without chemotherapy
  - surgery with postoperative radiotherapy or chemo-radiotherapy
- rehabilitation
- palliation:
  - general palliative care, symptom control and nutritional support
  - tracheostomy
  - palliative surgery
  - radiotherapy
  - chemotherapy
  - radiotherapy and chemotherapy.

Treatment by curative intent

The treatment of laryngeal cancer depends on a number of factors which are shown below.

Treatment factors

- Age
- Performance status
- Treatment preference of the patient
- Any previous treatment
- Patient's distance from the treatment facility
- Follow-up reliability
- Physician's preference for treatment
- Availability of high-quality imaging
- Skilled pathology
- Skill of the surgeon

The management of laryngeal cancer varies in different parts of the world. Even within one country, opinions about the best management of particular situations varies, both between the principal specialities involved and also among individual practitioners. However, in some circumstances there is remarkable agreement; controversies are limited to particular areas.

For example, a recent survey compared the policies of both otolaryngologists and clinical oncologists in the management of glottic carcinoma of various stages. In total, 1649 clinicians in the UK, Scandinavia, Australasia and in North America, from the Province of Ontario and the states of Massachusetts and New York, were surveyed. In all disease situations opinions varied significantly with respect to the treatment modality advised (radiotherapy or surgery) and in more advanced stage disease there was controversy about laryngeal conservation.

In $T_1N_0 M_0$ glottic cancer, radical radiotherapy was recommended by 94% of oncologists and 81%

of otolaryngologists overall, with the remainder advocating larynx-conserving surgery. Despite the overwhelming majority of those surveyed recommending radiotherapy, there was geographical variation among otolaryngologists, with radiotherapy being favoured by 91% in the UK but only 58% in New York.

For $T_3N_0M_0$ glottic cancer there was greater disparity between specialities. Radiotherapy was recommended by 89% of oncologists but only 59% of surgeons. 18% of surgeons favoured larynx-conserving surgery and 23% preferred laryngectomy. Again there was no geographical diversity. More than 95% of oncologists in Scandinavia, Ontario and the UK recommended radiotherapy, compared with only about 75% in the USA and 84% in Australasia. Among surgeons, preference rates for conservation surgery varied from only 3% in the UK to 62% in New York. Detailed responses are shown in Table 14.6.

The policy in many centres in the UK is to irradiate virtually all tumours and to carry out a total laryngectomy for recurrent disease. While for small glottic tumours this is excellent treatment as the cure rate is very high, there are no controlled prospective trials comparing radiotherapy with surgery and there is now evidence that as the size of the tumour increases, it is possible to predict which tumours may not do well with radiotherapy and where primary conservation surgery, i.e. surgery without total laryngectomy, may be advantageous.

In continental Europe and North America, there is a more enthusiastic approach to conservation surgery, although there are no controlled trials showing that primary conservation surgery is any better than radiotherapy followed by partial or total laryngectomy for recurrence.

In summary, in the UK and throughout the world, the most popular treatment for T_1–T_3N_0 glottic and supraglottic carcinoma remains radical radiotherapy. The management of T_4N_0 cancer is more controversial, with some physicians in North America favouring organ preservation over total laryngectomy, and similarly the place of postoperative radiotherapy is also controversial (Table 14.7). These are discussed in turn in the treatment strategy below.

In coming to any conclusions, however, it should be remembered that one should ask whether there is enough information in the literature to permit a rational decision to substantiate that one treatment plan is better than another. Do different doctors in different specialities have different information at their disposal, or do they maintain different beliefs in the face of identical information? Do they agree about the probability of treatment outcomes but disagree about their relative value or utility, e.g. survival versus quality of life outcomes? Do they integrate information differently from one another and therefore reach different conclusions despite having identical information at their disposal? The answer to these question is that there is a striking lack of level I (randomized control trial)

Table 14.6 Treatment preferences in the management of glottic cancer

(a) Early laryngeal (glottic) cancer

Geographic region	Speciality	$T_1N_0M_0$ radiotherapy	$T_2N_0M_0$ radiotherapy
Ontario	Surgeons	48 (81)	56 (93)
	Oncologists	53 (93)	56 (98)
Scandinavia	Surgeons	29 (69)	40 (93)
	Oncologists	13 (68)	19 (100)
UK	Surgeons	239 (91)	257 (97)
	Oncologists	126 (96)	132 (99)
Australasia	Surgeons	47 (80)	44 (76)
	Oncologists	72 (96)	75 (100)
Massachusetts	Surgeons	37 (70)	36 (67)
	Oncologists	47 (94)	48 (96)
New York	Surgeons	34 (58)	3 (52)
	Oncologists	70 (96)	74 (99)
Subtotals	Surgeons	434 (81)	466 (86)
	Oncologists	381 (94)	404 (99)
Total		815 (87)	870 (91)

(b) $T_3N_0M_0$ cancer of the glottic larynx

Geographic region	Speciality	Radiotherapy	Conservation surgery	Total laryngectomy
Ontario	Surgeons	47(80)	5 (9)	7 (12)
	Oncologists	55 (97)	0 (0)	2 (4)
Scandinavia	Surgeons	34 (79)	5 (12)	4 (9)
	Oncologists	19 (100)	0 (0)	0 (0)
UK	Surgeons	209 (80)	7 (3)	46 (18)
	Oncologists	127 (96)	0 (0)	5 (4)
Australasia	Surgeons	17 (30)	13 (23)	27 (47)
	Oncologists	63 (84)	0 (0)	12 (16)
Massachusetts	Surgeons	10 (18)	24 (44)	21 (38)
	Oncologists	38 (78)	4 (8)	7 (14)
New York	Surgeons	5 (8)	41 (62)	20 (30)
	Oncologists	55 (73)	9 (12)	11 (15)
Subtotals	Surgeons	322 (59)	95 (18)	125 (23)
	Oncologists	357 (89)	13 (3)	32 (8)
Total		697 (72)	108 (11)	157 (17)

Data are shown as *n* (%).

evidence for the majority of decisions in head and neck cancer management. Doctors' decisions, beliefs, values and thought processes remain principally influenced by their own personal experience and previous education, along with the descriptive reports and what their colleagues teach. Unless the profession of head and neck oncology attempts to answer these questions and perform some controlled clinical trials (e.g. in the management of T_1 laryngeal cancer) to generate the necessary level I evidence, then it may be required to face some regulation in its practice in the future.

Treatment of glottic cancer

The treatment of laryngeal cancer depends on physician, patient and tumour factors. The selection of initial therapy depends on a combination of all of these and this has

already been referred to. In the early stages of glottic cancer (T_1 and T_2) the preferred treatment in many centres around the world is radiotherapy, particularly in those instances where the primary lesions are exophytic, there is no significant subglottic or supraglottic extension and the tumour does not extend to either the anterior commissure or the arytenoid. In these situations, cure rates with radiotherapy exceed 90% 5 year survival rates and the patient's voice should return to normal or near-normal. However, radiotherapy can produce a severe reaction which may lead in some patients to cartilage necrosis (particularly in those who smoke heavily, or have chronic laryngitis, nasal sepsis or chronic bronchitis). In this situation, particularly if the patient lives in an industrial area, good radiotherapy is not available or through patient preference, surgery may be considered. Surgical excision of T_1 glottic cancer confined to the vocal cord (known as the midcord lesion)

Table 14.7   Curative treatment of squamous cell carcinoma of the larynx

Glottis	N_0	N_1	N_2	N_3
T_1	Radiotherapy, ?endolaryngeal surgery (cordectomy for recurrence)	NA or surgery	NA or surgery	NA or surgery
T_2	Radiotherapy, ?hemilaryngectomy or TL + ?RT	TL + ?RT	NA or surgery	NA or surgery
T_3	? Radiotherapy, ?surgery (STL or TL + ?RT)	TL + ?RT	TL +RT	TL +RT
T_4	TL + RT	TL + RT	TL +RT	TL + RT
Supraglottis	N_0	N_1	N_2	N_3
T_1	Radiotherapy or endolaryngeal surgery	SGL + ?RT	SGL + RT	NA
T_2	Radiotherapy or surgery (SGL or TL) + ?RT	SGL or TL + ?RT	SGL or TL + RT	TL + RT
T_3	?Radiotherapy or surgery (SGL or TL) +?RT	SGL or TL + ?RT	SGL or TL + RT	TL + RT
T_4	Surgery + RT	TL + RT	TL + RT	TL +RT
Subglottis	N_0	N_1	N_2	N_3
T_1	Radiotherapy	TL + ?RT	TL + RT	TL + RT
T_2	Radiotherapy or surgery (TL)	TL + ?RT	TL + RT	TL + RT
T_3	Surgery (TL) + ?RT	TL + ?RT	TL + RT	TL + RT
T_4	Surgery (TL) + RT	TL + RT	TL + RT	TL + RT

NA: not usually applicable; SGL: supraglottic laryngectomy; TL: total laryngectomy; STL: subtotal laryngectomy; + RT: with elective postoperative radiotherapy; + ?RT: with postoperative radiotherapy in selected patients.

has cure rates similar to radiotherapy and may be performed using the laser or endolaryngeal scissors. Frozen section is mandatory and a tracheostomy is not normally required.

For those tumours that are multifocal or extend on to the contralateral cord (T_{1b}) where both vocal cords are mobile, radiotherapy is the preferred treatment and cure rates are no different for those with T_{1a} lesions. However, bilateral vocal-cord lesions that are strictly exophytic and keratotic in nature involving only the mucosa are probably managed best by endoscopic laser excision, which therefore avoids the need to irradiate the entire larynx and can offer excellent cure rates for well-differentiated hyperkeratotic lesions and *in situ* squamous cell carcinomas. The choice of treatment depends on many factors, but where voice quality is of paramount importance, one study has shown that the best results for voice follow radiotherapy rather than endoscopic surgery or cordectomy (Hirano, 1994). This is because surgical tissue loss causes postoperative air escape. However, there are almost no prospective controlled data addressing comparative voice outcomes for radiotherapy versus laser excision.

For T_2 laryngeal cancer, similar cure rates·can be obtained (80–90% 5 year survival) using either radiotherapy or surgery. Radiotherapy offers the advantages of better voice preservation but there are now recognized prognostic variables which can predict those patients who may do well with radiotherapy. These are shown below.

> **Prognostic variables related to a favourable outcome with radiotherapy**
>
> - Low tumour volume (tumours <3 cm^3 do better)
> - Mobile cord
> - No involvement of the ventricle
> - No deep ulceration
> - No fixation of anterior vocal cord
> - Lack of spread to subglottis or anterior subglottic wedge
> - Only one site involved
> - Cessation of smoking

There is, therefore, no need to justify the use of conservation surgery over radiotherapy in the management of T_2 laryngeal lesions, but rather those patients (particularly in the young) who may do poorly with radiotherapy should be targeted and offered primary surgery to include either a vertical hemilaryngectomy, extended vertical hemilaryngectomy, frontolateral or extended frontolateral partial laryngectomy. A tracheostomy is usually required, the operation is usually performed under frozen-section control, and postoperative irradiation should be considered if there are positive margins or previously unrecognized thyroid cartilage invasion on subsequent paraffin section analysis. As with radiotherapy, patients undergoing partial laryngeal surgery are advised to stop smoking.

With regard to the neck, in general T_1 and T_2 glottic carcinomas are not usually associated with any neck metastases. The primary echelon of nodal drainage is usually included in the radiotherapy portals and if surgery is undertaken then there is no place for elective neck dissection. Very rarely, N_1 neck disease is associated with an early glottic primary and in this situation, if the primary neoplasm is being treated with radiotherapy, then as long as the nodal disease is low volume (<2 cm) radiotherapy to the neck may be considered with salvage surgery in reserve.

An alternative is conservation surgery to the primary site and surgery to the neck, which would include a modified radical neck dissection types I, II or III or in some instances selective neck dissection may be considered at levels II, III and IV with or without postoperative radiotherapy, depending on the number of positive nodes harvested.

For those tumours that recur following radiotherapy, conservation surgery may still be an option. Patients may be considered for vertical laryngectomy if the criteria below are satisfied.

Glottic carcinoma: recurrence after radiotherapy

- The vocal cord remains mobile
- There is no more than 5 mm of subglottic spread
- There is no supraglottic or transglottic extension
- There is no involvement of more than between one-fifth and one-third of the contralateral cord
- There is no associated lymphadenopathy
- There should be no arytenoid involvement
- The patient's age and general condition should be considered
- Adequate pulmonary function is essential

In experienced hands, voice preservation and 5 year survival rates of 75% can be achieved (Shah *et al.*, 1990). However, few patients following radiotherapy will be suitable for salvage hemilaryngectomy and most will lose their larynx.

The treatment of T_3 glottic cancer is controversial. It is important to realize that there are two scenarios: the patient who has a small glottic cancer with infiltration of the vocal cord causing cord mobility with a low tumour volume, and the patient who presents with a large tumour mass which is transglottic and may or may not have stridor.

In the first case, a review of large series showed that cure rates are equal whether primary radiotherapy with salvage surgery is used or whether a primary surgical option is preferred. Indeed, Mendenhall *et al.* (1992) showed a 5 year cause-specific survival rate of 74% with irradiation alone and 63% for patients treated surgically and in another series (Jones *et al.*, 1990) the 5 year survival rate for radiotherapy was 70%, compared with surgery which was 40%. Although the data are retrospective, these studies show that patients with this type of tumour are probably best treated with initial radiotherapy as long as there are no nodes in the neck, since the surgical option is either an extended partial or total laryngectomy which can only offer cure

rates that are less good than radiotherapy and the voice quality will be much worse.

The patient with a transglottic T_3 glottic tumour and significant tumour volume has a high incidence of tumour metastases and is best treated with surgery. This will usually be with a total laryngectomy, with or without neck dissection, but in some institutions conservation surgery is proposed for selected T_3 glottic carcinomas using extended vertical partial laryngectomy or subtotal laryngectomy with cricohyoid epiglottopexy. Chevalier and Peak (Smee and Bridger, 1994) reported 123 cases of subtotal laryngectomy with cricohyoid epiglottopexy for patients with glottic carcinomas, of which 16 had T_3 carcinomas. The survival rate for the whole group at 5 years was 79% and there was no difference between the different tumour size groups, although the numbers were too small for statistical analysis. The operative technique consists of removal of the thyroid cartilage, both true and false vocal cords, the paraglottic space and the epiglottis, with preservation of the cricoid cartilage, one arytenoid and the hyoid bone. After closure, the cricoid comes into contact with the base of the tongue and the term cricohyoid epiglotopexy explains the mode of reconstruction. This operation has some enthusiastic supporters but it is technically difficult, the oncological margins are small and further results are awaited to see whether this operation is superior to total laryngectomy with subsequent voice restoration.

Advanced glottic cancer (T_3,N_+ and T_4) is usually treated in the majority of centres by total laryngectomy. In other words, the operation is indicated for those tumours that are advanced with cartilage destruction of both the thyroid and the cricoid cartilages, where there is anterior extralaryngeal spread into the anterior subglottic wedge and where there is involvement of the posterior commissure, fixation of the arytenoid or bilateral arytenoid tumour distribution. It is also carried out for circumferential disease with or without bilateral vocal-cord fixation or paralysis along with involvement of the medial wall of the piriform sinus or postcricoid region and the tongue base. Treatment of a patient with stridor has already been discussed, so that the patient may or may not have a tracheostomy at the time of surgery.

An alternative to total laryngectomy in experienced hands is a near-total laryngectomy, which is a voice-preserving operation designed for resection of selected, advanced unilateral carcinomas involving the larynx. It may be performed for unilateral T_3 and T_4 glottic and transglottic carcinomas. It is a complex operative procedure, the patient has a permanent tracheostome and local control rates appear to match those of total laryngectomy. Despite the enthusiasm of certain workers who have popularized this work over many years, the operation has not been universally accepted and there is no evidence that it has any advantages over total laryngectomy and subsequent voice restoration. Aspiration and shunt stenosis are its major complications.

In those patients with advanced laryngeal cancer who do not want surgery, who wish to keep their larynx or who are not a surgical option, organ preservation may be used using radiotherapy alone or more recently radiotherapy with adjuvant or neoadjuvant chemotherapy. Radiotherapy alone (either conventionally fractionated or CHART) can give 3 year local control rates of approximately 50%. The well-publicised VA Laryngeal Cancer Study Group on Neo-adjuvant Chemotherapy for organ preservation has shown that approximately 30–40 % of patients can be expected to survive with a preserved larynx although, like previous neoadjuvant trials, the VA trial failed to demonstrate that the addition of two or three cycles of chemotherapy (cisplatin and 5-flurouracil) improved survival or disease-free intervals. In addition, chemoradiotherapy was not compared with radiotherapy alone. In this study, retrospective analysis determined that small tumour size, aggressive infiltrating histology and increased DNA content were associated with a response to chemotherapy and in the future, identification of these patients may select those who might benefit from treatment.

Supraglottic laryngeal cancer

In general, single-modality therapy using usually radiotherapy or sometimes surgery by partial laryngectomy is the usual treatment for stage I and stage II (T_1/T_2N_0) supraglottic cancer. In the UK, the majority of patients receives radiotherapy, although controversy exists throughout the world regarding the merits of either of these treatment modalities and patients should be made aware that cure is possible with either of them with cure rates that approach 80–90% 5 year survival. Single-modality treatment involves less morbidity and cost and is used in the majority of localised stage I and stage II supraglottic cancer. In the UK, radiotherapy is also usually used for the majority of T_3N_0 supraglottic laryngeal cancers. In certain instances, the role of radiotherapy may be considered in the treatment of N_1 disease, although this is controversial, as indeed is the ability of radiotherapy alone to offer adequate cure for T_3 supraglottic disease.

T_1 and T_2 epiglottic tumours should be treated by radiotherapy with careful follow-up and salvage total laryngectomy for recurrence. This policy gives results that are as good as primary surgery, with the advantage that two patients out of three retain their larynx unless the ini-

tial operation that was to be offered as an alternative to radiotherapy was a supraglottic partial laryngectomy. If there are palpable lymph nodes in the neck then the patient should be treated by surgery, either a supraglottic or total laryngectomy.

A supraglottic partial laryngectomy may be performed as long as the tumour does not involve the true vocal cords, as long as the true vocal cords are mobile and there is no cartilage destruction (Fig. 14.5). There should be no paraglottic space involvement but involvement of the pre-epiglottic space does not necessarily preclude partial laryngeal surgery. If the tumour extends into the tongue base, a total laryngectomy should be performed and this should also be done if the patient is over 70 years old and in those who have chronic obstructive airways disease since they will experience difficulty with postoperative aspiration and swallowing. A total laryngectomy will usually be necessary for those tumours that recur after radiotherapy.

Partial supraglottic laryngectomy: indications

■ No vocal cord involvement
■ Normal vocal cord mobility
■ No cartilage destruction
■ No paraglottic space involvement
■ No significant pre-epiglottic space involvement
■ Absence of tongue-base involvement
■ Not usually indicated after radiotherapy
■ Age 70 years or less
■ Good cardiopulmonary reserve
■ Experienced surgeon

In exceptional circumstances, a supraglottic laryngectomy may be considered if the primary lesion was, and

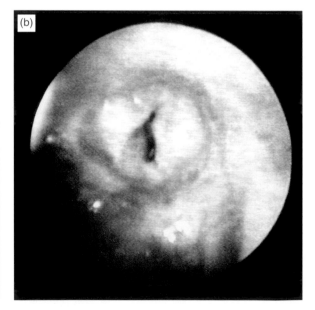

Figure 14.5 T_2N_0 squamous cell carcinoma of the supraglottic larynx. The CT scan shows no extension into the pre-epiglottic space. (a) Treatment was with supraglottic laryngectomy and left selective neck dissection (levels II–IV). (b) The final result.

still is, small and confined to the anterior laryngeal vestibule and was free of the anterior commissure at the start of radiotherapy. In addition, the lesion should be well differentiated, and the patient should have good cardiopulmonary reserve and be aged 70 years or less. Sometimes other factors dictate partial surgery, such as refusal of total laryngectomy in a borderline patient or a similar situation in a professional voice user (Shaw, 1991).

In summary, a supraglottic laryngectomy should only be advised if the conditions are ideal and the patient is suitable, since the results of total laryngectomy are excellent whereas the results of a partial laryngectomy performed on the wrong patient for the wrong reasons can be disastrous.

An alternative to radiotherapy in early supraglottic disease is endoscopic laser supraglottic laryngectomy. This may be done as a method to improve the airway of a patient with invasive squamous cell carcinoma prior to definitive treatment with radiotherapy. It is indicated in the treatment of T_{is} supraglottic tumours (carcinoma *in situ*), should be considered adequate treatment for T_1 disease only and should be viewed with caution for more advanced disease, although there are those who use endoscopic laser surgery for advanced T_2 and T_3 supraglottic laryngeal cancer with good results, but with quite high recurrence rates (approximately 20%) requiring further salvage surgery (Steiner and Ambrosch, 1996).

Tumours of the aryepiglottic fold will often extend into the pre-epiglottic space and many of these have lymph nodes in the neck. Radiotherapy is therefore not advisable in these situations and the patients should usually have surgery. These patients do well with a partial supraglottic laryngectomy including the removal of one arytenoid since the only alternative is a total laryngectomy and partial pharyngectomy. A horizontal supraglottic laryngectomy may be indicated in certain high-volume T_1 and T_2 supraglottic cancers (greater than 3 cm^3 in size) but also those T_3 supraglottic tumours without extension into the vocal cord and those with limited pre-epiglottic space involvement or extension into the piriform sinus above the level of the vocal cords. Once the arytenoid is involved, it has to be removed, which increases the risk of aspiration and subsequent local impairment. As previously stated, general health and good pulmonary reserve are essential for this sort of surgery, a tracheostomy is required, a preoperative percutaneous gastrostomy (PEG) is usually placed and the tumour should be assessed at endoscopy and with suitable radiology.

Tumours of the false cord are unfortunately increasing in incidence and are quite difficult to treat. They often involve the true vocal cords and are therefore seldom suitable for partial laryngectomy. Since the only surgical treatment available is a total laryngectomy, patients with these tumours are best treated with radiotherapy and should be followed very closely since they may develop an enlarged lymph node needing subsequent neck surgery; and if there is recurrence at the primary site, they will require a total laryngectomy. Using this policy, many patients retain their larynx. Many patients with advanced supraglottic laryn-

geal cancer (T_3 and T_4) require a total laryngectomy. This will include all T_3 supraglottic cancers which are not amenable to supraglottic laryngectomy described above and all T_4 supraglottic cancers exhibiting thyroid or cricoid cartilage invasion, extension to the soft tissues of the neck, the apex of the pyriform sinus or beyond the posterior third of the tongue base. A favourable T_3 supraglottic cancer that may be considered for conservation surgery, including those with vocal-cord fixation due to aryepiglottic fold involvement, some cases with pre-epiglottic space invasion and hypopharyngeal extension when the medial piriform sinus is minimally involved. Otherwise, radical surgery should be considered.

In certain instances when the tumour does not involve one vocal cord, a near-total laryngectomy is an appropriate alternative and, similarly, supracricoid partial laryngectomy may be used for a supraglottic transglottic tumour with one mobile arytenoid even when vocal-cord movement is decreased.

In patients with stage III and stage IV supraglottic laryngeal cancer who decline surgery, are not suitable for surgery or wish to retain their larynx, radiotherapy plus chemotherapy has been shown in a controlled randomized trial to provide survival which is equal to surgery plus postoperative radiotherapy. Such treatment should be carried out in the context of carefully controlled clinical trials.

There is a high incidence of occult metastases in cases of supraglottic cancer so that treatment of the neck should be considered for those tumours that are T_2 and above. If the primary tumour is being treated by radiotherapy, then the primary echelon nodes in levels II, III and IV should be treated prophylactically and, as there is a high risk of bilateral spread in these cases, treatment should include both sides of the neck. When a primary tumour is being treated surgically, in the N_0 neck a selective neck dissection should be performed at levels II–IV. Limited N_1 disease may be treated using usually a modified radical neck dissection, although selective neck dissection as described above may be used when there is only one node palpable in level II, III or IV and postoperative radiation is to be given. For N_2 and N_3 disease, a modified radical neck or radical neck dissection should be performed.

Subglottic tumours are relatively uncommon, forming approximately 5% of patients with laryngeal cancer. There has been some debate about whether these tumours actually exist, since on previous staging criteria many probably included direct extension from primary glottic cancer.

Although there have been attempts to perform infraglottic partial laryngectomy by removing the lower half of the thyroid cartilage and the cricoid cartilage, and later joining the trachea to the remaining thyroid cartilage, this operation is impractical and the only safe operation for a patient who has this uncommon tumour is a total laryngectomy and partial thyroidectomy. Because this inevitably means the patient loses their voice, it is preferable in early T_1 and T_2 subglottic cancer to treat these patients with radiotherapy, careful follow-up and salvage surgery, but with advanced disease, recurrent disease

who have had preoperative radiotherapy, the internal jugular vein may be encountered surprisingly early as it is often pulled forward by adhesions. The surgeon dissects posteriorly to identify the carotid artery and this is retracted laterally along with the internal jugular vein. The omohyoid muscle is divided (usually through its tendon) and the short middle thyroid vein is ligated. These manoeuvres allow access to the paracarotid tunnel, which should be dissected down to the clavicle and up to the hyoid bone. The branches of the anterior jugular veins are tied on the side on which the thyroid lobe is to be removed and the inferior thyroid artery is ligated. In the upper part of the dissection, the superior thyroid pedicle is identified and ligated, with care being taken to identify and preserve the hypoglossal nerve. This structure should not be confused with the superior laryngeal nerve, which is encountered 1 cm lower as it passes medially to the thyrohyoid membrane. The hypoglossal nerve is often pulled inferiorly in patients who have had radiotherapy. It lies very close to the greater horn of the hyoid bone and failure to identify it may lead to damage during laryngeal mobilization. Hypoglossal damage greatly reduces swallowing performance postlaryngectomy. The nerve is usually identified as it lies in close relationship to the common facial vein where it joins the internal jugular vein, and ligation of this structure leads one to the nerve.

Next, the strap muscles are divided inferiorly immediately above the sternum (Fig. 14.9) and superiorly just above the hyoid bone. Dissection continues through the fat lateral to the trachea until the tracheal wall is exposed. At this point it is important to perform a level IV and level VI dissection. The paratracheal chain of nodes is dissected out and followed down into the superior mediastinum. This is a common place for recurrence and one often finds occult nodal disease in nodes within the subsequent specimen at this point. It is also a good opportunity to practise exposure of the recurrent laryngeal nerve, lying as it does in the tracheo-oesophageal groove.

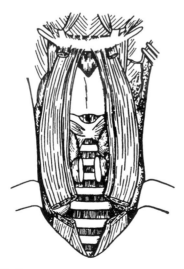

Figure 14.9 Total laryngectomy: division of strap muscles and thyroid isthmus.

The nerve is divided and the groove dissected separating the posterior membranous wall of the trachea from the oesophagus. It is important to do only as much dissection as is necessary here so to avoid damage to the oesophageal wall, creating any dead space or comprising the party wall lower down, which may be subsequently required for planned primary tracheo-oesophageal puncture.

In the upper part of the dissection, the hyoid bone is mobilized and its body grasped in a pair of Allis forceps. Having divided the muscles close above the hyoid bone, using traction and countertraction, the tongue base and pharyngeal mucosa are identified above the pre-epiglottic space. No attempt is made to preserve any part of the hyoid bone.

The inferior thyroid veins and both superior thyroid arteries and veins are ligated. The inferior thyroid artery on the side opposite from the tumour is preserved as this is the only blood supply to both the remaining thyroid lobe and parathyroids. This lobe is now mobilized by dividing the isthmus and peeling it laterally off the trachea, dividing the numerous small vessels that run into the thyroid gland here with cutting diathermy. Lastly, the surgeon divides the ligament of Berry which is the condensation of pretracheal fascia which tethers the thyroid posteriorly to the trachea and which is intimately related to the recurrent laryngeal nerve at this point. The strap muscles are dissected off the retained thyroid lobe and left in continuity with the specimen. This is the only point during the operation at which it is justifiable to dissect the strap muscles. If there is any doubt about whether or not the tumour may have spread into the contralateral thyroid lobe or if one is dealing with subglottic cancer, a total thyroidectomy should be performed. It is much easier to give the patient thyroid and calcium supplements then to salvage them from recurrent disease.

Division of the trachea (Fig. 14.10)

The surgeon ligates the inferior thyroid veins and the trachea is divided and the airway secured. The cervical trachea is then mobilized by dissecting in the plane between the trachea and the oesophagus. Care is taken not to mobilize these two structures from each other too far below the resection point as this can devascularize the remaining trachea. If a cervical neck 'H' incision is being used, the position of the skin flap for the final tracheostomy should now be estimated and a hole made at this site about 2.5 cm in diameter by developing the lower flap.

The anaesthetist must be ready to change the connections, the anaesthetic connecting tube stitched on the chest at the beginning of the operation must still be in a good position, and a tracheostomy or an endotracheal tube of appropriate size must be available with its cuff having been tested and then deflated. The trachea is then divided. In the past, surgeons were advised the trachea should be bevelled from below upwards so that the end of the trachea will be vertical when it is swung forwards. However, this technique cuts through cartilage, which often then becomes necrotic and is then expelled and can

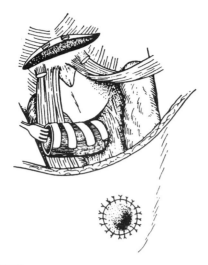

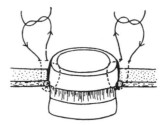

Figure 14.11   Method of suture for the tracheostome.

Figure 14.10   Total laryngectomy: the trachea is divided and the stoma may be created either within the incision line or separately using the a 'H' incision as shown above.

lead to stomal stenosis. It is much better to divide cleanly through one of the spaces between the tracheal rings, especially if there is plenty of trachea to deal with. The extent of tracheal resection should be determined by the extent of any subglottic spread. However, if there is disease in the subglottis and upper trachea, the trachea may be resected down to the level of the suprasternal notch. It may be then mobilised down to the carina to facilitate formation of the trachestome.

If the anaesthetist has removed the endotracheal tube and the oesophagus has been mobilized from the trachea, the trachea can be divided in one movement at this point. It may be pulled forwards through the hole in the lower skin flap or sewn to the lower flap if a Gluck–Sorenson incision is used. A small swab is placed in the laryngeal remnant to prevent contaminated secretions running down into the wound. A cuffed tube is placed in the trachea and linked to the corrugated anaesthetic connector that was placed on the chest at the start of the operation to continue ventilation.

Making the stoma is an important part of the operation and can be done in either one or two layers to ensure an airtight junction. Chromic catgut or vicryl sutures (3/0) can be used to stitch the peritracheal fascia to the subcutaneous tissues in the lower skin flap. This leaves a small excess of trachea projecting above the level of the skin which will provide an airtight closure of subcutaneous tissue to peritracheal fascia (Fig. 14.11). This can be sewn in with a non-absorbable suture [Ethilon or Prolene (2.0)]. Alternatively, a one-layer silk (2.0) closure may be performed.

Removal of the larynx

The larynx can be removed from below upwards or above downwards, but the latter is safer because the inside of the larynx can be seen and there is no danger of cutting into the tumour.

The body of the hyoid bone is grasped with a heavy artery or Kocher's toothed forceps and pulled forwards. With cutting diathermy, the surgeon cuts through the base of the tongue and enters the pharynx on the contralateral side to the tumour. Beginners are often surprised at how deep they have to go to enter the pharynx. Care is taken at this point not to open into the pre-epiglottic space. This is avoided by a high pharyngeal entry. As soon as the pharynx is opened, the tumour is inspected and the first assistant retracts the base of the tongue with a retractor placed through the hole in the pharyngeal mucosa. In supraglottic tumours with tongue-base extension, the tongue is retracted on the contralateral side and the tumour excised under direct vision. Then, the tip of the epiglottis is grasped with Allis forceps and pulled anteriorly and inferiorly. The pharyngeal mucosa is cut with scissors laterally on each side of the epiglottis, aiming towards the superior cornu of the thyroid cartilage.

The surgeon now changes position and stands at the head of the table, so that he or she can see downwards into the larynx. The epiglottis is held with the Allis forceps and pulled forwards by an assistant, and the larynx is released by dividing the constrictor muscles along the posterior edge of the thyroid cartilage with either cutting diathermy or scissors. Then, the pharyngeal mucosa is divided on each side in the region of the superior cornu of the thyroid cartilage, aiming downwards for the posterior part of the arytenoid cartilage.

These two cuts are joined posteriorly, inferior to the cricoarytenoid joint, where there is a good plane of cleavage on the posterior cricoarytenoid muscle. Care is taken to keep below the cricoarytenoid joint and its overlying mucosa, because cancer can spread posteriorly through this joint. By following this plane downwards between the trachea and the oesophagus the larynx can be removed. The lobe of the thyroid gland which it is intended to preserve must not be removed by careless dissection during this stage. The retained lobe of the thyroid gland must be well clear of the tracheostomy or it may cause tracheal stenosis.

If a sucker is put into the lumen of the pharynx during removal of the larynx, it should not be allowed it to be taken out since it prevents cancer cells being spilled into the tissues of the neck. Contamination of the wound with instruments or suckers that have been used during removal of the tumour can be avoided by placing them in a separate receiver and discarding after removal of the tumour.

If primary voice restoration is to be carried out, a posterior midline cricopharyngeal myotomy is now performed (Fig. 14.12). A fistula is made between the upper oesophagus and the tracheostome using a knife with a no. 15 blade and a Foley catheter (size 14) inserted to facilitate postoperative feeding. It is important at this point not to mobilize the upper oesophagus off the posterior tracheal wall as this leads to increased fistula formation and devascularization of the trachea.

Repair of the pharynx (Fig. 14.13)

After the larynx has been removed, gloves and instruments are changed. The wound is then irrigated.

Depending on the amount and length of the pharyngeal remnant, various types of pharyngeal repair are now possible. The simplest and most effective method is to perform a straight-line closure in three layers. Before starting to close the pharynx, if primary voice restoration has not been performed, a nasogastric tube is passed and confirmation is obtained that it is in the oesophagus. If the mucosal edges are lacerated or have holes in them, the edges are tidied up. Damaged mucosa must not be used for the closure. In the irradiated patient or if some pharyngeal mucosa has been removed, at this point consideration is given as to whether augmentation is required using either myocutaneous flap (pectoralis major or latissimus dorsi) or free flap.

For a simple pharyngeal closure the surgeon starts at the lower end of the pharyngeal defect using a 3.0 Vicryl suture (or alternatively catgut) and uses a running extra-mucosal Connell stitch which picks up the edges of the pharyngeal mucosa but does not pierce the mucosa, (so that the submucosal edges stick together) and provides an inverting suture. This is continued upwards and then may be tied a one-third of the way up and then continued; this repeated once more until the top is reached. One layer is now completed and the defect has been closed in a straight line with no three-point junction. This layer may be enforced using a second layer taking the fascia and then the third layer using the constrictor muscles. At this point, it is important to note that a tight, efficient closure reduces the fistula rate but may compound subsequent development of good oesophageal speech by creating a tight hypertonic neopharynx. In this situation, some surgeons advocate a one-layer mucosa only closure in the lower third of the defect.

Alternative techniques for closure include a T-shape repair, but this inevitably produces a three-point junction, which is poor surgical technique and may be one of the factors which causes a fistula. However, in some situations a T-shape closure is the only one possible and as long as it is repaired properly, there is no evidence that the fistula rate is any higher using this technique.

Finally, in patients with short necks and redundant mucosa, it may be possible to perform a transverse straight-line closure, which is reported to offer significant advantages for postoperative voice restoration within the neopharynx. In contrast to the other techniques, it does not create a neoepiglottis.

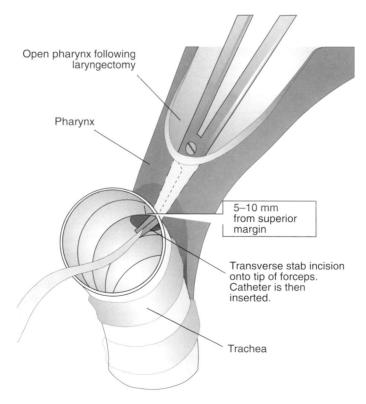

Open pharynx following laryngectomy

Pharynx

5–10 mm from superior margin

Transverse stab incision onto tip of forceps. Catheter is then inserted.

Trachea

Figure 14.12 Technique for primary voice puncture.

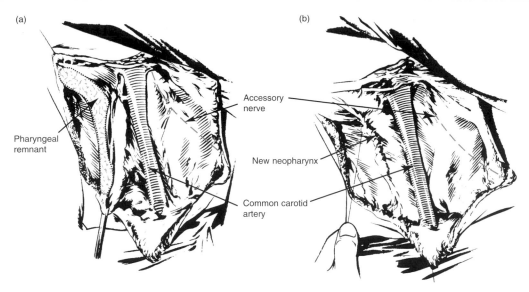

(a)

Pharyngeal
remnant

(b)

Accessory
nerve

New neopharynx

Common carotid
artery

Figure 14.13 Total laryngectomy: pharyngeal repair. (a) The pharyngeal defect; (b) the repair, using the straight-line technique. Alternatively, the defect may be closed in a 'T' fashion.

Closure

Two suction drains are placed without crossing the neopharynx and the skin is closed in two layers using Vicryl for platysma and either Ethilon or clips for the skin.

Total laryngectomy: handy hints

- Patients should be selected carefully
- The incision should be well thought out
- A good assistant is necessary
- The paracarotid tunnel should be entered early
- One should aim to encompass the whole tumour
- The inferior and superior thyroid arteries must be ligated
- The hypoglossal nerves must not be damaged
- The strap muscles are divided
- The hyoid is detached and the pharynx entered high away from the tumour
- The pre-epiglottic space must not be entered
- When dealing with the thyroid the parathyroids should be preserved if possible
- Levels IV and VI are dissected routinely
- The trachea is divided with minimal dissection of the tracheo-oesophageal wall
- Care is taken with tracheo-oesophageal puncture
- The tumour should be resected under direct vision
- Meticulous closure is important

Specific aftercare

Patients are covered with prophylactic antibiotics for at least 48 h after the pharynx has been entered and kept nil by mouth for 7 days, after which a soft diet is introduced. Feeding is done via the nasogastric tube or the stomogastric tube used for primary voice restoration.

One of the most important parts of rehabilitation of a patient after total laryngectomy is voice restoration. If primary voice restoration is not carried out, then this may be done by anticipated secondary tracheo-oesophageal puncture, oesophageal speech or by various artificial devices. Rehabilitation of speech is discussed in Chapter 18.

The majority of patients in the UK will undergo voice rehabilitation following total laryngectomy using either primary or secondary surgical voice restoration. However, in certain instances oesophageal speech will be the method chosen. Although the voice achieved by this method can be very good, it is naturally never as good as the normal voice and many women dislike it because it sounds gruff and masculine. However, many men who need their voice for work have successfully returned to full employment using this method. The principle of oesophageal speech is that the air is passed into the oesophagus either by swallowing or by pressing with the tongue, and is then regurgitated so that it causes the cricopharyngeus or other pharyngeal structures to vibrate, producing a sound that is modulated by the articulating mechanism in the usual way. It is thought that development of good oesophageal voice depends on the following factors: gender, age (elderly patients sometimes do not bother to develop this type of voice), motivation, intelligence, local factors in the pharynx (such as scarring), the formation of diverticula and the shape of the pharynx (a wide pharynx is thought to be necessary), and the condition of the oesophagus since if the patient has a hiatus hernia he or she may find it difficult to control the airstream in the oesophagus.

Good oesophageal speech depends on:

- Gender
- Age
- Motivation
- Intelligence
- Local factors in the pharynx
- State of the oesophagus

It is difficult to assess how many patients develop a satisfactory oesophageal voice. Although more than 60% may do so given intensive treatment, this is not the usual figure. Certainly very good results can be obtained by keeping the patient in hospital until he or she has developed satisfactory speech and giving lessons two or three times a day. This system is used in The Netherlands with extremely good results, but in countries with limited facilities, particularly in the UK, where this is not possible, the results are not nearly so good and probably no more than one-third develop really satisfactory speech. For these patients, various alternatives are available. These include external machines that produce a sound which the patient can then modify by articulation. Such machines include the Cooper Rand electronic speech aid, the Servox transcervical vibrator, the Tait oral vibrator mounted on a dental plate and the Bart's vibrator. Most of these devices consist of a machine held to the patient's throat which produces a buzzing sound. The theory is that the patient then modifies the sound by articulation to produce intelligible speech; in practice, the noise produced is monotonous, metallic and often scarcely intelligible to the unaccustomed listener.

Complications

■ Fistula: this is dealt with in Chapter 6
■ Stenosis of the pharynx: this usually responds to dilatation which may be by bouginage under general anaesthesia. In patients in whom recurrence has been excluded, good results can be obtained from balloon dilatation by an interested radiologist. On occasions, pharyngeal augmentation with either a pectoralis major or latissimus dorsi flap will be required. Residual or recurrent disease should be excluded
■ Stenosis of the tracheostome (see later)
■ Recurrence within the pharynx or the site of the tracheostomy: recurrence within the pharynx is unlikely to respond to radiotherapy and if resectable, patients should undergo a neopharyngectomy and free jejunal transfer
■ Stomal recurrence has four recognized causes:
 – implantation into the tract of a preoperative tracheostomy
 – inadequate incision
 – tumour in the paratracheal nodes
 – second tumour in the cervical trachea

If the recurrence invades the anterior part of the stoma, it is virtually always untreatable because the lesion on the surface is the tip of the iceberg wrapped around the great vessels in the mediastinum. If the lesion affects the upper, posterior part of the stoma it may rarely be managed successfully by a thoracotracheostomal resection (see later).

Operative technique of supraglottic laryngectomy

Anaesthetic

A general anaesthetic with endotracheal intubation is used for the prior neck dissection, a tracheostomy is performed just before the laryngectomy and the anaesthetic is continued through this. If the patient needs a PEG, this can be performed now.

Incision and neck dissection

Halfway through, this operation may need to be modified to a total laryngectomy and also a contralateral neck dissection may also be required. For these reasons, a collar incision with two lateral limbs is used, as described previously; this meets all eventualities. As the operation is not usually indicated following failed radiotherapy, this problem need not be considered.

The flaps are elevated and stitched in the usual way. The appropriate neck dissection is carried out, leaving the specimen attached by the superior lymphatic pedicle. The thyroid gland should not be included in the neck dissection as this is unnecessary, and exposes the recurrent laryngeal nerve to possible damage. Care is taken not to injure the vagus nerve, as paralysed vocal cords after a supraglottic laryngectomy are a tragedy that may well end with the patient requiring total laryngectomy because of aspiration.

Mobilization of the supraglottic larynx

The principle of this part of the operation is to mobilize all of the supraglottic larynx in continuity with the pre-epiglottic space and associated lymph nodes.

The strap muscles are divided (Fig. 14.14) on both sides at the level of the superior border of the thyroid cartilage and turned down to the lower border of the cartilage. In the midline, the lower border of the thyroid cartilage and the notch on the upper border are identified. This distance is measured and a mark made halfway between the two points with Methylene Blue. This marks the position of the anterior commissure in men. In women, the commissure is slightly higher, being one third of the distance between the two above points from the notch. From this point, a horizontal line is marked posteriorly along the cartilage perpendicular to the posterior edge of the thyroid cartilage, using needles soaked in dye. The surgeon cuts through the perichondrium along the upper edge of the cartilage and elevates it down to the level of the marks in the cartilage (Fig. 14.15). Care is taken not to tear the perichondrium, which is particularly likely to happen in the midline where it is very thin.

With a Stryker saw or dental fissure burr the cartilage is divided along the line marked with dye, taking care to divide only the cartilage and not the mucosa of the larynx. Both sides of the thyroid cartilage are divided. Next, the muscles attached to the upper border of the hyoid bone are divided. The superior thyroid artery and vein are divided and transfixed on either one or both sides, depending on the extent of the operation.

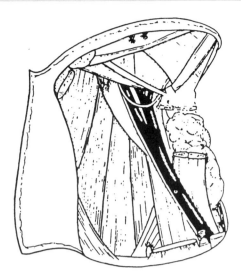

Figure 14.14 Supraglottic laryngectomy: division of strap muscles.

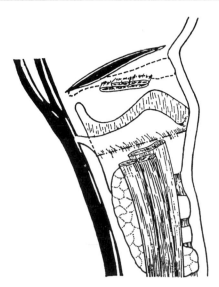

Figure 14.16 Supraglottic laryngectomy: entry to vallecula.

Removing the tumour (Figs 14.16 and 14.17)

This step is best carried out from the top of the table and it is wise at this stage to wear a headlight. The surgeon cuts down with scissors towards the vallecula, just above the hyoid bone, on the side of the neck dissection and enters into the pharynx. If there is a tumour in the vallecula then the pharynx is entered through the piriform fossa on the side of the neck dissection. The mucosa is divided at the base of the tongue with scissors, with the surgeon working from side to side through the vallecula, keeping well clear of the tumour. The base of the tongue is retracted and the epiglottis held forward with Allis forceps. Standing at the head of the table the surgeon can now look down into the larynx and assess the extent of the tumour accurately.

For an epiglottic tumour, each aryepiglottic fold is divided immediately anterosuperior to the arytenoid

cartilage, well clear of tumour; for a tumour on the aryepiglottic fold, the uninvolved side is divided above the arytenoid cartilage but, on the side of the tumour, incision is made through the cricoarytenoid joint.

It is now necessary to see the ventricles, so the assistant retracts the arytenoids laterally with two skin hooks. One blade of the scissors is placed inside the ventricle superior to the vocal cord and the other blade outside the thyroid cartilage opposite the incision in the cartilage. The cuts are carried forward through the ventricles and the specimen and the neck dissection are removed in continuity (Figs 14.18 and 14.19).

Cricopharyngeal myotomy (Fig. 14.20)

The next step of the operation is to divide the cricopharyngeus muscle. The surgeon passes a finger into

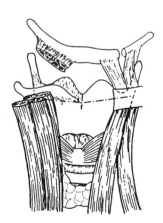

Figure 14.15 Supraglottic laryngectomy: cartilage cuts marked and perichondrium turned down.

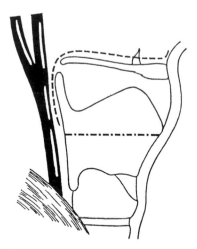

Figure 14.17 Supraglottic laryngectomy: extent of excision.

the oesophagus: the muscle will be felt in a spasm, which later causes difficulty in swallowing if it is not relieved. With a finger in the oesophagus the surgeon cuts down through the muscle fibres as far as the mucosa. The upper part of the oesophagus should then feel loose and capacious. The myotomy is carried out posteriorly to avoid damage to the recurrent laryngeal nerves.

Repair of the pharynx (Figs 14.21 and 14.22)

It is important to make absolutely sure that all bleeding has stopped. Any raw surfaces should be left to heal by granulation and no attempt is made to close any gaps with mucosal flaps, as this leads to laryngeal immobility from fibrosis.

The pharynx is closed in three layers, the first one of which is under some tension. Using 2/0 Vicryl, a stitch is placed at the apex of the wound on the opposite side of entry into the pharynx. This stitch is tied, tagged with an artery forceps and given to the assistant, who puts the handles over the point of another artery forceps. Then, stitches are placed about 8 mm apart, taking a large extramucosal bite tongue base above, and in the perichondrial flap. These stitches should not be tied, but tagged and stored in order, on the upturned artery forceps. After placing stitches over halfway across the defect, the order of the forceps is reversed by passing them on to another forceps, the last being passed first and so on.

The first stitch has been tied already and is left hanging on an artery forceps as a marker. Then the third stitch is crossed, but not tied taking the tension off the second stitch, which the assistant ties and cuts on the knot. He or she then takes the fourth stitch and crosses it to take the tension off the third stitch, which must not be released

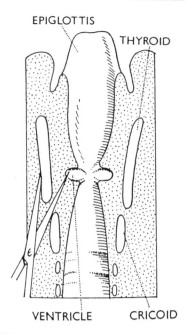

Figure 14.19 Schematic diagram to show division through the ventricle and the thyroid cartilage.

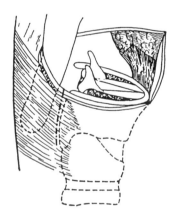

Figure 14.20 Cricopharyngeal myotomy.

until now; it is tied and the fifth stitch taken, taking the tension of the fourth held by the assistant. The proceedure continues in this fashion until over half the defect has been closed. The remainder of the defect on the side of entry into the pharynx is now nearly vertical; stay sutures are placed at the top and bottom of this and the rest of the defect is closed with extramucosal inverting sutures. While closing the lower end of this part of the defect, the surgeon is careful not to catch any of the mucosa over the arytenoid cartilage in the stitch. There should be no tension on these sutures.

A second row of interrupted sutures is placed from the base of the tongue above to the sternothyroid muscle remnant below, and finally a third row of interrupted

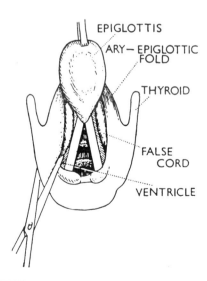

Figure 14.18 Larynx from above to show line of division through the ventricle.

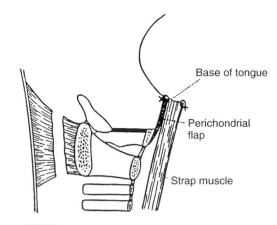

Figure 14.21 Pharyngeal repair.

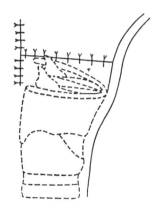

Figure 14.22 Pharyngeal repair completed.

sutures from the sternohyoid muscle below to the bellies of the digastric muscle above, using 2/0 Vicryl for each layer.

The skin is closed in the usual fashion leaving a suction drain in the wound, the tracheostomy left in place and a nasogastric tube is inserted unless the patient has already had a PEG.

Specific aftercare

The tracheostomy tube is corked as soon as this can be tolerated, usually between 7 and 10 days. When the tracheostomy has been fully corked and the patient breathes easily, feeding by mouth can commence. In the early postoperative period, when the patient experiences difficulty in swallowing saliva, he or she should be encouraged to sit forward and spit into a bowl to help mobilize the tongue base.

The patient has lost many of the protective mechanisms of the respiratory tract: the epiglottis, the aryepiglottic folds, the false vocal cords and the supraglottic sensory reflex. In order to be able to swallow without inhaling, he or she must, therefore, be able first to approximate the vocal cords, and secondly to develop a positive subglottic pressure.

Feeding begins with a semisolid diet such as rice pudding, icecream or jelly. The patient is instructed to take a deep breath before each mouthful, then bolt it in one rather than allowing it to trickle down.

During this early phase many patients have difficulty swallowing, inhale some of their food and cough. The dysphagia speech therapist must be prepared at this stage to sit with them and encourage them to persevere. Intake and output charts must be kept meticulously and fluid shortages made good with an intravenous infusion. The patient is weighed every 2 or 3 days to make sure that he or she is getting enough to eat. When the patient is taking a reasonable amount, the tracheostomy tube can be removed and the stoma allowed to close. This stage should be reached about a week after the patient starts feeding and thereafter the type and quantity of food that the patient can take is rapidly increased. Some patients take longer than this but most swallow eventually.

Specific complaints

Persistent oedema: this usually occurs over the arytenoid cartilage because the lymphatic drainage of the mucosa in this area is via the aryepiglottic folds, which are divided during the operation. If this completely occludes the airway the patient can often swallow well because he or she cannot inhale. In this case the patient can return home with the tracheostomy in place and the larynx will slowly open up.

Paralysis of the recurrent laryngeal nerve: this may occur during the cricopharyngeal myotomy. If it does the patient will almost certainly need a total laryngectomy because of inhalation.

Extensions and modifications of the supraglottic laryngectomy

Cord fixation in aryepiglottic fold lesions: if this operation is done for a tumour of one aryepiglottic fold, one arytenoid is removed, paralysing the vocal cord on that side. The cord remnant is sutured in the midline to ensure glottic closure. If this fails to close the gap, it can be closed by an injection of Teflon or a modified thyroplasty.

Suprahemilaryngectomy: this is an extension of the supraglottic laryngectomy in which an additional half of the larynx including the vocal cord is removed. Attempts have been made to reform this vocal cord by infracturing the upper half of the thyroid cartilage. If this is done very accurately and with a high degree of skill, the results can be very gratifying, but in the average otolaryngologist's hands if a tumour is so large as to require this operation then it is safer to perform a total laryngectomy.

Supraglottic laryngectomy for piriform sinus lesions: unlike the USA, it is very rare in the UK to find small piriform sinus tumours that can be safely removed by a supraglottic laryngectomy. This is discussed in Chapter 17. It is probably unsafe for the average otolaryngologist to consider supraglottic laryngectomy for this tumour and many of these patients should have a total laryngectomy and partial pharyngectomy.

Operative technique of vertical hemilaryngectomy

Anaesthetic

The patient is laid in the supine position on the operating table and a general anaesthetic begun through an oral endotracheal tube. A tracheostomy is made between the third and fourth tracheal rings, a size 36 cuffed tracheostomy tube inserted through which the general anaesthetic is continued. The skin is resterilized and new towels are applied.

Incision

If the strict criteria of selection for this operation are applied, a neck dissection will not be needed. For this reason, a collar incision about 8 cm long is used across the prominence of the thyroid cartilage (the incision is marked with Methylene Blue first to prevent an asymmetrical scar). The surgeon incises down to the platysma and elevates flaps up to the hyoid bone superiorly and down to the second tracheal ring inferiorly, taking care not to encroach on the tracheostomy wound.

Mobilization of muscle flaps

After raising the flaps, the skin surface is excluded from the wound with small towels and a Joll's clamp. Then, the anterior borders of both sternomastoid muscles are freed and identified. The sternohyoid muscle is freed on the involved side only down its whole length anteriorly and posteriorly, but not detached from either its insertion or its origin. A tape is passed round this muscle to retract it laterally and the thyrohyoid and sternothyroid muscles are freed (again on the involved side only) in a similar manner up to their attachments to the oblique line on the thyroid cartilage. The surgeon cuts them off the oblique line, using sharp dissection, as close to their insertion as possible, and retracts them laterally (Fig. 14.23).

Formation of the perichondrial flap

A finger is placed behind the posterior lamina of the thyroid cartilage and with a no. 15 blade, an incision is made along the superior border of the thyroid cartilage to the thyroid notch, then down the prominence at the midline and then along the lower margin to just in front of the posterior lamina (Fig. 14.24). The flap thus marked out is elevated using a Freer's elevator and non-toothed dissection forceps. The flap remains attached to the posterior lamina of the thyroid cartilage.

Removal of the tumour

With a Stryker saw or dental fissure burr the surgeon cuts the midline of the thyroid cartilage (Fig. 14.25) but does not enter the lumen at this point. The involved side of

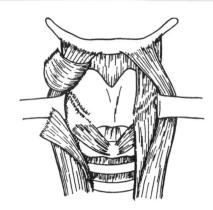

Figure 14.23 Vertical hemilaryngectomy: detachment of the strap muscles.

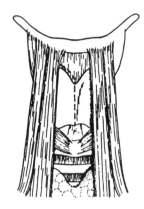

Figure 14.24 Vertical hemilaryngectomy: cartilage incisions.

the larynx is rotated forward and another vertical cartilaginous cut made just in front of the posterior lamina where the perichondrial flap is attached.

The point of entry into the larynx depends on whether the tumour affects the anterior commissure or not. If it does not come up to the commissure, then the surgeon opens into the larynx in the midline, either with scissors or with a knife blade passed through the thyrohyoid membrane in the superior thyroid notch. If the growth comes up to the anterior commissure, one-fifth of the opposite vocal cord is removed by making the laryngofissure slightly to the opposite side.

When the larynx has been divided, the healthy side is retracted and the involved side grasped with Allis forceps. The surgeon cuts through the cricothyroid membrane along the lower border of the thyroid cartilage on the involved side and ties the cricothyroid artery. Similarly, a cut is made along the upper border of the thyroid cartilage through the thyrohyoid membrane. If the growth affects the vocal process, the arytenoid cartilage is disarticulated from the cricoid and removed. If, however, the growth does not come up to the vocal process it is better to retain the arytenoid. One must not cut across the arytenoid cartilage, especially if the patient has been irradiated, as this causes mucosal oedema after the operation. The specimen

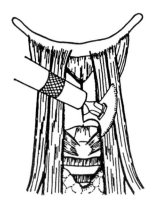

Figure 14.25 Vertical hemilaryngectomy: division of cartilage.

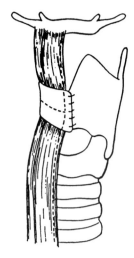

Figure 14.26 Vertical hemilaryngectomy: laryngeal repair.

is finally detached posteriorly by cutting with one blade of the scissors inside and one blade outside the posterior saw cut. Haemostasis is secured with coagulation diathermy after transfixing the superior laryngeal artery.

If there is a subglottic extension of less than 5 mm, the upper half of the ring of the cricoid cartilage is removed to increase the margin of clearance.

Closure (Fig. 14.26)

There is no need to perform a mucosal closure, but it is possible to do so by creating a flap of the mucosa of the piriform sinus, rotating it into the laryngeal defect and stitching it into the mucosal defect.

Next, the surgeon takes the thyrohyoid and sternothyroid muscles and brings their cut ends together, everting them into the larynx exactly opposite the remaining vocal cord. They are stitched into position with two vertical mattress sutures of 3/0 chromic catgut or Vicryl. The idea is to evert the ends into the form of a cord in the correct position. At this point the two sutured muscles will tend to point anteriorly but they can be rotated into the correct position by suturing them anteriorly to the remaining mucosa on the other side of the larynx and posteriorly to the mucosa that remains over the arytenoid area.

Then, the sternohyoid muscle is brought into add bulk to the newly formed vocal cord. The perichondrial flap is passed outside the sternohyoid muscle and sutured to the cartilage and perichondrium on the remaining side, holding the muscles in like a belt. Any gaps remaining above and below the closure are closed with pursestring sutures of 3/0 chromic catgut or Vicryl. The skin is closed in the usual fashion with suction drainage.

An alternative method to reconstruct the neocord is to use a revascularized free temporoparietal flap wrapped around a free cartilage graft from the contralateral thyroid ala. Early results using this technique are encouraging.

Specific aftercare

The tracheostomy is half corked at the end of a week, and can be fully corked and removed in about 10 days, earlier or later depending on the amount of swelling that occurs within the larynx and also on how much cord has been removed on the contralateral side.

The patient is not allowed to speak for at least a week and then is helped to speak by a speech therapist. The speech ought to be quite normal from quite early on.

Specific complaints

Air leak: if the closure has not been performed properly, surgical emphysema occurs (even after a week), every time the patient coughs or tries to speak. This usually settles well with a pressure bandage and voice rest.

Laryngeal stenosis: if more than one-fifth of the opposite vocal cord has been removed, a Silastic keel should be put in place and left there for at least 5 weeks. An alternative is a McNaught keel made from tantalum plate, which can be cut with heavy scissors. It has a vertical plate that lies in the laryngeal lumen, to separate the raw edges, and three flanges for fixation. Its design is shown in Fig. 14.27 and its use in laryngeal stenosis is also described in Chapter 10. It is often tempting to perform the closure without this in order to discharge the patient from hospital sooner, but this inevitably leads to a laryngeal stenosis if much of the opposite cord has been removed. If stenosis occurs, the larynx is reopened, the stenosis divided and a keel put in place for 5 weeks. There will be no need to perform another tracheostomy as the first one will still be in place.

Polyp formation: if the arytenoid cartilage has been cut, particularly in an irradiated patient, oedematous mucosa forms over the area. This looks like a large supraglottic polyp and it can be removed by direct laryngoscopy. Polyp formation on the newly formed vocal cord may occur but when this is stripped off at direct laryngoscopy (which is easy) a good fibrous cord is seen underneath it.

Extensions and modifications of vertical hemilaryngectomy

Cordectomy can be performed if the tumour does not involve either the vocal process of the arytenoid cartilage or the anterior commissure (Fig. 14.28). It is usually performed with the CO_2 laser and only carried out as an open

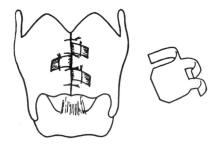

Figure 14.27 Vertical hemilaryngectomy: the use of the McNaught keel.

procedure when either the laser or quality radiotherapy is not available. The thyroid cartilage is split in the midline as described previously, but an external perichondrial flap is not developed and no cartilage is removed. Once the larynx is open, the sound side is retracted and the involved cord removed. The superior laryngeal artery is transfixed. A mucosal closure is performed and the sternohyoid muscle slid inside the larynx on the internal perichondrium of the thyroid cartilage to replace the lost bulk.

Frontal laryngectomy is performed for tumours that only affect the anterior commissure (Fig. 14.29).

The area to be removed is the anterior commissure and anterior one-fifth to one-third of both vocal cords with adjacent cartilage. If the laryngeal remnant is closed primarily, laryngeal stenosis will almost certainly occur and a McNaught keel should be used to prevent this occurrence.

Once the specimen has been removed, the keel is inserted and the cartilages are closed over the limb of the keel that enters the larynx, suturing the side arms of the keel on to the perichondrium of the thyroid cartilage. This is left in for 5 weeks, when the neck is reopened and the keel removed. During this time the tracheostomy is left in place.

Neoglottis procedures

The most common neoglottis procedure currently performed is voice restoration using the Blom–Singer valve and this is discussed in Chapter 18.

Near-total laryngectomy

The technique of near-total laryngectomy was introduced over 15 years ago. It initially did not achieve widespread acceptance because of doubts about its oncological effectiveness. Results are now beginning to emerge which show that the use of the procedure for T_3 carcinoma of the larynx is at least comparable to other surgical modalities, and that it has the advantage of voice preservation.

The technique is essentially an extended hemilaryngectomy. One-half of the larynx is completely removed together with about two-thirds of the other side, leaving an arytenoid on the unaffected side. This effectively removes both paraglottic spaces. Closure is via a small mucosal tube in which the arytenoid is integrated and the patient is usually able to speak without aspirating.

Although its place in the therapeutic spectrum is not yet clearly established, in view of recent good results more attention will have to be given to it than has been formerly.

Supracricoid subtotal laryngectomy with cricohyoidoepiglottoplexy (subtotal laryngectomy)

This operation is performed under tracheostomy cover but, unlike near-total laryngectomy, has the aim of restoration of speech and swallowing without a permanent tracheostomy. It consists of removal of the thyroid cartilage, both true and false vocal cords, the paraglottic space and one arytenoid, with preservation of the epiglottis, the cricoid cartilage, one arytenoid and the hyoid bone. The larynx is closed using three heavy absorbable (catgut or Vicryl) stitches (one midline and two lateral). These stitches encircle the cricoid, cross through the inferior edge of the epiglottis and the base of the tongue and finally encircle the hyoid bone. After the knots are tied, the cricoid comes into contact with the base of the tongue (cricohyoidoepiglottoplexy). Avoidance of damage to the hypoglossal nerve laterally is vital to postoperative function. Intravenous antibiotic treatment is administered for 10 days, a nasogastric tube remains in place (or alternatively a PEG) and the tracheostomy tube

(a)
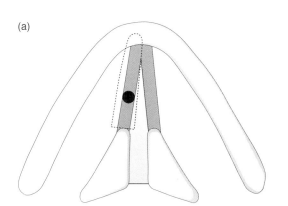

(b)
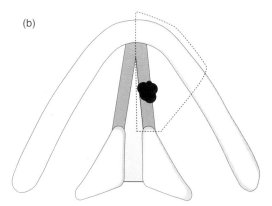

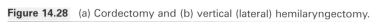

Figure 14.28 (a) Cordectomy and (b) vertical (lateral) hemilaryngectomy.

(a) Frontal partial laryngectomy

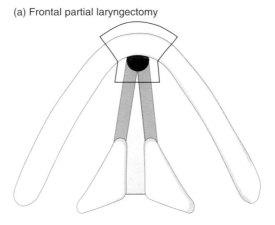

(b) Frontolateral partial laryngectomy

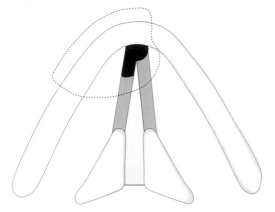

(c) Extended frontolateral partial laryngectomy

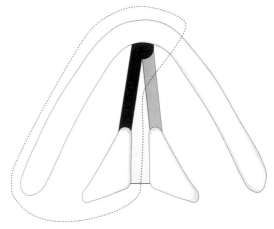

Figure 14.29 (a) Frontal partial, (b) frontolateral partial and (c) extended frontolateral partial laryngectomy.

is plugged as soon as can be tolerated by the patient, usually around the 8th day. Patients are urged to phonate early, oral feeding is begun as soon as the patient can swallow their saliva, which is usually around the 10th day. Then the nasogastric (or gastrostomy) and tracheostomy tubes are removed.

This operation allows the excision of extended T_2 glottic and some T_3 glottic and supraglottic tumours with local recurrence rates that are lower than partial and extended partial vertical laryngectomy. This is because of the total excision of the thyroid cartilage and the paraglottic space with the primary tumour. It may be indicated in tumours of the anterior two-thirds of the true vocal cords with earlier anterior commissure involvement, tumours of the entire vocal cord on one side with limited mobility and early anterior commissure tumour involvement and tumours that involve both vocal cords when radiotherapy is not appropriate. It should not be done when there is any pharyngeal extension, arytenoid cartilage fixation or subglottic extension greater than 7 mm and care should be taken when considering it in patients over 60 years of age.

Surgically and oncologically, it is a difficult procedure to perform and, like near-total laryngectomy, its place in the therapeutic spectrum is not yet clearly established, but based on published results, it may have a role to play in certain carefully selected cases.

Stomal recurrence

The incidence of stomal recurrence following total laryngectomy ranges from 5 to 15%. The causes are:

- inadequate resection with positive margins
- residual disease in the paratracheal nodes
- subglottic extension
- tracheostomy performed close to the tumour prior to resection.

Only 3% of patients with N_0 tumours develop stomal disease, compared with 8% of N_1 tumours and 33% of N_2 tumours. The risk of stomal recurrence after emergency tracheostomy ranges from 8 to 26%. This risk drops dramatically if a subsequent laryngectomy is performed within 48 h of the initial tracheostomy.

Classification

The classification is illustrated in Fig. 14.30. Sisson Type I is localized and usually presents as a discreet nodule in the superior aspect of the stoma. The prognosis is usually good if detected early. Sisson type II indicates involvement of the oesophagus but no inferior involvement. The prognosis for type II is fair to good depending on the amount of oesophageal involvement. Sisson type III originates inferior to the stoma and usually has direct extension into the mediastinum. Sisson type IV indicates that there is extension laterally and usually under either side of the clavicles. In one series (Gluckman *et al.*, 1994) the overall 2 year survival for patients undergoing surgery was 16% with a determinate survival of 24%. However, analysis by type of stomal recurrence revealed a 45% 5 year survival for type I and II lesions, compared with a 9% 5 year survival for types III and IV. The average survival for patients who are not operated on is 6 months and is accompanied by an extremely poor quality of life.

Surgery is the only viable treatment option, despite a growing experience in both radiotherapy and combination chemotherapy and radiotherapy techniques. Surgical candidates should be medically fit, with a negative metastatic workup, and the extent of local disease must have been evaluated with CT or MRI. Sisson types III and IV stomal recurrence are unlikely to benefit from surgery. It appears that in Sisson Types I and II, radical surgery can be justified in carefully selected cases. Reconstruction is usually completed with the use of regional skin flaps, regional myocutaneous flaps and, in some cases, free jejunal transfer for total pharyngeal reconstruction.

Technique of thorocotracheostomy

The lesion is excised in continuity with an ellipse of skin around the stoma (Fig. 14.31) and the incision carried down as for an upper medial sternotomy. Access into the upper mediastinum is facilitated by excising the whole of the manubrium and medial ends of both clavicles and the rest of both chest flaps are raised, giving access to the required area. The recurrent tumour is excised by mobilizing the trachea along with associated involvement of lymph glands, and extension into soft tissues, thyroid remnants, neopharynx and external skin. At this point, the left innominate vein is seen crossing the trachea and may be mobilized for access purposes as the trachea is mobilized down to the carina. If any further access is required, it may rarely be divided.

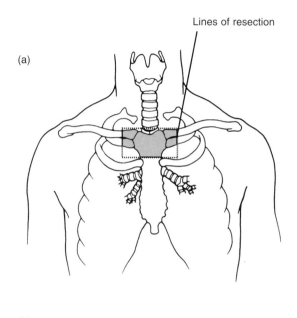

(a)

Lines of resection

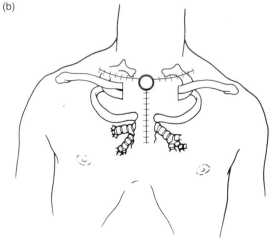

(b)

Figure 14.31 Technique of thoracotracheostomy. (a) The area for manubrial resection is marked out. (b) Final result with stoma.

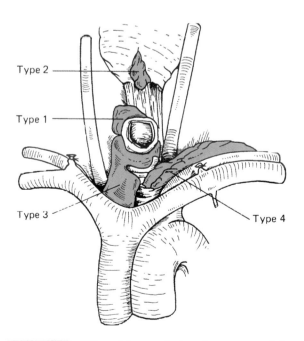

Figure 14.30 Different types of stomal recurrence (after Sisson).

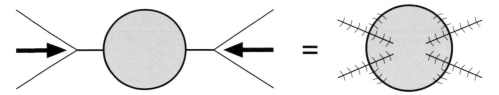

Figure 14.32 Technique of 'Y–V' advancement to facilitate stomal enlargement.

If there is significant extension into the upper oesophagus, then a neopharyngo-oesophagectomy and stomach transposition should be carried out rather than free jejunal transfer.

Following the resection, the removal of the upper manubrium facilitates the bringing forward of the trachea to form a new tracheostome and the upper skin flap will usually reach the upper posterior part of the tracheostome. This may be technically difficult in patients who have previously been irradiated but it is important as the suturing of these two structures helps to maintain the position of the tracheostome. Reconstruction of the gullet is completed by the free jejunal transfer or stomach pull-up and if sternal skin has taken, then the gap between the tracheostome and the upper flap is completed with either a pedicled pectoralis major or latissimus dorsi flap, or alternatively a free flap may be used. Closure is completed in two layers with the appropriate drains.

Complications

The most devastating complication of this operation is dehiscence of the tracheostome with disappearance of the trachea into the upper mediastinum. If this happens, particularly after radiotherapy, the outlook is gloomy.

Stomal stenosis

This may occur immediately after laryngectomy or may develop years later. Its occurrence is uncommon. It used to be taught that it was seen more often when the tracheostome was placed within a Gluck–Sorensen incision rather than in the lower skin flap when a cervical collar incision is used, but this has now been disproved. Stomal stenosis may be caused by excessive scar tissue from postoperative infection or fistula, keloid formation, excessive fat around the stoma, defective or absent tracheal rings, recurrent tumour or failure to wear a stoma button in 'the stoma at risk'.

Causes of stomal stenosis

- Excessive scar tissue
- Excessive fat around the stoma
- Defective or absent tracheal rings
- Recurrent tumour
- Failure to wear a stoma button

The condition may be less common nowadays due to the use of monofilament sutures, better humidification, prophylactic antibiotics and early removal of the tracheostomy or laryngectomy tube. The stenosis usually takes the form of a vertical slit or a concentric stenosis and is very difficult to treat, as is evident from the many operations that have been described. One operation may not be satisfactory for all patients but the two procedures described below will treat the majority.

Procedure no. 1

The simplest and easiest way to deal with stomal stenosis is to perform 'Y–V' advancement. A Y incision is made at 3 o'clock and 9 o'clock, the subsequent flap advanced into the stoma and closure is Y to V (Fig. 14.32). Closure is in one or two layers and this technique is extremely effective. Stoma buttons should be worn postoperatively for at least 3 months.

Procedure no. 2

Two circular incisions are made around the tracheal opening, the outer one incising skin outside the scar tissue and the inner one incising healthy tracheal mucosa (Fig. 14.33). The area between the two consecutive incisions is removed and discarded, since it consists of scar tissue. Then, four radial incisions about 5 cm long are made at 10, 2, 4 and 8 o'clock. The skin is undermined as far as possible creating four flaps. These flaps are sutured to the tracheal mucosa in two layers, one with 3/0 catgut or Vicryl and the other with 4/0 Ethilon or prolene. The contraction lines of these flaps tend to pull the tracheal mucosa upwards and outwards, thus preventing the formation of further stenosis.

There are other techniques described such as multiple Z-plasties around the stoma, but these are complicated and seldom used today.

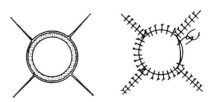

Figure 14.33 Revision of tracheostome using two consecutive circular incisions.

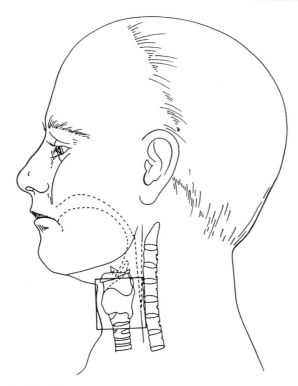

Figure 14.35 Radiotherapy field for early glottic carcinoma.

placement are, therefore, absolutely essential to ensure that the tumour is properly covered. The fields are centred on the vocal cords and extend up to include the thyroid cartilage and down to include the cricoid cartilage. Anteriorly, the skin of the neck is included. The posterior border is at the anterior margin of the vertebral bodies (Fig. 14.35). For most patients a set-up using directly opposed fields, wedged to ensure homogeneity, is suitable. In squat patients with short necks, or when longer fields are needed to cover subglottic extension, two anterior oblique fields may be more appropriate. Again, wedges are used to optimize the dose distribution. This set-up ensures that the patient's shoulders do not get in the way of the beam and enables sparing of the skin at the side of the neck. It is the practice is some centres always to use this type of field arrangement in preference to lateral fields, in order to minimize the high dose volume and avoid unnecessary treatment of normal tissues.

For advanced tumours, the field is extended up or down as necessary to encompass the full extent of the disease, as revealed at examination under anaesthesia and by radiography, with a margin of about 2 cm (Fig. 14.36). Accuracy of field placement is checked by the use of planning films from the simulator and portal verification films obtained from the treatment machine. The prescribed dose, beam energy and fractionation schedule are the same

In the second phase of treatment, the posterior border of the lateral photon fields is brought forward to take the cord out of the volume. An additional 26 Gy is given in 13 fractions to the primary tumour and any clinically involved nodes. At the same time the nodes in the posterior part of the neck overlying the cord are treated with lateral electron fields matched on to the posterior margins of the lateral photon fields. The appropriate electron energy is selected to treat the nodes while keeping the total cord dose below a total of 44 Gy (including the contribution from phase I). If these areas are clinically uninvolved, then an additional dose of 10 Gy in a further five fractions is adequate. If there was palpable disease then 26 Gy is given in 13 fractions.

The total dose in phases I and II to the primary tumour and clinically involved nodes is therefore 66 Gy in 33 fractions over 6.5 weeks. Uninvolved nodal areas being treated prophylactically will receive a total dose of 50 Gy in 25 fractions over 5 weeks, which is usually adequate to sterilize microscopic disease.

Glottic carcinoma

A shell to immobilize the patient and for beam direction is prepared as described above. For early tumours (T_1 or T_2), where there is no likelihood of occult nodal involvement, very small fields are used. These usually measure 5×5 cm. A perfectly fitting shell and accurate field

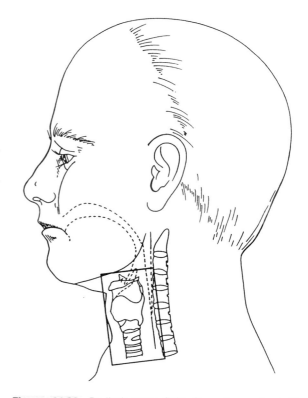

Figure 14.36 Radiotherapy field for advanced glottic carcinoma.

as those used for supraglottic cancer. While surgery is the preferred treatment for the minority of patients with obvious nodal involvement, primary radical radiotherapy is sometimes used. Under these circumstances, the whole neck should also be irradiated as described for supraglottic cancer.

Subglottic cancer

The treatment volume in cases of subglottic carcinoma encompasses the larynx and upper trachea, as well as the paratracheal and superior mediastinal lymph nodes. Because of the changing contour from the neck to the thorax, this is a relatively difficult area to irradiate satisfactorily. Patients are immobilized in a shell, which is also necessary for accurate alignment of treatment beams. A complex three-field technique is usually used. Left and right lateral fields have their posterior borders running through the vertebral bodies, anterior to the spinal cord, and extend anteriorly to include the skin of the neck. They cover the larynx and are angled downwards to include the superior mediastinum. Wedges are used in both longitudinal and transverse directions to even out the dose distribution. Alternatively, if facilities are available, this can be achieved by the use of individually prepared tissue compensators. In addition, a wedged or compensated anterior beam is also used. This covers the width of the neck and extends from the thyroid notch down to the manubriosternal joint. Its lower corners are blocked to shield the lung apices. Dosimetry is made easier if three-dimensional CT planning is available. The prescribed dose-fractionation schedule is the same as that used for supraglottic cancer.

Postoperative irradiation

For patients who have undergone primary surgery, postoperative radiotherapy is indicated to diminish the likelihood of local recurrence. It should be undertaken if there was histological evidence of lymph-node involvement, particularly if multiple nodes were involved or there was any degree of extracapsular spread, or if there was direct extension of the tumour beyond the larynx into the soft tissues of the neck, oropharynx or hypopharynx, or if there were positive resection margins. In these cases, the volume to be irradiated includes all soft tissues from the mandible to the clavicle. A full dose of 60 Gy in 30 fractions or its equivalent should be given. Treatment should be started as soon as permitted by wound healing, preferably within 3 weeks. If radiotherapy is delayed for longer, its chances of success are greatly diminished.

Indications for postoperative irradiation

- Extralaryngeal tumour extension
- Positive resection margins
- Lymph node involvement (particularly if there was multiple nodes or extracapsular spread)

References

Birchall M. (1988) Human laryngeal allograft: shift of emphasis on transplantation (commentary), *Lancet* **251**: 539–40.

Desanto L. W. (1994) Cancer of the larynx – psychosocial aspects, in: *Laryngeal Cancer, Proceedings of the 2nd World Congress on Laryngeal Cancer* (R. Smee and G. P. Bridger eds), Elsevier, Oxford, pp. 42–53.

Fagan J. J. and Loock J. W. (1996) Tracheostomy and peristomal recurrence. *Clin Otolaryngol* **21**: 328–30.

Glanz H. K. (1994) Further development of the TNM classification of laryngeal carcinoma, in: *Laryngeal Cancer, Proceedings of the 2nd World Congress on Laryngeal Cancer* (R. Smee and G. P. Bridger eds), Elsevier, Oxford, pp. 244–52.

Gluckman J. L., Righi P., Schuller D. and Hamaker R. (1994) Stomal recurrence following total laryngectomy, in: *Laryngeal Cancer, Proceedings of the 2nd World Congress on Laryngeal Cancer* (R. Smee and G. P. Bridger, eds), Elsevier, Oxford, pp. 621–4.

Hirano M. (1994) Video-stroboscopic advances, in: *Laryngeal Cancer, Proceedings of the 2nd World Congress on Laryngeal Cancer*, (R. Smee and G. P. Bridger, eds), Elsevier, Oxford, pp. 270–2.

Hirano M., Mori K. and Iwashita, H. (1994) Voice in laryngeal cancer, in: *Laryngeal Cancer, Proceedings of the 2nd World Congress on Laryngeal Cancer* (R. Smee and G. P. Bridger, eds), Elsevier, Oxford, pp. 54–64.

Hoare T. J., Thomson H. G. and Proops D. W. (1993) Detection of laryngeal cancer – the case for early specialist assessment, *R Soc Med* **86**. 390–2.

Jakobsson P. Å., Eneroth C. M., Killander D., Moberger G. and Martensson B. (1973) Historical classification and grading of malignancy in carcinoma of the larynx, *Acta Radiol Ther Phys Biol* **12**: 1–8.

Jones A. S., Cook J. A., Phillips D. E. and Soler Lluch E. (1992) Treatment of T_3 carcinoma of the larynx by surgery or radiotherapy, *Clin Otolaryngol* **17**: 433–6.

Kotwall C., Sako K., Razack M. S., Rao U., Bakamjian V. and Shedd D. P. (1987) Metastatic patterns in squamous cell cancer of the head and neck, *Am J Surg* **154**: 439.

Marks J. E. (1993) Larynx and hypopharynx radiation therapy, in: *Otolaryngology – Head and Neck Surgery*, 2nd edn, Vol. 3 (C. Cummings, J. M. Fredrickson, L. A. Harker, C. J. Krause, and D. E. Schuher, eds), Mosby, St Louis, MO.

Mendenhall W. M., Parsons J. T., Stringer S. P., Cassisi N. J. and Million R. R. (1992) Stage T_3 squamous carcinoma of the glottic larynx: a comparison of laryngectomy and irradiation, *Int J Radiat Oncol Phys* **23**: 725–32.

Olsen K. D., Lewis J. E. and Orvidas L. J. (1994) Verrucous carcinoma of the larynx, in: *Laryngeal Cancer, Proceedings of the 2nd World Congress on Laryngeal Cancer* (R. Smee and G. P. Bridger, eds), Elsevier, Oxford.

O'Sullivan B., Mackillop W., Gilbert R., Gaze M. N., Lundgen J., Atkinson, C. *et al.* (1994) Controversies in the management of laryngeal cancer: results of an international patterns of care survey, *Radiother Oncol* **31**: 23–32.

Robin P. E. and Olofsson J. V. (1997) Tumours of the larynx, in: *Scott-Brown's Otolaryngology*, 6th edn, Vol. 5, *Laryngology and Head and Neck Surgery*, Butterworth Heinemann, Oxford, Chap. 11, pp. 1–47.

Smee R. and Bridger G. P., eds (1994) *Laryngeal Cancer. Proceedings of the 2nd World Congress on Laryngeal Cancer* (R. Smee and G. P. Bridger, eds), Elsevier, Oxford.

Shah J. P. (1996) Larynx and trachea, in: *Head and Neck Surgery*, 2nd edn, Mosby-Wolfe, London, Chap. 8, pp. 267–353.

Shah J. P., Loreé T. R., Kowalski L. (1990) Conservation surgery for radiation failure carcinoma of the glottic larynx, *Head Neck* **12**: 326–31.

Shaw H. J. (1991) Role of partial laryngectomy after irradiation in the treatment of laryngeal cancer: a view from the United Kingdom. *Ann Otol Rhinol Laryngol* **100**: 268–73.

Shephard I., Glaholm J. and Watkinson J. C. (1998) Conservation surgery in head and neck cancer (Editorial), *Clin Otolaryngol* **23**: 385–7.

Steiner W. and Ambrosch, P. (1994) CO_2 laser microsurgery for laryngeal cancer, in: *Laryngeal Cancer, Proceedings of the 2nd World Congress on Laryngeal Cancer*. (R. Smee and G. P. Bridger, eds), Elsevier, Oxford, pp. 369–72.

Suárez C., Rodrigo J. P., Alvarez I. and Alvarez J. C. (1994) Postoperative radiotherapy in supraglottic laryngectomy, in: *Laryngeal Cancer, Proceedings of the 2nd World Congress on Laryngeal Cancer* (R. Smee and G. P. Bridger, eds), Elsevier, Oxford, pp. 481–4.

UICC (International Union against Cancer) (1997) *TNM Classification of Malignant Tumours* (L. H. Sobin and C. H. Wittekind, eds), 5th edn, Wiley-Liss, New York.

Weinstein G. S. and Laccourreye O. (1998) Supracricoid partial laryngectomy, in: *Advances in Head and Neck Oncology* (K. T. Robbins, ed.), Singular, San Diego, CA, pp. 83–98.

Wolf G. T., Hong W. K. and Fisher S. G. (1996) Neoadjuvant chemotherapy for organ preservation: current status, in: *Proceedings of the 4th International Conference on Head and Neck Cancer*. Society of Head and Neck Surgeons and the American Society of Head and Neck Surgery, pp. 89–97.

15 Tumours of the lip and oral cavity

'Make accurate incisions surrounding the whole tumour, so as to not leave a single root'
Galen, 129–200 AD

Introduction

Tumours of the lip and oral cavity often present a significant problem to the surgeon with regard to early diagnosis and staging, access for resection as well as reconstruction of both the soft tissues and bone. Tumours of the lip are now included within the International Union Against Cancer (UICC) classification for oral cavity tumours and will be discussed first.

THE LIP

Surgical anatomy

The lips represent the anterior boundary of the oral cavity and are covered with non-keratinizing stratified squamous epithelium. They appear red because this epithelium is transparent and contains no hairs, sebaceous glands or pigment in its substance. The mucosa of the lips covers the orbicularis oris muscle. On the vermilion border, the mucosa is closely applied to the muscles but on the lingual surface there are many mucous glands and supporting tissue within the muscle and the mucosa. The distance between the surface epithelium of the lip and orbicularis oris is only about 2 mm. An ulcerative squamous carcinoma can, therefore, fix the skin quite early to the deep substance of the lip.

The major blood supply of the lip comes from the facial artery, which gives off small submental arteries to the lower lip and then gives rise to the inferior and superior labial arteries. These vessels encircle the mouth between the orbicularis oris and the submucosa of the lip.

The upper and lower lips have a cutaneous and mucosal system of lymphatics. In the lower lip, there is one medial and two lateral collecting trunks. The medial trunk drains the inner third of the lip and the lateral trunks drain the outer two-thirds. The medial trunk drains to the submental lymph nodes (level 1) and the lateral trunks to the submandibular triangle of lymph nodes (level 1).

Numerous anastomoses account for the bilateral metastases seen in midline tumours. Collecting lymph trunks enter the mental foramen in 22% of normal subjects.

Drainage of the upper lip is to the preauricular, infraparotid, submandibular and submental lymph nodes.

The commissure of the mouth is a delicately formed structure that is difficult both to reconstitute and to remake. For this reason, it is better to keep the commissure if at all possible in any lip operation rather than attempting to refashion one later on.

Surgical pathology

The lip is the most common site of cancer in the mouth. In the UK, the incidence is 6 per million population and in the USA, 18 per million population, which reflects a greater exposure to sunlight. Approximately 93% of tumours present on the lower lip (Fig. 15.1) and the male to female ratio is 80:1. The most common tumour on the lower lip is a squamous cell carcinoma.

In contrast, in the upper lip the most common tumour is a basal cell carcinoma. This is more common in females than in males, with a ratio of 5:1. Lip cancer is most common in the White male smoker with a fair or ruddy

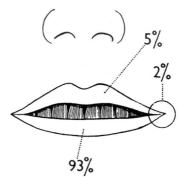

Figure 15.1 Site incidence of lip cancer.

complexion and light hair, who is often of Celtic descent and in the sixth decade of life. Lip cancer is 10 times more common in White people than in those with coloured skin.

Lip cancer is traditionally associated with the following risk factors:

- heavy cigarette smoking
- pipe smoking
- poor dental hygiene
- chronic alcoholism
- chronic erosive skin diseases, e.g. lichen planus
- immunosuppression.

Tumours occur on the lower lip on the exposed vermilion border just outside the line of contact with the upper lip, usually halfway between the midline and the commissure. More than 30% of patients with carcinoma of the lip have outdoor occupations. The effect of solar exposure is the loss of elastic fibres, atrophy of fat and glandular elements and hyperkeratosis with atypia. The lower lip receives the most solar irradiation and the upper lip, by comparison, is shaded. The lip is susceptible to actinic change because, in the White population, it lacks a pigment layer for protection

Ninety-eight per cent of tumours of the lower lip represent squamous cell carcinomas. The remainder are tumours of minor salivary glands, predominantly mucoepidermoid or adenoid cystic carcinoma.

There are three types of squamous carcinoma: exophytic, verrucous and ulcerative. Exophytic tumours are probably the most common and verrucous tumours are rare. Exophytic lesions become necrotic and ulceration occurs late, when the tumour is over 1 cm. The ulcerative type is minimally elevated and ulceration occurs early; it is usually of a more aggressive, poorly differentiated histological grade and fixes the muscle early. Carcinoma of the upper lip and commissure grows more rapidly, ulcerates sooner and metastasizes earlier than lower lip cancer. There is an increased incidence of metastases not only with this site, but also with increasing tumour size.

Clinically apparent cervical lymph-node metastases occur in fewer than 10% of patients with carcinoma of the lower lip. Approximately 20% of patients with commissure lesions will have lymph-node metastases. Some 5–15% of patients will develop lymph-node metastases at some time in the future. Not all lymphadenopathy represents metastases. Infection of the tumour, or poor oral hygiene may cause inflammatory adenopathy.

Rare tumours and 'tumour-like' lesions

- malignant melanoma
- sarcoma
- salivary gland tumours
- myoblastomas
- pyogenic granuloma
- keratoacanthoma
- granulomatous cheilitis.

Malignant melanomas are rare within the vermilion portion of the lip but may occur in the associated nearby skin. Sarcomas of the lip are extremely rare. Benign and malignant tumours of minor salivary gland origin are rare in the lip. They develop in the depths of the labial substance without any connection to the mucous membrane.

Myoblastomas have been reported in the lip but these usually remain below or beneath the mucosa. Pyogenic granuloma has a softer consistency than cancer and it can arise particularly during pregnancy.

Keratoacanthoma can occur on a cutaneous aspect of the lip and give the appearance of a carcinoma. It is usually circular with a central crater. It may grow rapidly but then tends to regress spontaneously after a number of weeks.

Syphilitic chancres, leprosy, sarcoidosis and Crohn's disease are other causes of granulomatous cheilitis.

The main distinction between carcinoma and other lip lesions, however, is that from hyperkeratosis and cheilitis. Leucoplakia, in association with carcinoma of the lip, has been reported to occur in up to 75% of cases. The frequency with which malignant change occurs in leucoplakia of the lip is unknown but it may approach 30%. Cheilitis may be associated with chronic dermatitis and eczema, or prolonged exposure to sunshine.

Investigations

History

The consultant should ask how long the tumour has been present and whether or not the patient has any other symptoms elsewhere to suggest a synchronous primary. Questions are also asked about their smoking and drinking habits and their occupation, since lip tumours are more common in outdoor workers. Some carcinomas of the lip (particular basal cell carcinoma) tend to have a protracted clinical course which still can be cured despite the long history. The history of lip crusting that bleeds regularly on removal of the crust is characteristic of these tumours, particularly squamous cell carcinoma. It is uncommon for carcinoma to arise *de novo* from an entirely normal lower lip. Three per cent of patients develop metastases very early, when the primary lesion is 1 cm or less, and this indicates very aggressive biological behaviour. In those patients with advanced disease, pain, swelling and tenderness can occur, particularly when infection is present.

Examination

The tumour is examined and its measurements are recorded. Accuracy can be improved by observing the tumour under magnification. Accurate recording helps in planning future surgery. A careful note is made of the degree of infiltration by bimanual palpation of the lip. It should be ascertained whether the lesion extends on to the alveolus, premaxilla or into the floor of the nose. This is important because it will completely change treatment policy. Hypoanaesthesia is checked for in the distribution of the mental nerve because some tumours may grow along the nerve into the medullary portion of the mandible. This is much more likely to occur in older patients who are edentulous. Finally, the rest of the lips and mouth are examined for areas of leucoplakia and erythroleucoplakia. It is also important to examine the rest of the head and neck for synchronous skin tumours feel the neck for metastatic nodes and finally examine the rest of the upper aerodigestive tract to complete the examination.

Radiology and laboratory investigations

Imaging is required only in advanced cases where extension of disease into the soft tissues, the lower and upper alveolus, the premaxilla and the floor of the nose or neck is suspected.

Laboratory investigations are of no great value unless syphilis is suspected.

Biopsy

This is mandatory prior to treatment to confirm the diagnosis because hyperkeratosis, cheilitis, keratoacanthoma and other such benign lesions can be confused with carcinoma. An incisional biopsy may be better than an excisional one. A biopsy at the centre of an ulcerative or exophytic tumour, however, may show only necrotic debris.

Staging

The anatomical sites for the lip (upper and lower lip, commissures) are shown in below. The 'T' and overall staging for lip cancer is shown later in Table 15.3.

Anatomical regions and sites of the lip and oral cavity (UICC, 1997)

Lip
- Upper lip, vermilion surface
- Lower lip, vermilion surface
- Commissures

Oral cavity
- Buccal mucosa
  - Mucosal surfaces of upper and lower lips
  - Mucosal surface of cheeks
  - Retromolar areas
  - Buccoalveolar sulci, upper and lower
- Upper alveolus and gingiva
- Lower alveolus and gingiva
- Hard palate
- Tongue
  - Dorsal surface and lateral borders anterior to vallate papillae (anterior two-thirds)
- Floor of the mouth

Treatment policy

The survival rates for lip cancer, treated with either radiation therapy or surgery, are very similar. Both modalities, particularly for early disease, are expected to give cure rates greater than 85%. As expected, the cure rate drops significantly as the size of the tumour increases. Curability falls to approximately 60% for lesions measuring 2–3 cm in diameter and to around 40% for tumours larger than 3 cm. There is also a close relationship between histological grade and curability: there is a 95% 3 year cure rate for grade I carcinomas but only 45% and 38%, respectively, for grades II and III. The advantage of surgical therapy is that it immediately eradicates the disease and provides information on both histology and clearance. It has no effect on adjacent normal tissue and the subsequent pathological examination of the specimen provides details of staging. It is particularly useful in the younger patient. In the elderly, radiotherapy can have obvious advantages and can be given as either interstitial, contact or external beam radiotherapy. Care should be taken to protect the adjacent uninvolved tissue by proper shielding to limit the amount of mucositis and radiodermatitis.

Leucoplakia of the lip or actinic cheilitis is best managed with a lip shave, which constitutes both diagnosis and treatment. Alternatively, in this condition and in some superficial tumours, the laser may be used (Fig. 15.2).

The majority of tumours are on the lower lip. In this situation, up to one-third of the lower lip can be resected and primary reconstruction achieved. For larger defects of the lower lip, reconstruction may require additional tissue from another location such as part of the upper lip.

The upper lip is slightly more complicated because its middle third constitutes the philtrum area which should not be violated unless absolutely necessary. This means that the amount of tissue that can be donated to the lower lip is less than can be donated from the lower lip to the upper lip and, where primary reconstruction is to be attempted, there is less tissue available in the upper lip.

Repair of lip defects

- Vermilion
  Mucosal advancement
- Lower lip
  - <1/3 – Primary closure
  - 1/3–2/3 – Abbe, Abbe Estlander or Karapandzic flaps
  - >2/3 – Bilateral Gillies fan flaps, axial scalp flap or free tissue transfer
- Upper lip
  - <1/3 – Primary closure or Abbe flap
  - 1/3 – 2/3 – Reverse Karapandzic or perialar advancement
  - >2/3 – Combination perialar advancement, reverse Karapandzic or Abbe flap
    - Rarely bilateral nasolabial flaps, Gillies fan flaps or free tissue transfer
- Commissure
  Abbe Estlander, double rhomboid flaps or free tissue transfer

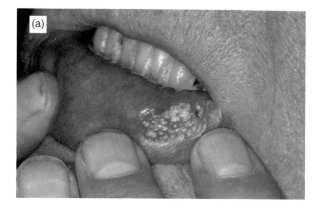

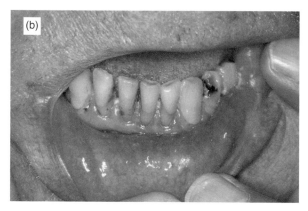

Figure 15.2 (a) Superficial squamous cell carcinoma of the left lower lip treated by laser peel excision. (b) The patient remains alive and well 4 years later.

In the lower lip, for tumours that are laterally placed and which measure more than one-third of the lower lip, reconstruction can be completed with an Abbe or Abbe Estlander flap from the upper lip. For tumours in the midline of the lower lip, particularly for those that approach two–thirds of the lower lip, the defect may be reconstructed using either the Bernard technique or the Karapandzic principle. The Bernard technique employs lateral advancement flaps where oral mucosa is preserved and used to restore the vermilion border. The main complaints of patients undergoing this technique are drooling, poor speech intelligibility, cracking and fissuring of the tissues, lack of sensation and inadequacy of stomal size. Because of this, a more pleasing functional result can be obtained in the reconstruction of large (particularly lower lip) defects using the Karapandzic principle, which consists of mobilizing arterialized, innervated flaps of skin and the orbicularis oris muscle from the surrounding network of suspensory muscles.

In the rare situation where a whole lower lip reconstruction is required, this may be done with local tissue using either Webster cheek advancement or bilateral Gillies fan flaps. The Webster cheek advancement flap results, not surprisingly, in a tight lower lip and a bulky upper lip with poor lower lip function. The best technique in this situation is the bilateral Gillies fan flap (or modified McGregor fan flap) with tongue flap reconstruction for the vermilion. It brings in new tissue for reconstruction and results in a lip that is bulkier and less tight than with other techniques.

If local tissue is not available, a lower lip may be reconstructed using either pedicled distant flaps such as the scalp, or free flaps in the form of a sensate free radial forearm flap. The advantage of the scalp flap is that it is hairy and can camouflage the reconstruction. Both techniques can be supplemented with subseqeuent vermilion reconstruction using the tongue; alternatively, tattooing can be equally effective.

In the upper lip, for defects greater than one-third which are laterally placed, a reverse Karapandzic flap is particularly useful. For tumours that involve up to two-thirds of the upper lip which are usually towards the midline and for those tumours that involve the collumella and extend into the upper lip (where this technique may be combined with a premaxillectomy), the technique of choice is the Webster bilateral perialar cheek advancement. This method makes use of the lax tissue in the nasolabial fold. Perialar incisions are made around each alar base extending upwards along the groove between the nose and cheek for approximately 1.5 cm. Lateral to this, a deep crescent of tissue is removed, the check is mobilized off the maxilla preserving the infraorbital nerve for sensation, and at the same time, the mucosa is freed along the upper buccal sulcus and the lip and cheek are advanced medially. Using this technique bilaterally large defects in the upper lip can be closed and where more tissue is required, the defect may be supplemented with an Abbe flap from the lower lip (Fig. 15.3). If the columella is to be reconstructed as well, an extended Abbe flap can be used.

It is uncommon to have to perform total upper lip reconstruction and, in many situations, a combination of techniques works best. Subtotal upper lip reconstruction is probably best achieved using a combination of bilateral perialar advancement and Abbe lip transfer from the lower lip supplemented by a reverse Karapandzic flap. In the rare situation of total upper lip reconstruction, this may be done using either simple nasolabial flaps based inferiorly or superiorly, or more formal Gillies fan flaps (or modified McGregor fan flaps), and both techniques can be supplemented by vermilion reconstruction using either the tongue or tattooing. Alternatively, a sensate radial free forearm flap may be used but this often has a poor cosmetic result and requires suspension in the correct position with a tendon fascial or synthetic sling.

Reconstruction of the commissure is a difficult problem. Mucosal defects may be dealt with using double rhomboid flaps from the buccal mucosa. A full-thickness defect of the commissure is best dealt with using double-skin rhomboid flaps for external reconstruction and double-mucosal rhomboid flaps for internal reconstruction. Large extensive defects may require free tissue

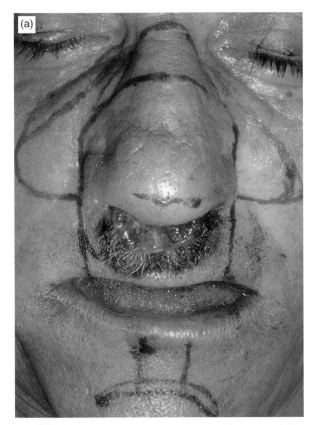

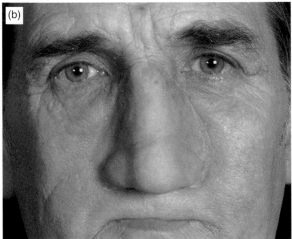

Figure 15.3 (a) Reconstruction of the upper lip following a two-thirds resection for a squamous cell carcinoma of the columella involving the upper lip. Reconstruction was with bilateral perialar cresentic advancement. The Abbe flap marked on the lower lip was not used. The patient also had a premaxillectomy and total rhinectomy. (b) The nose was reconstructed with an osseointegrated prosthesis.

transfer. In certain instances, a maxillofacial prosthesis may offer excellent cosmetic reconstructive results without recourse to major surgery.

Spread of carcinoma of the lip to the regional nodes is a poor prognostic sign and only 50% of patients in this situation are ultimately cured. It is impossible to achieve continuity between the primary excision and neck resection, which inevitably means that cancer-containing skin lymphatics are transected. This is borne out by the high incidence of recurrence in the upper incision line of the neck dissection. Consideration must, therefore, be given to planned postoperative radiotherapy to the chin and neck region for high-risk tumours.

Technique of lip operations

Wedge excision

Preparation

Great attention must be paid to the patient's teeth, as it is unwise to operate in the presence of gross dental infection. If tooth extraction is required, it is worth spending time doing this and the patient should be referred to a restorative dentist for an expert opinion. The alveolus should be allowed to heal prior to lip surgery. The patient's skin is prepared in the usual fashion, any moustache or beard should be shaved as appropriate and nasal sepsis is dealt with conventionally.

Anaesthesia

Many of the smaller tumours are ideal to be removed under local anaesthetic. Otherwise, patients should be anaesthetized with nasoendotracheal incubation and the anaesthetic tube brought out over the patient's head so as to be out of the way of the operating field. The oropharynx is packed off and the surgeon should remove the pack at the end of the operation to ensure limited trauma to the lip repair.

Excision

The majority of tumours encountered will either be squamous cell or basal cell carcinomas. For those tumours measuring less than 1 cm, a 5 mm margin is appropriate, otherwise a 1 cm margin is used unless one is dealing with minor salivary gland tumours. All tumours recurring after radiotherapy should be excised with a margin of at least 1 cm and consideration given to Mohs' surgery, frozen-section control or delayed reconstruction. The tumour is marked out with the appropriate margin on either side. If there is any doubt as to whether more than one-third of the lip will be excised when these marks are made, the lip is placed on the stretch and the distance measured accurately. No more than-one third of the lower lip should be removed and primarily repaired with this operation. Depending on the position of the tumour on the lower lip, the excision can be dealt with using a wedge, modified wedge, W-plasty or half W-plasty so as to avoid the bottom of the wedge encroaching on the crease line of the chin (Fig. 15.4). This avoids a scar crossing the crease line as well as a dog-ear at the lower end.

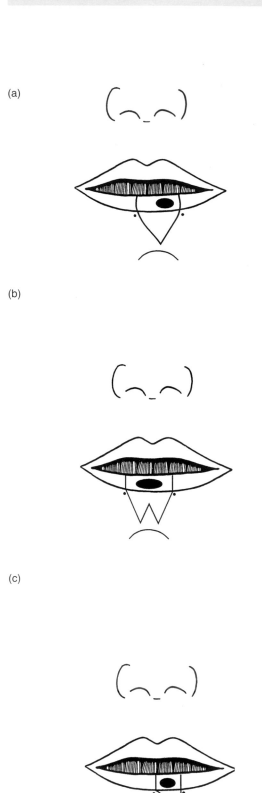

Figure 15.4 Lines of excision for a lip tumour using either (a) a wedge, (b) a W-plasty or (c) half W plasty.

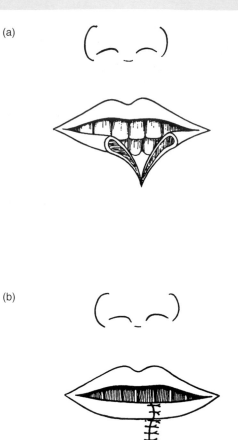

Figure 15.5 Wedge excision: (a) specimen removed: note the dot marking the vermilion skin junction; (b) repair: care is taken to achieve accurate apposition of vermilion edges.

The vermilion border should be tattooed accurately with Methylene Blue and this (as is marking out the tumour) is probably best done using loupes. This technique facilitates accurate repositioning at the end of surgery (Fig. 15.5)

If local anaesthetic is to be used, it should be administered at this point. A regional mental block is better than direct infiltration, which can cause significant tissue distortion. The assistant firmly holds the lip on either side between finger and thumb to control arterial bleeding. With the knife held exactly at right angles to the lip, the surgeon removes the tumour as the assistant releases one side of the lip slowly to facilitate the identification, clamping and tying of the inferior labial artery using an absorbable stitch. This is then repeated on the opposite side. Further bleeding is controlled using coagulation diathermy.

Lip repair

This should be done meticulously using either a two- or three-layer technique (Fig. 15.6). The intraoral mucosa

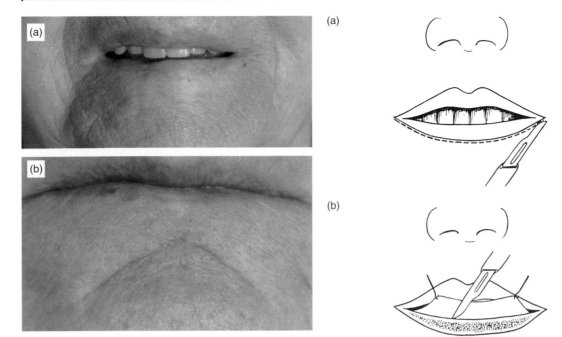

Figure 15.6 Final results following resection for carcinoma of the lower lip using (a) wedge excision and (b) 'w'-plasty technique.

Figure 15.7 Lip shave: (a) incision along the vermilion skin junction; (b) vermilion elevated off the orbicularis oris.

may be repaired primarily using an absorbable stitch (Vicryl or catgut) and then the orbicularis oris muscle repaired with a similar absorbable stitch. If this layer is omitted, there will be tension on the skin and mucosal suture lines producing an ugly thinning of the repaired portion of the lip. Alternatively, the orbicularis oris and the oral mucosa may be closed as one layer. It is important to match the vermilion border (using loupes) with 5/0 or 6/0 Ethilon and to use the same suture material to close the skin. The first few sutures on the vermilion can be closed with Ethilon. It is important not to tear the red margin on the lip on the surface as a necrotic area can form, causing a notch.

Aftercare

- General patient care
- The patient is not allowed to suck anything
- The wound is kept clean twice a day by removing crusts
- Antibiotic cream such as Bactroban or Fucidin may be applied
- Half of the external sutures may be removed at 3 or 4 days; the rest are removed at a week as appropriate

---

Lip shave and vermilion advancement

This operation can be performed on its own if the carcinoma is very superficial, or may be combined with a wedge excision. If it is combined, then it is easier to sew up the line of the muscle layer of the wedge before carrying out a lip shave.

An accurate incision is made, along the vermilion border (Fig. 15.7) with an assistant's finger in each corner of the mouth to keep the lip on the stretch. The mucosa is elevated off the orbicularis oris muscle, first with a knife (Fig. 15.7) and then with the blunt point of the scissors. At the back of the lip is a thicker layer of mucous glands. It is important just to elevate the mucosa, which must on no account be buttonholed as this causes crusting and a dip in the final repair. Elevation continues right down into the sulcus and on to the alveolus (Fig. 15.8). This is very important because if the mucosa is not elevated this far, retraction occurs later and after a year the lip will not be red. After full elevation of the mucosa, it is held on two skin hooks, brought forward out of the mouth and kept off the cheilitic portion with scissors, keeping the form of the lower margin of the vermilion, i.e. a gentle curve. Then, the remaining mucosa is reattached to the skin (Fig 15.8) with interrupted sutures of 5/0 Ethilon after haemostasis has been secured with adrenaline swabs. It is important to make a larger lower lip than is ultimately desired, because of subsequent wound contraction.

Aftercare

- General care including a soft diet.
- The area should be kept free of crusting with antibiotic cream.

(a)

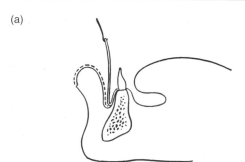

(b)

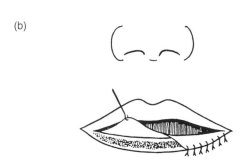

Figure 15.8 (a) Lip shave: mucosal elevation must be carried on down into the suclus. (b) vermilion advancement: once the leucoplakic lip has been trimmed off, the healthy mucosa is stiched forwards to form a new lip.

Abbe lip switch operation

This operation is indicated if more than one-third of the upper or lower lip has to be removed. It uses an axial flap consisting of skin, muscle and mucous membrane, pedicled on the superior or inferior labial artery. An Abbe lip switch from the lower to the upper lip will now be described.

The excision is outlined either as a shield or an conventional 'V' incision using Methylene Blue (Fig. 15.9). This is to allow the excision of a minimum of 1 cm of normal tissue on either side of the tumour. The vermilion border is also marked using Methylene Blue. The size of the excision is accurately measured using a ruler. Some of the local tissue in the upper lip will facilitate the repair,

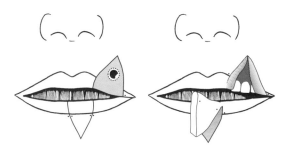

Figure 15.9 Abbe lip switch operation. The excision is marked out as shown on the upper lip and the flap repair is indicated on the lower lip.

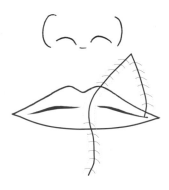

Figure 15.10 Abbe lip switch operation. The excision is completed and the flap from the lower lip is transposed into the upper lip.

so the size of the flap required from the lower lip is less than the defect in the upper lip; the rule of thumb is that it can be a half to two-thirds the size of the defect. This is important because for upper to lower lip transfer, there is less tissue to borrow in the upper lip than there is in the lower lip. The triangular donor site defect in the lower lip is marked out (Fig 15.9) so that its length is equal to that of the defect, while the base is one-half of the defect. This will give proportionate shortening of the upper and lower lips. The pedicle of the flap can be medial or lateral and contains the inferior labial artery, which runs 5 mm below the vermilion margin of the lip; it is better to leave a thick pedicle rather than risk damaging the artery. These flaps rarely die but if the artery is damaged, then they probably will and this will produce a horrendous defect to repair subsequently.

When all the marks have been made, the tumour is excised with a knife held at right angles to the skin and the lip. Then, the lower lip is cut and mobilized except for its lateral pedicle. It will be necessary to cut down to the muscles of the face and to incise the mucosa of the lower buccoalveolar sulcus. The flap is rotated into the defect (Fig. 15.10) and one 5/0 Ethilon suture placed through the needle marks at the vermilion edges. The flap is sutured to the defect in three layers as before, with considerable care being taken with the muscle layer sutures, and the external skin is closed meticulously.

Aftercare for Abbe lip switch

- General care
- The patient should be fed with a feeding cup or straw
- Keep the wound free of crusting with an antibiotic cream as described previously
- Three weeks later the pedicle is transected as a second stage and suturing completed

---

The commissure should be kept at all costs. If not, an Abbe Estlander flap is used. The final result is excellent (Fig. 15.11).

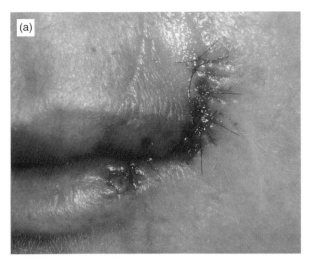

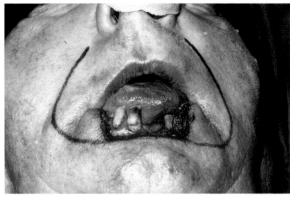

Figure 15.12 Defect in the lower lip following a two-thirds resection for a squamous cell carcinoma. Bilateral Karapandic flaps are marked out.

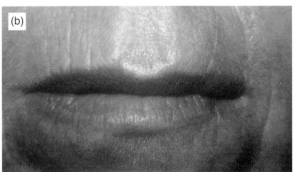

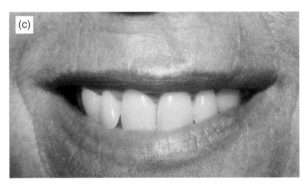

Figure 15.13 Defect in the lower lip following a two-thirds resection for a squamous cell carcinoma. The result is a competent, fully functional lower lip with good aesthetic result.

Figure 15.11 Patient who has undergone wide resection of the left upper lip for a recurrent basal cell carcinoma. Repair has been completed with an Abbe lip switch operation. (a) The pedicle connecting the blood supply from the lower lip to the flap in the upper lip has just been divided. (b,c) The final result.

Karapandzic flap

This technique can be used to reconstruct three-quarters of the lower lip. It is simple and quick to perform, and results in a functional, pleasing, acceptable and aesthetic lip. The tumour excision is marked out (Fig. 15.12) and either unilateral, or more usually bilateral, Karapandzic flaps are marked, extending up into the nasolabial folds.

Incisions are made transversly from the base of the postexcisional defect extending around the commissures into the upper lip. Using loupes, the orbicularis oris muscle fibres are spread apart longitudinally in the line of the skin excision down to the submucosal layer so that vessels and nerves remain intact. Intraoral mucosa is incised for 1–2 cm from the edge of the defect and then the lip reconstruction is sutured in layers. The result is a competent, sensate, fully functional lower lip with a good aesthetic result (Fig 15.13).

Bilateral Gillies fan flaps for total lower lip reconstruction

These fan flaps are constructed bilaterally as illustrated in Fig. 15.14. They are rotated on their pedicles and sutured

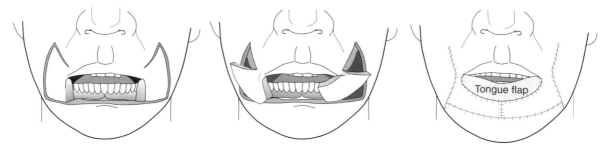

Figure 15.14 Total lower lip reconstruction with bilateral Gillies fan flaps. The flaps are designed as shown and rotated in to fill the defect.

end-to-end without tension to reconstitute a lip of considerable bulk. The vermilion is reconstructed with a tongue flap which is divided at 14 days.

Abbe Estlander flap for angle tumours

This flap is performed to reconstruct defects that require partial commissure reconstruction. The method is essentially the same as described above for the Abbe flap except that the medial pedicle becomes the commissure (Fig. 15.15a). The flap is marked out as shown, rotated and sewn in, and a new commissure is formed. Care should be taken not to damage the pedicle and the only major problem with this technique is that it results in a rounded commissure which often leads to postoperative asymmetry. This may be corrected with a commissureplasty performed 3 months after initial surgery. Full commissure reconstruction requires either double rhomboid cheek flaps with vermilion advancement or free tissue transfer.

Because of the difficulty in creating a new commissure, every attempt should be made to retain the angle of the mouth. It is sometimes possible to use an Abbe flap to repair the defect and sew the ends of the commissure to the bare area of the flap (15.15b and c). This can be corrected later as a second stage operation (Fig. 15.15d and e) and gives a better result than the Abbe Estlander in this situation since the position of the normal commissure is maintained.

Commissureplasty

This operation is based on the double Z-plasty principle (Fig 15.16). An incision is made exactly at the middle of the rounded corner of the mouth, about 2.5 cm long. At the end of this, two 2.5 cm incisions are made upwards and downwards and then lateral extensions are made from these for the same distance but angled at 60°. When the flaps are transposed and sutured, the angle of the mouth is sharpened. Further sharpening can be achieved using a modified vermilion advancement technique.

Perialar crescentic advancement for upper lip cancer (Webster's technique)

This is a most elegant technique which may be used unilaterally to reconstruct defects in one side of the lip

or, when combined bilaterally, may be used to reconstruct up to two-thirds of the upper lip that involve the philtrum, providing an excellent cosmetic result. Even larger defects may be closed when this is combined with an Abbe flap from the lower lip or a reverse Karapandzic flap.

The flap is outlined as shown in Fig. 15.17 and, with the crescents excised, the cheek is mobilized to facilitate advancement. Meticulous primary closure can easily be achieved. Postoperative care is as described previously.

Total upper lip reconstruction

This is rarely required but may be performed using either bilateral nasolabial or formal Gillies fan flaps (Fig. 15.18) supplemented with vermilion reconstruction using tongue advancement.

The conventional Abbe flap as described is used to reconstruct upper lip defects from the lower lip. Reverse Abbe flaps may be used from the upper lip to the lower lip but because of the problems of symmetry and the philtrum these are usually smaller and require more skill, and the outcome is not usually as good. They are rarely used.

Management of malignant change in actinic cheilitis

It is often difficult to know whether an area in a lip affected by actinic cheilitis has become malignant and is infiltrated by tumour. If during a lip shave an area of infiltration is found, frozen sections should be performed. The lip shave can then be accompanied by a wedge excision and primary closure.

Place of prophylactic neck dissection

The place of prophylactic neck dissection in patients with cancer of the lip has not been studied prospectively . The cure rate from therapeutic neck dissection for a subsequently occult metastasis compares favourably with the results of elective neck dissection. Some authors have recommended aggressive treatment including bilateral suprahyoid (level I) or supraomohyoid (levels I–III) neck dissection if the primary lesion is greater than 1.5 cm in

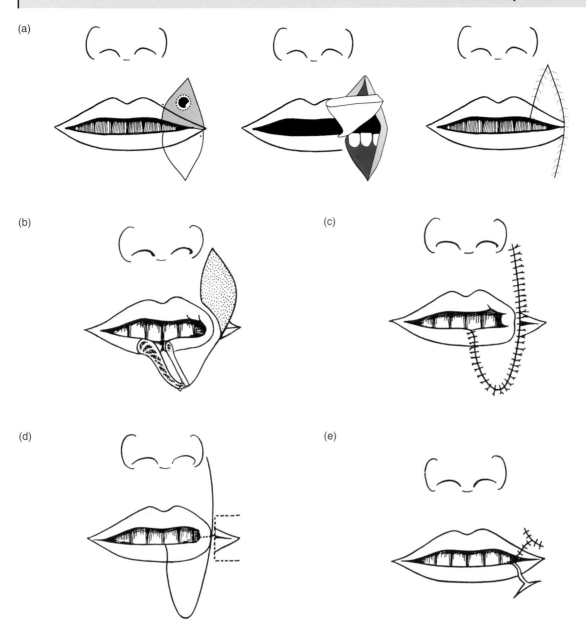

(a)

(b)

(c)

(d)

(e)

Figure 15.15 (a) Use of an Abbe Estlander flap to reconstruct tumours of the commissure. (b) Abbe lip switch operation: flap turned into defect leaving the commissure intact, and (c) repair, sewing the ends of the commissure to the bare areas on the flap. (d) Second-stage Abbe lip switch: solid line shows the healed initial incision. The pedicle is transected and vertical and horizontal incisions, and lateral incisions are made, all of the same length. (e) When the vermilion margins are reapproximated, the incisions are closed in a T.

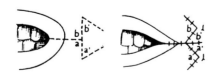

Figure 15.16 Commissureplasty.

diameter, if the cancer is in the upper lip, if it is recurrent or poorly differentiated. If tumour is found in a neck-dissection specimen, a full neck dissection may be completed or the patient given postoperative radiotherapy. Alternatively, a policy of 'wait and see' should be adopted. If the tumour is being treated with radiotherapy, then those with high-risk tumours can receive prophylactic neck irradiation.

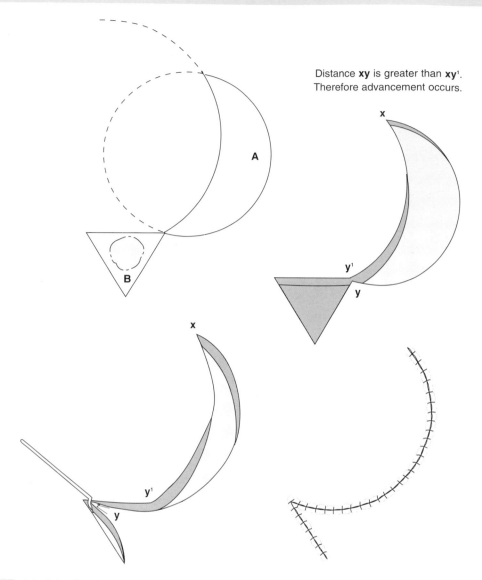

Distance **xy** is greater than **xy**¹.
Therefore advancement occurs.

Figure 15.17   Principle of perialar crescentic advancement.

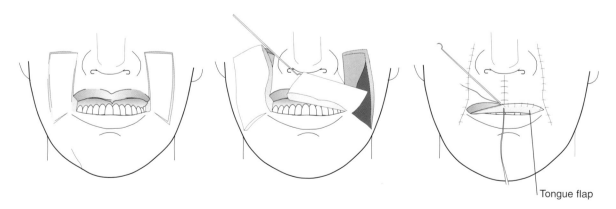

Tongue flap

Figure 15.18   Total upper lip reconstruction using bilateral Gillies fan flaps. The flaps are designed and rotated inwards as shown.

Radiotherapy techniques

External beam therapy

The lower lip remains one of the few ideal sites for orthovoltage (300 kV) X-ray therapy in the megavoltage radiotherapy era. The patient lies supine and the upper lip is protected by a shaped lead sheet which also enters the mouth and lies between the lower lip and the mandible, thus shielding the tongue and lower alveolus. A second sheet of lead overlies the lower lip, revealing the tumour with a 1 cm margin of healthy tissue through an appropriately sized semicircular aperture. Using a single anterior field, a fractionated course of 50 Gy in 15 fractions over 3 weeks or its equivalent is given.

Despite the suitability of this therapy for treating carcinoma of the lip, some radiotherapy centres no longer have orthovoltage facilities. It is considered an obsolete modality because the physical characteristics of the beam limit its usefulness in treating disease at other sites. Electron beams, generated by a linear accelerator, are increasingly being used instead of orthovoltage therapy in this setting. The set-up for treatment of lip carcinoma with an electron beam is similar to that used with orthovoltage equipment. It is, however, somewhat more cumbersome as the lead shielding needs to be thicker and the intraoral part of the posterior lead sheet has to be covered in a thick layer of wax to absorb the secondary X-rays generated when high-energy electrons strike heavy metals. In addition, because of the physical characteristics of electron beams, a wider margin of 2 cm of normal tissue around the tumour has to be included in the treatment volume. Electrons of 8–10 MeV should be used and the prescribed dose and fractionation schedule will be the same as that used for orthovoltage treatment.

Interstitial therapy

The accessibility of the lip and the relatively small size of most of its cancers, make this site suitable for interstitial treatment. The original technique, now less commonly used, entails implantation with rigid needles containing caesium which replaces radium, obsolete because of difficulties with radiation protection. Nowadays, techniques involving the use of hollow, fine, flexible plastic or rigid metal tubes which are subsequently loaded with iridium wire are usually employed. Whichever technique is used, the implantation is usually performed under general anaesthesia. Both the old and new methods are effective, but better results using iridium have been reported. However as these studies were not randomized trials but retrospective comparisons with historical controls, great caution is needed in interpreting the claimed superiority of iridium, since many other unidentified factors may have contributed to this apparent benefit. A genuine advantage of iridium wire afterloading is that because there is no radiation exposure to staff during the implant procedure, great care may be taken to ensure perfect geometry of the implant, and hence an optimal dose distri-

bution. In addition, the energy of the radiation emanating from iridium is lower than that from radium or caesium, making radiation protection easier. From the patient's point of view flexible tubes cause less discomfort. However, iridium wire is costly and has a half-life of only 74 days, whereas caesium needles, with a half-life of 30 years could be reused almost indefinitely.

The usual dose prescription for implants with caesium needles is 60–70 Gy over 6–7 days, calculated under the Manchester rules. With iridium, a slightly shorter overall time is often used; 60 Gy, calculated according to the Paris system of dosimetry, is given over about 5 days.

A rarely used technique for irradiation of lip cancers involves the preparation of a device which sandwiches the lip between two plates of Perspex, each loaded with a suitable distribution of an appropriate radionuclide. This double mould or surface applicator is worn intermittently, for example for 6 h each day for 8 days. The preparation of a good double mould requires certain technical skills and when lip cancer can effectively be treated in simpler ways, it is not surprising that its use is limited.

Whether external beam or implant irradiation is used, it is inevitable that there will be a brisk mucosal and cutaneous reaction. This will proceed to moist desquamation on the skin and formation of a fibrinous membrane within the mouth, both of which will take at least a couple of weeks to heal. Ultimately, however, a good functional and cosmetic result is usual (Fig. 15.19). Later, there may be some atrophy of the substance of the lip, and the skin will become depigmented and may show telangiectasia, but bad scarring is unusual. Atrophy of lip musculature in the irradiated field leads to close attachment of the vermilion to the underlying muscles and sometimes to general hardness in the area. It can therefore occasionally be difficult to diagnose recurrence. In the unusual case of doubt or deformity after irradiation, a wedge excision of the irradiated area may be considered. After radiation therapy there is permanent

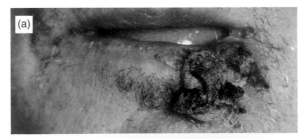

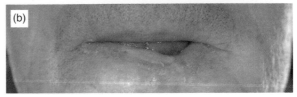

Figure 15.19 (a) Patient with a T_4N_0 squamous carcinoma of the lower lip treated with radiotherapy. (b) The patient remains alive and well 3 years later.

hypersensitivity to thermal and actinic stimuli. Patients who have outdoor occupations remain at a disadvantage, therefore, after such therapy and are perhaps better treated with surgery initially.

ORAL CAVITY

Surgical anatomy

The anatomical regions and sites forming the oral cavity under the joint UICC – American Joint Committee (AJC) classification (1997) were listed earlier (Staging section). Note that the soft palate and the posterior third of the tongue are excluded from the oral cavity and are part of the oropharynx.

The buccal mucosa is covered with non-keratinizing, stratified squamous epithelium. It covers the parotid duct and multiple minor salivary glands. It is generally fairly loose but tight over the buccinator muscle. It is also rather tightly fixed in the upper and lower sulci and for this reason it is very difficult to stitch a skin graft to these sites. The mucosa also covers the upper and lower alveoli, so that tumours of the buccal mucosa may well involve these sites. Lymph drainage from the buccal mucosa is to the submandibular lymph nodes and from there to the deep cervical chain. The rest of the mouth is covered by the same type of epithelium and there are multiple minor salivary glands in the hard palate and a few in the floor of the mouth. There are also collections of minor salivary glands at specific sites, as shown below. The interlacing muscle fibres of the tongue form an easy pathway for the spread of cancer, and the constant movement of the tongue with speech and mastication also facilitates the wide dissemination of malignant disease. For this reason, tongue tumours must always be assessed by palpation and excisional margins for the majority of tumours should be at least 2 cm.

Sites of minor salivary glands in the oral cavity

- Labial glands in the submucosa of the inner surface of the lips
- Retromolar glands in the vicinity of the opening of the parotid duct
- Buccal glands in the mucous membrane of the cheek
- Glands of the floor of the mouth
- Lesser sublingual glands near the major sublingual gland
- Glossopalatine glands, extending posteriorly from the lesser sublingual glands to the mucosa of the glossopalatine fold
- Palatine glands, some 400 in number, distributed over the hard and soft palates and uvula, but not in the midline or anterior to a line between the first molar teeth
- Lingual glands situated close to the inferior surface of the tongue on each side of the frenulum, and at the base and lateral borders of the tongue

---

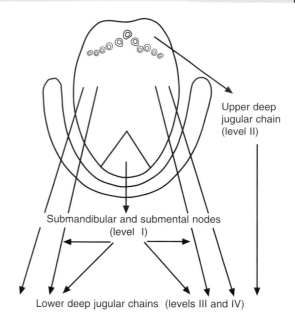

Figure 15.20 Lymph drainage of the tongue.

Lymphatic drainage from the tip of the tongue drains to the submental nodes and to the nodes in the deep jugular cervical chain (Fig. 15.20). The sublingual portion of the tongue usually drains to the submandibular nodes, and the rest of the anterior two-thirds of the tongue drains to the deep jugular chain from the level of the posterior belly of digastric to the omohyoid (level III). This is important because the only gland enlarged with the tumour on the lateral border of the anterior two-thirds of the tongue may be the jugulodigastric or jugulomohyoid node.

It is also important to realize that lymph from the anterior part of the mouth can drain via a fast-track pattern to the lower jugular chain (levels III and IV), making a suprahyoid neck dissection illogical. The tip and middle of the tongue have a rich bilateral capillary lymphatic network but this is less on the lateral margins. The U-shaped floor of the mouth drains mainly to the submandibular glands and the upper deep jugular chain (levels I, II and III). There is a moderate bilateral lymphatic drainage from the anterior parts of the floor of the mouth. The lymph drainage of the alveolus is much the same as that of the floor of the mouth but the capillary network is less extensive.

In any cancer of the mouth, nodes in front of and behind the facial artery as it crosses the mandible (prefacial and postfacial nodes) are often affected and should be included in the field of any modified radical or radical neck dissection.

The mandible is a key structure in intraoral malignancy. The pattern of invasion by tumour and the mechanisms of spread within the bone determine the surgical approach to many tumours. The blood supply of the mandible influences both excisional and reconstructive techniques. Loss of the teeth causes changes in the shape, structure and vascularity, as well as in patterns of tumour spread.

The body of the mandible can be divided into an upper part, which carries the teeth and is covered by mucoperiosteum (the alveolar segment), and the lower part, covered by periosteum alone. On its labial and buccal surfaces the line that separates the two runs along the lower buccal sulcus: on the lingual surface the line corresponds largely to that of the mylohyoid line on the bone.

The alveolar segment, with its covering of mucoperiosteum, is in direct contact with the oral cavity and it is the only part of the mandible which is, strictly speaking, intraoral.

These lines, along which mucous membrane and periosteum separate on each side of the bone, are approximately similar both in level and direction, running backwards and slightly upwards to meet behind the third molar where the pterygomandibular raphé is attached to the bone.

The mucosal surface behind the third molar up to the maxillary tuberosity is called the retromolar trigone. There the mucosa overlies the anterior border of the ascending mandibular ramus, separated from it by the pterygomandibular raphé, where the buccinator and the superior constrictor muscles decussate.

Running through the mandible on each side, transmitting the inferior alveolar nerve with its accompanying vessels, is the mandibular canal. The site of entry of the neurovascular bundle into the canal is marked on the medial surface of the ramus by a bony spur, the lingula. The nerve leaves the outer surface of the mandible below the first premolar tooth at the mental foramen.

The mandible has a comparatively small proportion of cancellous bone, which is concentrated in the body. Through this bone runs the mandibular canal and, as it has no lining of compact bone, the canal is in direct contact with the cancellous bone of the body. The ramus has very little cancellous bone and this is largely localized just behind the third molar tooth.

The tooth sockets are lined by a thin layer of compact bone, the lamina dura, and each is in continuity with the mandibular canal through the foramen opposite the apex of each root, which carries the vessels and nerves supplying the pulp of the teeth.

Considerable changes in the mandible occur after extraction of the teeth. The socket fills with blood clot which organizes rapidly to form cancellous bone, and the overlying mucosa heals extremely rapidly. Whilst the socket fills rapidly with bone, the projecting margins of the original socket are resorbed and the bone in this area is rounded down to produce the narrow ridge typical of the edentulous mandible. When there is extreme resorption, the bone is referred to as 'pipestem'. In such a mandible, the floor of the mouth, the occlusal surface of the alveolus and the buccal sulcus are all virtually on the same plane. The alveolus is reduced to a strip of mucoperiosteum between the mucosal surface on each side. The mandibular canal and its contained inferior alveolar vessels and nerve comes to lie much closer to the oral surface.

A further anatomical effect of losing teeth is the relative change in the site of attachment of the mylohyoid to the mandible. Resorption of the alveolar segment leaves the attachment much closer to the ridge. The rise of the mylohyoid line in passing backwards brings the muscle insertion alongside the ridge in the molar region. This is of major importance as a factor in the mechanism of mandibular invasion by tumour.

In addition to the general remodelling associated with the edentulous state, the tooth socket disappears, the line of teeth being converted into an occlusal ridge. All along the line of the crest, the bone is imperfectly sealed by cortex and, where the cortical deficiencies are present, the mucoperiosteum is in direct continuity with the cancellous bone of the medulla. These defects are usually small but some can be as large as 2 mm in diameter. At their most frequent, almost the entire ridge lacks a cover of cortical bone, the appearance being of a moth-eaten line, 2–3 mm broad, all along the crest where the surface consists of cancellous bone.

In the mandible, the absence of a protective cover of compact bone over the entire occlusal ridge means that virtually from the outset, tumour is free to infiltrate through into the medullary cavity and reach the inferior alveolar nerve, with the subsequent potential thereafter for perineural spread.

Blood supply to the mandible

The intact mandible derives its blood supply from the inferior alveolar vessels and from its soft-tissue attachments, which are therefore very important.

Inferior alveolar vessels

These vessels, in addition to the supplying the teeth, supply the surrounding bone. The calibre of the artery and, therefore, the proportion of the total blood supply of the mandible it carries decrease both with age and whether or not teeth are present. Blood flow may decrease with age and loss of teeth.

Soft-tissue attachments

The ramus has extensive vascular sources provided by the bony attachments of the pterygomasseteric muscle sling. The alveolar segment of the body of the bone is covered with mucoperiosteum and through this it is vascularized. This alveolar mucoperiosteum, in turn, derives its blood supply from the soft tissues attached to the bone below the lower buccal sulcus laterally and the mylohyoid line medially (Fig. 15.21).

On its lingual surface the mandibular body, below the line of reflection of mucosa, has no soft-tissue attachments and, hence, no vascular sources other than those provided by the linear attachment of mylohyoid and the genial and digastric muscles at the symphysis. In contrast, the entire labial and buccal surface below the lower buccal sulcus is covered by soft tissue firmly attached to the bone.

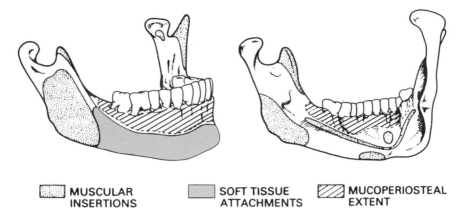

MUSCULAR INSERTIONS   SOFT TISSUE ATTACHMENTS   MUCOPERIOSTEAL EXTENT

Figure 15.21 Blood supply of the mandible.

This attachment ends at the lower border of the body, except on each side of the symphysis where the bone broadens for the attachment of the digastric muscle. Therefore the body of the mandible receives the bulk of its blood supply from its labiobuccal aspect and not from its lingual side.

In addition to the possibility of cancer spread along the inferior alveolar nerve and the inferior dental canal by squamous cell carcinomas and adenoid cystic carcinomas, there are other channels which facilitate rapid spread.

> *Other channels of spread*
>
> ■ Small bony canals in hard palate
> ■ Greater and lesser palatine foramina
> ■ Lateral incisive foramina

The duct of the submandibular gland runs submucosally on the mylohyoid muscle and tumours or scarring due to previous surgery or radiotherapy may obstruct this duct or its opening to cause swelling of the submandibular salivary gland.

Classically, in its early stages, this swelling is intermittent and occurs at mealtimes, but as the scarring or the tumour progresses the enlargement may persist and then may be confused with, and should be differentiated from, a metastatic lymph node in the submandibular triangle.

Surgical pathology

The relative incidence of different types of oral tumour is shown in Table 15.1. From the tables, it can be seen that squamous cell carcinoma forms the vast majority and this tumour is discussed first.

The incidence of squamous carcinomas of various sites is shown in Table 15.2.

Development of squamous carcinoma

Many carcinogenic factors have been proposed in the aetiology of squamous carcinoma of the oral cavity and these are listed below.

Table 15.1 Incidence of mouth tumours

Type of tumour	Incidence (%)
Ectodermal	
Miscellaneous benign (mainly neural tumours)	1.0
Benign salivary	2.0
Squamous carcinoma (verrucous carcinoma 5.0)	85.0
Malignant salivary	5.0
Melanoma	0.1
Mesodermal	
Haemangioma	1.5
Granular cell myoblastoma	1.0
Other benign	1.0
Malignant	
Non-Hodgkin's lymphoma	1.0
Hodgkin's lymphoma	0.1
Fibrosarcoma	0.5
Other sarcomas	1.0
Metastatic	1.0

Table 15.2 Site incidence of oral squamous carcinoma

Site of carcinoma	Incidence (%)
Retromolar	2
Buccal mucosa	10

Tongue
  Lateral border 31
  Tip 2
  Dorsum 2
	35

Floor of the mouth
  Anterior 25
  Lateral 5
	30

Lower alveolus	15
Upper alveolus	5
Hard palate	3

Risk factors for squamous carcinoma

- **Smoking**
- **High alcohol intake**
- Dental caries
- Alcoholic mouth washes
- Hot spicy foods
- Leucoplakia
- Avitaminosis
- Betel nut chewing (and smokeless tobacco)
- Chronic glossitis
- Malnutrition
- Syphilis
- Cirrhosis
- Plummer–Vinson syndrome
- Lichen planus
- Chronic hyperplastic candidiasis
- Human immunodeficiency virus (HIV)
- Xeroderma pigmentosa
- Dyskeratosis congenita
- Submucosal fibrosis

There is no evidence to show that these are all premalignant, but they are certainly associated factors. There is no doubt that smoking is associated with an increased incidence of oral cancer. Smoking and drinking alone increase the incidence of the disease and together they are synergistic, increasing the risk of a cancer in the oral cavity by about six-fold.

The only true premalignant lesions in the oral cavity are leucoplakia and erythroleucoplakia. Leucoplakia literally means a white plaque and it is used in different ways by different authors. For example, some authors include other white lesions in the mouth such as lichen planus, whereas most restrict the term to abnormal keratinization; the white appearance of lesions in this condition is usually caused by keratin becoming white when it is wet.

Furthermore, the term leucoplakia has no pathological significance. The interest in this lesion is due to the fact that a small proportion become malignant over time. In one study of patients with oral leucoplakia followed up 30 years, 6% of patients developed squamous carcinoma and there was a strong association between the type of leucoplakia and the potential for development of cancer. In those patients with histological evidence of dysplasia, 13% developed a carcinoma while in those with erosive leucoplakia, the risk increased to 26%. It seems that leucoplakia with severe epithelial dysplasia is the most likely one to undergo malignant change.

Clinical variants of leucoplakia

- Leucoplakia simplex
- Verrucous leucoplakia
- Erythroleucoplakia

There are various clinical appearances: an area of soft, white, velvety mucosa; a patch of white, resembling paint on the mucosa; an area of distinct pallor described as leucoplakia simplex; and verrucous leucoplakia, combining leucoplakia and erythroleucoplakia. Some leucoplakias show an irregular mixture of white and red areas. The erythroleucoplakias are the most dangerous lesions and the most likely to become malignant. Erythroleucoplakia is defined as an oral mucosal lesion which appears as a red velvety plaque that cannot be clinically or pathologically ascribed to any other predetermined condition.

About 80% of leucoplakias show the combination of hyperkeratosis, parakeratosis and acanthosis with no evidence of epithelial dysplasia. Moderate dysplasia is found in about 10% of specimens and severe dysplasia or carcinoma *in situ* in about 5%, many of which will be predominantly erythroleucoplakia. Leucoplakia most commonly occurs on the buccal mucosa, followed by the alveolar mucosa, tongue, lip, palate, floor of mouth and gingiva, in that order. In the buccal mucosa, the most common site is the occlusal line. The treatment of the suspicious 'premalignant lesion' is shown in Fig. 15.22.

Lichen planus is a keratin-producing disease that usually affects the buccal mucosa; it is easily recognized by the multiple narrow and grey, but slightly elevated, lines (Wickham's striae) that converge towards each other forming a mesh. The intervening mucosa looks rather oedematous. Another variety presents as elevated white spots and there is also a hypertrophic type resembling leucoplakia. Less frequent are the erosive and ulcerative varieties. If dyskeratosis is found in these lesions, they are premalignant but this is an exception rather than the rule. In one study of 725 patients with oral lichen planus followed up for up to 30 years, only 4% of patients developed subsequent oral squamous carcinoma.

Fordyce's disease consists of ectopic aggregates of sebaceous glands looking like clusters of greyish white or yellow nodules. It is not premalignant, nor is the white spongy naevus, which looks like leucoplakia and occurs in childhood.

Recent reports have shown that 80% of acquired immunodeficiency syndrome (AIDS) sufferers develop hairy oral leucoplakia. This is a unilateral corrugated lesion usually occurring on the posterolateral border of the tongue. However, it may occur on the floor of the mouth, buccal mucosa and palate. Histological examination shows a thick epithelium with hyperkeratosis, areas of koilocytes and pyknotic nuclei.

Squamous cell carcinoma

Pathology

Squamous cell carcinoma of the oral cavity is generally said to be exophytic, ulcerative or infiltrative on gross pathological appearance. However, as a general rule, the majority of cancers show more than one of these characteristics. Many are both ulcerative and infiltrative and the exophytic tumours are less common.

Initial histological grading by Broders (1941) used two intermediate grades, moderately well differentiated, and

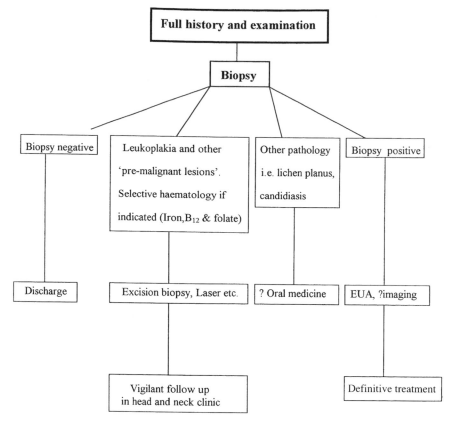

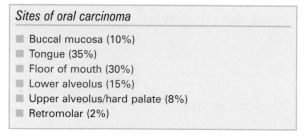

Figure 15.22 Treatment of the suspicious premalignant lesion.

moderately differentiated and a more sophisticated and detailed grading system was introduced by Jacobson *et al.* (1973) whereby the tumour cell population was graded I–IV depending on the degree of differentiation, the degree of nucleomorphism and the frequency of mitotic figures. In addition, the tumour–host relationship was estimated on a scale of I–IV by the mode and stage of invasion.

Some workers have found a positive correlation between grading and prognosis, although others have not. There is now ample evidence that the depth of invasion of the tumour is related to prognosis, with the incidence of cervical metastases increasing with increasing depth of tumour (Spiro *et al.*, 1986). Some recent work has suggested that if histological grading is applied to the invasive margin of the tumour, a more positive correlation may be obtained.

Variants of squamous carcinoma

The verrucous carcinoma represents a very well-differentiated squamous carcinoma. Within the oral cavity it forms a flat, warty tumour which is slow growing. It is a rare tumour comprising less than 5% of all squamous carcinomas within the oral cavity and consists of highly differentiated squamous cells with occasional mitoses. Histopathologically, the diagnosis may be difficult unless the biopsy specimen is large and deep enough to include

the deep margin. Within a verrucous carcinoma, there may be an area of a less differentiated squamous carcinoma and this can occur in up to 20% of cases. Verrucous carcinomas are slow-growing tumours, undoubtedly malignant, but this is a local phenomenon and they rarely, if ever, metastasize to local lymph nodes.

Squamous carcinoma at specific sites

Sites of oral carcinoma

- Buccal mucosa (10%)
- Tongue (35%)
- Floor of mouth (30%)
- Lower alveolus (15%)
- Upper alveolus/hard palate (8%)
- Retromolar (2%)

Buccal carcinoma

Buccal carcinoma affects men more than women, occurs in the older age group and has a definite geographic incidence, being most common in Indian communities, in Africa and south-east Asia (where it forms 40% of all cancers); in this region the chewing of betel nut and reverse smoking are common habits and possibly as a consequence, leucoplakia and submucosal fibrosis are more common. It is also fairly common in the USA, where a percentage of the population still chews tobacco. It is, however, uncommon in the UK. Buccal cancer is often diagnosed at a late stage, as this is the most insensitive part of the mouth.

The cheek forms the lateral wall of the mouth and consists of the buccinator muscle, external fibroadipose tissue and skin. The mucosal surface extends from the upper to the lower gingivobuccal sulci, where the mucosa is reflected over the upper and lower alveolar ridges, and forms the commissure of the lips and overlies the ascending ramus of the mandible. The most common sites for buccal carcinoma are the commissure of the mouth, along with the occlusal plane and in the retromolar areas.

There are three clinical types of buccal carcinoma, the exophytic, the ulceroinfiltrative and the verrucous, in that order of frequency. Most buccal carcinomas are well differentiated in type, and carcinoma of the buccal mucosa is the most common cancer in the mouth to be associated with pre-existing leucoplakia. Exophytic carcinomas are found most often around the buccal commissure, where ulceroinfiltrative carcinomas invade the buccinator muscle early and present a deep excavating ulcer with diffuse peripheral extension. Lesions lying posteriorly extend easily into the ptyerygomaxillary fossa and they can also invade the anterior tonsillar pillars, the alveolar ridges and the pterygoid fossa. The verrucous tumour most commonly occurs on the lower buccal sulcus and the lower alveolus. It can occur elsewhere in the mouth, but forms no more than 5% of all oral cancers. It has a characteristic papillary appearance: although it often appears relatively innocuous, it invades the soft tissues of the cheek, the maxilla and the mandible. It rarely metastasizes even to lymph nodes and almost never to distant sites.

Only 15% of buccal carcinomas are associated with palpable glands when first seen and it is said that 5% have microscopically positive lymph nodes when there are none to feel.

Carcinoma of the tongue

Carcinoma of the tongue is a disease of the middle aged and elderly, with an equal gender incidence. Fifty years ago it was predominantly a disease of men and there is no good explanation for this change in the gender ratio. Recent figures suggest a rise in the incidence of tongue cancer in young women.

Most squamous carcinomas are well differentiated, while poorly differentiated varieties are rare. Up to 40% of carcinomas in the mouth arise in the anterior two-thirds of the tongue and 85% of these arise from the lateral border (Fig. 15.23). Tumours arising from the dorsum, the ventral surface or the tip are very uncommon. The incidence of lymph-node metastases is shown in the box. The high number of occult metastases in the N_0 neck should be noted. Tongue tumours may be infiltrative or exophytic. The infiltrative types may appear to be quite small on the surface, but palpation often shows that they

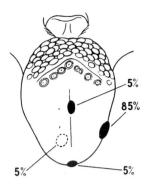

Figure 15.23 Site of incidence of tumours of the oral tongue.

have invaded most or part of the tongue. The behaviour of the tumour becomes more aggressive, the further posterior in the mouth the lesion lies.

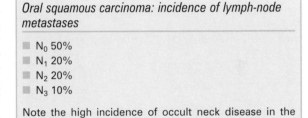

Oral squamous carcinoma: incidence of lymph-node metastases

- N_0 50%
- N_1 20%
- N_2 20%
- N_3 10%

Note the high incidence of occult neck disease in the clinically N_0 neck

Aggressive features of posterior tongue tumours
- The incidence of lymph-nodes metastases is increased.
- The tumour can spread to the tonsillar pillars, the retromolar area and the floor of the mouth.
- Large invasive carcinomas can extend beneath intact mucosa into the muscles of the posterior third of the tongue and thence into the pre-epiglottic space.
- The tumour extends within the musculature of the tongue, but particularly in a posterior direction beneath an intact mucosa.

Infiltration of the muscles ultimately causes immobility of the tongue. The tumour invades with ease through the midline septum of the tongue.

The incidence of lymph-node metastases is proportional to both the tumour T-stage and its depth, and there is also correlation between certain histological grades of the tumour and lymph-node metastases.

Carcinoma of the floor of the mouth

Tumours of the floor of the mouth are usually divided into those arising from the anterior part and those arising laterally. The reason for this distinction is the differing surgical problems that these two sites present. A common site in the anterior floor of mouth is around the papilla at the point where the submandibular duct opens. Remaining tumours are distributed evenly along the floor of the mouth. These tumours spread marginally in both medial and lateral directions. Regional spread is therefore into the ventral surface of the tongue and deep spread occurs to the tongue base, particularly into the hyoglossus and genioglossus muscles. Lateral spread on to the alveolus is more important. The point at which the tumour reaches the lingual surface of the mandible depends on two factors: firstly, the level of attachment of the mylohyoid muscle to the mandible, which rises steadily from the anterior floor backwards towards the molar region and, secondly, on whether the patient has teeth present or not. In the dentate mandible, the teeth form some barrier preventing spread from the lingual to the buccal surfaces.

Sometimes, patients with floor of the mouth tumours are edentulous, in which case the sequence of pathological events is different. The alveolar segment of the mandible has been resorbed, and the occlusal ridge does not have a complete covering of cortical bone but is penetrated by foramina, so that the tumour can readily spread into the mandible through these, gaining access to the medullary cavity and to the inferior alveolar nerve (Fig. 15.24). This nerve provides an important pathway for the spread of tumour which can spread relatively quickly along the nerve as far as the pterygoid fossa and the skull base.

Another important structure in the spread of a tumour in the floor of the mouth is the muscle floor formed by the mylohyoid muscle. Anteriorly, this presents a barrier to the inferior spread of tumour, but the muscle is deficient posteriorly and, in this area, the mucosa of the floor of the mouth lies very close to the overlying skin, separated only by subcutaneous tissue. Tumours here can spread relatively easy into the submandibular area, forming a palpable and ultimately visible lump.

Carcinoma of the lower alveolus

Carcinoma of the lower alveolus generally affects the anterolateral part and spread on to the floor of the mouth occurs readily. Thirty per cent of patients have radiological evidence of bone destruction.

For tumours affecting the lower alveolus, the site and frequency of lymph-node metastases are the same as for tumours of the floor of the mouth. Carcinomas of the gingiva generally affect the premolar and molar areas and quite often arise in an area of leucoplakia. These tumours may be ulcerating or exophytic. At least 50% of these tumours invade the underlying bone, by the same pathways as already indicated for tumours of the floor of mouth. These tumours usually metastasize first to the submandibular nodes and such a metastasis may be fixed first to the periosteum and then to the mandible.

A tumour arising from any of the common primary sites (floor of mouth and tongue) can invade the mandible, but this process is most important in alveolar tumours. Some aspects of mandibular bone invasion are worth considering in more detail. The spread of squamous cell carcinoma within the oral cavity is an infiltrative phenomenon through soft tissues and bone, but is embolic along lymphatics and permeative along nerves. At present, there is no evidence to suggest that tumour spread to the mandible is embolic along the lymphatic vessels or that tumour spread from the mandible to lymph nodes is by periosteal lymphatics. In fact, tumour can spread from primary mucosal sites within the oral cavity along the lymphatics, and if these vessels have a close anatomical relationship with the mandible, then tumour metastases will pass close to the periosteum on their way to the lymph nodes. As previously stated, such spread is embolic and, as such, periosteum is not involved and therefore bone and periosteum need not primarily be excised as part of the *en bloc* management regarding the lymphatic spread of intraoral squamous carcinoma.

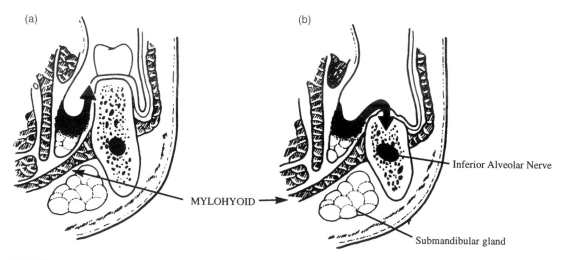

(a)   (b)

Inferior Alveolar Nerve

MYLOHYOID →

Submandibular gland

Figure 15.24 Pathways of spread of tumour into the mandible in the non-irradiated patient. (a) Dentate mandible, (b) edentulous.

How does tumour penetrate the mandible?

The two most important factors in the natural history of the spread of intraoral squamous carcinoma and the pattern of any bone invasion are:

- the presence or absence of teeth
- whether or not mandible has been previously irradiated.

Dental status. Under normal circumstances, periosteum is very resistant to tumour infiltration and the presence of squamous cell carcinoma can initiate periosteal new bone formation on the lingual, buccolabial and inferior surfaces. It does not occur on the alveolar aspect of the mandible which supports its susceptibility to tumour invasion. With age and lack of teeth, loss of vertical mandibular height due to progressive alveolar bone resorption brings the occlusal surface closer to the mucosa of the floor of the mouth. Tumour spread at this site initially tends to be superficial and radial and is therefore greatest in the edentulous mandible. The spread is by direct infiltration and not by metastasis, whether or not the patient has been previously irradiated. Non-occlusal foramina provide additional sites of entry, namely the mental, genial and mandibular foramina.

Effect of prior irradiation. In contrast, in the irradiated mandible, squamous cell carcinoma has been observed to penetrate any of the cortical surfaces with which it comes into contact during infiltrative spread through the soft tissues. This means that despite clinical examination showing tumour extending on to the alveolus, in the presence of previous irradiation, there may be other sites of deep tumour invasion into the mandible. In the irradiated mandible, although patterns of spread are similar within the bone, the fact that tumour could have entered the mandible at any site means that conservation surgery is not feasible and resection margins for mandibulectomy should be based on the soft-tissue extent of the tumour.

Once tumour has invaded the mandible, the pattern of spread is independent of previous irradiation. Two main routes have been described. The first is spread in the medulla between cancellous bony trabeculae and the second is spread in relation to the inferior alveolar nerve.

How does tumour spread with the mandible?

Medullary spread. The spread of squamous cell carcinoma along the medullary cavity of the non-irradiated mandible is associated with replacement by fibrous tissue and loss of haemopoesis. The presence of haemopoetic marrow at the lateral resection margin of the bone excision thus implies that clearance margins are adequate. Secondly, there is insignificant tumour extension in the marrow cavity beyond the superficial mucosal extent of tumour which means that the planning of excision margins usually relies on the mucosal and soft tissue extent of disease. The exception to this is spread from the horizontal to the ascending ramus. In the latter, there is no medullary cavity to guide the excision margins.

Neural spread. Spread of squamous cell carcinoma within nerves is seen in the endoneurium, perineurium and epineurium. It is important to be aware of such spread and examine for it because it may extend beyond the mandible and reach, for example, the infratemporal fossa and the trigeminal ganglion. Spread may occur in multiple nerves such as the lingual and hypoglossal and other unnamed nerves, and the presence of perineural spread is a poor prognostic sign. Its presence depends on the site of entry within the mandible and whether or not the patient has been previously irradiated, and it can occur in up to 50% of tumours in the retromolar area.

Barriers to mandibular invasion include not only periosteum but also the mucosa and submucosa overlying the sublingual gland, the submandibular gland and the mylohyoid. These structures appear to act as a significant barrier to deep infiltration and initial involvement of bone by direct spread in the previously non-irradiated patient is usually confined above the mylohyoid line. The height of this line varies in the dentate and the edentulous mandible and this means that the patterns of spread varies in these two types of patient.

It is striking how seldom, both in the dentate and the edentulous mandible, the bone is involved by direct extension below the mylohyoid line, even in the presence of extensive metastatic disease involving the submandibular nodes, as long as the patient has not been previously irradiated.

The proximity of the mucosa in the retromolar trigone to the bone, the presence of foramina behind the third molar, even in the dentate mandible, and an absence of cortex in the edentulous mandible result in early tumour invasion at these sites, with particular spread to the medullary bone that is present in the anterior part of the ramus in this region. On its buccal aspect, the level of the lower buccal sulcus corresponds largely to that of the mylohyoid line and the mechanism of spread from a buccal carcinoma into the mandible is largely similar to that of tumour spread from the floor of the mouth, whether the bone is dentate or edentulous.

Once the tumour enters the medullary cavity, the inferior alveolar nerve provides a ready pathway for perineural spread in a proximal and distal direction. This can occur unobtrusively with little involvement of the surrounding mandible and, until a relatively late stage, the nerve will look and function normally. Such spread may be discontinuous.

Carcinoma of the upper alveolus and hard palate

Squamous carcinoma of these sites is uncommon in the UK, where tumours are much more likely to be salivary gland in type. In certain parts of India, squamous carcinomas are very common on the hard palate owing to the curious habit of smoking chuttas with the burning end inside the mouth. Squamous carcinoma of the hard palate is a disease of elderly men, usually detected in the seventh decade of life and often preceded by leucoplakia.

Second tumours

The hallmark of mouth cancer is the propensity for second tumours. Mouth cancer is frequently multiple both in time and space. Up to 30% of patients with mouth cancer later develop another tumour, the most common sites again being in the mouth but also at distant sites such as the lung.

Such intraoral second tumours must be distinguished from recurrence at the primary site, which also is not that uncommon because of the way in which these tumours spread, necessitating wide margins at initial presentation.

'T' categories and overall staging

The definition of the 'T' stages and overall stage groupings of squamous carcinoma of the oral cavity (UICC–AJC) are shown in Table 15.3.

Nodal metastases

There is no difference in lymph-node metastatic rates between various sites but the rate increases with increasing T stage, increasing tumour depth (Fig. 15.25) and decreasing differentiation of the tumour. The level of the nodes in the neck is of prognostic importance. Overall, unlike most other head and neck sites, the submandibular group of nodes is usually invaded first.

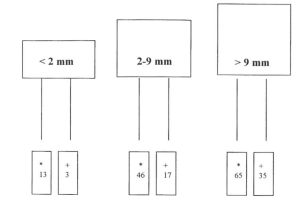

* % with lymph node metastases
+ % dead of disease

Figure 15.25 The incidence of lymph-node metastases and survival in relation to the thickness of the primary lesions for T_1 and T_2 squamous carcinomas of the oral tongue and floor of mouth (Shah, 1996).

Prognostic factors in oral carcinoma

- Tumour site
- Tumour depth
- Type of histology
- Degree of differentiation
- Presence of perineural spread
- Level and size of metastatic lymph nodes
- Mandibular invasion

Other tumours

Sarcoma

Fibrosarcoma and other soft-tissue sarcomas occur in younger patients and even infants. There are very few clinical features to differentiate them from carcinoma, although sarcomas tend to grow more quickly and ulceration is a later feature. The management of sarcomas is covered in Chapter 25.

Lymphoma

Both Hodgkin's and non-Hodgkin's lymphoma occur rarely in the mouth. The most common site is the palate and biopsy is mandatory. The classification and treatment of lymphoma are covered in Chapter 25.

Table 15.3 Lip and oral cavity: 'T' classification and overall staging

T: Primary tumour

T_X	Primary tumour cannot be assessed
T_0	No evidence of primary tumour
T_{is}	Carcinoma *in situ*
T_1	Tumour 2 cm or less in greatest dimension
T_2	Tumour more than 2 cm but no more than 4 cm in greatest dimension
T_3	Tumour more than 4 cm in greatest dimension
T_4	*Lip*: tumour invades adjacent structures, e.g. through cortical bone, inferior alveolar nerve, floor of mouth, skin of face *Oral cavity*: tumour invades adjacent structures, e.g. through cortical bone, into deep (extrinsic) muscle of tongue, maxillary sinus, skin (superficial erosion alone of bone/tooth socket by gingival primary is not sufficient to classify a tumour as T_4)

Stage grouping

Stage 0	T_{is}	N_0	M_0
Stage I	T_1	N_0	M_0
Stage II	T_2	N_0	M_0
Stage III	T_1	N_1	M_0
	T_2	N_1	M_0
	T_3	N_0, N_1	M_0
Stage IVA*	T_4	N_0, N_1	M_0
	Any $T_{1,2,3}$	N_2	M_0
Stage IVB*	Any $T_{1,2,3}$	N_2	M_0
Stage IVC*	Any T	Any N	M_1

UICC (1997). *New inclusion.

Other tumours

- Sarcoma
- Lymphoma
- Malignant melanoma
- Minor salivary gland tumours
- Granular cell myoblastoma

Malignant melanoma

Malignant melanoma is very rare and usually occurs on the upper alveolar ridge and palate. It often develops in a pre-existing naevus, usually in the young. Mucosal melanoma is considered in more detail in Chapter 25.

Minor salivary gland tumours

The pathology of salivary gland tumours is dealt with fully in Chapter 22. However, salivary gland tumours can occur in the mouth. The two most common types are the pleomorphic adenoma and the adenoid cystic carcinoma.

In reported series of minor salivary gland tumours, the incidence of malignancy varies from 32% to 88%. This depends on the type of department reporting the incidence and the difference in histological interpretation of highly cellular pleomorphic adenomas and mucoepidermoid tumours. The most common site of origin of these tumours is the posterior part of the hard palate. The cheeks, tongue, floor of mouth and retromolar region are rarely affected. The differential diagnosis includes other swellings such as a mucocoele, fibroma, sebaceous cyst, calculus and lipoma, as well as haemangiomas and lymphangiomas. They present as slow-growing, non-ulcerative masses in patients between the ages of 30 and 60 years, with no significant variation in gender or race incidence. Although a smooth palatal mass should always raise suspicion of a minor salivary gland tumour, it is reported that a correct clinical diagnosis is only made in about 10% of patients.

Granular cell myoblastoma

This is a smooth, sessile swelling on the tongue; the lesion arises from the voluntary muscle but may not be a true tumour and may merely represent a degenerative lesion. Radical treatment is not necessary. The most important point about this tumour is that the pathologist must recognize it; the epithelium covering it often shows changes described as pseudoepitheliomatous hyperplasia, which can be misdiagnosed as being malignant.

Investigation

History

The patient usually consults either a general medical or dental practitioner having noticed a mass or an ulcer in the mouth. Pain is a prominent feature, especially if the ulcer is touched; the pain may be referred to the ear owing to involvement of the lingual nerve. Alveolar or palatal tumours may be invasive and can interfere with the fitting of the patient's dentures or cause loosening of teeth. Sometimes the first sign is an enlarged neck node and, generally speaking, the more anterior the tumour the earlier the patient tends to seek advice.

Examination

The mouth should be examined with two tongue depressor blades. A standard routine must be followed in every case. First, the teeth and alveolar margins are examined. Then, the buccal mucosa is pulled outwards with the tongue blades and the sulci, the buccal mucosa and the parotid duct are examined. Next, the patient is asked to put out his or her tongue, which is examined for movement and mobility. When they place the tip of the tongue behind the upper alveolus the anterior floor of the mouth can be examined. The examination continues around the floor of the mouth on each side and then, at the posterior part of the fossa, where it meets the tongue and the anterior pillar, special attention is paid to the linguoalveolar sulcus or retromolar trigone 'coffin corner'. Tumours at this site can be missed if it is not properly examined with the tongue blades. The tonsil, the posterior wall of the oropharynx, and the hard and soft palate are examined. Finally, an indirect laryngoscopy is performed to examine the vallecula, epiglottis and aryepiglottic folds, and the posterior part of the soft palate is examined with a nasopharyngeal mirror. An accurate drawing is made of the tumour using the teeth as landmarks. Accurate measurements must be taken as it is very easy to get the margins of clearance wrong in a three-dimensional structure such as the mouth. Local examination is completed with the manual palpation of the tumour. Finally, the rest of the head and neck is examined, followed by a general examination.

It can be sometimes helpful to paint the tumour with 2% Toluidine Blue for 30 s or to use Orascreen (after which the patient must wash all of the dye out of the mouth). Although this is not an established technique, it appears that most malignant tumours in the oral cavity stain using this technique while other lesions, such as granulomas and papillomas, do not take up the stain and are washed clean with water. It may be useful for identifying sites of malignancy within areas of dysplastic tissue.

Radiology

Use of diagnostic algorithms

- To show the state of dentition and the position of the mental foramen (OPG)
- To show the site, size and extent of the primary tumour (CT/MRI)
- To assess tumour depth (CT/MRI/ultrasound)
- To assess mandibular invasion (OPG/CT/MRI/ scintigraphy)
- To assess the neck (CT/MRI)
- To assess the chest and abdomen (chest X-ray/ CT/liver ultrasound)

OPG: orthopantogram; CT: computed tomography; MRI: magnetic resonance imaging.

Laboratory studies

There are no special laboratory investigations other than those required in the routine preoperative work-up. If syphilis or HIV is suspected, after appropriate counselling, the relevant investigations may be ordered.

Biopsy

It used to be stated that it was unwise to perform a biopsy under local anaesthesia because of the increased risk of metastases related to a rise in tissue pressure, but there is no evidence that this occurs. In general, if tumours are large, then a biopsy can be taken in the out-patient department using punch forceps with or without the use of local anaesthetic. However, the majority of tumours will be biopsied under general anaesthetic during an examination under anaesthesia (EUA). When lesions are small (less than 1 cm), it is possible to carry out an excision biopsy with the appropriate margins under a general anaesthetic and if this turns out to be a carcinoma, and the margins are clear and the tumour is of minimal depth (less than 5 mm), then a 'wait and see' policy may be adopted. Tumours of greater thickness should receive prophylactic neck treatment, which in the postoperative setting with an N_0 neck will often be radiotherapy.

During an EUA, it is important to carry out another examination of the oral cavity, make an accurate drawing of the size and extent of the tumour using all available landmarks, take the appropriate biopsies and then carry out panendoscopy. The examination is completed by feeling both sides of the neck to include the midline.

Treatment policy

Surgery has no part to play, apart from biopsy, in the treatment of lymphoma within the oral cavity. Sarcomas (other than rhabdomyosarcoma) should be widely resected if possible and treated with a combination of postoperative radiotherapy and possibly chemotherapy. The treatment of head and neck lymphoma and sarcoma is discussed in Chapter 25.

The only issue to be discussed here, therefore, is the treatment of squamous carcinoma and salivary tumours. Virtually all of the latter require surgery in the first instance.

The modern-day management of oral cancer requires skills in assessment, access and ablative surgery along with an understanding of the appropriate techniques for reconstructive surgery. In addition, the help of a maxillofacial or plastic surgeon together with a prosthetic maxillofacial technician may be appropriate when dealing with difficult access, ablative and reconstructive surgery and prosthetic rehabilitation.

Points to assess in treatment planning

- Size and site of tumour
- State of dentition
- Presence or absence of mandibular invasion
- Age of the patient
- Elective treatment of the neck
- Appropriate form of reconstruction

Size and site of the tumour

T_1 and early T_2 tumours can be treated with either surgery or radiotherapy alone, with equal survival rates at around 80%. The advantages of surgery are that in small accessible lesions, surgical treatment is quick and efficient with often little need for reconstruction and it also provides tissue to assess the depth of tumour, which may indicate the need for prophylactic neck treatment. Radiotherapy may be given in the form of interstitial implants or as external therapy. In general, an implant is often preferable as it provides a high local dose with fewer complications than external radiotherapy, and the results are as good as surgery without, in some cases, the inevitable loss of function that accompanies surgical resection.

Early anterior lesions can safely be treated with implants, especially when there is no need to irradiate the neck. Although neck irradiation can be given to both sides of the neck, the problem with it is that, first, one can induce second primary tumours and, secondly, it is difficult to detect early recurrence so that subsequent disease in the neck is often deep seated and advanced when detected. Surgery is preferred for the more posterior lesions, those adjacent to the mandible or maxilla, or for those tumours that have recurred following implant therapy.

The larger T_2 and smaller T_3 lesions are often better treated with surgery and the larger T_4 tumours can do badly, so those that cannot be cured by surgery are dealt with by high-dose palliative radiotherapy with or without chemotherapy (or no treatment at all apart from palliation).

Dentoalveolar aspects of irradiation

If external beam radiotherapy is given to the mouth, this requires that the mandible will be irradiated to a greater or lesser extent. Despite advances in modern-day techniques, osteoradionecrosis to the mandible still remains a small but significant risk even if no further surgery is performed, but is an almost certain complication if anything other than wide resection of the mandible is carried out during subsequent salvage surgery. If the mandible has been irradiated, wide excision is necessary and reconstruction should be used in the form of a vascularized free tissue transfer of bone. This is important in lesions of the anterior floor of the mouth, where loss of the anterior arch of the mandible is totally disabling and causes the so-called 'Andy Gump' deformity (after the character in the American strip cartoon).

Radiotherapy causes xerostomia which leads to reduced oral clearance, increased plaque retention and periodontal disease and subsequently a greater dental caries rate. This is treatable if diagnosed early but, if untreated, will progress to pulpitis, root abscess and then osteoradionecrosis. Because of this, it is important that a restorative dentist or maxillofacial surgeon assesses the patient prior to treatment, and although dental extraction before radiation therapy is not mandatory, it may be necessary if future dental care cannot be regular and thorough. If, however, the teeth are initially in very poor condition and the patient is not dentally conscious, then all remaining teeth should be extracted, the sockets stitched and the patient put on antibiotics 10 days prior to irradiation.

Soft-tissue defect

Removal of soft tissue from the mouth has an important effect on functional ability and can significantly affect eating, drinking and speaking, especially if the tip of the tongue is immobilized. Advances in immediate free flap reconstruction mean that in the oral cavity the most popular way immediately to reconstruct soft tissue defects or isolate the mouth from the neck is free tissue transfer (usually a radial free forearm flap). This provides pliable vascularized tissue which can be tailormade to the size of the defect. Skin, vascularized tendon and nerve as well as bone can all be transferred.

Invasion of the periosteum of the mandible by tumour

It is important to consider the presence or absence of mandibular invasion prior to resecting an oral cavity tumour. The presence of mandibular invasion increases with the size of the primary tumour, its proximity to the mandible and whether or not there has been previous surgery or irradiation. Preoperative imaging (OPG/ scintigraphy/CT or MRI) can give an idea about the state of the mandible and the presence or absence of any invasion. In general, the absence of invasion negates the need for mandibular resection and the presence of gross invasion will usually dictate that wide resection is required with hemimandibulectomy and usually vascularized bony reconstruction.

The problem arises in the detection of early bony invasion which, in the absence of previous radiotherapy, will usually dictate that conservation surgery of the mandible can be safely carried out. In this situation, the best assessment of the mandibular periosteum is at the time of surgery and the surgeon has to have intraoperative flexibility to facilitate partial mandibular resection.

This may take the form of removing part of the mandible (upper or lower border), the lingual plate or the outer surface or any combination of these manoeuvres (Fig. 15.26).

Access to the oral cavity

Many smaller anterior tumours can be accessed by the mouth. Larger posterior tumours require adjunctive

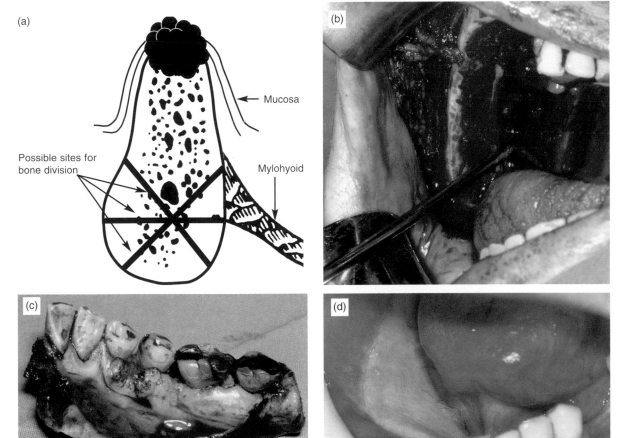

Figure 15.26 Partial conservative mandibulectomy. (a) The resection should include the mandibular canal and its contents. (b) Patient with a T_4N_0 squamous cell carcinoma of the lower alveolus treated via peroral access with rim resection and elective selective neck dissection (levels I–IV). (c) The specimen. (d) Reconstruction was with a radial free forearm flap.

techniques to provide appropriate access. When a neck dissection is being performed at the same time, access to the mouth may be through a pull-through technique whereby the tongue can be delivered into the neck. This technique is suitable for the more anterior tumours, particularly those on the lateral border of the tongue, and is not suitable for those that encroach towards or on to the mandible, or those that are placed more posteriorly. In this situation, best access is obtained by a lower lip split and paramedian mandibulotomy. Access to the upper alveolus and premaxilla can be facilitated with an upper lip split.

Access to the oral cavity

- Peroral
- Lip split with symphyseal or paramedian mandibulotomy
- Lateral mandibulotomy
- Mandibulectomy
- Pull-through procedure
- Upper lip split

Lymphadenopathy

If neck nodes are palpable, the patient should be treated by surgery. In the presence of a small T_1 or T_2 tumour with no palpable neck nodes (the N_0 neck), the treatment of the neck should be considered because of the high incidence of occult neck metastasis in this situation. If the primary tumour is being treated with an implant, then for all but the smallest tumours (less than 5 mm in thickness), the neck should receive prophylactic irradiation. For midline tumours, both sides of the neck should be irradiated and the site of the radiation should include the first-echelon lymph nodes (levels I–III). There is both prospective and retrospective evidence that using this technique, locoregional recurrence can be reduced but there is no evidence that it prolongs overall survival. If the primary tumour is being treated by surgery, then the neck should be treated surgically as well. For tumours with a thickness measuring greater than 5 mm, a selective supraomohyoid (levels I–III) or extended supraomohyoid (anterolateral neck dissection) which dissects levels I–IV should be utilized. This provides lymph nodes for staging, treats occult neck disease when present and provides access to the neck vessels for reconstruction.

Postoperative irradiation

Carcinoma of the oral cavity appears to be one of those tumours where survival can be improved using postoperative radiotherapy. In a study of postoperative radiotherapy using historical controls, Robertson *et al.* (1986) showed that the incidence of recurrent disease was reduced at 18 months using postoperative radiation. Despite the fact that at present there is no evidence that this improves survival, many centres around the UK routinely use postoperative radiotherapy for oral cavity

tumours measuring T_2 or greater treated with surgery. Although preoperative radiotherapy was popular in the past, and the disease responded and complications rates were not increased, subsequent survival rates at 2 and 5 years showed no improvement and this technique has now been almost universally abandoned.

Principles of reconstruction

- The reconstructive technique should not interfere with or limit any excisional surgery
- Form and function should be restored as quickly as possible
- Morbidity and mortality should not be increased unnecessarily by the reconstruction chosen
- A secondary cosmetic defect should not be produced unknowingly
- As a general rule, resection and reconstruction should take place as a one-stage procedure
- Procedures that involve soft tissue and bony reconstruction should not be used where a prosthesis would provide a better alternative

---

Treatment policies for each site

Leucoplakia

A biopsy should be obtained in every case and be taken if possible from what appears to be the most active part. Orascreen can be useful to identify potential biopsy sites, particularly if the lesion appears to be more like erythroplakia than a true leucoplakia. If histology shows little or no dysplasia, the patient probably requires no further treatment, although laser destruction can be used. Significant aetiological factors such as carious teeth and heavy smoking and drinking should be eliminated if possible and the patient reassured. Some patients will require long-term follow-up.

The patient with leucoerythroplakia is quite different. The histology report will usually show severe dyskeratosis or, more worryingly, carcinoma *in situ*. The entire affected area should be removed, usually with the laser and submitted to serial histological examination. The subsequent deficit may be left to granulate or covered with a split-skin graft using the quilting technique.

Buccal carcinoma

The buccal mucosa is very elastic, but cancers arising in the mucous membrane invade fairly early so that attempts at wide but superficial removal in this area run the risk not only of incomplete resection but, because of subsequent scarring, of causing fibrosis and restriction in opening the mouth. Therefore, the decision regarding assessment of tumours in this area, their resection and subsequent reconstruction is crucial.

Small T_1 tumours (less than 2 cm) can be removed locally, with a reasonably safe margin of normal tissue. The resultant defect can either be left to granulate, treated by primary closure or covered with either a split skin graft or buccal mucosal graft from the other cheek.

Another alternative is reconstruction using V–Y buccal advancement, either unilaterally or bilaterally. Interstitial radiotherapy provides a satisfactory and equally effective alternative to excision of small tumours at this site.

If the tumour is surrounded by a large area of leucoplakia and wide excision of buccal mucosa is needed, then skin grafting will definitely be required and the defect should not be left to granulate.

Tumours larger than this will often be managed with radiotherapy (as long as there is no encroachment on bone), with surgery being reserved for recurrence. Alternatively, surgery may be used as first-line management. Tumours of the buccal mucosa that involve the upper alveolar sulcus are difficult to access and quite difficult to graft. In this situation, access is important and, depending on which type of reconstruction is being employed, access to the lower alveolar sulcus can be achieved using a lip-split, and tumours of the upper alveolar sulcus may require an upper lip-split or Weber–Fergusson incision.

The large buccal cancers, by definition, often encroach on or involve the facial skin and this should be removed as part of the resection. If these tumours are near the lower alveolus they are removed together with adjacent cheek skin and the upper half of the alveolus. All that is required is soft-tissue reconstruction without attention to bone. The same applies with involvement of the upper alveolus. The resulting through and through defect may be reconstructed using a number of techniques depending on the age of the patient, the size of the defect, the nature and extent of the disease and the expertise of the surgeon.

Probably the best results here will be achieved with a bipaddled, de-epithelialized middle segment, radial free forearm flap but, alternatively, one or two flaps may be used to provide internal and external cover. These include:

■ Pectoralis major flap with internal skin graft
■ Deltopectoral flap turned in for both inside and outside cover
■ Pectoralis major flap for inside cover and deltopectoral flap (delayed) for outside cover
■ Axial island temporalis flap for outside cover and skin graft for inside cover
■ Cervicofacial rotation flap (external cover) with V–Y mucosal advancement for internal cover
■ In extreme situations, a forehead flap may be used for outside cover and a skin graft applied internally

Carcinoma of the tip of the tongue

These usually present early and can be excised as such. The tip of the tongue is excised in a V-shaped fashion and a new tongue tip made by primary reconstruction.

Carcinoma of the dorsum of the tongue

If the tumour is less than 2 cm in diameter, it is excised in an ellipse and the tongue defect closed primarily. Alternatively, small tumours may be treated by interstitial irradiation. Surgical treatment for larger tumours requires an extensive operation, and so radiotherapy is preferred in order to preserve the tongue. As large tumours cannot be treated by interstitial irradiation alone, external beam radiotherapy, perhaps combined with an interstitial implant, is used.

Carcinoma of the lateral border of the tongue

If no glands are palpable, then the choice lies between interstitial irradiation and partial glossectomy. If the tumour is greater than 2 cm in size (i.e. T_2) then usually surgery (hemiglossectomy) or, less often, external beam radiotherapy is the preferred technique. If glands are palpable, hemiglossectomy with neck dissection is preferable. This can usually be done without splitting the mandible (pull-through technique).

Carcinoma of the anterior floor of the mouth

When tumours of the anterior floor of mouth encroach on to the anterior alveolus, the mandible must be assessed for possible invasion. Often, the presence of invasion can only be confirmed during the operative procedure. The periostium is peeled up, and in the absence of any invasion, the tumour is resected and soft-tissue reconstruction completed using either a pectoralis major myocutaneous flap or, more commonly, the radial free forearm flap. If there is early bone invasion, in the absence of previous radiotherapy, then conservation mandibular surgery may be carried out to include rim resection and appropriate soft-tissue reconstruction as described above. If the patient has had previous irradiation or there is extensive tumour invasion, then the anterior segment of the mandible must be resected. Without reconstruction, this results in the horrible cosmetic appearance called the 'Andy Gump' deformity, so the bony contour of the lower jaw should be restored immediately by free tissue transfer if at all possible.

Radiotherapy in the form of external beam is not a preferred option in the primary treatment of tumours at this site since they do worse than those treated with surgery, as do those on the lateral border of the tongue. The optimum treatment for tumours at this site is therefore primary surgery with removal of the floor of the mouth, the anterior segment of the mandible and bilateral neck dissections as appropriate depending on the staging of each side of the neck. Exceptionally, interstitial radiotherapy may be appropriate for very early cancers at this site.

If no nodes are palpable, then a bilateral supraomohyoid or bilateral extended supraomohyoid neck dissection should be done. If any nodes are subsequently found to be positive, then postoperative radiotherapy may have to be administered. Palpable neck disease is treated on its merits.

Carcinoma of the lateral floor of mouth and lower alveolus

Tumours that encroach on to the lower alveolus are not usually suitable for interstitial radiation. As the results of surgery are better than for external beam radiotherapy at this site, these tumours are usually treated with surgical excision. Soft-tissue resection is completed, the mandible is assessed and any early invasion treated by rim resection. If the periosteum is not breached, then bony resection is not required. If there is extensive bony involvement or if the patient has had previous radiotherapy, then treatment should be a pelvimandibulectomy, which is removal of the floor of the mouth in continuity with a partial mandibulectomy, and as there are usually enlarged glands in this situation, a modified radical or radical neck dissection in continuity is also performed (commando procedure). In the absence of bony invasion or when a rim resection has been performed, soft-tissue reconstruction is completed using either a pectoralis major myocutaneous flap or free tissue transfer usually with a radial free forearm flap or lateral arm flap. If the mandible has been resected, then it should be replaced with one of the techniques described below.

Salivary gland tumours

Within the oral cavity, there is a 90% chance that a minor salivary gland tumour is malignant. The most common problem is the tumour on the hard palate, which is usually either a benign pleomorphic adenoma or, more commonly, a malignant adenoid cystic carcinoma. Both of these tumours are treated surgically by resection, which may involve bone if the tumours extend into the hard palate or the alveolus. This is discussed in Chapter 19 (Tumours of the nose and sinuses).

Salivary gland tumours also occur occasionally elsewhere in the mouth, usually on the floor of the mouth and the alveolus. These are invariably malignant and are either adenoid cystic or mucoepidermoid carcinomas. Very small tumours, 1 cm in diameter or less, may be controlled for long periods by using radiotherapy, but in the vast majority of cases, these tumours are best treated using surgery, which should be at least as extensive as that described for squamous carcinoma at the same site (see above) followed by postoperative radiotherapy.

Repair of the oral cavity

Many procedures have been described for repairing soft-tissue defects within the mouth. One should always 'replace like with like' and small defects without loss of tongue bulk can be left to granulate, primary closure can be considered or the defect can be covered with a split skin graft using the quilting technique. The possibilities of repair for larger defects within the oral cavity are:

- mucosal lining alone
- mucosal lining plus bulk
- mucosal lining plus bone
- mucosal lining plus bulk plus bone.

The reconstruction of the mandible is discussed in detail below. Soft-tissue defects may be closed as follows.

Closure of defects

- Primary closure
- Split skin grafts
- Flaps – buccal
  – lingual
  – nasolabial
  – distant

Primary closure

Although primary closure can be achieved within the oral cavity for many defects, the larger the defect that needs to be closed, the more function is compromised. Fixation of tissues such as the tongue to the floor of the mouth greatly impairs speech and swallowing and leads to severe drooling of saliva and food and, subsequently, an unsatisfactory cosmetic result. Whether or not primary closure is achievable depends on the amount of mobility remaining in the soft tissues of the mouth and tongue, the subsequent degree of fixation of the tongue that will result from primary closure and where the defect is located.

Because of these problems, most head and neck surgeons do not now use primary closure except for small defects where laxity of tissue allows a satisfactory functional and cosmetic result to be achieved. In these situations, consideration must be given, particularly in the absence of a through-and-through defect, to allow small defects to granulate as a secondary defect. This is often the simplest and easiest thing to do (particularly after laser resections) and can give a functional and cosmetic result as good as either primary closure or using the radial free forearm flap for larger defects, e.g. after hemiglossectomy.

Split skin grafts

These are now used rarely within the mouth and have their use in replacing lining alone. They are only appropriate if there is a vascular bed on which the graft can be sutured and are sewn in place using the quilting technique. They may be used to replace mucosa following excision of a superficial tongue tumour, or a small buccal or floor of the mouth tumour. However, they contract and scar, making future assessment of the site difficult.

Local flaps

The principles of local flap repair have been described in detail in Chapter 7. Small and moderately sized defects which require replacement of lining, and lining plus bulk may be replaced using the flaps below.

Buccal flaps. These are local flaps which can be designed from the buccal mucosa and rotated into small defects. They are of limited use but may be employed to reconstruct defects as single or double rhomboid flaps around the commissure or to replace moderately sized buccal defects with single or double V–Y advancement. They have a limited place in intraoral reconstruction. The position of the parotid duct must always be considered.

Lingual flaps. Lingual flaps can only be used to close a defect within the oral cavity or oropharynx when the excision does not involve the tongue. Otherwise, one of the cardinal rules of reconstruction is broken, i.e. 'thou must not unknowingly create a second deformity' and if part of the tongue has already been excised, the remaining soft tissue is vital to maintain residual function. Small lingual flaps may be used to repair defects in the lateral floor of the mouth and the oropharynx. The tongue is divided to one side of the midline and the resulting flap can be rotated into quite a large defect. In modern-day intraoral reconstruction, its use is limited to providing a mobile and satisfactory floor of mouth repair for small to moderate defects in that area and also for lip reconstruction.

Nasolabial flaps. Bilateral nasolabial flaps may be used to repair small to moderate defects in the anterior floor of mouth. They are quick and easy to raise and in the elderly, where this is plenty of lax skin in the nasolabial fold, they provide a rapid and reliable way to reconstruct the floor of the mouth. However, the tissue is thick and not as pliable as radial forearm skin, so that in the ideal situation their use in reconstruction of this area plays a secondary role to that technique. The patient should be edentulous.

Distant flaps

Cutaneous axial flaps. The two cutaneous axial flaps that may be used in intraoral reconstruction are the forehead flap and the deltopectoral flap. In the past, they have played a significant role in intraoral reconstruction. Although they are rarely used nowadays, one should remain conversant with them, for use in the occasional patient. For example, in the very elderly patient, where a rapid reliable source of vascularized skin is required for intraoral reconstruction (particularly in a salvage situation), the forehead flap remains a satisfactory source and can be used when a radial forearm flap fails in the anterior floor of mouth (Fig. 15.27). However, the donor site is cosmetically poor and the flap requires later division. Likewise, the deltopectoral flap is not the first choice of vascularized skin for intraoral reconstruction because it also requires later division but it may be used either for salvage or rarely in some specific situations, e.g. the through-and-through cheek defect, where it can provide outside cover when free tissue transfer is either inappropriate or unavailable.

Myocutaneous flaps. These flaps have been used extensively in intraoral reconstruction since the early 1980s. They are less commonly used nowadays owing to advances in microvascular reconstruction.

Myocutaneous flaps for intraoral reconstruction

- Pectoralis major flap
- Latissimus dorsi flap
- Sternomastoid muscle or myocutaneous flap
- Trapezius myocutaneous flap
- Platysma flap

These flaps can be particularly useful since they are usually extremely reliable and provide one-stage reconstruction with lining and bulk, which can be particularly useful if the mandible is not being replaced. However, their bulk

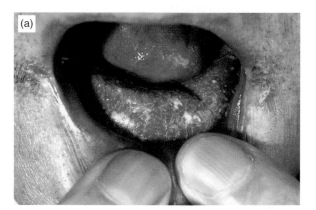

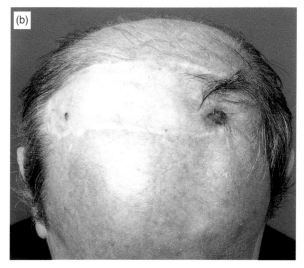

Figure 15.27 Repair of a defect in the anterior floor of mouth using a forehead flap following failed radial free forearm reconstruction after partial mandibulectomy, anterior floor of mouth resection and selective neck dissection for a T_4N_0 squamous cell carcinoma of the floor of the mouth.

---

may be a significant disadvantage within the oral cavity. Where three-dimensional soft-tissue reconstruction is required, a free flap such as the radial free forearm will usually give a superior result.

The pectoralis major flap has been one of the most widely used flaps in intraoral cavity reconstruction. Its main disadvantages are that is bulky and is not ideally suited to the reconstruction of small to moderate defects in the floor of the mouth. In addition, it violates the breast, which may be a problem particularly in women. The latissimus dorsi flap provides bulk and lining for intraoral reconstruction and may be used either as a myocutaneous pedicled flap or as a free flap for reconstruction following subtotal or total glossectomy. It is an easy flap to raise, does not violate the breast but does involve repositioning of the patient during the procedure. The sternomastoid and platysma flaps are rarely used these days but in certain situations may be of value and should not be forgotten.

Free tissue transfer options for intraoral reconstruction

- Radial free forearm flap
  - Vascularized fascia
  - Vascularized skin and fascia
  - Vascularized fascia, tendon or nerve
  - Vascularized skin, fascia, tendon or nerve
  - Vascularized skin, fascia, tendon or bone
- Lateral arm flap
  - Vascularized skin and fascia (with and without nerve)
- Latissimus dorsi flap
  - Vascularized muscle
  - Vascularized skin and muscle
  - Composite flap available with serratus anterior, rib and scapula
- Rectus abdominus
  - Vascularized muscle
  - Vascularized skin and muscle (and nerve)
- Deep circumflex iliac artery (DCIA) flap
  - Vascularized bone and muscle
  - Vascularized skin, bone and muscle
- Scapular flap
  - Vascularized fascia
  - Vascularized skin and fascia
  - Vascularized skin, muscle and bone
  - Vascularized muscle and bone alone
  - Vascularized double skin paddles, with or without muscle and bone
- Fibula
  - Vascularized bone
  - Vascularized skin and bone (and nerve)

Microvascular free tissue transfer. The majority of soft tissue repairs within the oral cavity require three-dimensional reconstruction with soft pliable skin often without significant bulk. This is easily achieved with the radial free forearm flap (Fig. 15.28) which, in addition to providing a tailormade flap to fill the defect, can provide vascularized nerve, tendon to lift the corner of the mouth and vascularized bone (see below). Where more bulk is

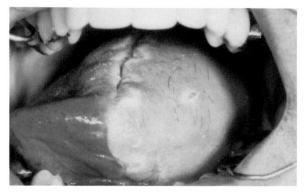

Figure 15.28 Radial free forearm flap for intraoral reconstruction following hemiglossectomy.

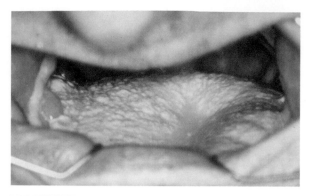

Figure 15.29 Free latissimus dorsi flap used for reconstruction following subtotal glossectomy.

required, the lateral arm flap is useful and for larger, bulky defects such as subtotal or total glossectomy a free latissimus dorsi or free rectus abdominus flap is of particular use (Fig. 15.29).

Mandibular reconstruction

The modern-day practice of head and neck oncology within the oral cavity dictates that wherever possible mandibular conservation surgery should be carried out and therefore it is now possible to conserve many mandibles which in the past would have been resected. Even when the tumour is on to and into the mandible, in the absence of previous radiotherapy, partial conservative resections may be carried out which leave a rim of mandible which functions adequately postoperatively and precludes the need for bony reconstruction.

However, there are instances where it is inevitable that the mandible must be resected. As a general rule, when mandible has been removed, it should be repaired remembering to replace like with like.

Essential points when assessing the need for mandibular reconstruction

- The age of the patient
- The expectations of the patient
- The size of the mandibular defect
- The site of the mandibular defect
- The surgical expertise available
- Was mandibular resection anticipated prior to surgery?
- Has the patient had previous radiotherapy?

Where small bony defects have been created without a soft-tissue defect and in the absence of previous radiotherapy, free bone grafts may be used from the iliac crest. These have quite a good success rate but in general their use is limited to quite small defects since larger ones are best replaced with vascularized bone and soft tissue.

In the elderly, particularly those with high-risk tumours that may recur, mandibular reconstruction may not be a priority and soft-tissue reconstruction may be achieved using a pedicled pectoralis major or latissimus dorsi flap. In this situation, the bulk of the muscle pedicle, together with the skin in the mouth, fills out the defect, making it cosmetically acceptable, although with time there is some atrophy and inevitable sinking in of the cheek. The main problem is that functionally the flap adds nothing to the repair and the contralateral remaining segment of mandible swings to the side of excision at rest whenever the patient opens his or her mouth, which functionally is less than ideal. This can be corrected, in part, if the patient wears a lower denture by using a dental prosthesis to provide reasonable occlusion.

If reconstruction is planned at a later date, then it is wise to place a titanium reconstruction plate spacer between the two cut ends of the mandible to maintain cosmesis and function, so that reconstruction can be carried out 6–12 months later when there is no evidence of recurrence. Alternatively, the mandibular fragments may be immobilized using external fixation.

Mandibular reconstruction in the ideal setting is carried out as a one-stage procedure and the choice of vascularized bone depends on the site and size of the defect, the requirements of the concomitant soft-tissue reconstruction, whether or not osseointegration is required and the skill of the surgeon. Immediate reconstruction should always be considered if the anterior arch is resected since the resultant defect is cosmetically and functionally unacceptable. In the past, defects confined to the horizontal ramus of the mandible have been repaired using vascularized radius. However, the bone is thin and not ideally suitable for osseointegration, and the donor site fractures. Better alternatives are now available.

Hemimandibular defects requiring reconstruction have been classified (Jewer *et al.*, 1989) based on a system that divides the mandible into a central segment (C) which includes the lower canines, a lateral segment (L) which does not include the condyle, and a lateral segment (H) which includes the condyle. This HCL classification of mandibular defects is useful but does not help you in planning the formal osteotomies required to conform the donor bones to the natural curvatures of the mandible. In addition, many patients are edentulous and this gives rise to difficulties in determining the limits of the central segment.

Soutar (1994) has therefore modified the HCL classification as follows (Fig. 15.30). C is the central segment extending from mental foramen to mental foramen and which is then divided at the midline into left (Cl) and right (Cr); 'L' is the lateral segment of the mandible from the mental foramen into the lingula preserving the condyle and posterior ascending ramus, and 'A' is the ascending ramus of the mandible. Using this system, a standard right hemimandibulectomy equates to ALCr and implies two changes in direction that the bony reconstruction will have to accommodate. A pure lateral defect (L) could be reconstructed using a straight bone, whereas LCl denotes reconstruction of the left mandible requiring an osteotomy to maintain chin prominence.

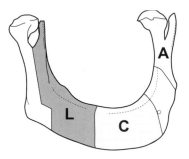

Figure 15.30 Classification of mandibular defects (after Soutar). L: lateral segment; C: central segment; A: ascending ramus of the mandible.

Because of the above, it is quite clear that depending on the size and site of the mandibular reconstruction, a number of donor sites will have important uses in different clinical situations.

Small hemimandibular defects (L) and LC defects requiring a single osteotomy can be repaired using vascularized radius with or without soft-tissue repair. The cortical nature of the bone is ideally suited to small cortical screw fixation but its thickness lacks the support for reliable subsequent osseointegration.

For larger hemimandibular defects (L and LA), the bone of the composite iliac crest flap based on the deep circumflex iliac artery (DCIA) is ideally suited to hemimandibular reconstruction because of the natural curve of the iliac crest. The upper portion of the crest usually forms the lower border of the mandible and it can be designed so that the vascular pedicle enters either at the angle for ipsilateral anastomosis or at its symphysis for contralateral anastomosis. While this flap is ideal for bony reconstruction, it is more difficult to use when combined with soft-tissue reconstruction. The external skin paddle has a precarious blood supply and its mobility is limited. This problem can be overcome by using the flap in combination with the internal oblique muscle which can be left either to re-epithelize or can be skin grafted. The bone of the iliac crest is predominately cancellous with a very thin cortex and is therefore fixed less rigidly with plate and cortical screws than the more cortical bones. Subsequent osseointegration of implants is not a problem.

When larger segments of bone are required for hemimandible reconstruction, at the symphysis, and where mobility of a skin paddle is needed and/or double skin paddles are required for inside and outside cover, the scapular osseocutaneous flap is extremely useful. The bone is good-quality corticocancellous bone but is relatively thin. It is straight and therefore requires an osteotomy to change direction but because of its cortical component, it is readily fixed by small plates and cortical screws allowing immediate rigid fixation. However, because of its thinness, subsequent osseointegration can be a problem.

For extensive angle-to-angle reconstruction or for the atrophic/edentulous mandible (with or without soft tis-

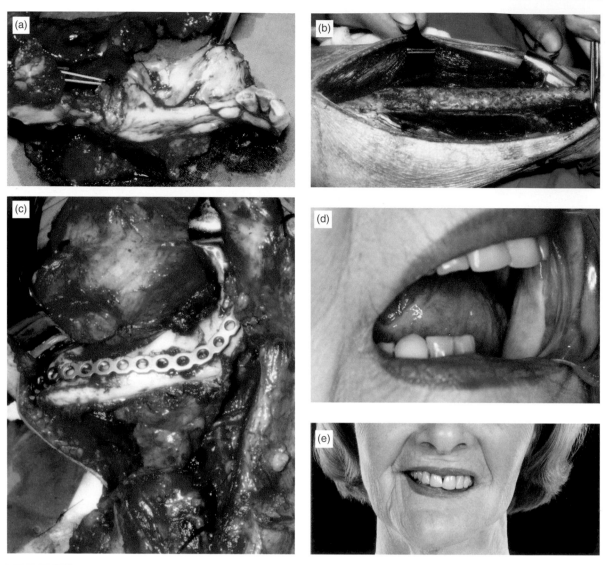

Figure 15.31 (a)–(e) Reconstruction of the left hemimandible following resection of a recurrent T₄ N₀ squamous cell carcinoma of the buccal mucosa invading the mandible. Bony reconstruction was with a free fibula transfer and soft tissue reconstruction with a radial free forearm flap. The donor sites for the radical forearm (f) and fibula (g) are shown opposite.

sue) the fibula flap has come into its own as a source of vascularized cortical bone (Fig. 15.31). It offers the longest length of bone that is available. It is extremely strong with a high cortical component but has a problem in that a number of osteotomies are required, which can be difficult because of the dense cortical nature of the bone. Closing wedge osteotomies are preferred to keep as much periostium as possible intact and to safeguard the vascular pedicle. The flap may be raised and left perfused on the leg while the osteotomies and plating are carried out, and although the island of skin centred over the centre of the fibula is more reliable, thin and pliable than the DCIA flap, it still suffers from some restriction in manoeuvrability.

The major disadvantage of the fibula is that is has a relatively short vascular pedicle. This can be overcome by the creation of an arteriovenous (AV) fistula at the donor site using a saphenous vein graft which can then be divided, creating increased pedicle length to facilitate anastomosis to the donor flap vessels. More usually, the distal bone is used, effectively lengthening the pedicle. Care must be taken when raising the flap to avoid the tibial vessels at the tripartite anastomosis relating to the origin of the peroneal artery and the common peroneal nerve must be preserved. The cortical nature of this long bone gives it tremendous strength and enables absolute rigid fixation with plates and screws. It is suitable for osseointegration and is the flap choice for extended angle-to-angle reconstruction.

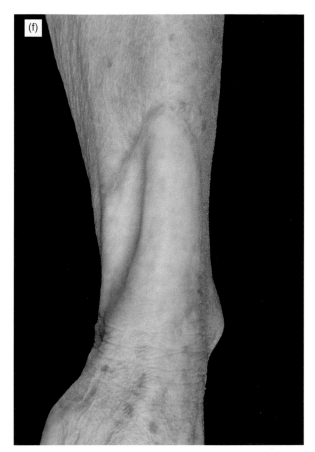

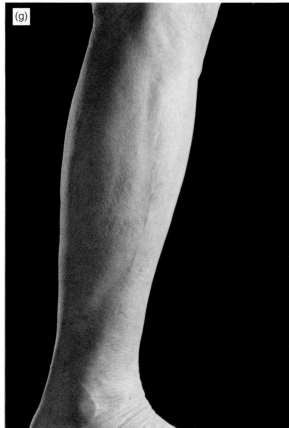

Figure 15.31 *Continued.* (f) and (g).

Technique of operations for tongue cancer

Local excision of mouth cancers

Many mouth cancers measuring 1.5 cm in diameter or less can be managed successfully by local excision using sharp dissection or laser. The operation is done under general anaesthetic and there is no need for a preliminary tracheostomy. The mouth is held open with a dental prop placed between the teeth and the area excised with a margin of at least 1 cm. The margins of the excised specimen are marked so that the pathologist will later be able to orientate it clearly and identify any resection margins that are not clear of tumour.

Then the surgeon changes his or her gloves and secures haemostasis. Defects that cannot be closed primarily are left to granulate or covered with a split skin graft using the quilting technique. A thin split-skin graft of appropriate size is taken from the thigh or the upper arm, and stitched it in place around the edge of the defect with interrupted vicryl sutures on a cutting needle. Then further interrupted sutures are placed through the graft and through the bed about 5–10 mm apart to achieve overall anchorage, thus ensuring that as the capillaries grow in they are not sheared off. Finally, a few small nicks are made in the graft between the sutures so that any serum or blood can escape. No dressing is necessary.

This operation is suitable for smaller tumours provided that invasion of the substance of the tongue is minimal. Larger tumours should be treated by at least a hemiglossectomy.

Hemiglossectomy

Attention must be paid to the assessment of the probable defect and the appropriate reconstruction. The surgeon tattoos around the tumour to define clearance margins. If the patient depends on the voice for their livelihood, then attempts must be made to leave a good tip to the tongue and to leave a sulcus so that the patient can wear dentures, either immediately or later.

The operation begins with a tracheostomy (if this is being performed) and a general anaesthetic is continued via this. The primary lesion may be excised via the mouth using either electrocautery or a laser. This is done as one procedure to include a 2 cm margin of surrounding tissue.

Incision and neck dissection

The incision used is either a Schobinger, a utility or a 'T on its side'.

Depending on the state of the neck, a selective supraomohyoid or selective extended supraomohyoid neck dissection is performed and, in the presence of palpable disease, the neck dissection will usually be either a modified radical or a radical neck dissection. The specimen is left attached at the submandibular region and the first question when the dissection is complete is whether or not a lip split and mandibulotomy is needed for access. It is usually possible in this operation to perform surgery without splitting the lip, which is preferable since it prevents oedema and subsequent scarring, and gives a better functional result.

Assuming that the operation can be done without a lip split and using a pull-through technique, the incision in the upper part of the neck is continued to the apex of the submental triangles and upwards to the mandible. The skin is elevated off the mandible, and at this point it is possible to cut the mucosa in the gingivolabial sulcus and thereby enter the mouth. When dealing with bilateral neck disease, in-continuity resections are not necessary.

Excision

Access to the tongue tumour can be obtained either by a mandibulotomy or using the pull-through procedure.

Mandibulotomy

This is best carried out as a paramedian mandibulotomy anterior to the mental foramen. The easiest, simplest and most effective way to divide the mandible here is in a straight line using a reciprocating saw. This also gives the best results. Alternatively, a step osteotomy or osteotomy incorporating a sagittal split can be used (Fig. 15.32). Siting the osteotomy in the edentulous patient to avoid injury to the mental nerve can be difficult, particularly as the nerve sometimes loops medially as it exits the mental foramen. In the dentate mandible, the presence of teeth can act as a landmark when correlated with radiological studies, and it is important to look at the OPG before surgery. Because a step osteotomy carries the risk of exposing the tooth roots and the sagittal split certainly does, then the wisest and simplest choice is vertical division of the bone. In this situation, the interdental tissues are divided down to bone, the mucoperiosteum is incised and mobilized and the mandible is preplated and divided. The usual site for this is usually between the second incisor and the canine where the roots diverge and this is usually visible on the OPG. In certain instances, an alternative site may be appropriate in the presence of previous dental extraction. Having previously sited the position for the titanium plates and screws, the incision is made with a reciprocating saw. If this procedure is carried out properly, the risks of non-union are minimal.

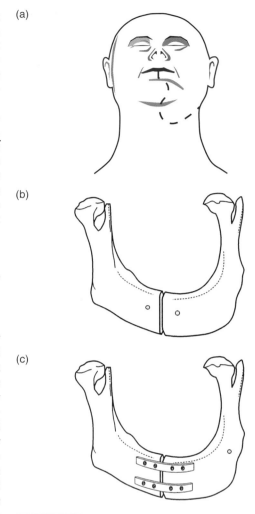

Figure 15.32 (a) Incision for a lip split; (b) technique for vertical paramedian mandibular osteotomy together with (c) replating using titanium plates and screws.

Key steps in mandibulotomy
■ The point of division is defined
■ The incision is marked
■ The interdental tissues are divided
■ The mucoperiostium is incised and mobilized
■ The bone is partially incised
■ The mandible is preplated
■ The plates and screws are retained
■ The bone is incised with a reciprocating saw

Pull-through procedure

The mandible and its periosteum are exposed with the first group of muscles, i.e. the anterior belly of the digastric muscle. An incision is made along the external surface of the inferior border of the horizontal ramus. The periosteum is lifted off the inner surface of the mandible using a periosteal elevator. The anterior belly of the digastric muscle is divided close to its attachment to the digastric fossa on the lower border (Fig.15.33). The second layer of muscle making up the floor of the mouth is the mylohyoid muscle. This is divided close to its attachment along the mylohyoid line on the mandible. The third layer of muscles is exposed, i.e. the geniohyoid muscle anteriorly and the hyoglossus muscle posteriorly. The geniohyoid muscle is cut close to its attachment to the inferior genial tubercle on the posterior aspect of the symphysis menti. Occasionally, it is necessary to divide the anterior margin of the hyoglossus muscle to aid exposure and mobilization. This exposes the deepest layer of

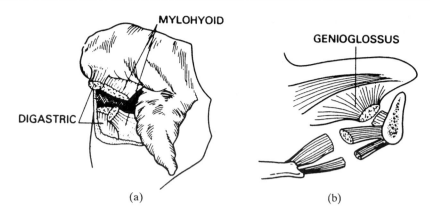

Figure 15.33 Pull-through procedure: (a) exposed digastric and mylohyoid muscles, (b) the genioglossus muscle divided.

the floor of the mouth, the genioglossus muscle and intrinsic muscles of the tongue. Division of the genioglossus muscle and the periosteum of the mandible is carried out at the apex of the alveolar ridge, which allows the tongue, the intervening lymphatics and the periosteum to be delivered into the neck, still in continuity with the neck dissection.

Excision of the tumour

The tip of the tongue is held in a towel clip or on a suture and pulled forward, and the tumour is removed using cutting diathermy along the tattoo marks. It will be necessary to stop and tie the lingual artery, but time must not be wasted in tying other bleeding points until the tumour has been removed. Margins should be at least 2 cm and the clearance margin must be in depth as well as width. The cutting diathermy goes through the muscles of the floor of the mouth and the whole specimen is removed, with the diathermy kept at right angles to the tattoo marks. If it is angled, then there will be poor tumour clearance in the deeper part of the resection. Haemostasis is secured with coagulation diathermy and 3/0 Vicryl ties, the wound is irrigated and the operator changes his or her gown and gloves.

If the tumour is greater than 3 cm in diameter or if there is deep invasion of the tongue, then extension beyond a hemiglossectomy is required to complete a subtotal glossectomy when, in its extreme, only a stump of tongue above the vallecula is spared, along with the base of the tongue on the contralateral side.

Repair

Following excision of very small tumours some defects can be closed primarily, but the larger defects can be left to granulate or repaired with a radial free forearm flap. In the very elderly, where the neck has not been entered, it is simplest to leave defects to granulate and the functional results are no worse than if a radial free forearm flap is used. Following subtotal glossectomy, larger flaps with bulk are required and these will usually include either pedicled pectoralis major or latissimus dorsi flaps, or free latissimus dorsi or rectus abdominus flaps.

Aftercare

- General care.
- The tracheostomy is kept in place for at least a week since this not only protects the airway but also facilitates any return to theatre and the administration of a further anaesthetic without the need to reintubate the patient and interfere with the oral cavity.
- Usually the patient will have a preoperative percutaneous gastrostomy (PEG). The patient is started on a soft diet after 10 days and can start to chew after 6 weeks.
- Dentures should not be worn for at least 2–3 months following surgery.
- If there is a poor sulcus after primary closure and the patient wishes to wear dentures, then an epithelial inlay is inserted after 3 months.
- If the patient who has undergone extensive surgery in the mouth wishes to have dental rehabilitation, then they should be considered for osseointegrated implants.
- Dental care is continued into, during and after postoperative radiotherapy.

Complications

Bleeding from the tongue. This must be stopped early and promptly because the whole tongue can swell and the suture line can burst. It can usually be managed by operating through the mouth, reopening the suture line, and catching and securing the bleeding points. This is the main reason why all patients undergoing major tongue operations should have a tracheostomy.

Non-union of the mandible. There are many reasons for this, the most common being that a tooth root has been damaged, so that a drill hole has gone through a tooth root, or that the mandible has been divided through a tooth root (Fig. 15.34). When splitting irradiated bone, rigid fixation should always be used because it is prone to non-union. If a fistula occurs owing to breakdown of the mouth wound, then saliva will penetrate the

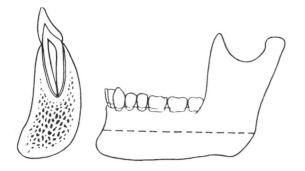

Figure 15.34 The roots of the teeth come halfway down the mandible, so that drill holes above the dashed line in the diagram will almost certainly go through a root. This is why it is wise to consider removal of the teeth prior to any mandibular surgery.

mandible and it will not heal subsequently. A common way to develop a fistula in the past was to leave the ends of the mandibular wires too long, so that they protruded into the mouth and acted as a track for saliva. The use of wires has largely been superseded nowadays by using plates.

The treatment of mandibular non-union depends on the cause. If the trouble is due to a tooth, then it should be removed under antibiotic cover. If the mandible still does not heal, it should be reopened, re-explored and rewired or re-plated with cancellous bone chips packed around the split.

If non-union is due to a fistula, then the fistula should be closed and the patient started on antibiotics; if the mandible still does not heal it is, reopened it and replated as before.

If the patient has been irradiated and osteoradionecrosis becomes established then, in the first instance, it should be treated conservatively with prolonged antibiotic administration, ultrasound therapy and the use of hyperbaric oxygen. If this fails then a wide segment of mandible must be resected and immediate vascularized bony reconstruction performed wherever possible.

Poor speech. The speech result depends on how much of the floor of the mouth and/or tongue has been removed, but matters can always be improved by providing a tip to the tongue, performing the appropriate reconstruction or facilitating an epithelial inlay to make a new sulcus. This allows the patient to wear dentures, which vastly improves the speech. Repairing the defect with a flap as a primary procedure allows the tongue to be freely mobile from the earliest stages. Improvement is facilitated by the appropriate speech therapy. If there is loss of sensation or function in the lower lip, this makes matters worse.

Recurrence in the primary site. When this occurs, if it is detected early, then a wide excision of the tongue, hemi-mandibulectomy and repair with a flap might be possible.

Recurrence in nodes. If the patient has had an involved gland in one side of the neck and has had a neck dissection, he or she may recur on the operated side or may develop recurrence in the midline or in the contralateral neck. Patients should be seen for follow-up as described in Chapter 2. Depending on the site, size and extent of the nodal recurrence, a form of neck dissection may be possible.

Operations for tumours of the floor of the mouth and alveolus

Pelvimandibulectomy

Tumours of this area are dealt with in a very similar manner by the operation of pelvimandibulectomy.

Anaesthetic, incision and neck dissection

A preoperative PEG has usually been carried out. A general anaesthetic is used, but a temporary tracheostomy is carried out and the anaesthetic continued through this. The incision for the neck dissection is either a Schobinger or a T on its side. Access to the oral cavity will usually be required by using a lip split. The incision is continued either around the chin or straight down and the lip is split either at an angle or in a straight line. Cosmetic results are better if the lip is not split and a pull-through procedure is performed. If the patient has an enlarged node in the neck, a modified radical or radical neck dissection is performed and left pedicled to the submandibular area, where it attaches to the mandibular periosteum.

Removal of the primary tumour

The superior cervical flap is raised well over the mandible, with or without splitting the lower lip. The oral mucosa is divided in the gutter lateral to the mandible, well away from the tumour.

It is usually necessary to remove a segment of the mandible but it may be possible in the previously untreated case to preserve either the lower border of the mandible or its outer plate, thus preserving bony continuity, which is superior to removal of the whole mandible and subsequent reconstruction. If implants are required or if the tumour dictates radical surgery, then mandibulectomy and immediate bony reconstruction will be necessary.

If the tumour affects the alveolar ridge, the superior part of the mandible (i.e. the alveolus) is removed in the appropriate involved area. The mandible is divided with a Stryker saw and the tumour visualized by working from outside through the access provided by elevating the cheek. The segment of mandible is left in continuity with the primary tumour and the whole segment of the mandible is excised; alternatively, if conservation surgery is possible and only the lingual plate is invaded, this can be removed in continuity leaving an outer rim (Fig. 15.35).

Repair

When there has been a full segment of bone removed, this is replaced as discussed previously under mandibular

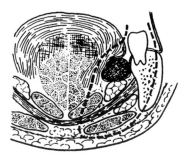

Figure 15.35 Removal of the lingual plate of the mandible in continuity with the tumour.

reconstruction. The soft tissues in this area must always be replaced after resection of a carcinoma of the floor of the mouth or of the alveolus in the following circumstances:

■ when part of the mandible has been resected leaving an area of raw bone, particularly if the patient has been irradiated, of if a full-thickness excision of the mandible has been carried out and a bone graft has been inserted to replace a small defect

■ when the anterior part of the floor of the mouth has been resected. Replacement with soft tissues of the floor of the mouth is necessary in this case, otherwise suturing of the anterior part of the tongue remnant to the labial mucosa leads to ptosis of the lower lip and interference with articulation.

Specific reconstructive techniques

These have already been discussed in some detail earlier in this chapter, and also in Chapter 7.

The lingual flap. In order to be able to use this flap satisfactorily, the greater part of the tongue must have been preserved, including its blood supply from the lingual artery. The tongue flap is marked using tattoo marks with a line extending along the dorsum of the tongue to define an area consisting of half the width of the tongue, so that the lingual artery is included in the base of the flap. The curled edge of the flap is opened up, transposed laterally and stitched into place over the exposed alveolus and the floor of the mouth. The edge of the anterior two-thirds or free portion of the tongue is closed primarily in two layers, using either 3/0 chromic catgut or Vicryl on a cutting needle to reconstitute the tip of the tongue. It is possible to leave the remaining part of the donor site on the central third of the tongue raw to granulate, but there is a danger that it will adhere to the flap. It is probably preferable, therefore, to stitch a split skin graft over this area. The lingual flap is extremely vascular and can provide a good result with regard to both cover of the defect over the bone and restoration of articulation, and may be useful in certain instances when a radial free forearm flap or another vascularized flap is not possible. Its disadvantages are mainly associated with poor donor site function.

Nasolabial flap. This still has a place in intraoral reconstruction. It is used primarily to repair the anterior floor of the mouth and is based inferiorly on the branches of the superior labial or facial artery, which pierce the subcutaneous tissues from its bed to supply a rich dense subdermal network of vessels. The flap may be used either as a normal pedicled flap, leaving a temporary fistula that is closed after division of the pedicle, or as a subcutaneous pedicled flap so that the operation can be completed at one sitting.

A flap is marked out based inferiorly and running in the nasolabial fold. The base of the flap lies approximately 1 cm inferolateral to the angle of the mouth, and the tip of the flap lies at the point where the nasolabial groove meets the nose. The flap is elevated, preserving all of the subcutaneous tissue within it and the perforating branches of the superior labial artery in its base. (If a radical neck dissection has been carried out, the facial artery should be preserved if at all possible.) Then a tunnel is developed beneath the buccal mucosa, emerging at the alveolus. If the flap is to retain its pedicle, it is pushed through this tunnel; it should be of sufficient length to reach to the opposite side of the defect. This flap is sewn into the anterior part of the defect and then a similar nasolabial flap is raised from the opposite side of the cheek. This is passed through a similar tunnel and sutured into the posterior half of the defect, suturing its anterior edge to the posterior edge of the first flap and its posterior edge to the edge of the ventral surface of the tongue (Fig. 15.36).

The primary defect is closed in two layers down to the point where the flap passes into the cheek, leaving a temporary fistula. Three weeks later, the base of the pedicle is divided and returned to the cheek and the defect closed, excising any part of the flap that is redundant or any tissue that will provide an unsightly scar.

With greater experience, the flap can also be used with a subcutaneous pedicle. After the flaps have been raised, the epidermis is taken off from the part of the pedicle that is to be buried, using either an electric dermatome or a scalpel. The flaps are passed into the

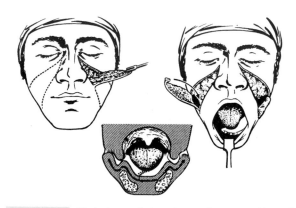

Figure 15.36 Technique of elevation and transposition of the nasolabial flap.

defect and sutured in place as before; the primary defect is closed completely in the nasolabial groove. The patient should be edentulous.

Bone grafts and composite reconstruction. As discussed previously, there is almost no place now for the use of the free bone graft in mandibular reconstruction. Often the recipient site is so unhealthy that it is surprising that non-vascularized grafts took at all in the past.

The majority of composite defects within the oral cavity are filled using free tissue transfer. There is thus little role for myo-osseocutaneous grafts unless the expertise of free tissue transfer is not available. The available choices are:

- the pectoralis major myo-osseocutaneous graft to include the fifth or sixth rib
- the trapezius myo-osseocutaneous graft containing the spine of the scapula
- the sternomastoid flap with clavicle.

Operations on the buccal mucosa

Local excision and primary closure

This operation can be performed for small tumours that are no more than 2 cm at their widest point. The line of incision and excision using a knife or laser should include a reasonably safe margin of at least 1 cm of normal tissue, and its edges and excision should be fashioned in the horizontal plane if possible to facilitate closure (Fig. 15.37). The incision is closed by interrupted sutures of 3/0 chromic catgut or Vicryl. If there is any tension on the suture line, a mattress suture may be used using either Vicryl or silk. Larger defects can be closed using V–Y advancement, either singly or bilaterally.

Local excision and skin grafting

This operation is used to remove a large area of leucoplakia or for a tumour which measures more than 3 cm in diameter. It is important that there is no need to compromise on the margin of safety of excisions because the defect will be closed by using a skin graft. The lesion is excised with a good margin (at least 1 cm), making certain that the lines of excision do not extend upwards or downwards into the sulci as it makes it very difficult to stitch a skin graft on to these areas. The depth of the excision can be gauged by the extent of infiltration; this operation should not be performed if the subcutaneous tissues of the cheek are involved, since flap repair will be involved using more bulky tissue. Very little attention need be paid to the position of the parotid duct, as cutting it does not usually lead to significant complications, although it is important to realize that the buccal branch of the facial nerve runs close to the duct.

The skin graft is taken from the inner side of the thigh and a template made of the size required from *tulle gras*. The skin is placed on this template and cut to size. With the *tulle gras* in place, the skin graft is stitched in with interrupted sutures of 3/0 Vicryl or chromic catgut, using the quilting technique.

Tumours of the superior gingivobuccal sulcus

In this area, surgical access is difficult and one of the most important features in the treatment of oral cavity tumours is access for excision and reconstruction. Skin grafts are almost impossible to suture into place and fix in a satisfactory manner. The best access is achieved by a Weber–Fergusson approach on the face (Fig. 15.38), which incorporates a lateral rhinotomy with an extended incision to include an upper lip split. The patient is prepared in the usual manner and anaesthetized with a

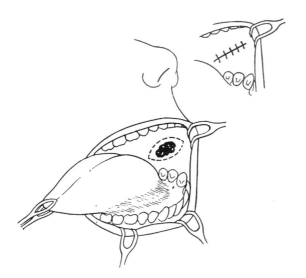

Figure 15.37 Local excision and primary closure of a buccal cancer with the excision line horizontal.

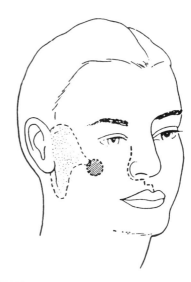

Figure 15.38 For access to tumours in the superior gingivobuccal sulcus, approach is via a Fergusson incision.

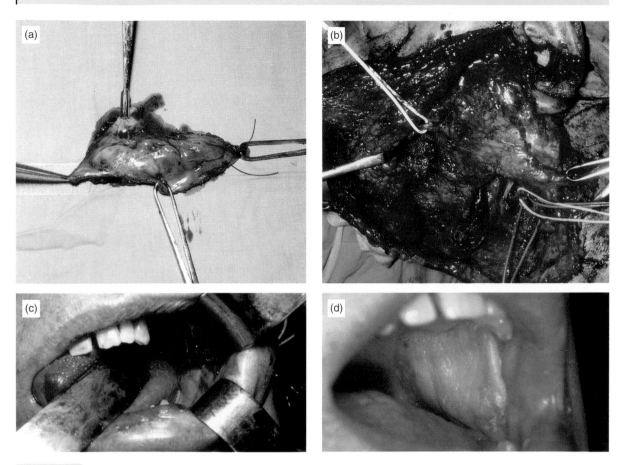

Figure 15.39 (a) Resection of an adenocarcinoma of the accessory lobe of the parotid gland invading the buccal mucosa. (b) Access was achieved by total conservative parotidectomy with facial nerve retraction which facilitated (c) wide buccal mucosa excision. (d) Reconstruction was with a radial free forearm flap.

nasoendotracheal tube, passed down the contralateral nostril. The throat is packed conventionally. A Fergusson incision is marked appropriately, extending from the lower border of the nasal bone into the nasobuccal sulcus, following and staying just lateral to the margin of the nose down to the ala, towards the midline of the columella and then down through the lip in an S-shape or a step-like fashion. The vermilion borders should be tattooed, and the incision made with a knife held at right angles to the skin. The cheek flap is elevated after injection with 1/200 000 saline with adrenaline and then the mucosa is cut in the upper sulcus.

Before making the incision, it is wise to tattoo a safe margin of the intended excision on the mucosa. When this point is reached, the elevation of the mucosal part of the cheek flap is stopped. The lesion is excised round the tattoo marks with a good, deep margin. Haemostasis is secured and the defect closed by approximation of the mucosal edges with 3/0 chromic catgut or Vicryl, making sure that the knots are inside the mouth. If the tumour is more than 3 cm in diameter, the defect will have to be filled with a flap as described in the next section.

For tumours of the parotid gland (usually adenocarcinoma) that involve the buccal mucosa from direct extension of either the deep lobe or accessory lobe of the parotid gland, access can be achieved by formal parotid exploration, total conservative parotidectomy with facial nerve retraction, which facilitates wide buccal mucosa excision. Reconstruction is facilitated with a radial free arm flap (Fig. 15.39).

Deeply infiltrating tumours of the buccal mucosa combined with neck dissection

As described previously, two operations are possible at this site, depending on whether the tumour is nearer to the lower or upper alveolus.

Tumours nearer the lower alveolus

A preliminary tracheostomy is performed, if required, through a small horizontal incision and general anaesthesia established via this route, so that the endotracheal tube is clear of the operative field.

Incision. For these advanced tumours, a neck dissection of some sort will be required not only to treat the neck but also for access providing the vessels for reconstruction. If the neck has previously been irradiated, conventional incisions may still be used or a McFee incision may be preferred. The neck dissection remains pedicled on the submandibular region, although this is not absolutely necessary.

Excision. These tumours are extensive by definition and will probably involve skin, and will almost certainly be larger on the inside of the mouth than on the skin of the cheek. Therefore, it is often useful to remember that the amount of skin of the cheek to be removed should be marked within the mouth. A safe margin may be marked around the tumour on the inside of the mouth, and a needle stuck through this circle at various points so that it comes out of the skin of the cheeks; the needle is painted with Methylene Blue and withdrawn sharply to identify the margin on the outside of the cheek. Using the marks on the outside of the cheek, the skin may be incised through and through, and the resection continues to leave the specimen attached to the lower alveolus. Using a Stryker saw, conservation surgery permits that, in the absence of previous irradiation, the upper half of the adjacent alveolus may be divided and the tumour excised along with the neck-dissection specimen. By extending the incision down the adjacent part of the floor of the mouth and through into the mandibular region, the specimen is removed in continuity. This last step often results in a loss of continuity but where possible remove the specimen *en bloc* if possible.

Repair. These large through-and-through defects are best repaired primarily. Bone is not usually required, so the principal needs are intraoral lining, associated bulk and extraoral skin cover. This may be achieved in a number of ways depending upon expertise available as previously discussed. Subsequent surgery may be required to allow the patient to wear a partial or complete denture. A lingual sulcus is required and for this, the technique of epithelial inlay is used. Prior to this a temporary denture for the patient must have been made so that it can be applied at the time of the operation. The intended area of the sulcus is infiltrated with local anaesthetic and an incision made around the alveolus. This is deepened into the lowest part of the sulcus and extended right back to the angle of the mandible. A prepared split-thickness skin graft is then draped over a piece of gutta percha which is fixed to the dentures by screws when it is hardened. The denture is then fixed in place using alveolar wires which can then be removed after a week. Subsequent dental restoration can either be with a denture or the use of osseointegration.

Tumours opposite the upper alveolus

For tumours in this area, the defects are similar and can be repaired in a similar way.

A summary of the curative treatment of oral cancer is shown in Table 15.4 and approximate 5 year survival rates (ultimate local control) are shown in Table 15.5.

Table 15.4 Curative treatment of oral cancer

	N_0	N_{1-3}
T_1	Surgery or implant brachytherapy	Surgery with postoperative radiotherapy
T_2	Surgery, (with or without postoperative radiotherapy) or implant brachytherapy (low volume $T_2 \leq 2.5$ cm)	Surgery and postoperative radiotherapy
T_3	Surgery and postoperative radiotherapy	Surgery and postoperative radiotherapy (if indicated)
T_4	Surgery and postoperative radiotherapy	Surgery and postoperative radiotherapy (if indicated)

Table 15.5 Curative treatment for oral cancer: approximate 5 year survival rates (ultimate local control)

Stage	5 year survival (%)
I	75–95%
II	65–85%
III	45–65%*
IV	10–35%*

Shah (1996).
*Combination treatment which includes surgery and radiotherapy.

Radiotherapy techniques

External beam irradiation

Before a beam-directing shell is made, an individualized bite block or gag is often prepared to hold the mouth open and depress the tongue. This has a central tube to enable the patient to breathe through the mouth if necessary. The purpose is to facilitate keeping the volume of healthy normal tissue irradiated to a minimum. The patient is treated supine, immobilized in the shell. It can sometimes be helpful for treatment planning if the margins of the tumour have been marked at EUA by the insertion of inert, radiopaque metal seeds, and for the position of any palpable nodes to be marked with wire.

Small node-negative tumours

For T_1 and small T_2N_0 tumours the treatment volume embraces the primary tumour with a margin of at least 2 cm and the first echelon of nodes. The precise arrangement of radiation fields to treat this volume is chosen to minimize the dose to the oral mucosa and salivary glands. With small lateralized tumours of the tongue, floor of mouth or buccal mucosa, this will most often entail the use of an anterior and a lateral field, appropriately wedged to ensure dose homogeneity. In the case of retromolar trigone tumours, anterior and posterior oblique lateral fields, similar to those used for lateral oropharyngeal tumours (Chapter 16), can be used. Treatment is with megavoltage photons from a linear accelerator giving 55 Gy in 20 daily fractions over 4 weeks or its equivalent.

Larger or node-positive tumours

Most patients with advanced oral cavity cancers are best treated with combined modality therapy involving excision of the primary tumour and neck dissection where appropriate, with planned postoperative radiotherapy. However, radical radiotherapy alone is still used for some patients. For larger tumours and those which cross the midline, parallel opposed fields may be necessary, at the expense of more mucositis and a greater likelihood of xerostomia. These fields will cover the primary tumour and the upper neck, and the spinal cord will be included in the treatment volume. Following an initial dose of 40 Gy in 20 fractions over 4 weeks using megavoltage photons, the patient should be replanned with the photon fields coming off the cord. Matched electron fields of an appropriate energy should be used to treat the nodes in the posterior part of the neck overlying the cord. When lower neck irradiation is necessary, an anterior field is used, the upper margin of which matches the lower margin of the fields treating the primary tumour. Irradiation of only one side of the neck is often appropriate, but if there is any likelihood of bilateral nodal involvement, both sides should be treated. This requires a split anterior field, that is one with a midline block to shield the spinal cord, larynx, hypopharynx and upper oesophagus.

If large volumes are included, it is preferable to give treatment over a period of up to 6.5 weeks, prescribing a total dose of 66 Gy in 33 daily fractions to the primary site and any clinically involved nodal areas, and a lower dose of 50 Gy in 25 fractions to clinically uninvolved nodal areas treated prophylactically.

A brisk mucositis is inevitable, regardless of the fractionation schedule chosen. It is therefore very important to ensure that oral hygiene is maintained. Simple, regular saline mouthwashes are often all that is required. Topical treatments such as Mucaine, Difflam or aspirin mucilage may help to alleviate the discomfort within the oral cavity, but often systemic analgesia with coproxamol or even oral morphine is necessary. It is equally important that the patient continues to receive adequate fluids and nutrition. Some patients will manage to eat and drink adequately, using liquidized food and high-calorie supplements, but the majority will require a gastrostomy.

Postoperative radiotherapy

Postoperative radiotherapy is given after primary surgery to diminish the likelihood of recurrence at the primary site or in the neck. Ideally, all the resection margins will be free of tumour, but the pathology report must be studied carefully and special attention given to areas of doubt. Radiotherapy is commenced as soon as wound healing is satisfactory. The primary site is covered with

an adequate margin (usually 2 cm) is enough, and the neck is also treated if more than one node was involved or if there was any evidence of extracapsular spread. If the primary tumour margins were pathologically involved then a full dose of 66 Gy in 2 Gy fractions should be given. Otherwise, a dose of 60 Gy in 30 fractions is adequate for the primary site and the dissected neck. When prophylactic treatment is given to the unoperated, clinically negative, contralateral side of the neck, a dose of 50 Gy in 25 fractions is appropriate. The cord dose should be kept within tolerance levels by a two-phase technique involving electrons as well as photons.

Care must be taken in the postoperative setting, as well as in the case of primary radical treatment, to avoid interruptions to treatment, as prolongation of the overall treatment time allows tumour cell repopulation and compromises the likelihood of cure. If unscheduled gaps occur, then they should be compensated for by the use of more than one fraction per day, with a minimum interfraction interval of 6 h, to keep the overall treatment time no longer than planned.

Interstitial therapy

The oral cavity is the most common site for interstitial implantation of radionuclides in the head and neck region. There are several reasons for this. First, many oral tumours are particularly suitable for this form of treatment, being small, relatively well demarcated and also anatomically easily accessible – by no means a trivial reason. Secondly, the fact that interstitial therapy treats a small, localized volume with a rapid fall-off of the dose remote from the implant enables a higher radiation dose to be given to tumours than would be tolerated by the larger volumes inevitably included by external beam irradiation. In addition, adjacent structures such as bone and salivary glands receive a lower dose from an implant than they would with external beam irradiation, diminishing morbidity and thereby making treatment more acceptable from the patient's point of view. Finally, clinical experience suggests that for suitable tumours control rates are better with interstitial therapy although, as in so many other settings, no comparative trials have been conducted to prove this.

Although radium needles were used very successfully for decades, they have now become obsolete, principally for reasons of radiation protection. Initially, they were replaced by caesium needles which were used in exactly the same way, but more recently iridium wire implants have superseded these. These are more versatile as the wire is flexible and can be cut to any length, enabling its use in situations where rigid needle implants were not possible. Another advantage, from the operator's point of view, is that radiation protection is easier. Firstly, the insertion of applicators into which the radioactive sources are subsequently put (afterloaded), when the accurate positioning of the tubes has been verified radiographically, means that there is no radiation exposure to staff in the operating theatre. Secondly, the radiation from iridium is far less penetrating than that from radium, making the shielding of nursing staff and visitors on the ward easier. The principal disadvantage of iridium is its relatively short half-life, making reuse impracticable and therefore increasing the cost.

There are two main techniques of iridium wire implantation. The choice between them is usually dictated by the site and size of the tumour to be treated. For small tumours of the floor of the mouth or lateral border of the tongue, iridium wire 'hairpins' may be used (Fig. 15.40). Under a short general anaesthetic, a steel applicator with two parallel slotted legs 12 mm apart is inserted into the tumour. Further applicators are then put in parallel with the plane of the first. When the position of the applicators is satisfactory, iridium wire hairpins, with their legs cut to an appropriate length, are slid down the slots in the applicator legs and sutured in place, and then the applicators are removed. The legs of the hairpins lie along a double plane and enable treatment of a slab of tissue approximately 2 cm thick. Further X-rays are then taken for dosimetric purposes, to determine the length of time for which the implant must remain in place for the prescribed dose to be delivered. The patient is able to eat and drink while the implant is in place, and it is removed at the end of treatment on the ward with no need for a second anaesthetic. Alternatively, flexible plastic tubes can be implanted percutaneously into the tumour using a steel introducer. Several parallel tubes about 1 cm apart will be used. For small tumours these will all lie in the same plane, but for larger tumours, a volume implant will be formed from two parallel planes. When treating small tumours of, for example, the buccal mucosa, the tubes will be more or less straight, but for larger tumours of the dorsum of the tongue or floor of mouth the tubes may be looped. The tubes are held in position by ball-shaped plastic washers and crimped lead discs. The tubes are not radiopaque, and are therefore loaded with inert wire before radiographs are taken for dosimetric purposes. Iridium wire, cut to appropriate lengths so that it will not protrude through the skin, is sealed inside finer plastic tubes and afterloaded into the outer plastic tubes (Fig. 15.41). At the end of treatment, the implant is easily

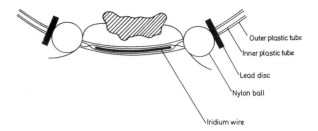

Figure 15.41 Iridium wire implant afterbladed into a flexible plastic tube.

removed on the ward. The skin punctures heal well and become almost invisible. The prescribed dose, calculated according to the Paris system, is the same whether hairpins or plastic tubes are used.

For small tumours where the risk of occult nodal disease is slight, radical radiotherapy can be given by interstitial therapy alone. For larger tumours an initial course of external beam therapy to the primary tumour and at least the first echelon of nodes is followed by an interstitial boost about 3 weeks later. Usually 60 Gy is given over 5 days when interstitial treatment alone is used. When external beam irradiation has been used first, giving a dose of 45–50 Gy in 20–25 fractions over 4 or 5 weeks, the prescribed dose from the implant will by 20–30 Gy over 2–3 days.

References and further reading

Broders A. C. (1941) The microscopic grading of cancer, *Surg Clin North Am* **21**: 947–52.

Gujrathi D., Kerr P., Anderson B. and Nason R. (1996) Treatment outcome of squamous cell carcinoma of the oral tongue, *J Otolaryngol* **25**: 145–9.

Hibbert J. (1997) Oral cavity, in: *Scott-Brown's Otolaryngology*, 6th Edn, Vol. 5, *Laryngology and Head and Neck Surgery*, Butterworth-Heinemann, Oxford, Chap. 3, pp. 1–32.

Hicks W. L., Loree T. R., Garcia R. I., Maamoun S., Marshall D., Orner J. B. *et al.* (1997) Squamous cell carcinoma of the floor of mouth: a 20 year review, *Head Neck* **19**: 400–5.

Inoue T., Inoue T., Teshima T., Murayama S., Shimizutani K., Fuchihata H. and Furukawa S. (1996) Phase III trial of high and low dose rate interstitial radiotherapy for early oral tongue cancer, *Int J Radiat Oncol Biol Phy* **36**: 1201–4.

Inoue T., Inoue T., Yamazaki H., Koizumi M., Kagawa K. *et al.* (1998) High dose rate versus low dose rate interstitial radiotherapy for carcinoma of the floor of mouth. *Int J Radiat Oncol Biol Phys* **41**: 53–8.

Jackson I. T. (1985) *Local Flaps in Head and Neck Reconstruction*, CV Mosby, St Louis, MO.

Jacobson P. A., Everoth C. M., Killander D., Moberger G. and Martensson B. (1973) Histological classification and grading of malignancy in cancer of the larynx, *Acta Radiol* **12**: 1–9.

Jewer D. D., Boyd J. B., Manktelow R. T., Zuker R. M., Rosen I. B., Gullane P. J. *et al.* (1989) Orofacial and mandibular reconstruction with the iliac crest free flap: a review of 60 cases

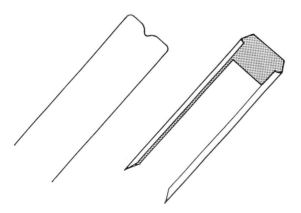

Figure 15.40 Iridium wire hairpin and applicator.

and a new method of classification, *Plastic Reconstruct Surg* **84**: 391–403, 404–5.

Matsumoto S., Takeda M., Shibuya H. and Suzuki S. (1996) T_1 and T_2 squamous carcinomas of the floor of the mouth: results of brachytherapy mainly using ^{198}Au grains, *Int J Radiat Oncol Biol Phys* **34**: 833–41.

Matsuura K., Hirokawa Y., Fujita M., Akagi Y. and Ito K. (1998) Treatment results of stage I and II oral tongue cancer with interstitial brachytherapy: maximum tumour thickness is prognostic of nodal metastasis, *Int J Radiat Oncol Biol Phys* **40**: 535–9.

McGregor I. A. and McGregor F. M. (1986) *Cancer of the Face and Mouth: Pathology and Management for Surgeons*, Churchill Livingstone, London.

Robertson A. G., McGregor I. A. and Soutar D. S. (1986) Postoperative radiotherapy in the management of advanced intra-oral cancers, *Chem Radiol* **37**: 173–8.

Sabroe S. (1998) Alcohol and cancer (Editorial). *BMJ* **317**: 827.

Shah J. (1996) Oral cavity and oropharynx, in: *Head and Neck Surgery*, 2nd edn, Mosby-Wolfe, London, Chapter 6, pp 167–234.

Soutar D. S. (1994) Mandibular reconstruction with vascularised bone, in: *Excision and Reconstruction in Head and Neck Cancer* (D. S. Soutar and R. Tiwari, eds), Churchill Livingstone, London, Chap. 5, pp. 59–78.

Spiro R. H., Huros H. G., Wong G. Y., Spiro J. D., Gnecco C. A. and Strong E. W. (1986) Predictive value of tumour thickness in squamous carcinoma confined to the tongue and floor of the mouth, *Am J Surg* **15**: 345–50.

UICC (International Union against Cancer) (1997) *TNM Classification of Malignant Tumours*, 5th edn (L. H. Sodin and Wittekind C. H., eds), Wiley-Liss. New York.

16 Tumours of the oropharynx

'Symptom severity provides an index of biological behavior
that cannot be discerned from the TNM cancer stage alone'

F. A. Pugliano, 1999

Introduction

Tumours of the oropharynx present a challenge to both the otolaryngologist and clinical oncologist. They usually present late and can be difficult to assess clinically because of their significant spread in three dimensions. Imaging is mandatory for staging and their close proximity to the oral cavity, mandible and supraglottic larynx means that any surgical resection has important considerations relating to access, reconstruction and functional rehabilitation. Some small tumours are suitable for conservation surgery and/or radiotherapy, but the majority of treatable squamous cell carcinomas require extensive resection and immediate reconstruction. This chapter outlines the current treatment of tumours of the oropharynx.

Surgical anatomy

The **oropharynx** extends from the level of the hard palate superiorly to the level of the hyoid bone inferiorly. Its anterior limit is the anterior faucial pillar, but this is contiguous with the retromolar trigone. It is divided into the following components:

1. the **anterior wall**, which is made up of the base of the tongue posterior to the foramen caecum, the vallecula and the lingual surface of the epiglottis; it is bounded by the pharyngoepiglottic folds
2. the **lateral wall**, which is made up of the anterior pillar (palatoglossus), posterior pillar (palatopharyngeus) and the pharyngeal palatine tonsil
3. the **roof**, which is formed by the soft palate containing the two heads of palatopharyngeus, the levator palati, the tensor palati and the palatoglossus. The oral surface of the soft palate is in the oropharynx and the nasopharyngeal surface is part of the nasopharynx
4. the **posterior wall**, which extends from the level of the hard palate to the level of the hyoid and is anterior to

the second and third cervical vertebrae. This consists of the superior and middle constrictors and the buccopharyngeal fascia, which separates it from the prevertebral fascia.

The lateral wall of the oropharynx is the **medial** wall of the parapharyngeal space. If a tumour extends through the lateral wall of the oropharynx, it enters this space and becomes contiguous with the carotid sheath, the symphathetic chain, the styloglossus, the stylopharyngeus and the pterygoid muscles.

Tumours of the posterior wall usually extend upwards into the nasopharynx and downwards into the hypopharyngeal region, and are probably best considered as parts of the contiguous regions, rather than separately as part of the oropharynx.

The most important area in the oropharynx, however, is the tongue base. This is made up of the genioglossus muscle, which is attached to the hyoid. Tumour infiltration into this muscle by definition almost always involves the whole of the tongue because the distance between the genioglossus at the base of the tongue, and the muscles of the anterior part of the tongue in the submental space is only about 2.5 cm. Furthermore, the base of the tongue is contiguous with the vallecula, which is the roof of the pre-epiglottic space. Early spread into the pre-epiglottic space means that a tongue tumour can very rapidly become a laryngeal tumour.

The lymphatic drainage from the oropharynx is mainly to levels II, III and IV, with an emphasis on the jugulodigastric node in level III. It also drains into the retropharyngeal and parapharyngeal nodes, which need to be considered in the assessment of disease in this area.

The area is lined with squamous epithelium and so squamous carcinoma represents the most common tumour. However, there is abundant lymphoid tissue in the palatine tonsil and also the lingual tonsil which can be affected in head and neck lymphoma; the soft palate is especially rich in minor salivary glands.

Surgical pathology

Epidemiology

The annual incidence of carcinoma of the oropharynx in the UK is between 6 and 8 per million, yet in the USA it is 60 per million. The maximum age incidence is in the seventh decade, and the male to female ratio for squamous carcinoma is 10:1. Recent trends have shown that patterns are changing, with patients presenting in the fourth and fifth decades of life, and the male to female ratio has lowered to approximately 4:1.

These small numbers make data collection difficult and hence there is a lack of published results. National survival figures are difficult to assess because some cancer registries use the International Classification of Diseases (ICD) system, which combines both oral cavity and oropharynx.

The most significant aetiological factor is **tobacco**, but tumours in this area are also seen in heavy drinkers and, as in the oral cavity, the cause is related to the synergistic effect of alcohol and tobacco intake, which increases the effect of either five times. In addition, the mixing of tobacco with lime, as in betel-nut chewing, causes well-differentiated tumours of the mouth, but also has an effect in the aetiology of oropharyngeal cancer. Other precursors and important contributory factors include ionizing radiation, iron deficiency anaemia, dental sepsis, submucosal fibrosis of the palatine arch and human papillomavirus (HPV) infection (types 8 and 16).

The incidence of non-Hodgkin's lymphoma is rather different. The maximum age incidence is in the sixth decade and the male to female ratio is 2:1. The management of non-Hodgkin's lymphoma is discussed in Chapter 25.

Tumour types

Because of the three types of tissue within the oropharynx which have previously been described, squamous cell carcinoma, lymphoma and minor salivary gland tumours can all occur. Squamous cell carcinoma is the most common malignancy and forms 90% of the tumours in this region. Non-Hodgkin's lymphomas account for 8% and minor salivary gland tumours for 2%. With regard to squamous cell carcinoma the most commonly affected site is the lateral wall (60%), then the tongue base (25%), the soft palate (10%) and finally the posterior wall (5%). Ninety per cent of lymphomas occur in the lateral wall or in the tongue base; minor salivary gland tumours have a predilection for the soft palate followed by the lateral wall, and then the tongue base.

The staging of oropharyngeal carcinoma is based on tumour size, with T_1 tumours measuring 2 cm or less at their largest diameter, increasing to T_4 tumours which are massive, measuring larger than 4 cm in size, and exhibit deep invasion into the maxillary antrum, the pterygoid muscles in the infratemporal fossa, the angle of the mandible or neck skin. The joint International Union

Table 16.1 TNM and overall staging of oropharyngeal tumours

T: Primary tumour

T_X	Primary tumour cannot be assessed
T_0	No evidence of primary tumour
T_{is}	Carcinoma *in situ*
T_1	Tumour 2 cm or less in greatest dimension
T_2	Tumour more than 2 cm but not more than 4 cm in greatest dimension
T_3	Tumour more than 4 cm in greatest dimension
T_4	Tumour invades adjacent structures, e.g. pterygoid muscles, mandible, hard palate, deep muscle of the tongue, larynx

Stage grouping

Stage 0	T_{is}	N_0	M_0
Stage I	T_1	N_0	M_0
Stage II	T_2	N_0	M_0
Stage III	T_1	N1	M_0
	T_2	N1	M_0
	T_3	$N0, T_1$	M_0
Stage IVA*	T_4	N_0, T_1	M_0
	Any $T_{1,2,3}$	N_2	M_0
Stage IVB*	Any $T_{1,2,3}$	N_3	M_0
Stage IVC*	Any T	Any N	M

UICC (1997).
*New inclusion.

Against Cancer (UICC)/American Joint Committee on Cancer (AJCC) T stages and overall stage groupings are shown in Table 16.1.

The presence or absence of lymphatic spread within the neck depends on the size and site of the primary tumour, the histology, the presence of perineural and vascular invasion, whether or not the patient has had previous surgery or irradiation and persistence of the tumour at the primary site following treatment. As in the oral cavity, the depth of tumour invasion is also directly related to the incidence of cervical metastases.

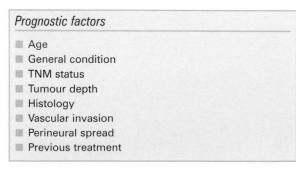

Prognostic factors
- Age
- General condition
- TNM status
- Tumour depth
- Histology
- Vascular invasion
- Perineural spread
- Previous treatment

Lymphatic spread is usually in a predictable, ordered fashion from superior to inferior, and in the N_0 neck, the first eschelon nodes are in levels II–IV, along with the retropharyngeal nodes. It is extremely uncommon to have metastases in level I or V in the clinically negative neck. What is odd in the spread of oropharyngeal tumours is the frequency with which they involve the nodes in the posterior triangle once there are palpable nodes in levels

Table 16.2 Incidence (%) of cervical lymph-node metastases in oropharyngeal tumours based on clinical examination of 1155 patients

Area	Primary tumour	N_0	N_1	$N_{2,3}$
Tonsillar fossa	T_1	29	41	29
	T_2	32	14	53
	T_3	30	18	52
	T_4	10	13	76
Base of tongue	T_1	30	15	55
	T_2	29	14	56
	T_3	25	23	51
	T_4	15	8	76
Soft palate	T_1	92	0	8
	T_2	63	12	24
	T_3	35	26	39
	T_4	33	11	56

Thawley and O'Leary (1992).

II, III and IV. The drainage is progressive down the lymph nodes and along the accessory nodes in the posterior triangle. In other head and neck tumours, nodes in the posterior triangle often herald a fatal outcome but, if properly treated, this is not necessarily the case in oropharyngeal tumours.

Spread of oropharyngeal tumours

- Local spread by continuity and contiguity
- Lymphatic spread
- Distant spread

Bilateral lymphatic metastases are often seen in tumours of the soft palate and base of tongue and contralateral metastases may occur if the patient has had previous neck surgery or irradiation. The incidence of neck metastases in oropharyngeal tumours is shown in Table 16.2.

One in three patients with oropharyngeal tumours will, at some time, develop a second primary, so it is important to consider the presence of a synchronous second primary, especially if contralateral nodes are found.

Again, as distinct from other head and neck tumours, as many as 8% of patients will have distant metastases which are apparent at presentation. This is probably due to the rich lymphatic drainage of the oropharynx, which leads to a higher incidence of local and hence distant metastases.

Tumour spread

Lateral wall tumours

These are the most common tumours (50%) and often involve the tonsil. They may spread anteriorly and upwards to the retromolar trigone and on to the buccal mucosa, as well as into the muscles of the tongue base. If they erode deeply, they involve the pterygoid muscles producing trismus. Lateral extension can involve the angle of the mandible and the inferior alveolar nerve, especially in elderly patients, since in the edentulous mandible the inferior alveolar nerve is more superior than usual. Inferiorly, these tumours can extend down the lateral pharyngeal wall into the piriform sinus, inferomedially on to the aryoepiglottic fold and hence into the paraglottic space, and posteriorly on to the posterior pharyngeal wall.

Lesions of the inferior pole of the tonsil are often difficult to see and sometimes primary tumours can lurk within the tonsillar crypts as the 'occult primary'. This group of tumours presents with a metastatic lymph node and an apparent occult primary site, and in this situation excision of the tonsil as a diagnostic procedure is crucial. If not identified in this way, they can remain occult for a number of years.

Fifty per cent of patients have palpable metastatic nodes at initial presentation, with another 25% having occult disease in a clinically N_0 neck.

Base of tongue tumours

These are the next most common oropharyngeal tumours (40%). Symptoms frequently do not appear until the lesions are at an advanced stage. They spread rapidly through the genioglossus muscle and across the midline, and can very quickly involve the entire tongue, pushing it upwards and forwards. Because of this, much of the tongue will often have to be removed for what appears to be a fairly small mucosal tumour at the base. Muscle contractions of the genioglossus help to propel the malignant cells not only into the lymphatic system but also through the potential spaces within the intrinsic tongue musculature. Spread can also be posterior and inferiorly into the vallecula, the epiglottis and hence into the supraglottis and the pre-epiglottic space.

Approximately 60–70% of these patients have a positive palpable cervical lymph node at initial presentation, and because of the propensity of bilateral spread within the tongue base, 20–30% will have bilateral nodes. It is important to assess the retropharyngeal nodes in both tongue base and lateral wall tumours. Twenty per cent of patients will present with nodes and no apparent primary.

Soft-palate tumours

Carcinoma of the soft palate occurs almost exclusively on the anterior surface. It may occur with leucoplakia and is common in heavy smokers, particularly in the elderly. Occasionally, several small primary tumours are seen in the same patient, of which a soft-palate tumour is one. As the tumour enlarges, it may involve the palatine nerves and the back of the maxillary antrum. It will certainly involve the nasopharynx and may go into the superior pole of the tonsil.

Posterior wall tumours

These are all extremely rare and in any one series, there will only be a small handful of cases. Very few definitive statements can, therefore, be made about this tumour except that it often involves contiguous submucosal spread in a superior and inferior direction to involve the naso-pharyngeal or hypopharyngeal posterior wall. In the un-treated patient, the prevertebral fascia often acts as a barrier to spread and bilateral metastases are common, as is spread to the retropharyngeal nodes.

Lymphoma

These consist almost entirely of non-Hodgkin's lymphoma. The histological classification, staging and relative site incidence of these lymphomas are described in Chapter 25.

Lymphomas particularly affect younger patients, who usually present with unilateral tonsil enlargement. Unless an adequate biopsy is taken, these are often reported as poorly differentiated tumours. Any poorly differentiated tumour reported from the oropharynx should be studied using immunocytochemistry in order to distinguish a lymphoma from a poorly differentiated or anaplastic carcinoma.

Minor salivary gland tumours

On the soft palate, most minor salivary gland tumours are benign pleomorphic adenomas. Elsewhere in the oro-pharynx, however, malignant tumours are the rule, with adenoid cystic and mucoepidermoid tumours being the most common. Adenoid cystic tumours invade perineural lymphatics and there is a rich source of tumour spread in this area along the greater and lesser palatine nerves and the inferior alveolar nerves. These tumours are discussed in more detail in Chapter 22.

Investigations

History

Presenting features of oropharyngeal tumours
■ Sore throat
■ Otalgia
■ Dysphagia
■ Ulcer
■ Pain
■ Trismus
■ Neck mass

The majority of patients present late and usually complain of a sore throat, otalgia or dysphagia. A small proportion will present because they have noticed an ulcer in the oropharyngeal region. About 20% will present with a metastatic node in the neck. Patients with lymphoid enlargement due to lymphoma may complain of muffled speech and difficulty in clearing food from the mouth during the first stage of swallowing. Patients with more advanced tumours may complain of more significant pain and/or trismus.

One of the most difficult groups to deal with is those patients who have tumours (particularly submucosal) of the tongue base. Nothing may be seen and they may present to a number of specialists for a diagnosis of their symptoms, which include cervical lymphadenopathy, throat pain, referred otalgia or pain on swallowing. The majority will have few clinical signs.

Examination

The whole oral mucosa should be examined systematically. Then the oropharynx is inspected using a tongue depressor to look at both tonsils, the posterior third of the tongue and the soft palate. A mirror is used to examine the tongue base, the vallecula and the postnasal space, so that the back of the soft palate can be inspected. Equally important is palpation, particularly of the tongue base. Squamous cell carcinoma tends to be hard, while lymphoma masses are firm and rubbery to palpation; salivary gland tumours are very often not ulcerated and have a firmer consistency than lymphomas but are not as hard as squamous cell carcinomas. Although palpation is of vital importance to assess the extent of tumour spread into the tongue base or the palate, extensive examination is not usually possible owing to the presence of pain in the conscious patient. The patient's dentition is also assessed and the advice of a restorative dentist is advisable prior to treatment, particularly if the patient is to receive radiotherapy. The dentition of some patients is too poor for conservative treatment and dental clearance is usually required.

Next, both sides of the neck are examined and the appropriate levels for palpable nodes assessed; if lymphoma is suspected, a general examination should be performed.

Radiology

The role of radiology in the assessment of oropharyngeal tumours is discussed in Chapter 3. It is important to assess the size, site and extent of the primary tumour with contiguous spread into the parapharyngeal space, tongue base, vallecula, epiglottis and supraglottis, the posterior pharyngeal wall and both sides of the neck. Particular attention should be paid to nodal enlargement in the retropharyngeal area, where positive disease will usually require surgical resection. Magnetic resonance imaging (MRI) is particularly useful for assessing tongue-base tumours.

It is important to assess the presence or absence and extent of any mandibular invasion, but this is thankfully quite rare in the majority of pharyngeal tumours. Far more sinister is perineural spread along the inferior alveolar nerve, but MRI is not yet at a stage where this can be detected reliably.

If the head and neck is being assessed by spiral CT, it will usually be practical to obtain a CT of the chest and upper abdomen as well, to complete the examination in high-risk patients. Otherwise, a chest radiograph is vital because of the higher incidence of distant metastases and secondary primary tumours in oropharyngeal index tumours than in any other primary site.

If a lymphoma is confirmed, then this is staged by a conventional whole-body CT scan.

Biopsy

All patients with oropharyngeal masses should be given a general anaesthetic and panendoscopy performed. This is carried out to assess the size, the site and the extent of the primary oropharyngeal tumour, to take a biopsy and to look for metastatic disease or synchronous primary tumours, as well as to assess the neck.

Incisional biopsy of all tumour masses should be performed but, if there is a smooth regular enlargement of one tonsil, then a tonsillectomy should be done if possible, because lymphoma is the most likely diagnosis and the pathologist will be able to evaluate the disease more accurately on whole-organ resection.

Obtaining a biopsy from the base of the tongue can be difficult. Many of these tumours are submucosal and a tissue diagnosis is only achieved by deep biopsies. In occasional circumstances, a deep incisional biopsy is sometimes rewarding, but the best way is to perform trucut biopsy of the tongue base under general anaesthetic. Many of these cases present not only with a hardness at the base of the tongue but also with a metastatic neck node, which is readily assessed by fine needle aspiration cytology (FNAC). In the presence of a positive biopsy from a primary pharyngeal squamous cell carcinoma, aspiration of palpable neck nodes is unnecessary.

At the time of endoscopy, if the primary site cannot be ascertained, and the patient has a metastatic node in either level II, III or IV and a primary pharyngeal tumour is suspected, then the tongue base on the side of the node should be biopsied. Any suspicious areas that bleed on contact endoscopy should also be biopsied. The tonsil should be palpated and even in the absence of any obvious disease, should be widely excised as in approximately 10–20% of cases an occult T_1/T_2 tonsillar tumour will manifest itself.

At the end of the examination and biopsy under anaesthesia, the surgeon should have a clear idea of the size and the extent of the tumour, and this information is combined with a diagram and the information obtained from preoperative imaging. It is always wise to perform preoperative imaging prior to biopsy as small incisional biopsy or even FNAC can affect the images. At the end of the procedure, the surgeon will usually know what treatment should be instigated and this should be written in the notes.

Treatment policy

Squamous carcinoma

To split and categorize the treatment of the oropharyngeal cancer into small anatomical sites is an intuitively attractive dogma. However, head and neck cancer does not conform to the rules of such a 'cookbook'. Tumours of the oropharynx usually arise from a common mucosal covering that has had a wide field change from significant exposure in the past to both alcohol and tobacco. These tumours frequently extend from one area to the next without any restriction, spreading by both continuity and contiguity, owing to the absence of formal barriers between the specific subsites of the oropharynx and the adjacent sites of the oral cavity and larynx. Frequently, it is impossible to say whether the tumour has arisen from the soft palate, the lateral pharyngeal wall, the tongue base or the tonsil.

Another problem is that many patients present late and are in a poor general condition with a low performance score. There is a high incidence of chronic smoking with related cardiac, pulmonary and vascular diseases, alcoholism, liver cirrhosis and occasionally oesophagitis with varices. These factors, taken in conjunction with poor nutritional status and the significant physiological effects and possible defects of the surgery, confound treatment decision making.

Not only is there a high incidence of second malignancies in oropharyngeal tumours, but there is also a significant incidence of early and bilateral metastatic neck disease due to the propensity of the tongue base to spread early on to both sides of the neck. In general, patients with bilateral neck disease have a 10% chance of long-term survival.

In many of these unfortunate patients, a surgical resection and subsequent reconstruction will inevitably interfere to some extent with their ability to swallow and to handle secretions, so consideration has to be given as to how the patient is going to manage the upper airway if they have a surgical resection and reconstruction. This is most evident in the difficult situation where a tongue-base tumour extends into the vallecula and resection is combined with a supraglottic laryngectomy. These patients experience considerable difficulty postoperatively, but some can return to near-normal swallowing given appropriate rehabilitation.

The following treatment policy should be viewed in the light of the previous comments and is inevitably, to some extent, an oversimplification of the problem.

Treatment options

■ Curative
 - Radiotherapy
 - Surgery
 - Surgery and post-operative radiotherapy
■ Palliation
 - Radiotherapy
 - Radiotherapy/chemotherapy
 - Tracheostomy
 - Pain relief

Access

Limited access to the oropharynx can be obtained via the oral cavity. Radical tonsillectomy can be performed using a tonsil gag, as can resection of tumours of the posterior pharyngeal wall and the soft palate. For larger tumours and those tumours which are more difficult to access, e.g. tongue-base tumours, a wider exposure is required.

Conservation mandibular surgery is usually feasible and access achieved using either a paramedian or lateral mandibulotomy. The problem with the latter is that the inferior alveolar nerve is divided, which renders the lower lip insensate and leads to drooling. For small tongue-base tumours, an elegant posterior approach is via a lateral pharyngotomy removing the ipsilateral hyoid.

Any incisions which relate to access must consider the levels required for neck dissection, which will usually be at least level II, III and IV for the N_0 neck, or otherwise a modified radical or radical neck resection. Such an operation facilitates exposure of the major vessels, which will provide the facility for microvascular free transfer. The oropharynx is a difficult area to reconstruct, given its three-dimensional complexity and the need for sensation. The principles for reconstruction have been discussed in Chapter 7.

Lateral wall tumours

Radiotherapy would be expected to give at least a 70% 5 year survival rate in T_1 and T_2, N_0 tumours but, unfortunately, squamous cell carcinoma of the lateral wall (in essence the tonsil) does not present in this way. Either the tumours are occult or, if they are obvious and either T_1 or T_2, they are usually associated with cervical lymph-node metastases. Radiotherapy for T_3 or T_4 tumours is less effective and patients would be fortunate to achieve 30–40% 5 year survival rates (Mak-Kregor *et al.*, 1996). Many authors have suggested that if there are nodal metastases, then radiotherapy has no place to play in initial management and surgery should be the prime modality followed usually by postoperative radiotherapy. However, a recent publication (Jones *et al.*, 1998) has shown that small oropharyngeal tumours with limited neck disease

(nodes measuring less than 2 cm) can be treated safely by external beam radiotherapy.

For small T_1 and T_2 lateral wall tumours in the absence of cervical lymphadenopathy, external radical beam radiotherapy can be given. Alternatively, conservation surgery may be practised. This can give equal if not better results by performing radical tonsillectomy (as well as simultaneous or delayed neck dissection in the presence of palpable disease) and then postoperative radiotherapy (Fig. 16.1). Surgery for the larger tumours is more extensive and can be achieved done by either conserving the mandible if the bone is not involved, or performing the commando operation. This consists of a modified radical or radial neck dissection, resection of the ascending process and part of the horizontal process of the mandible, the lateral pharyngeal wall, part of the tongue base and part of the soft palate. The subsequent defect requires three-dimensional reconstruction and the soft tissue can be repaired using either a pedicled or a free flap (Fig. 16.2). If bone is to be replaced, free tissue transfer

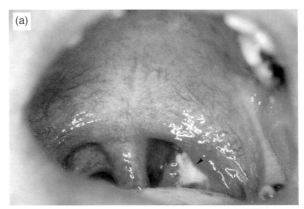

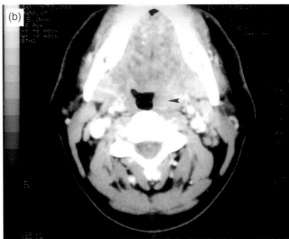

Figure 16.1 Patient a with a T_2N_{2a} squamous cell carcinoma of the left tonsil. (a) The primary tumour; (b) the extent of the disease is confirmed on CT imaging. Treatment was with localized resection of the primary site, discontinuous neck dissection and postoperative radiotherapy. The patient remains alive and well 3 years later.

involving bone and soft tissue together with skin may be required. Following this operation, postoperative radiotherapy is usually administered.

Tongue-base tumours

These tumours usually present so late that radiotherapy alone is of little value. However, if they are detected early, they can be treated with external radical beam radiotherapy with 5 year survival rates approaching 80%. For the not uncommon scenario of a relatively 'early' primary tongue-base tumour with bulky neck nodes, a neck dissection with postoperative radiotherapy to the primary tumour offers a good prospect of cure with minimum morbidity. Alternatively, conservation surgery gives equally good results using a lateral neck approach, resection of the hyoid on the ipsilateral side, lateral pharyngotomy and tongue-base resection without reconstruction. This operation carries minimum morbidity and is excellent in treating small tongue-base tumours (Fig. 16.3). For the larger tongue-base tumour, if cure is contemplated then wide resection is required with bulky reconstruction and postoperative radiotherapy. A unilateral or bilateral neck dissection is often required. Access to the mouth is usually from a lateral approach plus or minus a commando mandibular resec-

tion, or alternatively through a paramedian jaw splitting incision. Tumours that extend into the supraglottis may require supraglottic laryngectomy or even total laryngectomy, but in this situation careful consideration needs to be given as to whether oncological surgery is feasible.

An alternative approach in advanced (Stage III and IV) tongue-base tumours is to use chemoradiation. This technique avoids mutilating surgery (which is often futile) and early reports of some long-term survivors are encouraging (Robbins *et al.*, 1996). The results of controlled trials are awaited.

Reconstruction is usually needed in the form of bulk and this can be facilitated using either a pedicled pectoralis major or latissimus dorsi flap, or a free latissimus dorsi or rectus abdominus flap. This is a devastating operation for both the surgeon and the patient and there is an argument that given the poor chance of cure, the combined operation of total glossectomy with supraglottic or total laryngectomy is not a viable proposition. However, this means that a few potential curable patients may by denied a chance of cure on what are, in effect, purely emotional grounds.

Tumours of the posterior wall

These are described in Chapter 17.

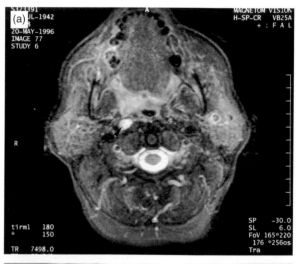
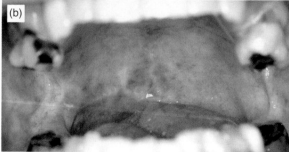
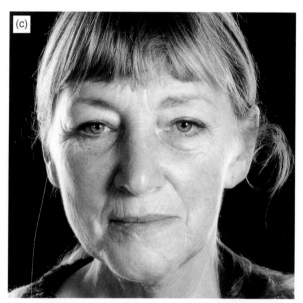
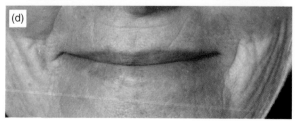

Figure 16.2 Patient with a T_3N_{2b} squamous cell carcinoma of the right tonsil extending into the soft palate. (a) Note the extent of the primary disease together with retropharyngeal lymph-node involvement (arrow) on MRI. (b) Treatment was with lip split and paramedian mandibulotomy, wide local resection, extended modified radical neck dissection and radial free forearm repair. (c and d) The patient remains alive and well 3 years later.

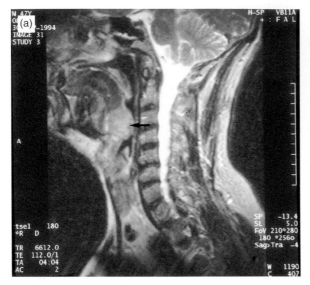

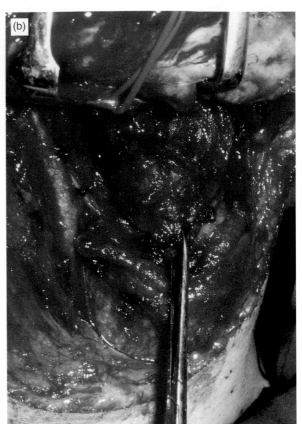

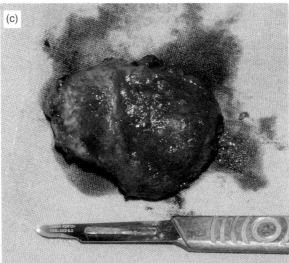

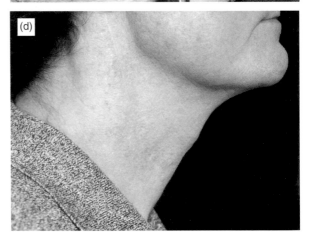

Figure 16.3 (a) MRI (sagital view) showing a T_2N_0 squamous cell carcinoma of the tongue base. (b) Treatment was with elective selective neck dissection, transhyoid pharyngotomy and wide local resection. (c) Excision was complete. (d) The patient received postoperative radiotherapy and remains alive and well 4 years later.

Soft-palate tumours

Very small soft-palate tumours of the uvula can be easily excised. The larger ones which involve a significant part of the soft palate are best treated with radiotherapy, reserving surgery for salvage since the morbidity of initial surgery is significant. However the radiotherapy often leaves a palatal defect when the tumour has disappeared which can cause nasal escape and regurgitation, but the size of the defect, the associated morbidity and postoperative function are usually better than if radical surgery and postoperative reconstruction were used initially.

Those patients that suffer nasal escape following radiotherapy to a soft-palate tumour should be assessed by a speech therapist and reconstruction initially should be

kept to the minimum using either a pedicled hard-palate flap or a pharyngoplasty. The alternative is a sensate radial free forearm palatal reconstruction but often this is too bulky, it does not function nor does sensation always return; therefore, this sort of repair should be reserved for larger defects, particularly those that extend on to the lateral pharyngeal wall and tongue base.

The best surgical approach for radical removal of the palate, which often encompasses the removal of the superior part of the lateral pharyngeal wall, is either a median or paramedian mandibulotomy, or alternatively a lateral angular mandibulotomy. In the short term, if a radial free forearm flap is not used to repair the defect, a dental prosthesis should be used until the patient has recovered

Table 16.3 Curative treatment of squamous carcinoma of the oropharynx

	N_0	N_1	$N_{2a/2b}$	N_{2c}	N_3
T_1	Conservation surgery and postoperative radiotherapy (or radiotherapy alone)	Conservation surgery and postoperative radiotherapy or primary radiotherapy for low-volume disease (one node less than 1 cm)	Surgery and postoperative radiotherapy	Surgery and postoperative radiotherapy	?Surgery, ?radiotherapy,
T_2	?Conservation surgery and postoperative radiotherapy or ? radiotherapy alone	?Conservation surgery and postoperative radiotherapy	Surgery and postoperative radiotherapy	Surgery and postoperative radiotherapy, or ?radiotherapy alone	?Surgery, ?radiotherapy
T_3	Surgery and postoperative radiotherapy	Surgery and postoperative radiotherapy	Surgery and postoperative radiotherapy	?Radiotherapy, or consider chemoradiation (see text)	?Surgery, ?radiotherapy. Consider chemoradiation (see text)
T_4	Surgery and postoperative radiotherapy, ?radiotherapy alone. If unfit for surgery, ?consider chemoradiation	?Surgery and postoperative radiotherapy, ?radiotherapy alone or consider chemoradiation	?Surgery and postoperative radiotherapy, ?radiotherapy alone or consider chemoradiation	?Radiotherapy, or consider chemoradiation	?Radiotherapy, ?chemoradiation (see text)

Table 16.4 Best achievable cure rates* for the treatment of oropharyngeal tumours (includes postoperative radiotherapy)

Stage	Pharyngeal wall	Tongue base	Tonsil	Soft palate
I	65	75	90	58
II	54	75	80	56
III	45	60	53	30
IV	8	55	45	20

Shah, 1996.
*Overall 5 year survival (%).

from surgery. If there is no evidence of residual or recurrent disease, local tissue can be used to good effect.

The current treatment philosophy of oropharyngeal tumours is shown in Table 16.3 and the best achievable cure rates (overall 5 year survival) are shown in Table 16.4.

Inoperability

This has been discussed in Chapter 2. It is important to consider in those patients where extensive surgery may be undertaken as to whether or not it is the correct course of action and to decide which patients might be better left alone.

Inoperability of oropharyngeal squamous cell carcinoma

- Poor general condition
- Advanced disease involving nasopharynx, tongue base, larynx and direct neck extension
- Distant metastases
- Second primary

Lymphoma

Once the diagnosis of lymphoma has been made, the disease should be staged and treatment may be with either chemotherapy or radiotherapy, or combined modality treatment. This is discussed in Chapter 25. Most recurrences occur within the first 18 months. If there is a recurrence, the patient has only a 10% chance of long-term survival.

Minor salivary gland tumours

The benign pleomorphic adenoma is probably the most common tumour on the soft palate. Once the diagnosis has been established by either FNAC or incisional biopsy, the tumours are excised and often the defect can be closed primarily, usually without any significant functional problems.

Minor salivary gland tumours occurring elsewhere in the oropharynx, however, are almost certain to be malignant. Adenoid cystic carcinoma should be treated similarly to squamous cell carcinoma, with a wide excision, appropriate reconstruction and postoperative radiotherapy from the skull base down to the clavicles. If it is treated primarily, no special attention needs to be given to the extensive resection of associated nerves, but if the patient has had previous treatment elsewhere, then the resection margin may need to be extended.

Mucoepidermoid carcinoma presents much the same problem but without the perineural spread. Although its biological behaviour is unpredictable and it is possible to divide tumours into high grade and low grade, in the oropharynx it is best to treat all tumours as high grade and as if they were squamous carcinomas. They should be treated with wide resection and consideration given to postoperative radiotherapy.

Failure of treatment

Reviews of current series suggest that one in five patients will die of recurrence of their primary tumour. Recurrence at the primary site may be difficult to detect, particularly when a myocutaneous flap has been put in place, but its presence is often heralded by an increase in swelling, pain and trismus. An alteration in the swallowing pattern is also ominous. It may sometimes be difficult to establish the diagnosis because tissue biopsy can be difficult. Postoperative CT or MRI will help to localize recurrent tissue masses, but again interpretation of films can be difficult owing to the distortion of the normal anatomical planes. The distinction between persistent oedema, fibrosis and recurrent tumour may be helped by a positron emission tomographic (PET) scan.

One in 10 patients will die of neck recurrence. In this situation, in the presence of palpable nodes and a non-dissected neck, the patient needs a modified radical or radical neck dissection and depending upon previous treatment, bilateral neck resection can be performed if there are bilateral nodes. At the time of primary treatment, in the presence of the N_0 neck, if the patient is being treated with irradiation, then the neck should be electively irradiated, including the posterior triangle because the incidence of occult neck disease here is significant.

Ten per cent of patients will die of distant metastases, 4% will die as a direct result of primary treatment and a further 10% will die of conditions unrelated to the tumour.

Overall, 25% of the 5 year survivors will develop a second primary, of whom approximately 70% will die.

Causes of death

- Primary recurrence
- Neck recurrence
- Distant metastases
- Second primary (synchronous or metachronous)
- Unrelated causes
- Result of primary treatment

Commando operation

As outlined in the treatment policy above, this operation is required for squamous carcinoma of the tonsil with a metastatic neck node, recurrent carcinoma of the lateral wall after radiotherapy and malignant salivary gland tumours of the lateral wall and soft palate. It is called the commando operation as an abbreviation for combined mandibular and oral cavity resection. This term does not relate to the extent of the operation or the bravery of either the surgeon or the patient.

The mandible is usually removed because it is involved with tumour, although some authors maintain that even if it is not involved, it should be removed to provide closure of the soft tissues. This is no longer necessary, owing to advances in free tissue transfer.

Preparation

Attention must be paid to oral cavity care and the teeth. All carious teeth must be removed and, if the patient has had previous radiotherapy, then it must be established that the remaining teeth are in good enough condition not to warrant complete extraction. When the mandible is divided, one must ensure that there are no tooth roots left near the divided edge, particularly in the irradiated mandible, as this will lead to problems with healing and subsequent malunion.

The operation is started by preparing the patient from above the ear, the face below the nose, and both sides of the neck and chest. Depending on the mode of reconstruction, the abdomen, arm, hip or lower leg may all need to be prepared. The operation begins with a tracheostomy and the anaesthetic is continued through this route.

Incision

The incision usually involves a lip split with paramedian mandibulotomy and access via a mandibular swing (Fig. 16.4). It is important to preserve the mental nerve to ensure that lower lip sensation remains intact. The incision can be extended into the neck as either a modified Schobinger or a 'T' on its side. This usually allows the upper skin flap to be taken over the mandible. It may not be necessary to bring the incision up to split the lip, but usually it is easier to do so as it makes access so much easier.

The neck dissection is carried out, making sure that the prevascular and postvascular facial nodes around the facial artery are cleared and paying particular attention to the corners of consternation relating to the subdigastric area and the posterior triangle. The neck dissection may be left pedicled on the posterior part of the submandibular gland at the angle of the mandible.

Excision

If conservation surgery is to be carried out in the previously non-irradiated patient, then partial mandibulectomy carried out at this stage. The periostium is incised over the mandible with a knife and the insertion of masseter is divided to allow access. The periosteum is elevated on the lateral and medial side of the bone up to the coronoid process, the sigmoid notch and the neck of the mandible. The mandible can then be divided partially using a reciprocating saw (Fig. 16.5) or for complete mandibulectomy, the neck of the mandible is divided using either the reciprocating saw or a Gigli saw, and the temporalis is divided to free the coronoid process using Mayo scissors. The mandible is next divided in its horizontal portion using the saw; this part of the operation should be left until after the coronoid process has been divided, since doing it before makes the coronoid process much more difficult to divide.

The oral cavity is entered and the tongue pulled forward with a stitch. The tumour is then identified and the extent of the tumour assessed, and the excision margins marked using either the diathermy or a tattoo. Then the

(a)

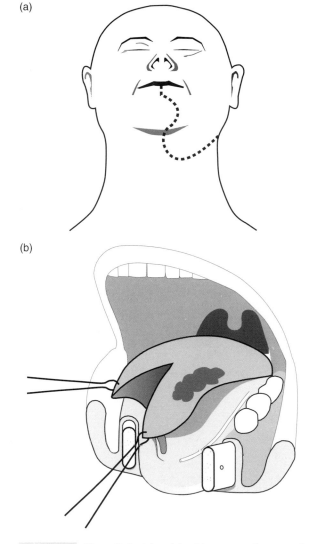

(b)

Figure 16.4 Lip split incision (a) with paramedian mandibulotomy and a mandibular swing (b).

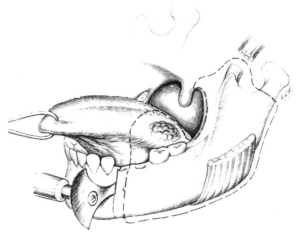

Figure 16.5 Temporalis attached; the mandibular neck is cut with either a Gigli or reciprocating saw. The anterior mandible is then divided with a reciprocating saw, medial to the mental nerve.

Local complications

Bleeding. This can occur during the extensive dissection, particularly during the resection of the primary tumour, and it should be controlled promptly. Postoperative bleeding is often venous from the pterygoid plexus. In the absence of significant wound swelling, it will usually decrease over time and can be compensated for by appropriate fluid and blood replacement without reopening the neck. Serious haemorrhage requires urgent return to theatre once the patient is resuscitated.

Wound breakdown. This is not uncommon, given the extent of the procedure and the fact that the oral cavity and oropharynx are contaminated areas. Patients are covered with prophylactic antibiotics for 48 h. Any subsequent wound discharge should be swabbed. Minor wound breakdown is easily managed using conventional wound toilet, but major breakdown requires packing so as to allow healing by secondary intention. In some instances, flap repair may be necessary. These problems are particularly common in irradiated patients.

Flap failure. All flaps should be monitored in the postoperative period (Chapter 7). It is uncommon for pedicled flaps to suffer significant problems in the postoperative period and it may even be difficult to monitor free flaps in the tongue-base region. Any cause for concern requires urgent assessment and return to theatre if the flap is compromised.

Fistula formation. Fistulae are not uncommon following surgery on the oropharynx. They are particularly common after extensive surgery with flap reconstruction or operations on the postirradiated patient, and also if the tonsil has been removed and a few weeks later a neck resection performed as a delayed procedure, when it is quite easy to enter the oropharynx or oral cavity during

tumour is removed using cutting diathermy and any significant branches of the lingual and external carotid artery should be ligated and tied. At this point of the operation, care should be taken not to retract too hard in an upper direction because the facial nerve can be traumatized.

At the end of the excision, the wound is irrigated and a warm pack inserted. The surgeon should then change his or her gown and gloves.

Complications

- General
- Local
  - Bleeding
  - Wound breakdown
  - Flap failure
  - Fistula formation
  - Recurrent disease

---

dissection of the submandibular triangle. The majority of fistulae will heal spontaneously by secondary intention, but where there are major problems including major vessel exposure, immediate flap reconstruction to provide cover will be required.

Recurrent disease. Recurrent disease at the primary site is often detected late and is usually a disaster. Very few patients are salvaged, although following conservation surgery for the lateral pharyngeal wall, further conservation surgery is possible by wide intraoral excision. Neck recurrence is treated on its merits. If the neck has not previously been dissected, the patient should undergo a neck dissection. Resection for recurrence in the dissected neck is often a dismal sign, with deep disease wrapped around major vessels, and is usually unresectable.

Reconstruction

The reconstruction of the oropharynx is one of the most difficult areas to treat and one of the most difficult challenges for the head and neck reconstructive surgeon. Following the resection, the defect is assessed and it is important to replace like with like. Skin and soft tissue need to be replaced, and consideration should be given as to whether a sensate flap is required. If mandible has been resected, it may or may not be reconstructed and replacement of the external skin is rarely required. The choices in reconstruction are:

- local flaps: lingual and temporalis flaps
- distant pedicled flaps: pectoralis major or latissimus dorsi myocutaneous flaps
- free tissue transfer: latissimus dorsi or rectus abdominus flaps
- deep circumflex iliac artery (DCIA), scapular and fibula flaps: for soft-tissue and bone reconstruction.

Local flaps

Lingual flap. If the defect is relatively small, for example, just involving the lateral wall without any palatal tongue excision, then the size of flap required is measured and a lingual flap, based posteriorly, is cut just anterior to the circumvalate line. It must include the lingual artery at the base, and the base of the flap should probably be the width of half the tongue. The surgeon cuts well down to the substance of the tongue and rotates the flap into the defect. It should be sewn in place in two layers using vicryl. The defect on the lateral side of the tongue is closed by primary suture. This flap can cause significant problems with tongue tethering when it is used for all but the smallest defect. It is seldom used nowadays.

Temporalis flap. This is an easy flap to raise and may be rotated into a unilateral soft-palate defect. The muscle is raised and divided superiorly; it is pedicled inferiorly and access to the mouth gained by going under the zygomatic arch. It is usually necessary to divide the temporalis tendon from the coronoid. The flap is sewn in place and allowed to granulate.

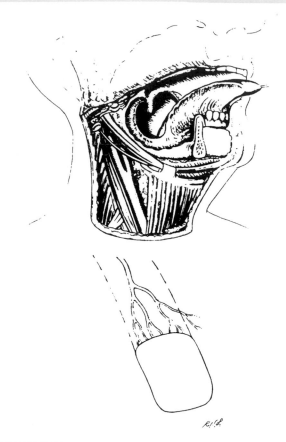

Figure 16.6 Defect following hemimandibulectomy and oropharyngeal resection with neck dissection. Repair may be completed with either a mycutaneous flap (pectoralis major flap in this case) or free tissue transfer.

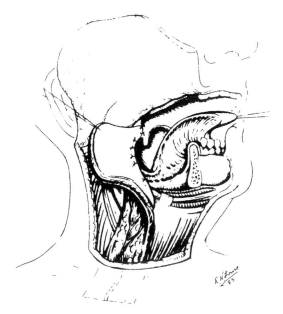

Figure 16.7 Flap is elevated and sewn in place.

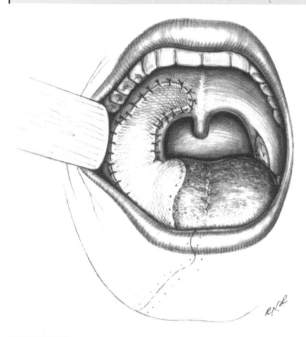

Figure 16.8 Final result.

Pectoralis major and latissimus dorsi myocutaneous flaps. These flaps are raised as described in Chapter 7. Their muscle pedicle fills the defect left by the neck dissection and they easily reach to the tongue base (Figs 16.6–16.8), but when used to reconstruct the lateral pharyngeal wall, care needs to be paid to hitching them up as they often pull away superiorly and lead to a fistula in the postoperative period. There is little use for other pedicled flaps (such as the deltopectoral flap) in modern-day oropharyngeal reconstruction.

Free flaps. Depending on the defect and the requirements of the skin, soft tissue and bone, a number of free flaps (e.g. radial forearm, DCIA, scapula and fibula) can provide large areas of insensate or sensate skin, soft tissue and bone (Fig. 16.2). These have been described above and their harvesting is described in Chapter 7.

Total glossectomy and supraglottic laryngectomy

This operation is rarely carried out today. Many of the patients are incurable and, even when a cure is contemplated, the morbidity is such that all but the bravest surgeons and patients decline the operation.

However, certain tumours of the tongue base and lateral pharyngeal wall that extend into the vallecula and on to the lingual surface of the epiglottis (with or without minimal invasion into the pre-epiglottic space) can be treated with localized tongue-base excision and supraglottic laryngectomy.

Preparation

The patient is prepared as described previously for the commando operation. A tracheostomy is performed first and the neck dissection is completed.

Excision

This is usually achieved via a paramedian mandibulotomy approach with mandibular swing. Alternatively, a lateral mandibulotomy or occasionally the commando operation will be necessary. The tumour is excised from the tongue base and lateral pharyngeal wall and then extended round so that the epiglottis can be grasped in Allis forceps and the supraglottis excised to include the vallecula and pre-epiglottic space (Fig. 16.9). If a total laryngectomy is contemplated, it is completed at this point in the conventional manner.

Closure

The large soft-tissue defect is easily closed using either a pedicled pectoralis major or latissimus dorsi flap, or a free latissimus dorsi or rectus abdominus flap. Given the extent of the operation, the former often suffices. If a supraglottic laryngectomy is performed, care must be taken to achieve meticulous closure when suturing the flap to the laryngeal remnant.

Complications

Complications of this operation are similar to those in the commando operation. In addition, these patients suffer significant postoperative problems with swallowing and aspiration and require the care of a dedicated speech therapist in the postoperative period, but with care and dedication many can be rehabilitated.

Palatectomy

Many soft-palate tumours can be excised intraorally. For larger tumours the palate may need to be almost totally resected.

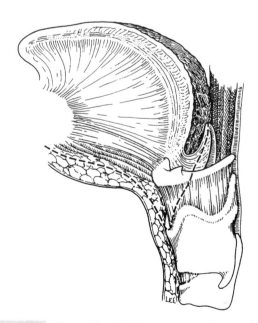

Figure 16.9 Extent of total glossectomy and supraglottic laryngectomy.

Preparation

The neck and face are prepared and a tracheostomy conducted in the conventional way. The neck resection is performed and pedicled at the angle of the mandible.

Excision

This can be done using either a paramedian or lateral mandibulotomy approach. In the latter, the mandibular periosteum is divided and the periosteum elevated off the ascending process of the mandible on both sides. At the angle, an oblique line is drawn in the dentate patient and a mandibulotomy made between the angle and the retromolar area. Prior to complete division, the mandible is preplated using plates and screws. These are then removed and the bone is divided. This makes realignment and subsequent reconstruction easy. In the edentulous patient, a mandibulotomy may be sited in the same place or along the ramus of the mandible as in the conventional mandibulotomy.

Either way, these incisions give access to the lateral wall of the oropharynx and direct access to the soft palate. The lateral wall and soft palate can then be removed (Fig. 16.10). The wound is then washed and gloves are changed.

Closure

The problem with this resection is that often the whole of the soft palate is removed along with the part of the lateral pharyngeal wall. Owing to the complex three-dimensional nature of this defect, bulk is not required and reconstruction is not served by using a pectoralis major myocutaneous flap.

The ideal reconstruction is a tailor-made contoured sensate radial free forearm flap, which may be sutured anteriorly and posteriorly, folded upon itself and sutured to

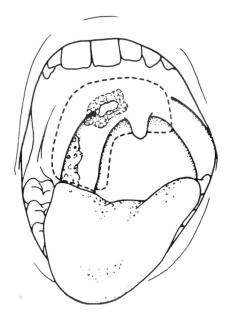

Figure 16.10 Extent of the excision required for removal of a palatal tumour.

the midline posteriorly to give support and close off the posterior choana into two channels. This technique results in an excellent functional reconstruction (Fig. 16.2).

Radiotherapy techniques

The radiotherapeutic technique chosen depends on whether or not the tumour is well lateralized. If there is a central tumour, or a large, lateral one which either crosses or even encroaches on the midline, there is a high probability of bilateral nodal involvement. In such cases, the whole width of the neck must be irradiated, whereas for small, laterally placed tumours, treatment of a limited volume can be effective. Such a set-up enables the contralateral mucosa and parotid gland to be spared, and therefore it causes much less morbidity.

Carcinomas of the tonsil or lateral wall

Small tumours without nodes

Before considering small-volume treatment for a lateral oropharyngeal tumour, it is essential that its limits have been precisely identified at examination under anaesthesia, and that any clinically occult extension has been excluded by a CT scan. As in the case of oral cavity tumours, it can be helpful for treatment planning if the tumour margins are marked by the insertion of inert metal seeds, which are used to indicate the position of the tumour on radiographs. For T_1 or T_2 squamous carcinoma of the tonsil or fauces which do not extend significantly into the base of tongue or parapharyngeal area, and where there is no lymphatic spread, small volume treatment is appropriate. Two ipsilateral fields are used (Fig. 16.11), a posterior oblique and an anterior oblique. Wedges are used to ensure that a homogeneous dose distribution is achieved (Fig. 16.12).

The fields extend from the level of the hard palate superiorly down to the hyoid. Their anterior border is through the central part of the tongue and their posterior limit is through the vertebral bodies. The volume encompassed therefore includes the primary tumour with an adequate margin and the jugulodigastric and parapharyngeal nodes, and extends to the midline. For $T_{1-2}N_0$ tumours it is not necessary to irradiate the lower neck prophylactically. The patient is planned lying supine in a shell with the mouth closed. A simulator check film is taken as a permanent record of the intended treatment, and portal verification films are taken or megavoltage imaging is performed to ensure that treatment is executed as planned. A dose of 55 Gy in 20 fractions over 4 weeks or its equivalent is given, using 4–6 MV X-rays from a linear accelerator.

Extensive lateral tumours and smaller ones with nodes

To embrace the primary tumour adequately and upper deep cervical nodes bilaterally a pair of lateral parallel opposed fields is used. Their margins are essentially the same as described for more limited tumours. Care is taken

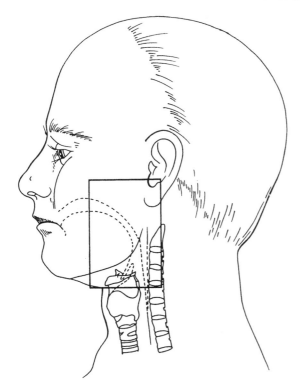

Figure 16.11 Volume to be irradiated in a patient with a small carcinoma of the lateral oropharynx without nodal involvement.

to ensure that these are extended if necessary to cover any direct tumour extension or nodal involvement. Although in most circumstances radiotherapists attach great importance to achieving a homogeneous dose

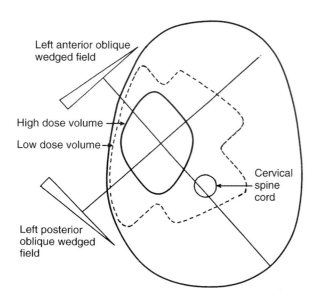

Figure 16.12 Plan of the radiotherapy field arrangement for a small lateral oropharyngeal tumour without nodal metastases.

distribution, the oropharynx provides an exception. If the tumour is confined to the tonsillar region and does not infiltrate the base of tongue or extend on to the palate, it is possible to weight the treatment, giving a greater dose to the affected side and an adequate prophylactic dose to the contralateral nodes. If there is palpable nodal enlargement, the lower neck is also treated. An anterior field is used, the upper border of which matches the lower border of the parallel opposed fields. If the lymphadenopathy is bilateral, then both sides of the lower neck are treated. A single anterior field covering the width of the neck is used and a midline block is required to shield the cervical cord. If there is extensive or bulky nodal disease, primary surgery with postoperative radiotherapy is usually preferred. Nonetheless, primary radical radiotherapy is sometimes appropriate, in which case it may not be possible to achieve adequate coverage without including the spinal cord in the high-dose volume. A two-phase technique, similar to that described for piriform fossa carcinoma (Chapter 17), enables the dose to the cord to be kept within safe limits. In such circumstances the likelihood of cure is slim, but radical treatment may be attempted as it is sometimes successful. A dose of 55 Gy in 20 fractions over 4 weeks is often given, but for the reasons set out in the section on supraglottic carcinoma (Chapter 14), many radiotherapists prefer a more protracted fractionation schedule.

Carcinoma of the base of tongue

The technique here is similar to that described above for bulky lateral wall tumours, or those with nodes. The inferior margin of the lateral fields should, however, be lower to cover actual or potential spread into the supraglottis. In addition, if the tumour is confined to the tongue base, the upper margin is placed below the level of the hard palate and the patient is treated with the mouth open and the tongue depressed. This enables the mucosa of the roof of the mouth to be spared to some extent. Treatment of nodal disease and selection of a fractionation schedule are as indicated above.

Sometimes a brachytherapy boost can be given to the primary tumour using looped iridium wires as described in Chapter 15.

Carcinoma of the soft palate

In most cases this is treated by evenly weighted parallel opposed lateral fields, as described for extensive lateral wall tumours. In the rare event of finding a small T_1 squamous carcinoma, interstitial therapy alone may be chosen. The principal advantage of this approach is that because the treatment volume is small, the reaction will be minimized. Implantation is a particularly valuable treatment method when irradiation of a previous primary tumour has limited the scope for further external beam radiotherapy.

Lymphoma

Lymphoma may be treated by chemotherapy alone, radiotherapy alone or planned combined chemotherapy and radiotherapy. Treatment options in lymphoma are discussed more fully in Chapter 25. If radiotherapy alone is used for stage IE (localized involvement of a single extralymphetic orgen or site) tonsillar lymphoma, it is routine to treat not only the involved site, but also the whole of Waldeyer's ring and the cervical lymph nodes. Large parallel opposed fields, similar to those needed for nasopharyngeal carcinoma, are used to cover the lingual and palatine tonsils, the adenoid area and the upper cervical lymph nodes. An anterior field with midline shielding is used to treat the lower neck. Lymphoma requires a lower radiation dose than that used for carcinoma. A 4 week course giving 40 Gy in 20 fractions is usually prescribed.

References and further reading

Gwozdz J. T., Morrison W. H., Garden A. S., Weber R. S., Peters L. J. and Ang K. K. (1997) Concomitant boost radiotherapy for squamous carcinoma of the tonsillar fossa, *Int J Radiat Oncol Biol Phys* **39**: 127–35.

Harrison L. B., Zelefsky M. J., Pfister D. G., Carper E., Raben A., Kraus D. H. *et al.* (1997) Detailed quality of life assessment in patients treated with primary radiotherapy for squamous cell cancer of the base of the tongue, *Head Neck* **19**: 169–75.

Henk J. N. (1978) Results of radiotherapy for carcinoma of the oropharynx, *Clin Otolaryngol* **3**: 137–43.

Henk J. N., Ahern R. P. and Tailor K. (1993) Carcinoma of the oropharynx in the United Kingdom, in *Head and Neck Cancer*, Vol. 3 (J. T. Johnson and M. S. Didolkr, Manni J. J., Hart A. A., Visser O. *et al.*, eds), Excerpta Medica, London, 779–84.

Jones A. S., Beasley N. J., Houghton D. J., Williams S. and Husband D. G. (1998) Treatment of otopharyngeal carcinoma by irradiation or by surgery, *Clin Otolaryngol* **23**: 172–6.

MacCragar S., Hilgers F. J. N., Levendag P. C. (1996) Disease-specific survival and loco-regional control in tonsillar carcinoma, *Clin Otolaryngol* 550–6.

Mak A. C., Morrison W. H., Garden A. S., Ang K. K., Goepfert H. and Peters L. J. (1995) Base of tongue carcinoma: treatment results using concomitant boost radiotherapy, *Int J Radiat Oncol Biol Phys* **33**: 289–96.

Mohr C., Bohndorf W., Carstens J., Harle F., Hausamen J. E., Hirche H. *et al.* (1994) Preoperative radiotherapy and radical surgery in comparison with radical surgery alone. A prospective multicentric, randomised DOSAK study of advanced squamous cell carcinoma of the oral cavity and the oropharynx (a 3-year follow-up), *Int J Oral Maxillofac Surg* **23**: 140–8.

Nason R. W., Anderson B. J., Gujrathi D. S., Abdoh A. A. and Cooke R. C. (1996) A retrospective comparison of treatment outcome in the posterior and anterior tongue, *Am J Surg* **172**: 665–70.

Perez C. A., Patel M. M., Chao K. S. C., Simpson J. R., Sessions D., Spector G. J. *et al.* (1998) Carcinoma of the tonsillar fossa: prognostic factors and long-term outcome, *Int J Radiat Oncol Biol Phys* **42**: 1077–84.

Shah J. P. (1996) Oral cavity and oropharynx, in *Head and Neck Surgery*, 2nd edn, Mosby-Wolfe, London, Chap. 6, pp. 167–234.

Spiro R. (1993) Less can mean more. The Hayes Martin lecture, *Am J Surg* **166**: 322–5.

Thawley S. E. and O'Leary M. O. (1992) Malignant neoplasms of the oropharynx, in *Otolaryngology – Head and Neck Surgery* (C. W. Cummings, J. Fredrickson, L. A. Harker, C. J. Krause and D. E. Schuller, eds), Mosby, St Louis, MO, Chap. 74, p. 1313.

UICC (International Union against Cancer) (1997) *TNM Classification of Malignant Tumours* (L. H. Sobin and C. H. Wittekind, eds), 5th edn, Wiley-Liss, New York.

Wang C. C., Montgomery W. and Efird J. (1995) Local control of oropharyngeal carcinoma by irradiation alone, *Laryngoscope* **105**: 529–33.

17 Tumours of the hypopharynx

'Be radical early and conservative late'

Introduction

The hypopharynx is a highly important anatomical site since physiologically it is a component of the upper areodigestive tract and, in its upper part, it represents a common conduit for both respiration and deglutition. Hence, any treatment of tumours in this area will by definition produce disturbances in swallowing with inevitable aspiration. Tumours arising in this region often present in an advanced state and the key to cure lies in early and accurate diagnosis and subsequent staging, and, in the majority of cases, treatment by curative intent using surgery and postoperative radiotherapy.

Surgical anatomy

The hypopharynx represents the lowermost part of the pharynx, beginning as it does at the level of the epiglottic tip or the floor of the vallecula, and ending at the level of the lower border of the cricoid cartilage. It consists of the piriform fossae (or sinuses) on each side, the posterior pharyngeal wall and the postcricoid region where the upper areodigestive tract continues into the cervical oesophagus.

The hypopharynx lies below and posterior to the base of the tongue, and behind and on each side of the larynx. It extends from the level of the hyoid bone superiorly down to the lower border of the cricoid cartilage inferiorly and is divided into three distinct sites:

■ the posterior pharyngeal wall
■ the piriform sinus
■ the postcricoid space.

The joint International Union Against Cancer (UICC) – American Joint Committee (AJC) definition of these sites is shown in Table 17.1.

The piriform fossae represent channels formed on either side of the larynx which are open posteriorly. The lateral walls are continuous with the posterior pharyngeal wall and the medial wall on each side forms part of the aryoepiglottic fold which then subsequently merges posteriorly with the postcricoid mucosa. Superiorly, the upper part of the fossa is bounded laterally by the thyrohyoid membrane and medially by the aryoepiglottic fold. The deepest and most inferior portion of the pyriform fossa is known as the apex and is related laterally to the thyroid cartilage, medially to the cricoid cartilage and inferiorly to the paraglottic space.

The posterior hypopharyngeal wall is less well defined. It should be regarded as the part of the hypopharynx that lies between two lines projected posteriorly from the vocal cords when they lie in the cadaveric position. It extends superiorly from the level of the hyoid bone which clinically is described as representing either the tip of the epiglottis or the base of the vallecula. It ends inferiorly at the level of the arytenoids and is separated from the prevertebral muscles by a fascial space. Laterally, it extends from the apex of one piriform sinus to another.

Table 17.1 Hypopharynx subsites

1. Pharyngo-oesophageal junction (postcricoid area) extends from the level of the arytenoid cartilages and connecting folds to the inferior border of the cricoid cartilage, thus forming the anterior wall of the hypopharynx

2. Piriform sinus extends from the pharyngoepiglottic fold to the upper end of the oesophagus. It is bounded laterally by the thyroid cartilage and medially by the hypopharyngeal surface of the aryepiglottic fold and the arytenoid and cricoid cartilages

3.* Posterior pharyngeal wall extends from the superior level of the hyoid bone (or floor of the vallecula) to the level of the inferior border of the cricoid cartilage and from the apex of one piriform sinus to the other

UICC (1997).
*New inclusion.

The postcricoid region lies behind the larynx and extends from the level of the arytenoid cartilages to the inferior border of the cricoid cartilage where it becomes continuous below with the upper end of the cervical oesophagus.

The cervical oesophagus is regarded as extending from the inferior border of the cricoid cartilage to the level of the thoracic inlet.

It can be seen from the above definitions that the boundaries of these subsites are somewhat arbitrary and it is sometimes difficult clinically to ascertain, for example, the upper limit of the posterior pharyngeal wall where it joins the oropharynx, or to define the lateral limits of the posterior pharyngeal wall where it merges with the piriform sinus.

Physiologically, the hypopharynx acts as a conduit for oral intake, participating in the complex neuromuscular co-ordination of the second stage of deglutition, and tumours in this area can impair this activity either by a mass effect or by interference with muscular co-ordination or nervous innervation.

The hypopharynx is lined throughout by squamous epithelium. The piriform sinus has a rich underlying network of lymphatics but this is less extensive in the other subsites. In general, the lymphatics in this area drain to the deep cervical chain in level IV, but the inferior part of the piriform fossa and the postcricoid area also drain to the paratracheal nodes in level VI, and the posterior pharyngeal wall also drains to the retropharyngeal nodes.

Surgical pathology

Squamous carcinoma

The overall site incidence varies from series to series but there is no doubt that tumours on the posterior wall of the hypopharynx are the least common tumour, forming approximately 10% of all these tumours. The most common tumour is that of the piriform sinus, which forms between half and two-thirds of the total; postcricoid tumours make up the remaining 40% or so. Primary tumours of the cervical oesophagus are extremely uncommon. Almost all carcinomas of the hypopharynx are squamous cell in type.

Therefore, it can be seen that tumours of the piriform sinus constitute the largest group of hypopharyngeal tumours, bearing in mind the difficulties in ascertaining the precise subsite of origin. Tumours of the piriform sinus can be divided into those which primarily involve the lateral wall or those which primarily involve the medial wall (the marginal lesion), although when first seen, some of these tumours are often extensive and there is often no practical value in subdividing them.

Those tumours which arise on the medial wall are often more extensive than they would appear at clinical examination. They extend through the aryepiglottic fold to invade the paraglottic space and can therefore fix the

hemilarynx on that side (Figs 17.1 and 17.2). They can also extend into the pre-epiglottic space and occasionally backwards into the postcricoid area, where vocal cord paralysis can occur if the cricoarytenoid joint is invaded or where the recurrent laryngeal nerve is involved, although this is more likely with postcricoid carcinomas than it is with piriform sinus tumours.

Approximately two-thirds to three-quarters of these patients have palpable neck-node metastasis at presentation which usually affects the upper and mid-deep cervical groups (levels II–IV) and 5% will have bilateral enlarged lymph glands at presentation (Fig. 17.3). Tumours arising laterally extend through the thyroid cartilage and through the thyrohyoid membrane to produce a palpable mass in the neck, should be differentiated from a separate lymph-node metastasis by its movement on deglutition. When such tumour spread occurs, invasion in this direction will involve the carotid sheath and the thyroid gland in about 25% of cases. Any large tumour in the piriform fossa can extend superiorly across the pharyngoepiglottic ligament, into the tongue base, often infiltrating beneath the mucosa.

Tumours of the postcricoid space are the next most common hypopharyngeal tumour. When first seen, they are seldom confined to the postcricoid space and extend down the cervical oesophagus to some degree. As in oesophageal tumours, submucosal extension is important and work by Harrison (1970) showed that this extension measured 10 mm on average. Hoe *et al.* (1996) studied the pathological basis for the resection of hypopharyngeal cancer and showed that maximal mural extensions in the upward, medial, lateral and downward directions were 14, 25, 17 and 20 mm, respectively. They recommended 2 cm upper and lateral resection margins, with 2.5 cm at the lower margin being sufficient. Submucos-

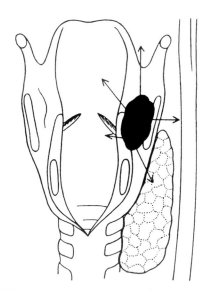

Figure 17.1 Routes of spread of tumours of the piriform fossa.

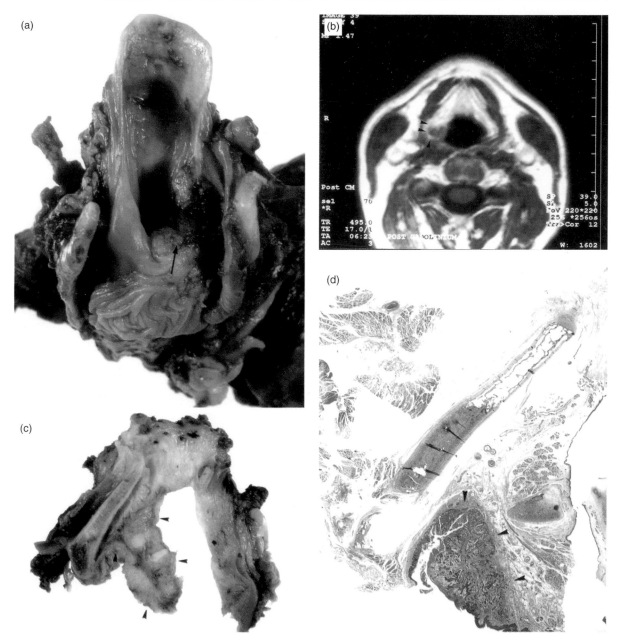

Figure 17.2 (a) T_3N_1 squamous cell carcinoma of the medial wall of the piriform sinus (marginal lesion) treated with total laryngectomy and partial pharyngectomy. (b) Note the tumour on MRI extending into the paraglottic space which is confirmed on both (c) pathological and (d) histological examination.

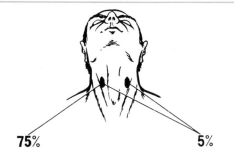

Figure 17.3 Lymph-node metastases in carcinoma of the piriform fossa.

al spread is particularly important when considering the membranous tracheo-oesophageal wall where post-cricoid tumours often occur. When first seen, approximately 20–30% of these cases have enlarged glands in the neck but only one in 20 will have bilateral nodes (Fig. 17.4). About 20% of patients will develop an involved lymph node in the mediastinum involving the paratracheal nodal chain. Extension can also readily occur in an anterior direction to involve the party wall between the oesophagus and the trachea, and laterally to involve the thyroid gland.

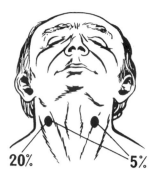

Figure 17.4 Incidence of cervical nodes in postcricoid carcinoma.

About 10% of patients with a postcricoid carcinoma have an immobile vocal cord. The causes of this include invasion of the tumour outside the pharynx into the tracheo-oesophageal grove to involve the recurrent laryngeal nerve, invasion of the cricoarytenoid joint and, very rarely, extension of the tumour into the larynx itself.

Carcinomas of the posterior hypopharyngeal wall are often symmetrical, and are exophytic in nature rather than infiltrative. They do not usually invade anteriorly into the larynx and their lower limit is usually just above the arytenoid cartilages. About half of these patients have a palpable lymph node in the neck which will usually involve the upper deep cervical chain and about 5% of patients will have bilaterally enlarged glands at presentation. These tumours also involve the retropharyngeal nodes and these need to be assessed prior to treatment.

Tumours of the cervical oesophagus are uncommon, but behave in exactly the same way as postcricoid tumours and indeed it is very often impossible to tell whether a tumour has arisen primarily in the postcricoid space or in the cervical oesophagus. In the remainder of this discussion, the term postcricoid carcinoma will be used to include tumours of the cervical oesophagus since their management, in essence, follows the same general principles.

As a general rule, at least 75% of patients with primary hypopharyngeal tumours will have regional nodal metastases at some time during the course of their disease (Table 17.2). At least 60% of these will present with clinically apparent palpable disease, but it is interesting to note that just under half of the patients undergoing elective regional lymph-node dissection will have micrometastases and that a quarter of those untreated necks will go on to develop subsequent nodal disease during treatment. It therefore becomes apparent that a crucial part of the treatment of this disease involves careful assessment and appropriate therapy to the neck and upper mediastinum.

The joint UICC–AJC definition of the 'T' categories and overall staging for hypopharyngeal tumours is shown in Table 17.3 (UICC, 1997).

This staging classification is new and now includes tumour size, which was not included in previous staging systems. This is particularly important for postcricoid tumours where the vertical length of the tumour is an important prognostic factor (less or more than 5 cm). The staging system now comes into line with current and previous classifications for the cervical oesophagus, which included tumour length (UICC–AJC, 1992).

Table 17.2 Incidence of lymph-node metastases at presentation

	N_0 (%)	$N_{1/2/3}$ (%)
Piriform fossa	35	65
Postcricoid area	70	30
Posterior pharyngeal wall	60	40
Overall	55	45

Stell and Swift (1987); Shah (1996).

Table 17.3 'T' and overall staging of hypopharyngeal tumours

T	Primary tumour
T_X	Primary tumour cannot be assessed
T_0	No evidence of primary tumour
T_{is}	Carcinoma *in situ*

Hypopharynx

T_1*	Tumour limited to one subsite of hypopharynx and 2 cm or less in greatest dimension
T_2*	Tumour invades more than one subsite of hypopharynx or an adjacent site, or measures more than 2 but not more than 4 cm in greatest dimension, **without** fixation of hemilarynx
T_3*	Tumour measures more than 4 cm in greatest dimension, or **with** fixation of hemilarynx
T_4*	Tumour invades adjacent structures, e.g. thyroid/cricoid cartilage, carotid artery, soft tissues of neck, prevertebral fascia/muscles, thyroid and/or oesophagus

Stage grouping

Stage 0	T_{is}	N_0	M_0
Stage I	T_1	N_0	M_0
Stage II	T_2	N_0	M_0
Stage III	T_1	N_1	M_0
	T_2	N_1	M_0
	T_3	N_0, N_1	M_0
Stage IVA*	T_4	N_0, N_1	M_0
	Any $T_{1,2,3}$	N_2	M_0
Stage IVB*	Any $T_{1,2,3}$	N_2	M_0
Stage IVC*	Any T	Any N	M_1

UICC (1997).
*New inclusion.

Rare tumours

Benign

Leiomyomas are probably the most common benign mesenchymal tumours of the hypopharynx and upper oesophagus, although they affect the lower third of the oesophagus more commonly. These tumours are more common in men than women, with an estimated ratio of 2:1, and have a maximum incidence in the third, fourth and fifth decades. They are usually rubbery and firm in consistency and, when small, present as an intramural swelling. As they grow, however, they tend to be dragged down into the oesophagus by the normal process of swallowing and then form a polypoid swelling which may reach considerable size. These tumours can usually be removed by dividing their pedicle via a pharyngotomy or oesophagotomy.

Lipomas and fibrolipomas occur occasionally in the hypopharynx and usually present as a well-defined clinical entity. They are virtually always polypoidal and can arise at any site in the pharynx or upper oesophagus. They too tend to be dragged downwards by the normal process of swallowing and thus can form a large pedunculated mass hanging down the oesophagus. A typical presenting symptom is dysphagia, although they may present with choking sensations, and if the tumour is displaced upwards it can fall into the larynx and cause dyspnoea. These tumours have a very small pedicle and, as they are not malignant, can often be removed endoscopically using a snare to divide the pedicle. If there is any difficulty with this removal, they can easily be removed through a lateral pharyngotomy.

Malignant

As described previously, malignant tumours of the hypopharynx are almost exclusively squamous cell carcinomas. Moderately and poorly differentiated tumours predominate, especially those affecting the piriform fossa. In one report (Jones, 1992), it was suggested that only 20% of hypopharyngeal tumours are well differentiated.

A carcinosarcoma, which may also be called pseudosarcoma or a spindle cell carcinoma, is probably a rare variant of squamous carcinoma. It occurs as a polypoid tumour, predominantly in men and the elderly, being only occasionally reported before the age of 45 years. Histologically, the stroma consists of spindle cells; scattered

through the stroma or on its surface are smaller islands of squamous carcinoma. There is considerable controversy as to the importance and origin of the stromal element: many think that it is a reaction to the squamous carcinoma, while others think that it is a true sarcoma. Whatever the truth, and despite its histologically bizarre appearance, this sarcomatous element is relatively unimportant and metastases bearing a resemblance to this part of the tumour do not occur. Indeed, a distant metastasis from this type of tumour is rare. These slowly growing tumours are relatively benign, but late in the disease the squamous element metastasizes to the lymph nodes in the neck in approximately half of the patients.

These tumours usually arise in the region of the pyriform fossa or from the mouth of the oesophagus, are always polypoidal and are usually radioresistant. They should be treated surgically but not radically: removal of the tumour, its pedicle and an area of normal surrounding mucosa is usually all that is needed.

Leiomyosarcoma is the malignant variant of the leiomyoma. It usually also presents as a polypoid swelling hanging down the oesophagus by a pedicle, arising in the region of the arytenoid. The presenting symptoms are usually dysphagia or a feeling of choking. This tumour is not aggressively malignant but usually relatively radioresistant and often responds well to removal, with an area of normal mucosa surrounding its pedicle, through a lateral pharyngotomy. The management of sarcomas is dealt with in Chapter 25.

Other non-squamous hypopharyngeal malignancies are usually either minor salivary gland in origin (usually adenoid cystic carcinomas) or reticuloendothelial lesions such as plasmacytomas. They are dealt with in a similar manner.

Epidemiology

This is discussed in principle in Chapter 1 and only a few extra salient points will be made here.

In general, reports on the descriptive epidemiology of hypopharyngeal cancer in the past have been somewhat unhelpful because it is an uncommon tumour. In addition, the two principal subsites (pyriform fossa and postcricoid area) give rise to tumours with different patterns of behaviour and yet many reports amalgamate these subsites in relation to epidemiological data.

Age-specific incidence rates for pharyngeal cancer show an increased risk of developing the disease with increasing age for both men and women. Postcricoid carcinoma remains the only squamous cancer of the head and neck that is more common in women than men, and it has wide geographical variations in its frequency (relative to other tumours in the hypopharynx). For example, postcricoid cancer forms up to half of pharyngeal cancers diagnosed in the UK and Canada, but is uncommon in the USA and Australasia. Possible reasons for this are discussed below. The incidence in the UK is approximately 1–3 per 100 000.

Alcohol and tobacco remain the two principal carcinogens implicated in tumours of the upper aerodigestive tract, to include the hypopharynx. The evidence is that alcohol and tobacco are major risk factors for oral and pharyngeal cancers and that there is a causal demonstrated relationship for alcohol in oesophageal cancer (Morton and McIvor, 1997).

In relation to postcricoid carcinoma, a major dietary risk factor (iron deficiency) has been described particularly in patients with the Plummer–Vinson syndrome. This syndrome (also called the Paterson–Brown–Kelly syndrome) is associated with anaemia (either microcytic or macrocytic), glossitis, oesophageal web, splenomegaly, koilonychia and achlohydria. Some also have a history of radiation to the neck (either external or internal as radioiodine for thyrotoxicosis) with a long latent interval of 25–30 years. This syndrome should be enquired about in the history and it should be ascertained whether or not the patient has had any previous radiotherapy.

Recent reports from Sweden and America have suggested that the incidence of both Plummer–Vinson syndrome and hypopharyngeal cancer has decreased with improvements in nutrition, replacement iron therapy and a better health service.

Clinical presentation and investigations

Patients with hypopharyngeal carcinoma usually present with a combination of symptoms which will include dysphagia, pain or discomfort on swallowing, referred pain to the ipsilateral ear, hoarseness or a neck mass. The characteristics of each of these symptoms is shown in Table 17.4.

Table 17.4 Symptoms suggesting a possible pharyngeal tumour

• **Dysphagia**	Often persistent and progressive. Patients who complain that food sticks on swallowing should be investigated for a tumour
• **Pain**	Usually lateralized and more prominent on swallowing. May radiate to the ipsilateral ear
• **Hoarseness**	When it occurs in association with dysphagia or referred otalgia usually means extension of tumour into the larynx
• **Neck mass**	Likely to be due to nodal metastases but may represent direct extension through the thyrohyoid membrane
• **Haemoptysis**	An unusual symptom, but can occur with tumours of the piriform sinus and tumours of the posterior pharyngeal wall
• **Weight loss**	Often occurs in the presence of significant disease

The clinical picture caused by a large tumour is often unmistakable, but in the early stages the symptoms may be indefinite. Whilst the feeling of a lump in the throat, which is worse on swallowing saliva, is rarely of serious significance (e.g. globus pharyngeus), vague symptoms, such as the feeling of a crumb in the throat or a persistent soreness, should always be treated with extreme suspicion, especially in older patients who smoke and drink. As it is impossible to examine the postcricoid space and the apex of the piriform fossa by indirect laryngoscopy or flexible nasopharyngoscopy, all patients with persistent throat symptoms, however non-specific, should have a barium swallow and pharyngo-oesophagoscopy. This policy will inevitably mean that some endoscopies will have normal findings but this is inevitable; by adopting strict criteria in the history and examination, they can usually be kept to a minimum.

Globus pharyngeus usually presents in younger women as a sensation of a lump in the throat in the midline, usually between the hyoid and the suprasternal notch but generally at the cricoid level. It is intermittent, typically occurring between meals, when swallowing saliva, in the evening or during times of stress and, although uncomfortable, is never painful. It is usually possible to differentiate these patients from those who have a hypopharyngeal tumour, but if there is any doubt further investigation is always warranted.

Persistent pharyngeal pain is nearly always a sinister symptom and should be investigated further. When associated with malignancy it reflects deep invasion of the laryngeal and pharyngeal structures, usually with associated perineural infiltration. It is often associated with referred pain to the ipsilateral ear. The presence of hoarseness is usually due to fixation of the hemilarynx and occasionally in postcricoid tumours it can reflect direct extension of tumour outside the gullet and invasion of the recurrent laryngeal nerve.

Always enquire about the general health but in particular, weight loss, chest symptoms and aspiration. It is important to take a detailed history of smoking habits and alcohol intake. Also enquire about the history of Paterson–Brown–Kelly syndrome.

Examination

All patients presenting with a throat complaint or a mass in the neck require a full head and neck and general examination. The pharynx and larynx may be examined in the out-patient clinic using either indirect laryngoscopy, a rigid endoscope through the mouth or a flexible nasopharyngoscope passed through the nose. Particular attention should be paid to obvious swelling or ulceration and also to the presence of pooling in the piriform fossa (Chevalier Jackson's sign) and oedema of the arytenoids. Pooling in the piriform fossa indicates failure of passage of secretions down the oesophagus, whereas oedema of the arytenoids may be the only obvious evidence on indirect laryngoscopy of a tumour, either of the medial wall of the piriform fossa or the postcricoid space.

With flexible nasopharyngeal endoscopy, the piriform fossae may be distended by the patient performing a Valsava manoeuvre with the glottis open, and the nostril is pinched. In a small percentage of patients who will not tolerate the above, examination under general anaesthesia is required. In patients where hypopharyngeal tumours are suspected, flexible oesophagogastroscopy is not enough and these patients require examination under general anaesthesia using a rigid laryngoscope and pharyngoscope by an ear, nose and throat (ENT) surgeon. This is because hypopharyngeal tumours may be missed on flexible gastroscopy (Fenton *et al.*, 1995).

Examination of the larynx involves assessment of the movement of both vocal cords, assessment of any supraglottic or subglottic disease, assessment of the airway and visualization of direct extension of a tumour of the piriform fossa through the aryoepiglottic fold into the supraglottic area.

The remainder of the upper aerodigestive tract is examined to exclude a second primary tumour and the presence or absence of laryngeal crepitus (the clicking sensation of the laryngeal cartilages over the prevertebral tissues) is also assessed. This may indicate any postcricoid or posterior pharyngeal wall involvement. Tenderness in the subglottic and upper tracheal area may indicate direct extension of the postcricoid tumour into the posterior tracheal wall. The neck is examined in the conventional manner. Any masses that are close to the larynx and pharynx should be carefully assessed as to whether or not they are enlarged lymph nodes or represent direct extension of a tumour. The neck should be examined bilaterally.

The patient's dentition is assessed and if there is any case for concern, particularly if the patient is due to have (or has had) radiotherapy, then the advice of a restorative dentist should be sought. It is important to carry out any imaging studies prior to endoscopy and biopsy if possible, since fine needle aspiration cytology (FNAC), endoscopic and open biopsy can all create artefactual features on both computed tomography (CT) and magnetic resonance imaging (MRI). The neck should be examined bilaterally.

Laboratory investigations

In many patients with hypopharyngeal cancer, haematological investigations are extremely important. Many of these patients, particularly if they have suffered from the Paterson–Brown–Kelly syndrome, are anaemic. About one-third of them are deficient in electrolytes, particularly potassium, and many of them have deficiency of the serum proteins. It is extremely important that these deficiencies are identified, assessed and if possible corrected prior to surgery. The patients, if possible, should undergo a formal nutritional assessment prior to treatment. Institutional guidelines in relation to preoperative laboratory investigations will vary from hospital to hospital but the following should be considered essential:

- full blood count (with B_{12} and folate if macrocytosis present)
- iron stores
- urea and electrolytes
- liver function tests
- serum calcium
- thyroid function.

Radiological assessment

Many patients with hypopharyngeal tumours will require some form of imaging for assessment and treatment planning. The contributions of various types of imaging modalities and their relative merits are discussed in Chapter 3.

Barium swallow

This is an extremely useful investigation in these tumours. Whilst it is well known that tumours of the cervical oesophagus and postcricoid space may not be demonstrated by this technique and further investigation is mandatory with rigid endoscopy, a barium swallow is of particular value in the following situations:

- to assess tumour length
- to rule out a synchronous primary tumour of the oesophagus
- to ascertain the presence or absence of aspiration
- to assess tumour mobility on the vertebral column during deglutition.

Computed tomography and magnetic resonance imaging

> **Specific uses of imaging**
>
> - To assess the extent of the primary tumour, its relation to the larynx, and extension into the paraglottic space, the postcricoid region and direct extension by continuity and contiguity into the surrounding structures to include the neck and the prevertebral fascia
> - To exclude a second primary or distant metastases (skull base to liver CT)
> - To assess the presence or absence of cartilage invasion
> - To assess the neck (see Chapter 12)
> - To assess the stomach prior to gastric transposition for reconstruction
> - To confirm or refute the presence of a pharyngeal pouch

In patients with throat symptoms who have no abnormality found on examination and investigation, and who have an apparent low risk of malignancy with the absence of major risk factors, barium videofluoroscopic swallow examination may be useful to diagnose pharyngo-oesophageal motility disorders.

The following points are important when examining a patient with a hypopharyngeal tumour under anaesthetic.

In a patient with a posterior pharyngeal wall tumour, it is particularly important to assess the lower and lateral limits of the tumour as encroachment below the level of the arytenoid cartilages or laterally into the piriform sinus indicates that a total pharyngolaryngectomy will be required. In addition, the mobility of the posterior pharyngeal wall on the prevertebral fascia is assessed with the scope and by palpation.

When examining a patient with a piriform fossa tumour, the main point to establish is whether the tumour can be removed leaving enough pharyngeal mucosa to close the pharyngeal defect. In general, once the whole piriform sinus is removed on one side with encroachment on to the posterior pharyngeal wall (i.e. two-thirds of the available mucosa) then consideration needs to be given as to whether the resulting defect requires augmentation with some form of pedicled or free flap. This is particularly pertinent if the patient has received previous radiotherapy.

In the situation where half of the available mucosa is to be removed, it is best to proceed to a total pharyngolaryngectomy. In addition, not only should the exact extent of the tumour be assessed (including the presence of invasion of the larynx), but particular care should be paid to the area close to the mouth of the cervical oesophagus, posterior to the arytenoid cartilages. Extension beyond this point usually indicates that total pharyngolaryngectomy will be required because removal of the tumour will necessitate excision of the entire pharyngeal lumen. At the same time, one should feel for extension into the tongue base, which is often more easily felt than seen.

Finally, in patients with a tumour in the postcricoid region or cervical oesophagus accurate assessment by endoscopy may be difficult. Thus, whilst it is easy to see the top end of the tumour, it is often difficult, and frequently impossible, to pass an oesophagoscope through the tumour to assess its lower limit. This difficulty can be overcome in a number of ways. The tumour can be dilated with bougies, a filiform bougie is left in the oesophageal lumen and it may then be possible to pass a narrow bronchoscope over this and down the oesophagus. Alternatively, a paediatric bronchoscope or oesophagoscope may be used. It is essential to examine the posterior wall of the trachea with a bronchoscope to include invasion of the party wall between the trachea and the

oesophagus. As the patient is under anaesthetic, try moving the oesophagus and pharynx over the prevertebral fascia to detect any degree of fixation. This information will be supplemented by that obtained by using a barium swallow.

Treatment policy

Approximately 25% of patients with hypopharyngeal carcinoma are not treatable at presentation. The most important causes of untreatability include advanced age, poor general condition, local tumour inoperability and extensive neck disease. Distant metastases are also a contraindication but are much less common at presentation than the above-mentioned factors.

Advanced age and poor general condition are difficult to define. Those patients over the age of 75 years or those with some generalized disease that has rendered them incapable of working or running a household (low performance status) should not be offered surgery, both because of its morbidity and because of the poor chances of long-term survival. Tumours of the piriform fossa which extend into the tongue base are rarely cured by surgery. A postcricoid tumour which is fixed to the prevertebral fascia is usually inoperable but this is an uncommon event. A more common event indicating inoperability is a vocal-cord paralysis due to extension of the tumour outside the oesophagus to invade the recurrent laryngeal nerve in the tracheo-oesophageal groove. Once tumours are extensive as this, they will usually be found to be both unresectable and incurable.

Patients with extensive nodal disease are rarely cured. This is because not only is nodal disease significant because of the size and number of the nodes involved, but also prognosis is affected by their position. Extension of disease into the tracheo-oesophageal groove and the upper mediastinum represents an ominous sign. It used to be thought that bilateral neck nodes indicated incurability but more recent studies have shown that this is not true if the nodes are small (i.e. less than 3 cm) in diameter on both sides. Bilateral nodes which are larger than this, and in particular when they are fixed on one side, usually indicate incurability.

Patients who are deemed surgically untreatable on the basis that the disease is unresectable may be considered for radiotherapy with paliative intent. Chemotherapy has no established role. Patients who are deemed unsuitable for surgery on the grounds of extreme old age or poor general condition may also be considered for radiotherapy. However, many such patients will be too frail for this to be a wise and humane treatment.

Long-term results for treatment are either by surgery or by radiotherapy (Table 17.5) and are not good. Results from famed institutions quote overall 5 year survival figures of approximately 35% for hypopharyngeal tumours, with the majority of tumours being treated with surgery with or without postoperative radiotherapy (Shah, 1996). Some rare stage I and II tumours of the

Table 17.5 Curative treatment of hypopharyngeal tumours

	Piriform sinus	Posterior pharyngeal wall	Postcricoid
Stage I (T_1, N_0)	Primary radiotherapy or surgery (PP or PPPL)	Primary radiotherapy or surgery (PP)	Primary radiotherapy or surgery (TLP)
Stage II (T_2, N_0)	Primary radiotherapy or surgery (PPPL or TLP)	Primary radiotherapy or surgery (PP or TLP)	?Primary Radiotherapy or surgery (TLP) and postoperative radiotherapy
Stage III (T_{1-2}, N_+: T_3, N_0; N_+)	Surgery (TLPP or TLP) and postoperative radiotherapy	Surgery (PP or TLP) and postoperative radiotherapy	Surgery (TLP or TLPO) and postoperative radiotherapy
Stage IV (T_4; N_0,N_+)	Surgery and (TLPP or TLP) and postoperative radiotherapy	Surgery (TLP) and postoperative radiotherapy	Surgery (TLPO) and postoperative and radiotherapy

LR: local resection; PP: partial pharyngectomy; PPPL: partial pharyngectomy and partial laryngectomy; TLPP: total laryngectomy and partial pharyngectomy; TLP: total laryngopharyngectomy; TLPO: total laryngopharyngoesophagectomy.

piriform sinus and posterior pharyngeal wall can be treated successfully with irradiation with very good results (50–90% 5 year overall survival; Jones, 1992; Mendenhall, 1996). For postcricoid carcinoma, some series quote 5 year survival rates with radiotherapy of about 30% provided that certain inclusion criteria are observed, although figures from other centres are less optimistic (20%; Axon *et al.*, 1997).

Inclusion criteria for primary radical radiotherapy

- Vertical length of the tumour should not exceed 5 cm
- The vocal cords must be mobile
- N_0 neck

If a tumour does not fulfil all three criteria, the patient should be submitted to surgery as long as age and general condition permit such a treatment policy. A patient who undergoes radiotherapy and subsequently suffers a recurrence should also be considered for surgery.

In the Liverpool series, the 5 year tumour-specific survival for hypopharyngeal tumours treated by surgery and/or radiotherapy was 28% and the observed survival 16% (Jones, 1998). Survival decreased with increasing T and N staging. Patients with piriform fossa cancer had a 31% 5 year survival and in those with postcricoid cancer 29% survived for 5 years. The figure for posterior pharyngeal wall tumours was 20% and the median survival for those with cervical oesophageal cancer was only 18 months. Multivariate analysis showed that age affected survival (patients under 60 years fared better) and advanced disease at the primary site and neck along with poor physical condition all adversely affected survival.

The outlook is not so good for those treated with radiotherapy alone. Only 16% of patients were alive at 5 years and only 4% retained their larynx. Analysis of the data shows that radical radiotherapy is not sufficient treatment for large hypopharyngeal tumours, and is associated with unacceptable failure rates and a greatly reduced chance of survival.

However, as previously stated, if radiotherapy is used for small volume disease, it is an excellent form of radical treatment and has the added advantage of sparing the patient a laryngectomy. In the management of early hypopharyngeal cancer with radiotherapy and salvage surgery (Jones, 1992) the 5 year tumour-specific survival rate was 41% in 106 previously untreated patients. Of these, half recurred and were successfully salvaged with surgery.

One of the great difficulties with hypopharyngeal tumours occurs in the patient who has been irradiated and who then develops ulceration of the postcricoid space but the subsequent biopsy is negative. In the authors' experience, virtually all of these patients die if they are not treated and post mortem examination usually shows recurrent tumour. The presence of ulceration in the postcricoid space after radiotherapy should be assumed to represent recurrent disease irrespective of the biopsy findings, and appropriate action should be taken and surgery given careful consideration.

Because the piriform fossa is a distendable space, tumours in this region are almost always large before they produce symptoms. Although the space is poor in sensory nerves, it is rich in lymphatics, so that these tumours are not only large at presentation but also usually associated with significant lymphadenopathy. Therefore, most of these patients do not do well with radiotherapy, and surgery is often advised as the primary form of treatment. In many patients, it is possible to resect the involved part of the pharynx, together with the larynx, and preserve enough pharyngeal mucosa to obtain a primary repair. This is usually possible when two-thirds of the pharyngeal mucosa remains, as long as the patient has not had previous radiotherapy; however, in this case, or if there is extensive mucosal resection, careful consideration should be given to pharyngeal augmentation using either a pedicled or free flap.

However, in approximately one-third of patients where there is extension of the tumour behind the arytenoid cartilages into the mouth of the cervical oesophagus, it is necessary to remove the entire pharynx, which must then be reconstructed, usually with a free jejunal graft. As these tumours do not extend for an appreciable distance down the oesophagus, a stomach transposition is not usually required.

Tumours that arise on the medial wall of the piriform sinus may exhibit limited extension on to the aryoepiglottic fold (the marginal lesion) and also show limited extension to other adjacent sites of the hypopharynx. These are candidates for consideration for a partial laryngopharyngectomy as long as their pulmonary function is satisfactory. These tumours should be carefully assessed, and as long as the primary tumour of the piriform sinus is limited to that site without any extension into the apex of the piriform fossa, conservation surgery can be considered. The tumour may involve the adjacent supraglottic larynx and in some patients may even cause vocal cord fixation. Invasion of the thyroid cartilage is usually considered a contraindication for a partial laryngopharyngectomy and invasion of the postcricoid region is a definite contraindication, as is deep invasion into the musculature of the tongue base. In carefully selected cases, this operation allows conservation surgery and laryngeal preservation for piriform sinus tumours with survival rates similar to those patients undergoing total laryngectomy and partial pharyngectomy (Spector, 1996).

Tumours on the posterior pharyngeal wall can be resected via either a lateral transhyoid or midline suprahyoid pharyngectomy with laryngeal preservation. This operation is only feasible if the larynx is completely uninvolved and if there is no extension of the tumour below the level of the arytenoid cartilage. However, if the larynx is involved, or if the tumour extends laterally into the piriform fossa or inferior to the arytenoid cartilages, this operation cannot be done and a total pharyngolaryngectomy must be performed, followed by some form of visceral repair.

Based on the above, approximately two-thirds of patients with a piriform fossa tumour only require a partial pharyngectomy and total laryngectomy, and some tumours on the posterior pharyngeal wall may be treated by partial pharyngectomy alone. For all other tumours, including those in the postcricoid region, the mainstay of surgical treatment is total pharyngolaryngectomy, which on occasion has to be combined with a total oesophagectomy. Total pharyngolaryngectomy is restricted to the neck and is indicated for those tumours of the piriform fossa which extend into the postcricoid space and those tumours which arise in the neopharyngeal remnant after total laryngectomy carried out for laryngeal carcinoma some years previously. In the past, for postcricoid tumours and for those tumours which arise primarily in

the cervical oesophagus, a total pharyngo-oesophagectomy has been performed. The evidence for this comes from Harrison's paper (1970) suggesting significant submucosal spread (greater than 1 cm) in the majority of cases and also because a small proportion of patients will have synchronous oesophageal tumours lower down. These recommendations were also made when gastric transposition was the only feasible method of one-stage pharyngeal repair.

Modern-day surgery dictates that many of these tumours can be successfully managed as long as 2.5 cm clearance can be achieved beneath the lower limit of the tumour. This means that the smaller (T_1/T_2) postcricoid tumours can be treated by pharyngolaryngectomy and free jejunal transfer, with the larger tumours receiving pharyngolaryngo-oesphagectomy and gastric transposition. In the former case, synchronous oesophageal primary lesions can be excluded by on-table flexible or rigid oesphagoscopy.

Results from large series show that the operative mortality for gastric transposition approaches 20% in some cases, whereas for free jejunal transfer the operative mortality is usually below 5%. For extensive postcricoid tumours of the cervical oesophagus an alternative to total pharyngo-oesophagectomy and gastric transposition is manubrial resection, extended pharyngolaryngectomy with frozen section control and a free jejunal transfer with oesophagojejunal anastomosis down to the level of the aortic arch. This operation in expert hands can achieve results that are better than stomach transposition since the extent of surgery in the chest and abdomen is less.

It used to be said that it was safer to perform a total pharyngolaryngo-oesophagectomy and gastric transposition rather than a pharyngolaryngectomy and free jejunal transfer for patients who suffer a recurrence of a postcricoid tumour following irradiation, for those who have an irradiation-induced tumour or those with tumour perforation, but there is little evidence to support this.

In rare situations, total pharyngolaryngectomy plus or minus oesophagectomy is also required when tumours of the thyroid gland invade the pharynx and upper oesophagus and in this situation reconstruction can be with either gastric transposition or free jejunal transfer, depending on which techniques are available locally.

The long-term results for treating hypopharyngeal tumours are shown in Table 17.6.

Neck dissection

The majority of these patients undergoing surgery will require a neck dissection. In the N$_0$ neck, a selective neck dissection will suffice. For tumours of the posterior pharyngeal wall levels II, III and IV should be dissected, along with the retropharyngeal space. For tumours of the piriform sinus, levels II, III and IV should be dissected. The retropharyngeal space will be accessed, palpated and dissected as part of the surgical resection, as will level VI. For postcricoid tumours levels II, III, IV, and VI should

Table 17.6 Published results for the treatment of hypopharyngeal tumours (disease-free 5 year survival) by staging and primary site

	5 Year disease-free survival (%)
Stage	
I	40–90
II	28–82
III	20–58
IV	15–18
Overall	28–56
Site	
Piriform sinus	31–55
Pharyngeal wall	44
Postcricoid	29
Hypopharynx NOS	37–45

Jones (1992, 1996); Mendelhall *et al.* (1996); Shah (1996); Spector (1996); Czaja and Gluckman (1997).

be dissected. Level VII should be palpated and any suspicious disease dealt with accordingly. Palpable disease requires either a radical, modified radical or extended radical neck dissection. These operations may be performed unilaterally or bilaterally depending on the size and site of the primary tumour, and the extent of the nodal disease.

Techniques and complications of operations on the hypopharynx

Pharyngeal resection

- Endoscopic excision: laser or diathermy
- Partial pharyngectomy
- Partial pharyngectomy and supraglottic laryngectomy
- Total laryngectomy and partial pharyngectomy
- Total pharyngectomy
- Total pharyngolaryngoesophagectomy (see page 343)

Surgery is performed under prophylactic antibiotic cover, which is continued for 48 h. The antibiotics used are either metronidazole and cefuroxime or co-amoxiclav.

Laser or diathermy excision

With this technique, it is possible to resect locally small accessible tumours along with small recurrences. This applies particularly to small, relatively superficial, primary tumours of the posterior pharyngeal wall and limited recurrences. The lesions are excised orally with the use of either diathermy or a laser but it should be stressed that these are highly selected patients in the hands of a small group of enthusiasts and there are few studies with significant long-term results. Access is either peroral (Fig. 17.5) or through a lateral pharyngotomy.

Partial pharyngectomy and total laryngectomy

Mobilization of the pharynx and larynx

The patient is anaesthetized and prepared as described for total laryngectomy in Chapter 14. The larynx and pharynx are mobilized as described using this technique by dissection medial to the sternomastoid muscles and the carotid sheath; the lobe of the thyroid gland with its intrinsic parathyroid glands on a non-involved side should be preserved if at all possible.

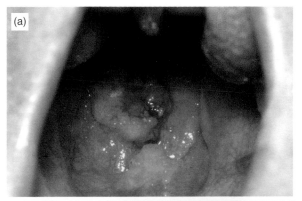

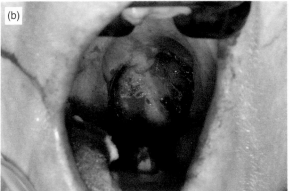

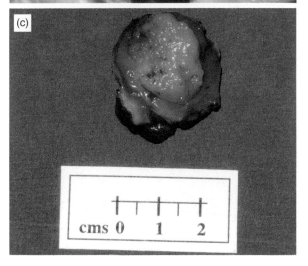

Figure 17.5 (a) Patient with a T_2N_0 squamous cell carcinoma of the posterior pharyngeal wall. (b) The tumour was resected perorally and (c) the excision was complete.

Removal of tumour

The subsequent operation is made much easier if the tracheostome is made before removing the tumour so that the endotracheal tube can be removed; this is done as in a total laryngectomy. To remove the tumour, the pharynx is entered through the vallecula on the contralateral side and the pharyngeal mucosa divided from side to side immediately above the hyoid bone externally, and immediately anterior to the epiglottis internally. At this point, the pre-epiglottic space must not be entered. Care is to taken to have a sufficiently wide margin around the superior edge of the tumour (at least 1–2 cm) and to excise widely into the tongue base as and when necessary. In order to obtain maximum exposure of the tumour, the lateral pharyngeal wall is divided on the non-involved side, carrying the incision down through the opposite piriform

fossa immediately posterior to the superior cornu of the thyroid cartilage; great care is taken at this point to preserve as much pharyngeal mucosa as possible. The larynx is rotated laterally using some form of retractor or hook around the posterior edge of the thyroid lamina so that the tumour in the piriform fossa can now be seen easily. The incision continues round it down the posterior pharyngeal wall with a margin of at least 2 cm of normal pharyngeal mucosa (Fig. 17.6). Externally, the incision is made posterior to the superior cornu of the thyroid cartilage. Finally, the incisions are joined across the anterior oesophageal wall immediately posterior to the arytenoid cartilages (provided this area is not involved by tumour), taking care to preserve the continuity of the oesophageal lumen. The specimen is removed in continuity with the neck dissection as appropriate, by divid-

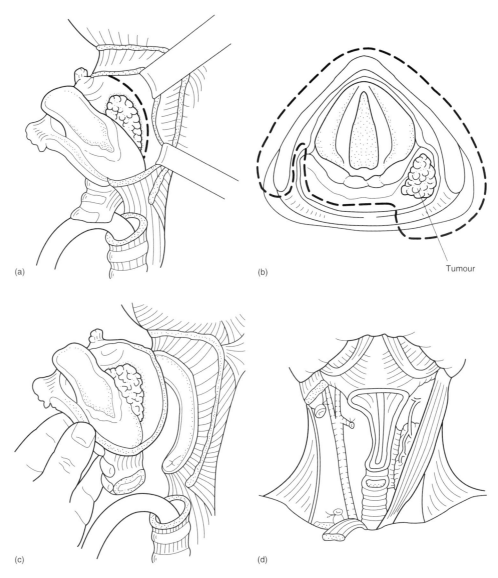

(a) (b) Tumour (c) (d)

Figure 17.6 The extent of pharyngeal resection when performing total laryngectomy and partial pharyngectomy. A right piriform fossa tumour, together with its resection margin is shown in (a) and (b). The laryngectomy and partial pharynectomy specimen has been resected in (c) and the defect which will be closed by primary reconstruction is shown in (d).

ing the few remaining fibres which attach the trachea to the oesophagus.

Repair

A cricopharyngeal myotomy and primary voice restoration are performed at this stage as appropriate. The pharyngeal mucosa is closed as described under the technique for total laryngectomy. Finally, the skin is closed with suction drainage in the conventional way.

Complications

These have been discussed in Chapters 6 and 14, and can be either general or local complications. The latter include stricture formation and recurrence.

Stricture formation is more common after this operation than after total laryngectomy for laryngeal cancer because the pharyngeal remnant is much smaller. It usually results when more than half of the pharyngeal mucosa is removed. In this situation (particularly after radiotherapy), primary augmentation using flap repair should be carried out. This improves both swallowing and voice postoperatively. A common site for a stricture is at the upper end of the pharyngeal repair where it meets the tongue base. This will usually respond to a few dilatations at monthly intervals, but if not, it will require repair later with augmentation using either a pedicled pectoralis major or latissimus dorsi flap, or a free radial forearm flap. Alternatively, excision of the neopharynx may be carried out and repair facilitated with a free jejunal transfer.

Recurrence in the pharynx should be managed as long as it is operable by total pharyngectomy and repair, preferably with a free jejunal transfer. Alternatively, a gastric transposition can be performed following additional oesophagectomy.

Total pharyngolaryngectomy

This operation is indicated for patients with extensive carcinoma of the piriform fossa where primary pharyngeal repair is not possible, for tumours of the piriform fossa or the posterior pharyngeal wall which extend into the mouth of the cervical oesophagus, and for those smaller postcricoid tumours which are not suitable for radiotherapy and where gastric transposition is not required.

Resection

The technique is similar for that of a laryngectomy. The incisions are made and the flaps are elevated. For palpable neck disease a neck dissection is carried out as appropriate and in the presence of the N0 neck, levels II, III and IV are dissected, level VI is dissected and level VII is palpated and dealt with in the appropriate manner. Any neck dissection is usually left attached by a large pedicle involving the superior and inferior laryngeal neurovascular bundles.

The larynx and pharynx are mobilized by dissection medial to the carotid sheath on each side (Fig. 17.7). The superior thyroid artery and vein are divided on each side, as is the inferior thyroid artery on the side of the tumour. By convention, both lobes of the thyroid gland should

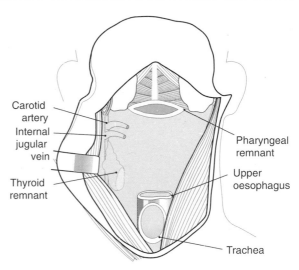

Figure 17.7 Defect following total laryngopharyngectomy.

Labels: Carotid artery; Internal jugular vein; Thyroid remnant; Pharyngeal remnant; Upper oesophagus; Trachea

be removed in continuity for postcricoid tumours, but for piriform fossa tumours it is perfectly acceptable to preserve one lobe of the thyroid gland as described for total laryngectomy. Non-involved parathyroid glands may be preserved with their vascular supply intact or, if not, they may be autotransplanted.

After warning the anaesthetist, the trachea is divided at the level of the fourth ring and a permanent stoma fashioned through which ventilation is continued.

The upper end of the oesophagus is palpated to feel the lower end of the tumour. Three centimetres below this point, vicryl stay-sutures are placed through the oesophageal muscular wall and the oesophagus is divided immediately above them. The specimen is opened and the surgeon checks that clearance is at least 2.5 cm beyond macroscopic evidence of disease. If there is any cause for concern, a frozen section is taken from the upper oesophageal remnant to check that clearance is complete.

The pharynx is divided at its upper end in the conventional manner as described for total laryngectomy and then the incision extended posteriorly to complete circumferential excision. This manoeuvre may be completed either before or after the lower resection is done.

The wound is washed, haemostasis is completed and gowns and gloves are changed.

Repair of the pharynx

As long as a stomach pull-up is not necessary for oncological clearance, the best method currently available to repair the pharynx is a free jejunal transfer. The flap is raised as described in Chapter 7, taking care to identify a long pedicle with plenty of jejunum. The mesenteric vessels are usually anastomosed using the artery end-to-end on to the superior thyroid or facial artery, or alternatively end-to-side on to the external carotid. The vein, which is often flimsy, is anastomosed most conveniently end-to-side to the internal jugular vein. If the internal jugular vein has been sacrificed, then interpositional jump grafts may be necessary to other veins low in the neck such as the stump of

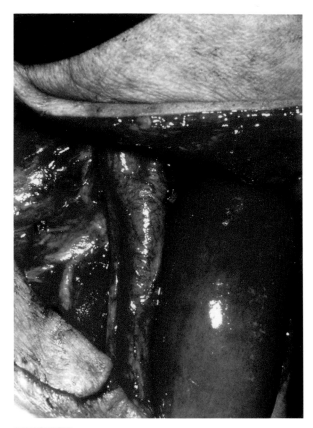

Figure 17.8 Free jejunal transfer in place.

the internal jugular vein or an anterior jugular vein on the other side, but since it is extremely rare for both internal jugular veins to be sacrificed it is usually possible to position the jejunal loop so that access to one internal jugular vein is possible. Once the vascular anastomoses are complete, the jejunal loop is anastomosed above and below to the oropharyngeal and oesophageal stumps using a running 3/0 prolene suture. The loop should be under some tension, since laxity can lead to functional dysphagia (Fig. 17.8). A nasogastric tube is left *in situ* or a feeding jejunostomy is used. Preoperative percutaneous gastrostomy (PEG) should be used with caution in these patients since the stomach may be required for gastric transposition.

Using this reconstructive technique, only about 5–10% of patients develop satisfactory oesophageal speech. The remainder will require some type of electronic vibrator, although early experience shows that some patients do well with secondary surgical voice restoration.

In the rare situation where a partial pharyngectomy and total laryngectomy is planned, but on table a total pharyngolaryngectomy is deemed necessary and one has not planned to do a free jejunal transfer, a number of other techniques are available to establish pharyngeal continuity. Although the pectoralis major flap has been proposed as a means of total pharyngeal reconstruction, in the authors' experience this flap is impossible to tube, invariably stenosis results and its use is not recommended. However, it is possible to tube a pedicled latissimus dorsi

flap in extreme circumstances, particularly in thin individuals with little muscle; alternatively, a large radial forearm flap may be tubed. However, it should be emphasized that both of these techniques are inferior to free jejunal transfer and inevitably lead to some degree of neopharyngeal stenosis.

Complications

Both general and local complications may occur. The latter include fistula and stricture formation, as well as flap necrosis.

Fistulae can occur after this operation, but as a general rule are often small and often close spontaneously.

Stricture formation occurs in at least 30–50% of patients undergoing skin flap repair, but is uncommon following free jejunal transfer. Periodic dilatation may be required but when this becomes required on a frequent basis, it is worthwhile training the patient to dilate the neopharynx and upper oesophagus with a Hurst Mercury bougie, or considering some form of secondary repair to augment the neopharynx.

Between 5 and 10% of free flaps fail as a result of an occlusion of either the arterial or venous anastomosis. The monitoring of free flaps in this setting is difficult and can be done either expectantly, by inspection using the flexible nasopharyngoscope or by bringing a separate segment of vascularized tissue to the surface as an independent monitor. However, this latter technique often leads to an increase in false-positive and false-negative results and an inevitable increase in the re-exploration rate.

In the clinical setting, with regard to the venous obstruction of the jejunal loop in the presence of, the fact that the flap is congested may be detected early since there is rapid sloughing of the jejunal mucosa which then leads to the production of dark blue–brown frothy saliva.

However, most commonly, flap failure is related to arterial occlusion and is detected by established necrosis. This usually presents at between 5 and 7 days but maybe suspected earlier by a fluctuating pyrexia, a rise in the white count and increasing erythema in the Gluck–Sorenson flap. Once necrosis is established, in all but the earliest cases, the jejunum is not salvageable and as long as infection is not established the best way to treat this is by a further free jejunal transfer, which can be carried out up to three times in the same patient.

If the flap is necrosed and there is significant infection present then subsequent management is difficult. If the infection is not too bad, then immediate reconstruction can be performed using either further free jejunal transfer or gastric transposition, but where infection is extensive, the best course of action is to leave the neck widely open, pack it and when it is clean, replace the pharynx by one of the methods described above. The outlook is not good in these cases.

Total pharyngolaryngoesophagectomy and replacement with stomach transposition

The technique consists of resection of the pharynx, larynx and oesophagus; the oesophagus and pharynx are then

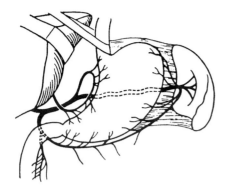

Figure 17.9 Left triangular ligament of liver divided and left lobe retracted to show the abdominal oesophagus.

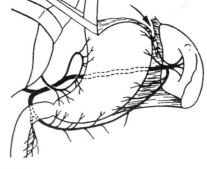

Figure 17.10 Upper end of gastrosplenic omentum is divided as shown.

replaced by the stomach, which is mobilized through an abdominal incision, and is drawn up through the oesophageal bed into the posterior mediastinum and anastomosed to the pharynx.

Anaesthetic and preparation

A general endotracheal anaesthetic is used, as already described. The patient is cleaned and towelled from the chin above to the suprapubic region below.

Neck incision

The operation is usually performed through a Gluck–Sorenson incision with appropriate side-arm extensions to facilitate a neck dissection. If the patient has previously been irradiated, the same incision is usually used. Alternatively, two horizontal incisions may be used with side-arm extensions forming an 'H' to facilitate neck dissection as appropriate and the stoma is brought out through the inferior skin flap. The appropriate neck dissection is performed on one or both sides as indicated, the specimen is left attached at this stage and then the pharynx, larynx and the whole thyroid gland are mobilized in the conventional manner.

Abdominal incision

The stomach and oesophagus are mobilized through a left upper paramedian incision. This reduces the morbidity of the procedure since the chest is not violated and the pharynx and larynx can be mobilized at the same time. A left thoracoabdominal incision is therefore avoided.

A left paramedian incision is made extending well up on to the rib margin and the peritoneal cavity opened. The stomach is most easily mobilized by working from above downwards so that the abdominal oesophagus must first be exposed. To achieve this, the left triangular ligament of the liver is divided to mobilize the left lobe of the liver, and the latter is retracted to the right until the abdominal oesophagus is clearly seen (Fig. 17.9). The abdominal oesophagus is mobilized by blunt dissection and retracted with a tape. This clearly displays the gastrosplenic ligament with the vasa brevia on the left side, and the lesser omentum with the oesophageal branches of the left gastric artery on the right side. The gastrosplenic

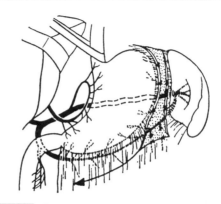

Figure 17.11 Greater omentum is now divided.

ligament (Fig. 17.10) with the vasa brevia is divided and the vessels are tied. The greater omentum is divided away from the stomach, preserving the marginal vessel originating from the right gastroepiploic artery (Fig. 17.11). As the omentum is divided, the omental vessels are stitched on the stomach side to prevent the suture being pulled off as the stomach is later drawn up through the mediastinum. Mobilization is continued down to the first inch of the first part of the duodenum, and the second half of the duodenum mobilized by Kocher's manoeuvre.

The lesser omentum is divided and the left gastric artery divided and transfixed. An anomalous hepatic artery may rise from the left gastric artery and should be detected before dividing the vessels.

A pyloromyotomy is performed by invaginating the pylorus between finger and thumb, rupturing its fibres. This allows adequate drainage of the stomach, but if there is any doubt a formal pyloroplasty should be carried out.

The stomach is now fully mobile. Next the oesophagus is mobilized by passing a hand up through the oesophageal hiatus and dissecting carefully with a finger in the plane next to the oesophageal wall; the fibres of the vagus nerve are ruptured by digital dissection whilst doing this (Fig. 17.12).

At the same time the oesophagus is mobilized from above through the neck incision. The surgeon takes great care whilst doing this, again by keeping strictly next

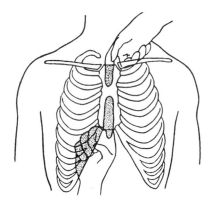

Figure 17.12   Digital mobilization of the entire oesophagus.

to the oesophagus. The posterior wall of the trachea, in particular, must be carefully preserved during this manoeuvre and it is important during this part of the operation to deflate the cuff of the endotracheal tube to avoid stretching, and damaging the posterior tracheal wall.

Once the oesophagus has been mobilized, a long tube drain is introduced into the mediastinum through the hiatus. This is done before the stomach is drawn up into the chest, because it is difficult to place the drain afterwards. This drain is brought out through a stab-wound on the left side of the abdomen. By traction on the pharynx and oesophagus, the stomach is drawn up into the mediastinum to lie in the oesophageal bed, at the same time guiding it from below. The bulk of the stomach acts as a plug to stop any bleeding vessels in the mediastinum, so that there is surprisingly little bleeding at this stage. The abdominal incision is closed in the conventional way in layers with deep tension sutures as appropriate.

The fundus of the stomach will now be lying in the neck. The oesophagus is divided at the oesophageal opening into the stomach and closed. The pharynx, larynx and entire oesophagus are removed and the tracheostomy is sutured at this stage.

After washing the wound and changing gowns and gloves, a separate horizontal incision is made in the fundus of the stomach using cutting diathermy and a two-layered pharyngogastric anastomosis fashioned using an outer layer of interrupted vicryl or silk (2/0) and an inner layer of interrupted vicryl (2/0). The outer posterior layer is sutured first, then the inner posterior layer, next the inner anterior layer and finally the outer anterior layer. The skin incision is closed with suction drainage in the customary fashion. Two prophylactic chest drains are placed and the patient is ventilated overnight on intensive care.

Postoperative care

This includes:

- **general care**
- **radiography**: a chest radiograph is taken immediately after the operation to exclude a pneumothorax
- **feeding**: patients may have an ileus lasting for at least 4 days so that full nasogastric tube feeding cannot be started for 5–6 days. Because of this and because of

their poor general condition, it is sometimes better for the patient to be fed through a feeding jejunostomy sited at the time of the initial surgery. Otherwise, the patient is fed intravenously. Nasogastric tube feeding can be started when bowel sounds return, and once the neck wound is healing satisfactory, feeding by mouth can be started on the seventh day
- **sutures**: neck sutures are removed between 7 and 10 days and stomal sutures between 10 days and 2 weeks. Abdominal sutures are removed between 10 days and 2 weeks
- **drains**: suction drainage on the abdominal drain is continued until it is minimal and then removed, usually after about 5 days. Chest drains can be clamped for 24 hours and removed 24 hours later in the absence of any significant haemopneumothorax. Neck drains are managed conservatively
- **thyroid and parathyroid replacement**: this is discussed in Chapter 6
- **speech therapy**: these patients rarely develop oesophageal speech and should be given the opportunity for secondary voice restoration. The insertion of a valve presents no special difficulty and hypertonicity is never a problem.

Complications

Both general and local complications may occur. The latter include pneumothorax, bleeding, fistula formation and regurgitation.

A chest radiograph should be taken immediately at the end of the operation to detect pneumothorax. As long as chest drains are placed prophylactically significant haemopneumothoraces are prevented. If chest drains have not been placed, and a chest radiograph demonstrates a pneumothorax or haemopneumothorax, then underwater drains should be immediately placed in the pleural cavity.

One would expect that as the oesophagus is mobilized by blind resection (which does not allow bleeding points to be found and tied) excessive bleeding might be encountered following this operation. Surprisingly, this is not the case, presumably because the torn vessels retract and are plugged by the bulk of the stomach lying in the posterior mediastinum. Haematoma formation in the mediastinum should be prevented by the use of a long suction drain passing through the stomach bed and the hiatus into the mediastinum.

Occasionally a small fistula forms which heals spontaneously but, in view of the high vascularity of the stomach, large areas of necrotic breakdown causing significant fistulae are not usually seen with this operation. Strictures do not occur.

Most of these patients swallow well, but a few suffer regurgitation due to minor hold-up at the pylorus. This can be overcome by instructing the patient to eat small meals every 2 h, taking food slowly, and the use of a prokinetic agent such as cisapride may be worth a therapeutic trial. Patients should avoid stooping low if at all possible and elevate the head of the bed by 15 cm at night. Regur-

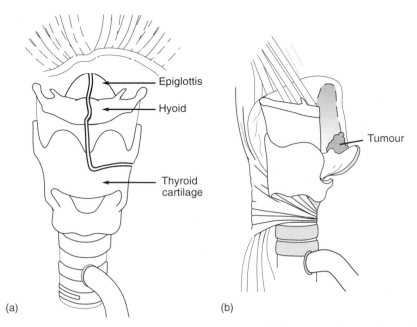

Epiglottis

Hyoid

Thyroid cartilage

Tumour

(a)   (b)

Figure 17.13 Partial pharyngectomy and supraglottic laryngectomy. (a) The extent of the incision; (b) tumour excision.

gitation of acid does not occur because of the vagotomy which, by necessity, is undertaken during dissection of the oesophagus.

Partial pharyngectomy and partial supraglottic laryngectomy

For successful partial pharyngolaryngectomy for piriform fossa or posterior pharyngeal wall squamous carcinoma:

- the primary tumour should be confined to the anatomic site of origin
- the tumour should not extend to the piriform fossa apex
- the ipsilateral hemilarynx should be fully mobile
- there should be no upward extension into the tongue base
- the tumour can involve a supraglottic larynx but there should be no transglottic extension.

Anaesthesia

The patient is intubated under general anaesthesia using an endotracheal tube. The tumour is assessed again endoscopically to confirm its extent and a preliminary tracheostomy performed. The surgical approach is similar to that for a supraglottic partial laryngectomy (see Chapter 14).

Surgical technique

A transverse neck incision is made at the level of the thyrohyoid membrane, just caudal to the hyoid bone and joining the sternomastoid muscles. Upper and lower skin flaps are developed to expose the hyoid bone and the upper half of the thyroid cartilage. The strap muscles are detached from the hyoid bone and retracted laterally and superiorly, the tongue base musculature on the side of the tumour is similarly detached and the hyoid is divided in the midline. Using a reciprocating saw, the upper end

of the thyroid cartilage on the ipsilateral side is divided from the midline up to its posterior margin and approximately 5 mm is resected (Fig. 17.13). Entry is then made into the oropharynx in the midline via the mucosa of the glossoepiglottic. The epiglottis is grasped and divided in its full thickness in the midline from the top down to the infrahyoid portion, which then meets with the cut through the thyroid notch. This permits rotation of the surgical specimen to view the tumour of the piriform sinus, which can then be excised along with half of the supraglottic larynx. Adequate mucosal and soft-tissue margins should approach 1 cm. The bleeding is controlled in the conventional manner and clearance ensured under frozen section control. A larger raw area remains at the lateral pharyngeal wall area where the primary tumour is removed (piriform sinus) and this is allowed to heal by secondary intention. Postoperative feeding is via a nasogastric feeding tube or preoperative PEG, and although no mucosal closure or skin flaps are necessary to provide lining for the lateral pharyngeal wall, pharyngeal closure is completed by reapproximation of the tongue-base musculature to the rest of the remaining ipsilateral half of the hyoid bone and associated strap muscles.

Postoperative complications

The patient is managed as for a supraglottic laryngectomy (Chapter 14).

Lateral pharyngotomy for tumours of the posterior pharyngeal wall

Because of their size and frequent association with enlarged lymph nodes, tumours on the posterior pharyngeal wall do not do well with radiotherapy. In the past this method of treatment was preferred to surgical resec-

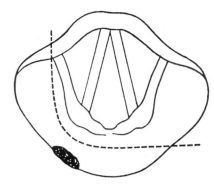

Figure 17.14 Area of resection of tumour on the posterior pharyngeal wall.

tion because the only operation commonly performed was a total pharyngolaryngectomy. However, if a tumour has not extended below the arytenoid cartilage into the cervical oesophagus, or laterally into the piriform fossa, then these tumours can be resected through a lateral pharyngotomy and laryngeal conservation achieved.

For the very occasional tumour of the posterior pharyngeal wall with extension into the piriform fossa or downwards into the oesophagus, a total pharyngolaryngectomy will be required with visceral reconstruction of the pharynx as described previously.

Anaesthesia

The operation is done under general endotracheal anaesthesia and a conventional tracheostomy fashioned. Once in place, the patient is retowelled, excluding the tracheostomy from the operation field.

Incision

The skin incision required will usually necessitate access for some form of neck dissection and because of this a modified Schobinger or 'T' on its side incision is usually sufficient. If a neck dissection is not being done, then the operation can be carried out through a skin crease incision on one side of the neck, extending from the midline to the posterior border of the sternomastoid at the level of superior border of the thyroid cartilage. Nowadays, no modifications are usually necessary to the excision if the patient has had previous radiotherapy, but if the surgeon so wishes the incision may be modified to incorporate such previous treatment.

Neck dissection

A modified radical neck dissection is carried out as appropriate. The specimen is left attached by a pedicle extending from the hyoid bone above to the lower border of the tumour below.

Pharyngotomy

If a neck dissection has not been performed, then access to the larynx and pharynx is achieved by retracting the sternomastoid muscle laterally and dissecting medial to the carotid sheath. Using cutting diathermy, the surgeon divides the muscles attached to the upper border of the hyoid

bone just above its lateral end; the mucosa is divided with scissors and the pharynx entered through the vallecula. This procedure can be facilitated and exposure of the pharynx increased by resecting the ipsilateral half of the hyoid bone. A retractor is inserted through this incision into the pharynx and the epiglottis retracted anteriorly. The incision continues downwards to open up the lateral wall of the pharynx, the incision running immediately posteriorly to the superior cornu of the thyroid cartilage.

Once the lateral pharyngotomy incision has been completed and the epiglottis retracted in a forward direction, the tumour of the posterior wall of the pharynx can be easily seen, inspected and resected (Fig. 17.14). Clearance should be with a 2 cm margin and if possible should be done in continuity with the neck dissection.

Repair

The most satisfactory form of repair of a defect following this excision is to use a revascularized free forearm flap. Otherwise, a split skin graft can be used or defects can be left to heal by secondary intention. This is harvested as described in Chapter 7. The flap may be raised while the excision of the primary tumour is being performed, preferably from the contralateral arm.

At the end of the excision, great care is taken to ensure that the bleeding points on the edge of the pharyngeal mucosa have been dealt with and the skin flap may be introduced, sutured initially into place and the microvascular anastomosis performed under no tension. Once the vascular supply is established, the final suturing in of the flap can take place. The remarks made regarding access to recipient vessels for anastomosis with regard to the jejunal loop similarly apply here.

Post-operative care

This includes:

- routine care
- tracheostomy: remove as soon as possible, usually after about a week
- tube feeding: in order to allow the graft on the posterior pharyngeal wall to take properly, the patient should be fed either via a nasogastric tube or by a PEG and oral feeding not commenced for 2 weeks following surgery.

Complications

Both general and local complications may occur.

Graft failure

If spotted early, the graft may be replaced. However, given its site, early failure may be missed and as a general rule, this is not as catastrophic as might first be thought. The denuded posterior pharyngeal wall following removal of the dead tissue can be left to heal slowly by secondary intention over many weeks.

Transhyoid partial pharyngectomy

Extensive primary squamous cell carcinomas of the posterior pharyngeal wall (with or without extension into the piriform sinus) are best dealt with by pharyngolaryngectomy. Small tumours in the upper part of the posterior pharyngeal wall can be excised transorally, whereas those small tumours in the lower part can be excised via a transhyoid partial pharyngectomy.

This can be performed through a transverse incision made at the level of the hyoid bone to expose the supra-hyoid musculature. This is detached from the superior surface of the hyoid bone using cutting diathermy. An anterior pharyngotomy gains access to the oropharynx and hypopharynx by incision of the vallecula mucosa on one side and through the glossoepiglottic fold to the vallecula on the opposite side. The defect is closed using absorbable sutures placed through the musculature of the base of the tongue and around the hyoid bone. Care should be taken not to damage either the lingual artery or the hypoglossal nerve, both of which are at the lateral aspect of the incision.

What is the best method of pharyngeal replacement?

Recent advances in head and neck reconstructive head and neck surgery to include microvascular free transfer mean that the head and neck surgeon now has a wide variety of techniques available to reconstruct any one defect. There is no one single best way to reconstruct the pharynx and each defect and reconstruction is tailored to the individual patient, the pathology, the size of the defect and the available surgical skills.

Currently, pharyngeal replacement can be assessed by various criteria which include procedure, morbidity and mortality, length of hospital stay and quality of life relating to the patient's swallow.

Pharyngeal replacement is, par excellence, one head and neck reconstructive procedure which, if it goes wrong, can lead to the untimely death of the patient. Various criteria are used for operative mortality. These include: death occurring during the operation, death occurring during the first 24 h; and death within the first week. Most authors, however, do not state the time interval after the procedure that they include in the period of operative mortality.

In a confidential review by the Royal College of Surgeons some years ago, the definition of a surgical death was one that occurred within the first 30 days after the operation. By this criterion, the mortality from gastric transposition is between 10 and 20%, while that for skin flap repair or jejunal transfer is around 5%. Recent studies have shown that both the median length of stay in hospital and the time taken to restore normal swallowing have reduced significantly. The median length of stay in hospital using a deltopectoral flap repair was around 3 months, with the time taken to restore normal swallowing around 8 months. This fell to around 40 days in hospital for a pectoralis-major flap repair and 3 months to restore swallowing. Nowadays, a reasonable figure for a hospital stay for gastric transposition would be about 21 days and about 14–21 days for free jejunal transfer and, with both operations, time taken to restore normal swallowing is about 2–3 weeks (Shah, 1996).

As regards the quality of the swallow, gastric transposition gives a near-normal swallow and in the majority

Table 17.7 Postoperative enteral feeding protocol (Queen Elizabeth Hospital, Birmingham, UK)

Feeding day 1	Commence full-strength standard polymeric feed (Nutrison) at 50 ml/h and increase the rate 6 hourly (e.g. in 25 ml increments) as tolerated up to 100 ml/h. Feed over 20 h (additional i.v. fluid is usually required)
Day 2	Adjust the feed rate to meet fluid and nutritional requirements as recommended by the dietician (based on the Schofield Equation, 1985)
Day 3	When full feed rate is achieved monitor nutritional status by regular checks on: fluid balance (daily) bowel habits (daily) serum biochemistry (twice weekly) U&E, LFT, glucose (twice weekly) weight (twice weekly)

Feed composition and/or volume is then altered as appropriate. If using specialized or hyperosmolar feeds then the regimen may be different. U&E: urea and electrolytes; LFT: liver function test.

of free jejunal transfers, the swallow is equally as good. However, in a small proportion of patients, dilatation is required and in a few others, if the loop is too long, functional dysphagia can result.

Given the above criteria, all things being equal, and as long as local expertise dictates, the best form of pharyngeal reconstruction at present would appear to be free jejunal transfer, but if pathology or expertise dictates that gastric transposition is necessary, this is an acceptable alternative.

A recent study of British otolaryngologists provided a good indication regarding current UK practice of reconstruction following resection for hypopharyngeal carcinoma. It appears that the stomach pull-up remains the most commonly used method of reconstruction, but the jejunal free flap is becoming increasingly popular because of its lower morbidity and mortality (Ayshford et al., 1999).

Nutritional factors

The average weight loss of a patient presenting with a hypopharyngeal cancer is 10 kg. In response to weight loss, the normal person mobilizes peripheral protein to the liver. Tumours alter normal metabolic responses and it is possible that the lean body mass is preserved by insulin.

Each patient should be examined and assessed on their merits, and a consultation should take place between medical and nursing staff and a dietician. In those patients who are nutritionally depleted (more than 10% loss of body weight) and where time dictates, preoperative total parental nutrition may be given 5–7 days before surgery. Otherwise, enteral feeding may commence after the resumption of bowel sounds following surgery. The mode of access is either via a nasogastric tube or by feeding jejunostomy. Preoperative PEG are not usually utilized since the stomach is violated and may be required for gastric transposition. Detailed various enteral feeds are available and vary from institution to institution (Table 17.7). Patients are started on water and then either osmolar enteral feeds and then full-strength feeds if started before recommencing oral intake. Exact details of other regimes are available in the literature (Morton and McIvor, 1997).

Radiotherapy techniques

Piriform fossa carcinoma

A beam-directing shell, similar to that used for patients with supraglottic carcinoma, is prepared with the patient lying supine and the neck straight.

Localized disease

In the rather unusual case of T_1 or T_2N_0 disease, a single-phase technique using relatively small parallel opposed wedged fields is possible. The fields extend from the level of the second cervical vertebra down to 1 cm or so below the cricoid cartilage. Anteriorly they cover the skin of the neck and their posterior limit lies over the vertebral bodies, great care being taken to ensure that the spinal cord is not included. The upper anterior corners of these fields are blocked to shield the submandibular gland and oral cavity. The treatment volume is therefore slightly larger than that required for supraglottic tumours. By including the entire larynx and laryngopharynx, the upper deep cervical nodes at the angle of the jaw and the upper oesophagus, both the primary tumour and possible areas of occult extension are covered. Check films are taken on the treatment machine or portal imaging is used to verify the accuracy of set-up and field placement. Treatment is with 4–6 MV X-rays; a dose of 55 Gy in 20 daily fractions or its equivalent is prescribed.

Advanced disease

In the more common case of locally advanced tumours and where there is lymph-node involvement, a two-phase technique is preferred. Essentially the same technique is used whether the patient is receiving primary radical radiotherapy or postoperative treatment. Even if only unilateral nodal disease is palpable, it is wise to treat both sides of the neck because of the high incidence of occult bilateral nodal metastasis.

The shell for the first phase holds the patient with the neck straight. The position of any palpable nodes is marked with wire on the shell. Initially large parallel opposed lateral fields are used to treat the whole of the upper part of the neck above the shoulders. This volume includes both the primary tumour and nodes in the upper neck. The upper anterior corner of the field may be shielded to spare part of the oral cavity and some salivary gland tissue. The lower neck is treated by a direct anterior field. The upper border of this anterior field is matched on to the lower border of the lateral fields. If possible, the fields

should not be junctioned through palpable nodal disease. The lower border of the anterior field extends down to the suprasternal notch and the area below the clavicles is shielded on both sides to spare the lung apices. Laterally, the field extends to cover the nodes in the supraclavicular fossae. Midline shielding is used to reduce the dose to the spinal cord and to spare the trachea only if one can be absolutely certain that it will not shield the tumour. Simulation is used to ensure that all nodal disease, as indicated by the wire markers, is included in the target volume. The dose that may safely be given to such a large field is limited by the tolerance of the spinal cord. A dose of 40 Gy in 20 fractions over 4 weeks is within safe limits.

The second phase follows immediately after the first phase has finished. The posterior border of the lateral fields is brought forward to lie through the middle of the vertebral bodies, anterior to the cord. The nodes in the posterior part of the neck overlying the cord are treated by electron strips matched on to the posterior margin of the lateral fields. An appropriate electron energy is selected to ensure adequate treatment of nodes while sparing the underlying cord. Treatment of the lower neck continues with an anterior field as before. If in phase I the junction between the lateral and anterior fields lay unavoidably through bulky nodal disease, it is wise to move the level of the junction for phase II.

For primary radical radiotherapy, a further 26 Gy in 13 fractions over 2.5 weeks is given to the primary tumour and palpable nodes. This takes the maximum tumour dose to 66 Gy in 33 fractions over 6.5 weeks. At the end of phase II, a further small volume boost using electrons may be given to any residual palpable nodes, to bring the total dose to 70 Gy in 35 fractions over 7 weeks. Any nodal areas which were clinically uninvolved at the start of treatment should receive a phase II dose of 10 Gy over five fractions, bringing the total dose to areas treated prophylactically to 50 Gy in 25 fractions. Careful planning ensures that the total dose to the cord throughout the whole treatment does not exceed 44 Gy.

The principal acute adverse effect of this treatment is mucositis, and feeding via a gastrostomy is usually necessary to ensure adequate nutrition. The pain of the reaction should be treated adequately, using morphine if necessary. Smoking exacerbates the mucosal reaction and so, for this reason as well as others, should be discouraged. One should resist the temptation to allow a break in treatment to allow the acute reaction to settle, as this significantly compromises the already slim chances of cure. If unplanned gaps in treatment occur, these should be compensated for by giving two fractions per day with a minimum interfraction interval of 6 h to keep the overall treatment time as originally intended.

Postcricoid carcinoma

Accurate delineation of disease extent is necessary for the radical radiotherapy of all head and neck cancers, and postcricoid carcinoma is no exception. Of particular importance here is the lower limit. The treatment volume encompasses the primary tumour and extends 3 cm below this point to cover any occult submucosal spread. The lower cervical nodes are also included, but because of the large area that would need to be covered, no attempt is made to treat prophylactically all possible areas of lymphatic spread. Several field arrangements may be used to irradiate this volume satisfactorily. The choice depends on the length of the tumour and the build of the patient. In a thinner patient with a long neck or short tumour, two lateral fields extending from the level of the hyoid bone to 3 cm beyond the macroscopic limits of the tumour are used. These are angled downwards to avoid the shoulders and ensure adequate coverage of the lower part of the volume. In squatter patients or if the tumour is more extensive, a third field may be added anteriorly, using a similar arrangement to that recommended for subglottic tumours. Alternatively, a pair of appropriately wedged anterior oblique fields may be used. The prescribed dose with any of these arrangements is as described for supraglottic carcinoma.

Carcinoma of the posterior pharyngeal wall

As is the case for postcricoid carcinoma, the patient is treated lying supine, with the neck fixed in a shell with the spine straight. The treatment volume for carcinoma of the posterior pharyngeal wall includes the primary tumour with a margin of 2–3 cm and the first echelon of nodes in the deep cervical chain. Usually a parallel pair of lateral fields is adequate, but sometimes they may need to be angled inferiorly, as described for postcricoid carcinoma. Again, no attempt is made to treat the whole neck. The dose fractionation schedule is selected as for supraglottic carcinoma.

Postoperative radiotherapy

It has been indicated that the preferred treatment for many patients with carcinoma of the hypopharynx is with primary surgery. For the majority of patients, adjuvant radiotherapy is appropriate. It has been shown that postoperative irradiation results in significantly better local control than preoperative radiotherapy. Whether this is translated into better survival is not clear, but improved local control is a worthwhile achievement on its own. In addition, there are fewer surgical complications in patients receiving postoperative irradiation. Probably all but those exceptionally few patients who have undergone surgery for a T_1N_0 carcinoma, for whom the chances of cure by surgery alone are excellent, should receive postoperative radiotherapy. The usual technique treats the primary site and areas of likely nodal spread in the manner described above for piriform fossa cancer. If excision has been complete, then a dose of 60 Gy in 30 fractions over 6 weeks should be adequate to the tumour bed and involved nodal areas. If the pathology report indicates that the margin was involved in any area, then 66 Gy should be used. For clinically uninvolved nodal areas requiring prophylactic treatment, a dose of 50 Gy in 25 fractions is enough.

References and further reading

Ayshford C. A., Walsh R. M. and Watkinson J. C. Reconstructive techniques currently used following resection for hypopharyngeal carcinoma, *J Laryngol Otol* 113: 145–8

Axon P. R., Woolford T.J., Hargreaves S. P., Yates P., Birzgalis A. R. and Farrington W. T. (1997) A comparison of surgery and radiotherapy in the management of postcricoid carcinoma, *Clin Otolaryngol* 22: 370–4.

Czaja J. M. and Gluckman J. L. (1997) Surgical management of early-stage hypopharyngeal carcinoma, *Am Otol Rhinol Laryngol* 106: 907–13.

Elias M. M., Hilgers F. J., Keus R. B., Gregor R. T., Hart A. A. and Balm A. J. (1995) Carcinoma of the pyriform sinus: a retrospective analysis of treatment results over a 20 year period, *Clin Otolaryngol Appl Sci* 20: 249–53.

Fenton J. E., Hone S., Gormley P., O'Dwyer T. P., McShane D. P. and Timon C. I. (1995) Hypopharynx tumours may be missed on flexible oesophagogastroscopy (Lesson of the week), *BMJ* 311: 623–4.

Garden A. S., Morrison W. H., Clayman G. L., Ang K. K. and Peters L. J. (1996) Early squamous cell carcinoma of the hypopharynx: outcomes of treatment with radiation alone to the primary disease, *Head Neck* 18: 317–22.

Hoe C. N., Lamb K. H., Ng W. F. and Wei W. I. (1996) Pathological basis for hypopharyngeal cancer, in *Proceedings of the IVth International Conference on Head and Neck Cancer*, The Society of Head and Neck Surgeons, Arlington, VA and The American Society of Head and Neck Surgery, Pittsburgh, PA, pp. 149–55.

Jones A. S. (1992) The management of early hypopharyngeal cancer: primary radiotherapy and salvage surgery, *Clin Otolaryngol* 17: 545–9.

Jones A. S. (1998) Tumours of the hypopharynx, in *Diseases of the Head and Neck, Nose and Throat* (A. S. Jones, D. E. Philips and F. J. M. Hilgers eds), Arnold, London, Chap. 15, pp. 230–49.

Jones A. S., Roland N. J., Husband, D. and Gati I. (1996) Free vascularised jejunal loop repair following total pharyngectomy for carcinoma of the hypopharynx. A report of 90 cases. *Br J Surg* 83: 1279–3.

Lefebvre J. L. (1996) Cancer of the hypopharynx: strategies for larynx preservation, in *Proceedings of the IVth International Conference on Head and Neck Cancer*, The Society of Head and Neck Surgeons, Arlington, VA and The American Society of Head and Neck Surgery, Pittsburgh, PA, pp. 170–4.

Lefebvre J. L., Chevalier D., Luboinski B., Kirkpatrick A., Collette L. and Sahmoud T. (1996) Larynx preservation in pyriform sinus cancer: preliminary results of a European Organisation for Research and Treatment of Cancer Phase III trial, *J Nat Cancer Inst* 88: 890–9.

Mendenhall W. N., Parsons J. T., Stringer S. P. and Cassisi N. J. (1996) Radiotherapy in the treatment of squamous cell carcinoma of the hypopharynx and cervical oesophagus, in *Proceedings of the IVth International Conference on Head and Neck Cancer*, The Society of Head and Neck Surgeons, Arlington, VA and The American Society of Head and Neck Surgery, Pittsburgh, PA, pp. 175–80.

Morton R. P. and McIvor N. P. (1997) Tumours of the hypopharynx, in *Scott-Brown's Otolaryngology*, 6th edn, Vol. 5, *Laryngology and Head and Neck Surgery* (J. Hibbert, ed.), Butterworth-Heinemann, London, Chap. 15, pp. 1–17.

Okamoto M., Takahashi H., Yao K., Inagi K., Nakayama M. and Makoshi T. (1996) Combined therapy for hypopharyngeal cancer, *Acta Otolaryngologica – Suppl* **524**: 83–7.

Razack M. S., Sako K. and Kalnins I. (1978) Squamous carcinoma of the pyriform sinus, *Head and Neck Surg* **1**: 31–4.

Sabroe S. (1998) Alcohol and cancer (Editorial), *BMJ* **317**: 827.

Shah J. (1996) Hypopharynx and cervical oesophagus, in *Head and Neck Surgery*, 2nd edn, Mosby-Wolfe, London, Chap. 7, pp. 235–65.

Spector G. J. *et al.* (1994) Pyriform sinus carcinomas in *Laryngeal Cancer* (R. Smee and G. P. Bridger, eds), Excerpta Medica, Amsterdam, pp. 602–5.

Spector J. G. (1996) Conservation surgery for laryngeal cancer: an overview, in *Proceedings of the IVth International Conference on Head and Neck Cancer*, The Society of Head and Neck Surgeons, Arlington, VA and The American Society of Head and Neck Surgery, Pittsburgh, PA, pp. 316–25.

Stell P. M. (1984) Replacement of the pharynx after pharyngolaryngectomy, *Ann R Coll Surg Engl* **66**: 388–90.

Stell P. M. (1988) The present status of surgery in the treatment of carcinoma of the hypopharynx and cervical oesophagus, *Adv Otorhinolaryngol* **39**: 120–34.

Stell P. M. and Swift A. C. (1987) Tumours of the hypopharynx, in *Scott-Brown's Otolaryngology*, 5th edn, Vol. 5, *Laryngology* (A. G. Kerr and P. M. Stell, eds), Butterworths, London, pp. 250–63.

UICC (International Union Against Cancer) (1992) *TNM Classification of Malignant Tumours*, 4th edn, 2nd rev. (P. Hermineck and L. H. Sobin, eds), Springer, Berlin.

UICC (International Union against Cancer) (1997) *TNM Classification of Malignant Tumours* (L. H. Sobin and C. H. Wittekind, eds), 5th edn, Wiley-Liss, New York.

Vries E. J. de, Stein D. W., Johnson J. T., Wagner R. L., Schusterman M. A., Myers E. N. *et al.* (1989) Hypopharyngeal reconstruction: a comparison of two alternatives, *Laryngoscope* **99**: 614–17.

Willatt D. J., Jackson S. R., McCormick M. S., Lubsen H., Michaels L. and Stell P. M. (1987) Vocal cord paralysis and tumour length in staging postcricoid cancer, *Eur J Surg Oncol* **13**: 131–7.

Zelefsky M. J., Kraus D. H., Pfister D. G., Raben A., Shah J. P., Strong E.W. *et al.* (1996) Combined chemotherapy and radiotherapy versus surgery and postoperative radiotherapy for advanced hypopharyngeal cancer, *Head Neck* **18**: 405–11.

18 Rehabilitation of speech and swallowing

'Speech created thought, which is the measure of the universe'
Percy Shelley, 1820

Introduction

The process of rehabilitation of function begins with counselling before the patient undergoes treatment. Some patients are left with chronic problems and long-term rehabilitation. In contrast, others having a course of primary radiotherapy for an early lesion may find that this rehabilitation is complete in a functional sense if not a psychological sense, almost as soon as therapy is terminated. Rehabilitation is a team enterprise, requiring not only a dietitian, but also a speech and language therapist with a particular interest in swallowing problems and a therapist with a particular interest in dysphonia rehabilitation and surgical voice restoration. Some form of liaison worker who can carry therapy over into the community is also vital where hospital in-patient stays are short.

Surgical voice restoration after laryngectomy

Surgical voice restoration following total laryngectomy remains one of the most conspicuous of therapeutic challenges. Understandably, depriving a patient of their ability to communicate verbally is considered the greatest of the difficulties which can confront a head and neck cancer patient. Nowadays, not only do most units encourage preoperative visits to the laryngectomee by the speech and language therapist, but usually a contact is made with a fellow patient who has already undergone the procedure. Such visits can be supplemented by booklets produced for example, in the UK, by the National Association of Laryngectomy Clubs, or by the International Association of Laryngectomies (IAL).

> ### Surgical voice restoration after laryngectomy
> - Oesophageal speech
> - Primary tracheo-oesophageal puncture
> - Secondary puncture
> - Other aids to communication

Oesophageal speech

The earliest form of speech rehabilitation was oesophageal speech, which is produced by compressing air into the oesophagus and then releasing the air, causing the pharyngo-oesophageal segment to vibrate which then produces the oesophageal tone used for speech. A pharyngo-oesophageal segment replaces the larynx as the generator of a vibrating column of air upon which the articulators and resonators in the oral cavity, nose and sinuses superimpose the individual's voice quality. A number of different methods may be used to encourage the patient to be able to inject air rapidly into the oesophagus and to expel it in a controlled manner, thus producing fluid speech. The most efficient method for teaching oesophageal speech is the consonant injection method. This injects air into the oesophagus during speech rather than just during periods of rest or breaks between phrases. The typical consonants which allow for compression and insufflation of the oesophagus with this method include plosive consonants: /pa/, /ka/, etc. In the glossopharyngeal press method, the patient pumps the tongue by moving the posterior tongue against the hard palate until it approximates the pharyngeal wall.

Finally, the inhalation method can also be used to supplement oesophageal air on the principle that the air will enter the oesophagus when the pharyngo-oesophageal segment is relaxed during pulmonary inhalation. Acquisition of oesophageal speech is therefore quite a complex and rehabilitation-intensive procedure and it is not surprising that only around 50% of laryngectomees are able to develop an adequate oesophageal voice. Older patients and women appeared to have particular difficulties with the technique.

> ### Advantages of tracheo-oesophageal valves
> - Increased intelligibility
> - Increased fluency
> - Easier to acquire
> - Enhanced intensity
> - Improved fundamental frequency

Primary tracheo-oesophageal puncture

The tracheo-oesophageal puncture method was introduced by Singer and Blom in 1980 and is currently the surgical method of choice for voice restoration. At laryngectomy, a small fistula is created between the posterior tracheal wall and the oesophagus, prior to the pharyngeal repair. A heavy curved artery forcep can be inserted into the oesophageal lumen and used to indent the posterior tracheal wall, and an assistant can then cut down on to the artery forceps. A stomogastric tube is fed through this fistula which can be used for feeding purposes until the wounds are healed. At this point, or a week or two thereafter, a small silicone valve prosthesis is inserted.

This prosthesis allows the diversion of pulmonary air from the trachea (Fig. 18.1). The vibrating pharyngo-oesophageal segment thus generated is lung powered rather than powered by small volumes of insufflated air. This is one of the principal reasons for the superior qual-ity of tracheo-oesophageal speech over oesophageal speech for the majority of users. Most patients acquire speech very rapidly following the fitment of the valve.

Contraindications for tracheo-oesophageal puncture

- Inability to care for the stoma
- Poor manual dexterity
- Stenotic stoma
- Poor eyesight
- Oesophageal stenosis
- Poor motivation

Secondary puncture

In cases where patients have not had a primary oesophageal puncture, a secondary procedure can be carried out using a specially designed endoscope. A puncture technique was initially introduced as a secondary method of

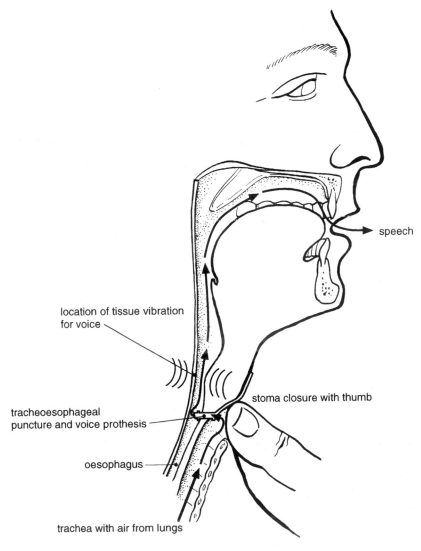

speech

location of tissue vibration for voice

stoma closure with thumb

tracheoesophageal puncture and voice prothesis

oesophagus

trachea with air from lungs

Figure 18.1   Lung-powered speech for tracheo-oesophageal valve phonation.

voice restoration, although the majority of surgeons now using the technique employ it as a primary method. The principal complication of tracheo-oesophageal puncture is one of leakage. Around 10% of patients have problems with this, which can sometimes circumvented by the insertion of a larger valve.

Choice of valves

The original Blom Singer valve was a hand-made prosthesis with a slit in its tip forming a one-way duckbill valve with an outer retention collar. The first commercially available Blom Singer valve was a 16 FG duckbill device which was followed by a prosthesis of similar diameter with a bevelled tip incorporating an internal one-way hinged flap valve (Fig. 18.2).

A 20 FG diameter counterpart has now been produced (Fig.18.2b, c). The latest development is an extended wear indwelling device which incorporates larger tracheal and oesophageal retention collars. This eliminates the need to teach the patient to change the prosthesis, which can be instead replaced intermittently in the clinic. The tracheo-oesophageal puncture requires preliminary dilation to a size 22 FG prior to insertion of the indwelling valve.

With the indwelling device there is no strap, so that there is an improved tracheo-oesophageal valve to neck seal and a reduction in skin irritation. It is available in

lengths ranging from 1.4 to 3.3 cm and replaced at 6 monthly intervals or earlier if needed. It is cleaned *in situ*, for example by tweezers, to take off any dried mucus on the tracheal surface and a pipette is used to flush particles into the oesophageal lumen. Valve failure is indicated by leakage of air through the valve. A recent development is the use of a tracheostoma valve, which eliminates the need manually to close off the tracheostoma with a finger during speech.

The Provox company has now produced a low-resistance indwelling voice prosthesis system. It contains a one-way hinged valve moulded in one piece with the prosthesis to form an integral part of the device (Fig. 18.2d) and is available in three lengths, 6, 8 and 10 mm. The original Provox device had to be inserted transorally. The acceptability of the Provox system was greatly enhanced by the newer system, which allows its replacement directly through the stoma.

Prevention of fungal infection

Patients prefer to have an indwelling valve which they do not have to change every 3 or 4 days. These indwelling valves also take some of the pressure off the valve-support service in the hospital out-patient department as increasing numbers of laryngectomees opt to use a tracheo-oesophageal prosthesis.

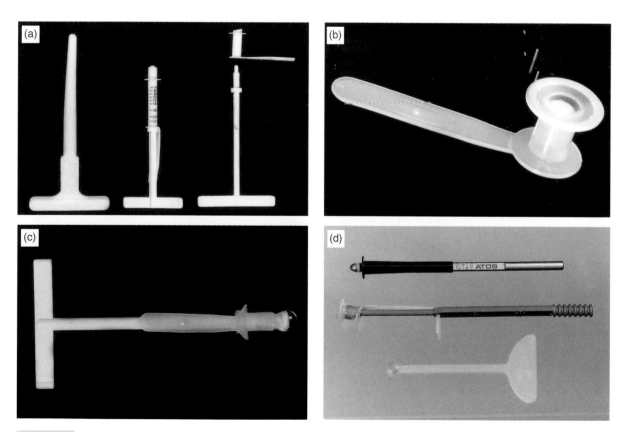

Figure 18.2 Selection of tracheo-oesophageal puncture valves: (a) conventional Blom Singer valve with dilator, sizer and introducer; (b) indwelling Blom Singer valve; (c) indwelling Blom Singer valve mounted on introducer, with a gelcap inserter; (d) Provox indwelling valve mounted on introducer, sizer and occlusive cap for use in the event of leakage.

One regularly encountered problem is however, *Candida* colonization of the indwelling valve. Fungal infection damages the prosthesis, and causes incomplete closure and a leakage through the prosthesis resulting in a shortened lifespan. Only a minority of subjects will never encounter this problem which can usually be prevented by a twice-daily protocol of Nystatin oral suspensions swilled around the mouth for a minimum of 3–4 min and either swallowed or expectorated. The patient is instructed to set a timer to ensure adequate contact time with the oral mucosa. An alternative is one 10 mg lozenge of Amphotericin dissolved slowly in the mouth four times daily. Some patients also benefit from soaking their dentures daily in 3% hydrogen peroxide to eliminate denture yeast. An alternative to regular Nystatin suspension is the use of a buccal bioadhesive slow-release tablet containing miconazole nitrate (Weissenbruch *et al.*, 1997).

Prevention of pharyngeal spasm

At an early stage in the development of tracheo-oesphageal speech methods, it became apparent that a number of patients failed to achieve good voice because of oesophageal distention and secondary spasm of the pharyngeal constrictor muscles. There are two methods for reducing pharyngeal segment hypertonicity. One is to perform a cricopharyngeal myotomy at the time of surgery, but this carries at least a theoretical risk of mucosal dehiscence and fistula formation. An alternative is therefore to identify the pharyngeal plexus by direct electric stimulation and to perform a peripheral denervation. The neurectomy preserves the blood supply to the pharyngeal wall and may enhance the quality of phonation due to residual elastic tone, with resulting increased fundamental frequency.

Heat moisture exchangers

The use of an external heat moisture exchanger (HME) reduces the amount of cough and sputum. The exchanger is a disposable filter cassette containing HME foam and may include a speech valve with a spring for airtight digital closure of the stoma (Balle *et al.*, 1997). The latter eases occlusion of the stoma from phonation. Modern adhesives such as colloid allow the external units to be applied within 1–2 months of surgery and changed without the former problems of skin pain and irritation.

The Kapitex Trachi-Naze system not only acts as a source of moist warmth but, by increasing functional airway resistance, also improves oxygenation.

Voice outcome of tracheo-oesophageal puncture

Some of the enthusiasts for tracheo-oesophageal puncture claim massively high success rates for tracheo-oesophageal speech. It is fair to say that as indwelling valves become more available, the rates of success for long-term phonation using tracheo-oesophageal prosthesis are gradually likely to increase. However, at present a figure of around 70% of patients achieving functional spoken communi-

cation seems realistic. The predictors of voice outcome seem to be as follows.

- **Prelaryngectomy communication status**: the evidence suggests that a patient with a major pre-existing communication disorder is most unlikely to achieve any postlaryngectomy oral communication, as might be predicted.
- **Age** seems to be a very substantial predictor of outcome, with the younger patients more likely to acquire good communication skills postoperatively.
- **Acute local complications** in some series occur in almost 50% of subjects. The occurrence of such a complication is an adverse prognostic factor for the long-term acquisition of good tracheo-oesophageal puncture speech.

Swimming for laryngectomy patients

The first demonstration of postlaryngectomy swimming took place at Lake Geneva in 1974. The device shown then, the Larkel breathing device, remains popular (Nigam and Samuel, 1997). It provides the option of either breathing through a snorkel or attaching the stoma via tubing to a mouthpiece; however, the latter requires nasal respiration, to which many subjects have become unaccustomed. The cuffed tracheal tube end may be inserted without removal of the speaking valve.

Other aids to communication

Cervical vibrators

Until recently, the artificial larynx was considered to be the method of choice only for patients who were unable to learn oesophageal speech. However, the use of an artificial larynx such as a transcervical (Servox) vibrator includes immediate and relatively intelligible speech, even when hospitalized. It is easy to imagine that from a patient's point of view, not having to write down every single thought or difficulty experienced when in hospital has a huge advantage. The former concern that this temporary use of an artificial larynx would somehow deter a patient from making the effort to acquire oesophageal speech probably never had any basis in reality, and has now been rendered obsolete by the development of tracheo-oesophageal prostheses which have a very short learning curve. The use of an artificial larynx gives a higher intensity voice than oesophageal speech, and this can also be useful at times for high noise environments. It is a useful fallback for patients who experience an acute problem with a valve.

Lip-reading classes

Otolaryngologists can be reluctant to recommend lip-reading classes for the relatives of the patients on whom they have performed total laryngectomy because this course of action appears like an admission of failure from the perspective of voice rehabilitation.

It must be remembered, however, that many of the patients undergoing total laryngectomy are fairly elderly and that their partners and relatives may have a degree of hearing impairment, which makes it difficult for them to pick up the sounds emanating from the tracheo-oesophageal fistula, artificial larynx, etc. Particularly during the early phases of rehabilitation, attendance at a lip-reading class by the relatives of these patients can be beneficial.

Effect of radiotherapy on voice quality

It is generally accepted that compared with the impact of surgical treatment for laryngeal cancer, radiotherapy results in significantly superior voice quality. The advent of objective methods of acoustic analysis has allowed the impact of radiotherapy on voice quality to be quantified objectively. Because of the dysphonia which precedes treatment for laryngeal cancer, radiotherapy produces a significant improvement in features such as intelligibility and sound perturbation. Studies also suggest that those with non-laryngeal tumours do not have a recordable change in measured voice parameters such as fundamental frequency, perturbation or intelligibility following irradiation.

Vocal-cord paralysis

Surgical anatomy

Phonation is initiated by area 4 in the Sylvian fissure of the cerebrum. Fibres pass down the internal capsule and, in the lower pons, some fibres decussate to the opposite side before entering the medulla, terminating in the nucleus ambiguus. The vagal nuclei are thus bilaterally innervated. The peripheral vagal trunk forms from roots emerging from the lower pons and upper medulla. It passes through the jugular foramen beside the jugular vein, posterior to the ninth cranial nerve and anterior to the 11th cranial nerve. High in the neck, the vagus produces the superior laryngeal nerve that is motor to the cricothyroid muscle and sensory to the laryngeal mucosa above the vocal cords. The vagus nerve then passes through the neck in the carotid sheath between the carotid artery and the jugular vein, and enters the chest where it gives off the recurrent laryngeal nerves.

The recurrent laryngeal nerves are motor to all of the intrinsic laryngeal muscles and sensory to the mucosa below the level of the vocal cords. On the left side, the recurrent laryngeal nerve passes anteriorly, under and then behind the aorta, beside the ligamentum arteriosum. It then passes in the tracheo-oesophageal groove and enters the larynx near the cricothyroid joint. The right recurrent laryngeal nerve passes into the chest anterior to the subclavian artery, loops around it and returns to the neck in the tracheo-oesophageal groove. Ortner's syndrome is said to be due to cardiomegaly pressing on the recurrent laryngeal nerve, thus causing paralysis. In order to do this, the left atrium would have to rise to the level of the arch of the aorta and thus pass completely behind the pulmonary arteries. While not impossible, it cannot be a very frequent occurrence.

Relations of the left recurrent laryngeal nerve
- Aortic arch
- Oesophagus
- Left mainstem bronchus
- Mediastinal lymph nodes
- Left atrium

Relations of the right recurrent laryngeal nerve
- Right subclavian artery
- Apex of the right upper lobe of the lung
- Supraclavicular lymph nodes

The glottis consists of approximately 60% membranous vocal cord, and 40% vocal process and medial border of the arytenoid body, i.e. there is a mobile soft portion and a hard cartilaginous portion. These behave in different ways when the recurrent laryngeal nerve is paralysed, and therefore subsequently rehabilitate in different ways.

Pathophysiology of vocal-cord paralysis

Vocal-cord paralysis may be unilateral or bilateral, abductor or adductor. The latter terminology relates to the movement that the cord cannot make when paralysed. The cord is often described as being either in the median position, or in the lateral or cadaveric position. It is impossible to record accurately the position of a paralysed vocal cord and no theory fully explains its position.

Semon's theory proposes that the abductor fibres are more susceptible to pressure than adductor fibres. Thus, a postcervical surgery haematoma provokes abductor paralysis and an adducted cord, whereas a fully transected recurrent laryngeal nerve paralyses the adductors as well, leaving the cord abducted. Semon's theory is difficult to refute and impossible to prove.

The theory put forward by Wagner and Grossman implies that the superior laryngeal nerve has an adductive effect through the cricothyroid muscle. This means that if there is a low lesion of the recurrent laryngeal nerve, the cricothyroid muscle will keep the cord in the midposition, whereas if the vagus is paralysed high in the neck then the adductive effect will be lost and the cord will be in the cadaveric position. This theory is clearly wrong: nearly every patient with vocal-cord paralysis secondary to lung cancer has an abducted vocal cord and a breathy voice. Modern thinking suggests that the final position of the vocal cord is not static and results from a number of forces such as the degree of muscle atrophy, the degree of re-innervation and the extent of synkinesis (mass movement).

Consequences of vocal-cord paralysis

The effect of a vocal-cord paralysis is dual. If the laryngeal sphincter is incompetent, then phonation will be poor and aspiration will be possible. Furthermore, loss of sensation, either in the upper or lower laryngeal compartment, will result in this aspiration being undetected and an aspiration pneumonia will be the result. Inability to obtain a positive subglottic pressure disorganizes the swallowing reflex and also makes it difficult to achieve an adequate cough to clear the lower respiratory tract.

Because of its longer course, the left recurrent laryngeal nerve is paralysed more often than the right; the ratio is about 4:1 and bilateral paralysis occurs in about 6% of cases. Men are affected eight times more than women, but this gender incidence will probably change as the incidence of lung cancer rises in women.

Causes of vocal cord paralysis

Causes of vocal-cord paralysis

- Malignant disease (25%)
- Surgical trauma (20%)
- Non-surgical trauma (15%)
- Idiopathic causes (15%)
- Neurological causes (15%)
- Inflammatory causes (5%)
- Miscellaneous causes (5%)

- **Malignant disease.** This is due to bronchial carcinoma (50%), oesophageal carcinoma (20%), thyroid carcinoma (10%) and nasopharyngeal carcinoma, glomus tumours and lymphomas (20%).
- **Surgical trauma.** This can occur in oesophageal and lung surgery for carcinoma, in carotid artery surgery, congenital heart surgery, thyroid surgery, partial laryngectomy, radical neck dissection, removal of pharyngeal pouch and anterior approaches for cervical spine fusion.
- **Non-surgical trauma.** This is an increasing cause of vocal-cord paralysis because of road traffic accidents and increasing violence in society, and on the sports field. Ortner's syndrome from cardiomegaly can be considered part of this. It is seen more often in horses than in humans!
- **Idiopathic causes.** If a viral neuritis affects the nerves, it is usually on the right side. The influenza or infectious mononucleosis viruses are often incriminated.
- **Neurological causes.** Not only can the well-known neurological diseases, such as multiple sclerosis, amyotrophic lateral sclerosis, syringomyelia and Parkinson's disease paralyse the vocal cords, but small-vessel disease can also affect the brainstem, causing vocal-cord paralysis. It is seen as the result of head injury and neuropathies that occur in alcoholism, diabetes and the Guillain–Barré syndrome.
- **Inflammatory causes.** These used to be a much more common cause of vocal-cord paralysis, but as the incidence of pulmonary tuberculosis and syphilitic aortitis has decreased, so has the incidence of paralysis due to these causes.
- **Miscellaneous causes.** These include haemolytic anaemia, thrombosis of the subclavian vein and various collagen diseases.

History

Voice quality

A forced whisper suggests an organic adductor paralysis, whereas a faint whisper is often a sign of functional adductor paralysis. A voice which is normal in the morning and tires as the day goes on occurs in a unilateral abductor paralysis. Stridor occurs in bilateral abductor paralysis, whereas aspiration implies bilateral adductor paralysis.

Paralysis due to surgical trauma is usually seen shortly after the operation, but is often diagnosed later. For example, it is possible for a bilateral abductor paralysis to be caused by a thyroidectomy and the patient to have few or no symptoms immediately afterwards. Only several years later, when the cricoarytenoid joint becomes fixed or the vocal cords become oedematous due to an upper respiratory infection, does the patient develop stridor.

Other symptoms

These include hoarseness, dysphagia, sore throat, pain in the ears, cough, haemoptysis and any newly noted neck lumps. The patient's smoking habits should be recorded, together with any recent illnesses, especially of the viral type. In the case of a patient with a vocal-cord paralysis secondary to an operation such as thyroidectomy, it is very important to know the patient's occupation and vocal demands.

Examination

Consideration of the causes gives an indication of what to look for in general examination of the patient. The neck and thyroid gland are examined carefully, paying particular attention to the tracheo-oesophageal groove because of the possibility of thyroid cancer paralysing the nerve, either directly or via a metastatic node.

Laryngoscopy should include fibre-optic and/or videostroboscopic assessment of the vocal cord position and of the mucosal phonating wave. It is difficult to report paramedian or cadaveric positions reliably. The best indication is the width of the membranous glottic chink on phonation. In the paramedian position it will only be about 1–2 mm. In the cadaveric position not only will the gap be greater but the tip of the vocal process will be directed medially as a definite prominence. A paralysed cord becomes bowed and atrophic and lies at a lower level than the normal cord with anterior rotation of the arytenoid. Preoperative evaluation includes a variety of subjective and objective voice parameters, such as maximum phonation time, amplitude perturbation (shimmer), pitch perturbation (jitter), or vocal profile analysis by an expert listener. Electromyography is the only test that will provide information on the integrity of laryngeal innervation.

Investigations

- CT scan from skull base to diaphragm
- Flow–volume loop
- Endoscopy

Radiology

The gold standard of imaging for vocal-fold motion impairment of unknown cause is now a computed tomographic (CT) scan from the skull base to the diaphragm. If a lung cancer is strongly suspected in the out-patient clinic, however, it may speed up the immediate management of the patient to request a wet film chest X-ray. Lung cancers with recurrent laryngeal nerve involvement are not amenable to curative treatment, however, and the CT will still be required to assess the mediastinum. The most important test in a bilateral paralysis is the flow–volume loop, which quantifies the degree of upper and lower respiratory obstruction.

Endoscopy

If the diagnosis is made clinically or radiologically, endoscopy will usually be required to confirm it. If the diagnosis remains obscure then endoscopy is mandatory. The endoscopy may consist of a bronchoscopy if there is a pulmonary tumour, or panendoscopy, which comprises nasopharyngoscopy and biopsy, direct laryngoscopy with mobility tests of the arytenoid to determine whether the immobility is due to muscle paralysis or to joint fixation, oesophagoscopy as well as a bronchoscopy.

Treatment policy

In addition to the operations described, all of these patients may be helped by speech therapy, particularly the patient with a unilateral abductor paralysis. Speech therapy should also be used postoperatively.

Unilateral abductor paralysis

This paralysis, in which one vocal cord is fixed in the paramedian position, may cause no symptoms at all, or only slight hoarseness; with the passage of time, any hoarseness usually disappears spontaneously as the mobile vocal cord compensates. Such a paralysis, if on the left side, is often due to a carcinoma of the left lung. With a paralysed vocal cord, the carcinoma is inoperable.

Unilateral adductor paralysis

A unilateral adductor paralysis causes both dysphonia due to air wastage and aspiration of food because the laryngeal sphincter is incompetent and part of the larynx is insensitive. If unilateral failure of adduction is due to bronchial carcinoma then the distress of altered voice and inefficient cough can be alleviated almost immediately by an injection of the vocal cord. Teflon has the unpredictable ability to produce a brisk granulomatous reaction associated with stridor. When these reactions occur, the airway may be compromised, and the Teflon is effectively irremovable as it is not encapsulated so that the subsequent granuloma is disseminated throughout the thyroarytenoid muscle.

Disadvantages of medialization by injection

- Cord changes in mass, stiffness and volume
- Hard to estimate amount/distribution
  - potential for long-term resorption: collagen
  - requirement for overcorrection
- Irreversible
- Local reactions – Teflon granuloma
  – hypersensitivity (30% with ZCI collagen)

Collagen

Injectable bovine collagen has been used in glottic insufficiency since 1983 and has superior bioimplant qualities when only a minor degree of medialization is required, particularly in cords which are atrophic, scarred or vocally defective. Some of the resorbed implant is replaced by the deposition of new host collagen from the metabolically active invading host fibroblasts, while the existing scar tissue softens, probably as a result of collagenase production by fibroblasts. ZCI (Zyderm collagen 11; Collagen Corp, Palo Alto, CA, USA) was the first injectable preparation used for clinical work. This is a highly purified suspension which remains stable for at least 3 years but has some disadvantages as it is not cross-linked and is sensitive to collagenase in the long term. In addition, at least 60% of the volume injected is water, which requires initial overinjection.

An alternative preparation from the same manufacturers, hypoallergenic GAX collagen, which contains a 0.0075% glutaraldehyde cross-linked collagen and is almost insensitive to collagenase. Its use may obviate the need for overcorrection. Unlike fat or Teflon, collagen cannot be injected transcutaneously under direct vision.

Injection with alloplastic or bioimplant material remains the quickest and least expensive method of medializing a paretic vocal cord and is associated with a useful improvement in glottic efficiency, particularly in the prevention of aspiration and allied complications. Nonetheless, there is some stroboscopic and voice analysis evidence that the results of more complex procedures may produce a superior phonatory quality.

Fat injection

It is usually stated that fat is eventually absorbed, and so lipoinjection may not be the best method of rehabilitation for patients with irreversible pathology and a reasonable life expectancy. Many unfortunate patients with vocal-cord paralysis have a short life span, however, and the use of lipoinjection has thus gained in popularity in recent years.

Thyroplasty

The two principal alternatives to cord injection are thyroplasty and nerve transfer, or other reinnervation procedures. The Isshiki type 1 thyroplasty was introduced in 1974 and involved the insertion of a block of Silastic through a window in the thyroid cartilage. The basic principle therefore is similar to the mechanism of cord injections but it requires an external approach. Proponents favour the greater degree of control over the vocal-cord position by adjusting the thickness and position of the block, and also the greater degree of reversibility in the event of airway insufficiency.

As with cord injection the procedure medializes only the membranous vocal cord, however, and can only partially resolve the problem of chronic aspiration because of the persistence of a posterior glottic chink. Histologically, there is no evidence of intralaryngeal scarring when dissection is kept lateral to the inner perichondrium of the thyroid cartilage.

Postoperative findings include an increase in fundamental frequency and intensity of the voice and a significantly longer maximum phonation time. The procedure has the advantage of preserving normal relationships between the vocal-fold mucosa and its substance, together with the associated potential for allowing recovery of normal motor function in the event of later neuromuscular regeneration. However, laryngeal framework medialization not only tends to leave a posterior glottic chink, however, but also fails to allow for changes in vocal cord tension.

Advantages of laryngeal framework surgery

- Intraoperative feedback (local anaesthetic)
- Volume, mass and stiffness of cord unaffected
- Level of implant correct
- Reversible: no tissue reaction

Arytenoid adduction

At one time it was believed that arytenoid adduction was indicated only for patients who had evidence preoperatively of a posterior glottic chink. Later studies indicated that arytenoid adduction as an adjunct to thyroplasty can improve voice quality. It may be particularly helpful in high vagal lesions where the cricothyroid is also paralysed. The posterior glottis cannot be closed by thyroplasty because of the superior projection of the cricoid cartilage medial to the thyroid lamina.

Reinnervation

Early studies in the 1960s and 1970s of the reanastomosis of the severed ends of the recurrent laryngeal nerve or transposition of an extrinsic nerve to its main trunk were found to result in misdirected reinnervation with subsequent synkinesis of the laryngeal muscles. This then rendered the organ functionally useless. Tucker has described a procedure for vocal-fold reinnervation using the ansa hypoglossi with an omohyoid neuromuscular pedicle. This reinnervation technique restores not only gross movement of the vocal cord, but also the ability to tense the muscles and therefore to control pitch. Theoretically at least, it therefore offers a return to normal function, although it has a built-in delay of 2–6 months before any improvement may be noted postoperatively. Histochemical and excitability studies following nerve–muscle pedicle implantation have demonstrated the feasibility of

laryngeal reinnervation, although there is residual controversy about the clinical success achieved by the average phonosurgeon.

The direct reanastomosis of the ansa hypoglossi to the recurrent laryngeal nerve has the advantages of being entirely reversible and not interfering with the structure of the vocal cord. However, it requires a cervical incision and is somewhat more costly to perform than other abduction procedures such as injection or thyroplasty. Reinnervation also offers the most 'natural' voice outcome in the right hands, but is not recommended in the presence of aspiration as it does not cause significant medialization.

The most recent development in laryngeal reinnervation has been the development of pacing by electrical stimulation. Such electrical pacing of implanted nerve pedicles allows selective dynamic control of cord abduction and elongation. These techniques seem in future more likely to restore simple laryngeal functions (respiratory or deglutitive) than the more complex phonatory function.

Bilateral adductor paralysis

This is fortunately very rare. It causes severe dysphonia and nearly all patients suffer aspiration leading to bronchopneumonia. In the acute phase, while natural resolution may be anticipated, it may be valuable to carry out a temporary vocal-fold augmentation, e.g. with fat or Gelfoam. Long-term solutions for persistent aspirators include a narrow field laryngectomy or, if resolution may be anticipated or there is a pressing reason to retain laryngeal function, epiglottic plication, surgical approximation of the vocal cords or tracheal diversion (tracheostomy) may be considered.

Bilateral vocal fold motion impairment

- Direct blow to the neck
- Surgery
  - thyroid surgery
  - carotid endarterectomy
  - anterior cervical fusion
  - cervical oesophageal surgery
- Traumatic endotracheal intubation
- Infiltration: tuberculosis, amyloid, sarcoid
- Parkinson's disease
- Amyotrophic lateral sclerosis

Bilateral abductor paralysis

This sometimes causes stridor. In particular in a slightly built woman who is relatively inactive, there may be little or no stridor, at least for the first few months or years after the onset of paralysis. Because the vocal cords are in the paramedian position, the voice is usually good. Sooner or later, however, all patients with this problem will have stridor, which may be precipitated by an upper respiratory tract infection. In the absence of ankylosis of the cricoarytenoid joints, the compromised airway may occlude completely during forced inspiration. The immediate problem is to provide a satisfactory airway, and therefore a tracheostomy should be performed.

It must be remembered that a patient with a tracheostomy has a drive for inspiratory abduction and the tracheostomy should be occluded at the time of assessment. A patient with a tracheostomy has a choice – either to keep the speaking tracheostomy tube, in which case there is a good voice but a hole in the neck, or to have the tracheostomy removed which results in inevitable deterioration in voice quality. In performing vocal cord lateralization surgery, the surgeon draws a fine line between improving the airway and keeping a serviceable voice. What is certain is that the patient cannot have both a good airway and a good voice. Retention of the tracheostomy for nocturnal use, with occlusion using a flesh-coloured obturator by day, may allow the best compromise for those patients whose principal dyspnoea is nocturnal. The flow-volume loop documents airflow rate and volume, the site of obstruction and the nature and severity of the obstructing lesion.

Vocal cord lateralization

■ Laser arytenoidectomy/cordotomy
■ Cordopexy, with or without arytenoid removal
■ Woodman's operation
■ Reinnervation

The first alternative to tracheostomy (Chevalier Jackson, 1922) involved removal of the whole of one cord including the ventricle. The most popular traditional operation became the external removal of one arytenoid, as described in 1946 by Woodman. Before any lateralization procedure, the patient should be appraised that the success rate is only about 70%.

Laser cordotomy/arytenoidectomy

The posterior one-half to one-third of the vocal cord can be obliquely vaporized, if necessary with the ablation of the body of the arytenoid, leaving a remnant of the muscular process. Partial arytenoidectomy may, however, risk postoperative infection. Total arytenoidectomy with the laser causes sufficient scarring on occasion to move the vocal cord medially rather then laterally. Methods are also described of using the laser to debulk the cord, and then retain the lateral position with fibrin glue. There have been no randomized trials of vocal fold lateralization, but in one cohort comparison of laser cordectomy with arytenoidectomy, the respiratory improvement was similar in both groups, with a wide intersubject variation in voice outcomes being observed with each procedure. The cordectomy was felt to be an easier procedure to perform correctly (Eckel et al., 1994).

The principal risk with extensive resection of the arytenoid area is of aspiration. It has been claimed that this risk can be reduced by performing a 'subtotal arytenoidectomy' (Remacle et al.,1996). The modification involves an initial transverse cut separating the membranous vocal cord from the vocal process, followed by a sub-

stantial resection of the arytenoid but with preservation of a thin posterior shell providing good postoperative fixation of the arytenoid region. One of the difficulties encountered in practice with any of these endolaryngeal procedures is, however, the grossly distorted position and angulation of the arytenoid in some longstanding paralyses, which can make it surprisingly difficult to match the endoscopic view with anatomical illustrations of the normal arytenoid.

External arytenoidectomy is best performed from a lateral approach (Woodman's operation), which avoids the disruption of the anterior commissure that results if an anterior approach is used. The arytenoid is removed with the exception of the vocal process, which is then lateralized using a submucosal suture anchored to the inferior horn of the thyroid cartilage.

Cordopexy, i.e. suture laterofixation of a cord, involves passing a wire around the vocal process and tightening it on the outside of the thyroid ala (see Fig. 18.5). Cordopexy may be combined with arytenoid removal if performed via an open approach. If the arytenoid is to be retained then the procedure can be performed endoscopically by excising a portion of the thyroarytenoid muscle and holding the mucosa of the cord back into the gap, hoping that during a 6 week period it will heal. This procedure mimics laser excision of the posterior part of the cord.

Reinnervation

Successful attempts have been made to reinnervate the posterior cricoarytenoid muscle selectively, thus restoring abductor function to a larynx with bilateral abductor paralysis. In order to achieve the normal cyclical inspiratory abductor movement of the vocal cords, the ideal nerve for reinnervation should have a spontaneous inspiratory signal. The best signal at present is in the phrenic nerve, which in animal experiments produces good abduction. The technique has never become very popular in humans because of the obvious risk of respiratory catastrophe if there is pre-existing damage to the contralateral phrenic nerve. Recently, the preganglionic sympathetic neurons have been used in dog posterior cricoarytenoid muscle reinnervation, and the results confirmed by direct laryngoscopy, electromyography and histological studies. The ansa hypoglossi is also said to demonstrate inspiratory activity and its sacrifice leaves very little deficit.

Phonosurgical techniques

Vocal cord medialization

Vocal cord medialization

■ Injection: Teflon, fat, collagen
■ Thyroplasty
■ Arytenoid adduction
■ Reinnervation

Injection

Transoral laryngoscopic injection may be performed under general anaesthetic or under Propofol sedation with cophenylcaine spray to the pharynx and larynx in the frail, high-risk patient.

A Bruning-Arnold syringe is charged with collagen or Teflon. The syringe has a very long needle and is controlled by a pistol grip with a ratchet handle, so designed that closure of one notch on the handle delivers 0.1 ml collagen paste. After charging the syringe, the surgeon exposes the larynx by direct laryngoscopy. On the paralysed side the upper surface of the vocal cord is exposed by retracting the false cord laterally with the end of the needle (Fig. 18.3). Then the needle is pushed into the soft tissues immediately lateral to the vocal cord and the handle closed one notch. The operator waits for several seconds as the paste only extrudes slowly; during this period the vocal cord will be seen to move slowly towards the midline. Once the position becomes stationary the patient is asked to say 'E' and, if the mobile cord does not approximate to the paralysed cord, another 0.1 ml is injected and again the surgeon waits. It should only be necessary to repeat the procedure at the most three times.

The two most important points about this procedure are, first, one must appreciate how slowly the paste extrudes from the needle, so that it must be kept in place after the handle has been closed for several seconds to allow the paste to enter the tissues, and secondly, the injection must be put in exactly the right place, that is immediately lateral to the vocal cords. An injection should not be put into the subglottic space, into the edge of the vocal cord or too far laterally.

Transcutaneous Teflon injection may be performed in one of two ways. The Bruning's needle may be introduced in the midline, through the cricothyroid membrane, and angled upwards and laterally into the cord, at an angle of 30° in a woman and 45° in a man. Some surgeons prefer to keep the course of the needle submucosal, but it can be simpler deliberately to pass the needle intraluminally, and then enter the vocal cord under endoscopic control. Alternatively, others prefer direct lateral penetration of the larynx through the thyroid ala.

Fat for injection may be harvested from a small periumbilical incision, either by an open method or with a liposuction cannula if one is available. If collected by lipo-

suction, it can be placed directly into the Bruning syringe. Otherwise, it should be mechanically crushed before injection. Overhomogenization is probably not advisable as it may overdebulk the implant. The sites and method of injection are as for Teflon injection but a degree of overcorrection is required to allow for subsequent water absorption (Oluwole *et al.*, 1996).

> ### Complications of injection
>
> - **Pain** is usual. It is often mild and should be treated with simple analgesics
> - **Infection** occurs occasionally and should be treated by antibiotics
> - **Laryngeal obstruction** can occur if too much collagen has been injected, particularly if infection supervenes. Treat the obstruction with antibiotics, steroids and humidification, and if necessary a temporary tracheostomy. Because of the danger of laryngeal obstruction, and because it is impossible to remove the collagen once it has been injected, it is better to inject too little than too much. This is because it is always possible to return later and give a further injection

Isshiki thyroplasty type I

The procedure is ideally performed under local anaesthesia with intravenous sedation. If the patient is oversedated or has a floppy tongue base, it may be necessary to pass the flexible endoscope through a laryngeal mask, which stents open the supraglottis and improves the view of the vocal cord throughout the procedure. Ideally, there should be three people present: surgeon, a surgical assistant to retract and another assistant to perform the endoscopy.

A block of silastic is cut in a wedge before the start of the procedure (Fig. 18.4). The plug may be fixed in the cartilage window with a protruding flange. Alternatively, it may fit tightly into the window, in which case it will need to be about 3 mm thick anteriorly and 5 mm thick posteriorly. The posteroinferior corner should be sliced off to prevent impingement on the cricoid ring.

The procedure after laryngeal entry, in particular, should be performed with the minimum of delay to reduce the risk of swelling. A 5 cm horizontal incision is made at the midpoint of the thyroid ala on the paralysed

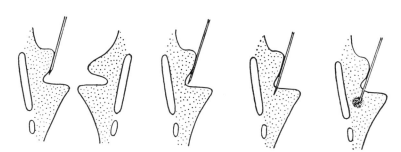

Figure 18.3 Correct location of vocal-fold injection.

(a)

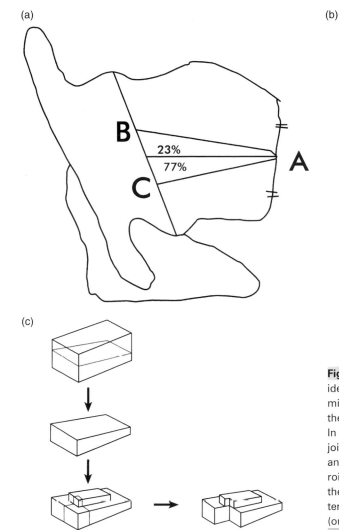

(b)

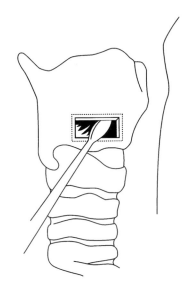

(c)

Figure 18.4 Medialization (Isshiki) thyroplasty. (a) External identification of the position of the vocal cord. A represents midpoint of the anterior thyroid prominence; while B–C is the middle third of the oblique line of the thyroid cartilage. In the majority of people, AC, the line of the vocal cords, joins the oblique line at the junction of the upper-two thirds and lowest third; (b) completion of the window in the thyroid lamina; (c) wedge-shaped prosthesis is fashioned using the excised piece of cartilage as the template with posteroinferior resection to prevent abuttment on the arytenoid (or concomitant nerve muscle pedicle).

side. The strap muscles are retracted and partially dissected off the oblique line and the outer perichondrium is reflected from the anterior ala. A line is marked out on the exposed ala from the midpoint of the anterior thyroid prominence (level of the anterior commissure) running posteriorly and slightly downwards, to join the junction of the upper two-thirds and lowest third of the oblique line (Fig. 18.4a, line AC).

A window is cut out of the thyroid ala below the anterior half of the marked line. The anterior wall of the window is 5–7 mm posterior to the midline, and its dimensions are 5–6 mm high in the male, 4–5 mm in the female; 12 mm wide in male and 10 mm in female patients. The inferior margin is 3 mm above the lower edge of the thyroid lamina. The inexperienced surgeon may find it helpful to make a small 'scout' perforation at what seems to be the surface marking of the vocal cord and verify this by applying a lacrimal probe through the hole under videolaryngoscopic control. In a calcified larynx, formation of the window is less traumatic if marked out with a fine rose head or fissure burr on an electric drill.

The safest method is to fashion a series of miniholes and then join these up, preserving the inner perichondrium by drilling only 80–90% of the thickness, leaving a paper-thin layer which can finally be divided with a fine elevator. Use of the middle ear (Rosen's) set of instruments can be helpful. There is nothing to be gained by retaining the cartilage window deep to the implant: indeed, this manoeuvre probably restricts the degree of medialization.

Care should be taken to stay outside the internal perichondrium of the thyroid ala. The inner perichondrium is then dissected off the remaining ala as far posteriorly as possible. It may well help the outcome to divide the perichondrium so as to free up the graft position, but this is better done around the vertical and superior limbs of the window. If possible, the inferior perichondrium should remain intact to prevent inferior extrusion.

The prosthesis should be positioned posteriorly if possible, to medialize the vocal process of the arytenoid. The final position is determined by a combination of auditory and endoscopic feedback. A degree of over-medialization in anticipation of at least a degree of intraoperative oedema is recommended. As the body of the arytenoid is not accessible from a lateral thyroid approach, and since it is a medial relation of the piriform fossa, it is impossible to move it medially with an Isshiki operation or an injection.

Complications of type I thyroplasty

- Airway obstruction
- Extrusion
- Late failure: as a result of intraoperative oedema, one may fail accurately to estimate the extent of medialization required. Thus, the early results are excellent, but the late result is disappointing as the reactive oedema settles. This problem is minimized not only by the administration of intraoperative steroids but also by keeping the duration of surgery as brief as possible once the larynx has been opened.

Thyroplasty with nerve muscle pedicle to the thyroarytenoid muscle. This procedure may be used in combination with thyroplasty (Tucker, 1990). A nerve–muscle pedicle is harvested from the branch of the ansa hypoglossi to the anterior belly of the omohyoid muscle and implanted through the window in the thyroid lamina. The posteroinferior corner of the silastic is resected to allow access for the pedicle.

Arytenoid adduction

The posterior margin of the thyroid cartilage is exposed by separating the inferior constrictor from the thyroid lamina. The mucosa of the piriform fossa is elevated until the muscular process of the arytenoid cartilage is identified. If the mucosa is perforated, the procedure will have to be abandoned. This identification is made much easier by removal of the central posterior margin of the thyroid ala. Partial opening up of the cricoarytenoid joint is sometimes used, but excessive opening will simply result in shortening of the vocal cord. A 4/0 prolene or a 5/0 Gore-tex suture is placed through the muscular process and surrounding soft tissue (to prevent fracture of the muscular process). The suture is fed through through a 16 G angiocath, or even a needle placed through a hole in the anteroinferior aspect of the ipsilateral thyroid cartilage and immediately medial to the thyroid ala. The suture is tied over a two-hole microplate, used as a bolster, under laryngoscopic control. If too much tension is applied the cord will bow.

It helps to put in two sutures to pull the process in the line of the thyroarytenoid and lateral cricoarytenoid muscles. The holes in the thyroid ala are positioned approximately as follows:

- vertical distance: three-quarters of the distance from the thyroid notch to the inferior border of the thyroid cartilage
- horizontal distance: one-third to one-half of the distance from the midline to the oblique line (insertion of the inferior constrictor).

Both arytenoid adduction and type I thyroplasty have a similar effect in reducing the patency of the upper airway but, at least in one study, show little difference in the degree of improvement in voice quality (Bielamowicz et al.,1995).

Ansa hypoglossi: recurrent laryngeal nerve anastomosis

Neural anastomosis allows reinnervation of the whole hemilarynx rather than just selective reinnervation of a muscle implanted with a neuromuscular pedicle. The technique medializes the ipsilateral thyroid lamina owing to loss of the lateral pull of the sternothyroid on the thyroid ala, giving an initial slight voice improvement. After complete neural regeneration of the motor axons from the ansa into the recurrent laryngeal nerve there is a low-level, tonic, non-cyclical innervation of the ipsilateral hemilarynx.

A collar incision is made from the midline at the level of the cricoid cartilage across the sternomastoid muscle. The platysma is divided, the sternomastoid retracted laterally and a nerve stimulator used around the internal jugular vein. The ansa is identified when strong twitches of the strap muscles occur. The most inferior branch is used in the anastomosis and is transected immediately proximal to its entry into the sternothyroid muscle. The great vessels are retracted laterally and the injured recurrent laryngeal nerve identified. The stimulator can be used to confirm its position if there is any doubt. The integrity of the distal recurrent laryngeal nerve should be confirmed. If it has been damaged then an alternative method, e.g. thyroplasty or collagen injection, should be considered. Neuroanastomosis is carried out with 10/0 Nylon and the wound is closed in layers. As the procedure induces a paramedian cord without abduction, it is contraindicated in any patient with reduced abduction of the contralateral cord.

Vocal cord lateralization

Laser cordectomy/arytenoidectomy

CO_2 laser resection of part of the vocal cord and/or arytenoid is usually undertaken with the laser on 4–10 W superpulse mode, preferably with a spot size no greater than 0.8 mm. The usual laser precautions are undertaken, particularly the protection of the patient's head and neck skin with saline soaks, and the used of metal-guarded endotracheal tubes. (If a tracheostomy is not in place, the anaesthetist may succeed in achieving very gentle spontaneous respiration under Propofol, without Venturi, using only a supply of oxygen via a postnasal space cannula. This allows paticularly good access to the posterior larynx/arytenoid region in this situation.)

Traditional cordotomy involves removal of a wedge of the posterior half of the cord, usually including the medial arytenoid, tapering the resection anteriorly so that the narrowest end of the wedge is in the membranous (phonating) cord, with the broad bulk of the resection in the posterior respiratory area of the glottis. The Kashima method of **transverse laser cordotomy** circumvents these difficulties through placement of a transverse incision through the vocal fold immediately anterior to the vocal process.

In **medial arytenoidectomy**, first the mucosa over the superior and medial portions of the arytenoid is lasered. Then the cartilage of the arytenoid body posterior to the vocal process is carefully shaved, taking care to protect the posterior commissure soft tissues with saline-soaked strips of cotton. Care must also be taken not to produce injury below the level of the arytenoid, which risks ankylosis of the cricoarytenoid joint (Crumley, 1993). The procedure may be carried out contralaterally at a later sitting. Perioperative dexamethasone and antibiotic cover may be helpful, especially in the minority of patients who do not have a pre-existing tracheostomy.

Cordopexy

Cordopexy (endoscopic laterofixation) appears to have a higher overall success (decannulation) rate than more traditional operations such as Woodman's procedure (below). Cordopexy is performed under general anaesthesia, ideally by two surgeons, one working endoscopically using the Kleinsasser suspension, and the other working on the laryngeal framework. A 3 cm collar incision is made over the thyroid ala. The point 4 mm anterior to and 2 mm below the midpoint of the oblique line is identified. The position of a needle inserted at this point is checked by the endoscopist: it should be above the tip of the vocal process (Fig. 18.5). If the needle is thus correctly positioned, a second needle is inserted 5 mm below it (Ejnell *et al.*, 1984). An 0 diameter monofilament thread (Nylon or Prolene) is inserted down the inferior needle, and the end retrieved internally by the endoscopist, who then manipulates it into the lumen of the upper needle, feeding it through so that it can be withdrawn. The suture is then tightened by the external surgeon, and knotted when the endoscopist is satisfied with the internal configuration (aim = 5 mm airway approximately). The skin incision is closed in two layers.

The difficult part of the operation is trying to feed the suture back out through the second needle. A modification to simplify this step is described by Moustafa *et al.* (1992), in which the needles used are epidural needles, and where the 0 Nylon suture is fed down the lower needle, and the 19 G epidural catheter down the upper one. Both structures are then withdrawn from the mouth by the endoscopist, who inserts the Nylon into the catheter, producing a snug fit. Withdrawal of the epidural catheter then automatically feeds the thread down the second needle. These steps are much more reliable than trying to guide the thread directly up the end of the needle.

Woodman's operation

The patient will have a tracheostomy via which the anaesthesic is applied. The head is slightly extended and turned away from the paralysed side. To access the crico-

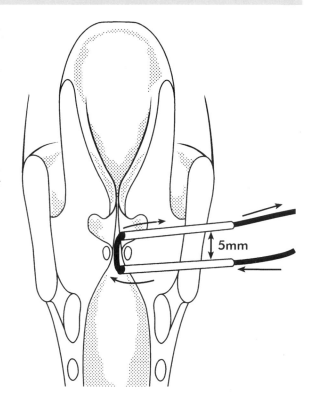

Figure 18.5 Vocal cord lateralization: cordopexy. The simplest way to feed the thread into the second needle is first to pass an epidural catheter down it and bring both it and the thread out through the mouth. Then, the thread is fed down the cannula and the cannula withdrawn through the neck.

thyroid joint, a horizontal skin-crease incision is made at the level of the cricoid cartilage. Skin flaps are raised and the sternomastoid is retracted. The surgeon cuts through the constrictor muscles on the back of the thyroid lamina and, with a finger behind the thyroid lamina, then rotates the larynx. This will allow the surgeon to work directly on the cricothyroid joint, which should then be disarticulated.

With a Langenbeck retractor, the thyroid cartilage is pulled forwards and the cricoid rotated so that the posterior cricoarytenoid muscle can be seen clearly. This gives access to the arytenoid, which should be disarticulated from the cricoid by entering the cricoarytenoid joint. This is done submucosally. The whole arytenoid is not taken out at this point. It is dissected submucosally and the vocal process identified. Before removal of the arytenoid, a 3/0 Nurolon suture is passed through the vocal process and tied round the inferior horn of the thyroid. The body of the arytenoid can then be removed. If it is removed too early, then it is very difficult to identify the vocal process and very difficult to achieve a good bite with any stitch. Another two sutures are inserted to lateralize the cord, if under laryngoscopic control, to create a posterior gap of 4–5 mm. The wound is drained and closed in the usual fashion.

The patient is allowed to recover for a few days from the procedure, and then the tracheostomy tube is corked to determine whether there is an adequate airway to allow decannulation.

Controversies in management

How does one know where the cord is?

Although some patients present with the cord definitely either in the midposition or in the cadaveric position, in at least half of cases it is difficult to say exactly where the cord lies. The best way of studying this is with videoendoscopy, but even on videotape review it can be hard conclusively to determine cord position, especially in the presence of synkinesis. In late cord paralysis, one can see how far the arytenoid is dipped forward and how far the vocal process has come to lie below the glottic line. One can see how much atrophy there has been in the thyroarytenoid muscle and, with a study of these videos, it is possible to design the best rehabilitative measure.

How does one know whether the arytenoid is fixed?

It is sometimes difficult to tell whether the cord is paralysed or whether the arytenoid is fixed. The apparent simplicity of the arytenoid mobilization test is misleading. It is difficult to move any arytenoid when the patient is asleep. Interarytenoid fibrosis is indicated by movement of one arytenoid towards the midline when the other is deflected laterally; normally, there should be no such contralateral associated movement. Certainly, gross degrees of fixation can be identified but it cannot be said that an arytenoid is fixed or mobile in every case.

How long should one wait to operate?

The timing of surgery depends on the cause of the paresis. Six to 12 months is taken as an arbitrary time for recovery of vocal-cord function, in potentially reversible or self-limiting pareses, but there is only anecdotal support for this convention. For a patient seen, e.g. with lung cancer or following pneumonectomy, there is nothing to be gained by delay and surgery should be performed as soon as possible to enhance voice quality and improve the cough.

Why is there a 30% failure rate with a Woodman's operation?

This is an intriguing question because the operation is a simple one with very few variables. Perhaps the most important technical point in doing a Woodman's operation is to insert the stitch in the cartilage of the vocal process prior to removing the arytenoid. If the arytenoid is removed before a stitch is put into place, then the soft tissues of the larynx fall medially and the stitch may be placed too laterally to achieve decent traction. Furthermore, the stitch may well cut out and allow the cord to drift back into the midposition. Scarring may also drag the cord back into that position, and there should be a commitment on the part of the surgeon to correct the airway in this operation rather than to preserve voice.

What can be done when a collagen injection goes wrong?

If a collagen operation goes wrong then too much has been inserted, in which case a tracheostomy is required; or the collagen has been put into the wrong place and a curious diplophonia arises. In either case, the collagen has to be removed, perhaps preceded by a tracheostomy. There is no good way to remove it other than to perform a laryngofissure and to enter the thyroarytenoid muscle. This will cause gross scarring and make the dysphonia worse.

Dysphagia

Causes of dysphagia following treatment for head and neck cancer

The functional causes of post-treatment dysphagia are listed below. Some of the dysfunction may be due to denervation, while oedema, scarring, stricture and loss of bulk (notably at the tongue base) also contribute.

> *Causes of dysphagia following treatment for head and neck cancer*
>
> ▪ Oral incompetence/loss of articulators
> ▪ Loss of tongue propulsion
> ▪ Aspiration
> ▪ Pharyngo-oesophageal hold-up
> ▪ Gastro-oesophageal reflux

Radiation effects

Postradiotherapy, xerostomia is a major additional cause of dysphagia, affecting the mastication and oral manipulation of food bolus, but not apparently the pharyngeal phase. Radiation-induced salivary gland dysfunction also causes tooth decay, altered taste sensation and a change in oral microflora. In one survey of patients following chemoradiation for oropharyngeal and hypopharyngeal tumours (Lazarus *et al.*, 1996), commonly observed abnormalities included reduced tongue base posterior pharyngeal wall contact and reduced laryngeal closure. The addition of postoperative irradiation following oral resection has been shown (Pauloski *et al.*, 1998) to increase pharyngeal residue and to reduce the following.

> *Postoperative irradiation following oral resection reduces:*
>
> ▪ oral transit
> ▪ oropharyngeal swallow efficiency
> ▪ cricopharyngeal opening.

Aspiration after partial laryngectomy

Prior to vertical partial and supraglottic horizontal laryngectomy, the patient should be well motivated to embark on intensive postoperative rehabilitation and should also have a sufficient respiratory reserve to withstand a degree of aspiration. With vertical hemilaryngectomy, the incidence of aspiration is unavoidably increased if the ipsilateral arytenoid has to be resected. Partial arytenoid resection is not feasible as the remnant is affected by refractory perichondritis. If excessive tongue base has to be resected, then it unlikely that a horizontal partial laryngectomy is the procedure of choice. If one arytenoid has to be resected, the risk of aspiration is higher. The cord should be tacked in the midline with a permanent submucosal suture. Prophylactic cricopharyngeal myotomy is advisable.

Assessment of the dysphagic patient

> *Assessment of the dysphagic patient*
>
> ▪ Bedside assessment
> ▪ Videofluoroscopy
> ▪ Videoendoscopic swallow study

Bedside assessment

Bedside assessment is the simplest method of assessing a swallow performance. A trained speech and language therapist with a particular interest in dysphagia carries out a clinical assessment which includes evaluation of the gag reflex, voluntary and reflex cough, vocal quality and volume, reflex and volitional swallow, posture, oral motor strength and range of motion, and respiratory quality during inspiration and expiration. Vocal quality may be classified as normal, wet–hoarse, breathy, harsh or nonassessable.

Following these preliminary physiological assessments, swallowing is observed during a standardized dysphagia evaluation protocol. This usually includes liquids, puréed and soft-texture foods and solids. The food assessment is usually started with the soft-consistency foods, which are less likely to provoke aspiration than thin liquids. Starting from a 2.5 ml volume a progressive sequence of increasing volumes is embarked on, limited obviously by the patient's tolerance and swallow performance. During the swallow performance assessment patients are evaluated for vocal quality, throat clearing, cough, colour changes and signs of respiratory distress. Swallow reflex, bolus control and manipulation after the introduction of food are also documented. A complete formal assessment such as this will take at least 30–45 min per patient.

Classification of swallow performance following bedside assessment

▪ **Within normal limits**
▪ **Mild:** slight delay in swallow reflex, but good apparent oral pharyngeal motor function
▪ **Moderate:** delayed swallow reflex, suspected pooling before swallow, heavy coating in the pharynx postswallow
▪ **Severe dysphagia:** trace of aspiration with delayed swallow reflex and probable pooling
▪ **Profound dysphagia:** absent swallow reflex and probable poor oral pharyngeal motor function

Aspiration is defined as the entry of food or barium below the vocal cords, which is sometimes inferred indirectly from the appearance of coughing or wet–hoarse voice quality. If the patient has a tracheostome, however, food may be seen appearing in the tracheal aspirate or expectorated mucus, providing conclusive proof of aspiration. It is very difficult to quantify aspiration at the bedside, however, unless it is clearly massive. The speech and language therapist may still therefore be left with the dilemma as to whether or not to encourage continued oral feeding.

Videofluoroscopy

The videofluoroscopic swallow study (VFSS) was introduced in the early 1980s by Jeri Logemann's team in Chicago. The methodology revolutionized the contribution of radiology to the diagnosis of swallowing disorders. In contrast to the traditional barium swallow, where the aim is to obtain a full column of barium to examine the tubular oesophagus and gastro-oesophageal junction for mucosal abnormalities, the focus of videofluoroscopy is on oropharyngeal function. Very small volumes of barium-containing substances of different consistency are swallowed during the procedure and the recording is videotaped for subsequent combined analysis by the speech and language therapist and radiologist. Views are taken in both the anteroposterior and lateral plane and barium-containing substances starting with pudding, thick liquids, thin liquids and solids are assessed. The average videofluoroscopy requires up to 120 s of fluoroscopy time. Aspiration into the lower respiratory tract can be viewed directly. It must be remembered, however, that the proportion of a bolus which is aspirated can, even using this direct visualization, only be estimated. Thus, attempts to distinguish between quite small percentage differences in bolus aspiration are unrealistic. It is, however, possible to quantify aspiration as mild, moderate or severe using videofluoroscopy and perhaps more importantly, to gain an estimation of the phase of the swallow cycle during which aspiration occurs (Fig. 18.6).

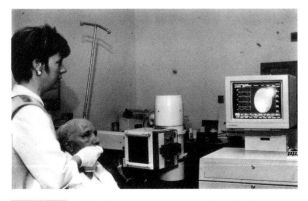

Figure 18.6 Videofluoroscopy combined with videoendoscopic swallow study.

The floor of the nasal cavity is formed by the hard palate; the floor of the maxillary antrum is the alveolus. The premolar and molar teeth are in intimate relationship to the floor of the maxillary sinus. Attached to the posterior wall of the maxillary antrum are the pterygoid plates. The space between the pterygoid plates and the maxillary sinus is the pterygomaxillary fissure, through which travels the maxillary artery.

The infratemporal fossa is the space behind the maxillary antrum, bounded medially by the pterygoid plates and laterally by the zygomatic arch, coronoid process and ascending ramus of the mandible. Inferoposteriorly it connects to the parapharyngeal space and superiorly lie the sphenoid bone, the foramen ovale and the foramen spinosum. It contains the mandibular branch of the fifth cranial nerve, the pterygoid muscles, the maxillary artery and the venous plexus. Tumours can be primary or metastatic, or spread from contiguous structures.

The nasal septum consists of the quadrilateral cartilage, the vomer and the perpendicular plate of the ethmoid. Anteriorly it is contiguous with the medial crura of the lower lateral cartilages. Tumours in the anterior part of the nose not only involve the nasal septum but readily escape from the nasal cavity via the gingivobuccal sulcus to involve the muscles of the upper lip and the mouth.

Surgical pathology

Epidemiology of carcinoma

Neoplasms of the sinuses and nasal cavity account for 0.2–0.8% of all carcinomas, and only 3% of those in the upper aerodigestive tract (Osguthorpe, 1994).

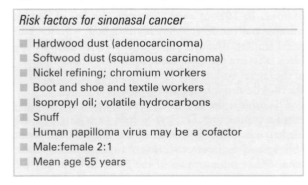

Risk factors for sinonasal cancer

- Hardwood dust (adenocarcinoma)
- Softwood dust (squamous carcinoma)
- Nickel refining; chromium workers
- Boot and shoe and textile workers
- Isopropyl oil; volatile hydrocarbons
- Snuff
- Human papilloma virus may be a cofactor
- Male:female 2:1
- Mean age 55 years

In the USA and the UK, the incidence of nasal tumours is about 10 per million population per year. In Japan and parts of Africa, the rates are more than twice that. Up to 44% of sinonasal neoplasms are attributed to occupational exposure. The best recognized aetiological factor in the UK is the wood industry. People working with hardwoods run the same risk of developing adenocarcinomas of the ethmoids as do smokers of developing lung cancer.

Retrospective cohort studies of nickel-refining workers in Wales, Norway and Canada show that the risk is increased 100 times, and rises with the length of exposure and in inverse proportion to the age at first exposure. There is also epidemiological evidence that there is

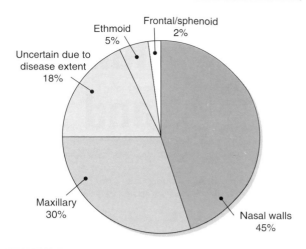

Figure 19.1 Site incidence of cancer of the nose and sinuses.

an increased risk in boot and shoe workers. It has been reported in people working with mustard gas, isopropyl oil and hydrocarbon gas, as well as in people who have had the radiological contrast medium thorium dioxide (Thorotrast) injected into the sinus. Snuff is a well-recognized aetiological factor in the Bantu.

Sites of origin of cancer of the nose and sinuses

Almost half of all sinonasal tumours arise from the lateral nasal walls (Jacobsen *et al.*, 1997) (Fig. 19.1).

Benign tumours

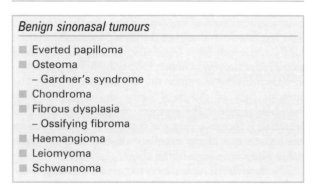

Benign sinonasal tumours

- Everted papilloma
- Osteoma
  - Gardner's syndrome
- Chondroma
- Fibrous dysplasia
  - Ossifying fibroma
- Haemangioma
- Leiomyoma
- Schwannoma

Everted papilloma

Most everted sinonasal papillomas arise from the septum. They are usually single, although occasionally diffuse in the vestibular region. The stratified squamous epithelium ranges from predominantly basal cell to the keratinized form. Where microcysts are present, these do not express the macrophage marker PG-M1.

Osteomas

An osteoma is a benign osteogenic tumour of slow growth containing mature bone. Osteomas are found most frequently on the mandible but, when they occur in the upper jaw, they are most common in the frontoethmoid region. When they fill the entire frontal sinus they extend into the ethmoid labyrinth through the inferior portion of the frontal sinus. When located away from the sinus ostium they are silent and are only discovered incidentally during radiographic examination. When they block the sinus drainage, a mucocoele can develop, requiring removal of the osteoma with an osteoplastic flap or external frontoethmoidectomy.

Osteomas in the ethmoid sinuses present a very different problem. They frequently cause proptosis and have almost always invaded the orbit. If they extend posteriorly they can be contiguous with the sphenoid bone, and thus close to the optic nerve. Unlike frontal sinus osteomas, they cannot be removed simply by severing a stalk. They require a full frontoethmoidectomy, preferably under direct vision. The very large compacted ones are better removed via a craniofacial approach.

Gardner's syndrome is an autosomal dominant syndrome of osteomas with other soft-tissue tumours and intestinal polyposis. The incidence of malignant degeneration of the intestinal polyps is 40%.

Chondromas

Chondromas can develop anywhere in the nose and sinuses. The difference between the benign and malignant varieties is difficult to predict histologically. In general, cartilaginous tumours eventually have a malignant potential, but in the final analysis, those that metastasize are malignant and those that don't probably are not. They have an aggressive nature and tend to recur, thus requiring more extensive resection than do osteomas.

Fibrous dysplasia

Fibrous dysplasia has a female preponderance. It is often first diagnosed in infancy or childhood and growth may slow or cease after puberty. It presents as a painless, slow-growing swelling, typically of the maxilla, and progresses to deformity. Ossifying fibroma is a variant of fibrous dysplasia. It belongs to a range of benign fibro-osseous lesions that occurs in the jaws, and is closely related to cementifying fibroma, benign cementoblastoma, periapical fibrous dysplasia and true fibrous dysplasia. Both ossifying and cementifying fibromas occur in the mandible and maxilla, and present as painless swellings. There is an equal gender incidence with peak age in the third and fourth decades.

Haemangioma

This very often occurs on the nasal septum, thus presenting with epistaxis. It is a cavernous haemangioma with a propensity to recur if resection is not adequate. Haemangiomas elsewhere in the upper jaw are extremely rare. They have been reported in the frontal bone, the nasal bones and the maxilla. They seem to occur between the ages of 20 and 50 years and females predominate. If the teeth are associated with the haemangioma, copious bleeding ensues on their removal. Haemangiomas are nearly always benign, so a policy of non-intervention is probably the best one.

They have a characteristic radiographic appearance. The soap-bubble appearance may represent a giant cell tumour of the jaws, but in haemangiomas the lacunae are smaller and interspersed with a fine fibrillar network which may show a sunray or sunburst appearance in profile.

Leiomyoma

Sinonasal leiomyomas are very rare: only around 20 have been described (Trott et al., 1994). They present as purplish masses causing nasal obstruction and do not recur if completely excised.

Schwannoma

Around 45% of benign peripheral nerve tumours occur in the head and neck region. Sinonasal schwannomas (neurilemmomas) account for only 4% and are reported from the age of 12 years up to the eighth decade. (Hasegawa et al., 1997). Almost all show positive S-100 protein staining. Unusually, they tend to lack a capsule, and thus can appear to the pathologist as suspicious of malignancy. Because of their rarity they also simulate a large number of other nasal masses, and can present as massive lesions with bony erosion.

Intermediate tumours

Intermediate tumours
■ Inverted papilloma
■ Cylindric cell papilloma
■ Haemangiopericytoma
■ Meningioma
■ Oncocytoma

Inverted papilloma (transitional cell papilloma)

Inverted papilloma
■ Up to 4% of all nasal neoplasms
■ 4 per million population; very rare in Black races
■ Male:female ratio varies from 3:1 to 10:1
■ Peak sixth decade: < 10 cases described in children
■ 60% symptoms < 1 year; 20% symptoms > 5 years
■ 25% misdiagnosed at initial consultation

The papillomas present as firm, bulky, red and vascular masses, usually on one side of the nose. Histologically they show patterns of inversion or papilliferous outgrowths, and are covered with squamous or transitional epithelium. There is an intact basement membrane and microcysts are present. The absence of microcysts should suggest low-grade squamous carcinoma. There are cellular atypia in 10%. There is a lot of confusion regarding the biological nature of inverted papilloma. The transitional cell carcinoma with which some are associated can be regarded as a form of non-keratinizing squamous cell carcinoma. The incidence of metachronous malignancy is only 1%, but that of synchronous malignancy may be up to 15%. This distinction may have led to some overtreatment of inverted papilloma in the past, as recent clinical studies support a very low rate of delayed malignant transformation in lesions that were entirely benign *ab initio*. Multiple sections must therefore be examined to define the initial tumour type as precisely as possible.

Cylindric cell papilloma

This unusual neoplasm arises in the antrum and lateral nasal wall. It more often arises in the antrum without involvement of the lateral nasal wall than does the inverted papilloma. The appearance to the naked eye is of a finely granular surface. Microscopically, the epithelium is columnar, oncocytic and deeply crenellated, and with large PG-M1-negative microcysts. These lesions appear to bear a similar relationship to malignancy as the inverted papilloma.

Haemangiopericytoma

The head and neck is the third most common site of origin for these tumours. It is found wherever there are capillaries. Histologically, there is perivascular hyalinization, reflecting the presumed origin in the pericyte (Catalano *et al.*, 1996). Cellular processes arise from the pericyte along its long axis and grip the vessel 'like fingers'. The proliferating fusiform and spindle cells are condensed around medium-sized vascular spaces. The haematoxylin and eosin (H&E) findings are thus fairly characteristic. If immunohistochemistry is used, however, Vimentin and CD34 stains are positive and a number show positive stains for the clotting factor XIIIa, which is expressed by pericytes. It is not clear why the sinonasal haemangiopericytoma has a lower metastatic potential than other axial–skeletal lesions which have a more sarcomatous behaviour. Preoperative embolization may help in the wide local excision, which is the treatment of choice (Rabosa *et al.*, 1997).

Sinonasal haemangioperiocytoma

- Rare lesion of low-grade malignant potential
- Painless grey to tan coloured polypoidal, spongy, haemorrhagic mass
- Presents with epistaxis, nasal obstruction, facial swelling, proptosis
- Mean age 55 years; range 4–80 years; male:female 1:1
- Recurrence rate 18%, 2.5% metastasize, 3% die of disease
- Occasionally causes paraneoplastic syndromes

Extracranial meningiomas arise from ectopic arachnoid tissue but can also spread to the frontal sinuses. Radiotherapy is sometimes beneficial for patients with inoperable or recurrent meningiomas. They are locally recurrent and difficult to eradicate surgically, which is the principal modality of treatment. Oncocytoma (oncocytic adenoma of minor salivary glands) is extremely rare in the nasal cavity. The biological behaviour is determined by local growth rather than histological features (Comin *et al.*, 1997). The cells resemble those of other oncocytomas, with abundant, acidophilic granular cytoplasm and many mitochondria, reflecting the probable origin of the oncocyte as an epithelial cell with mitochondrial hyperplasia.

Malignant tumours

Most neoplasms of the nose and sinuses are squamous. The principal types are listed below, in approximate order of frequency (Spiro *et al.*, 1995).

Malignant sinonasal tumours

- Basal cell carcinoma
- Squamous carcinoma
- Tumours of minor salivary glands
- Sarcomas
- Malignant melanoma
- Esthesioneuroblastoma
- Lymphoreticular neoplasms
- Plasmacytoma
- Adenocarcinoma
- Undifferentiated carcinoma
- Malignant fibrous dysplasia
- Malignant neurogenous tumours

Ohngren (1933) attempted a theoretical classification of sinus tumours into anteroinferior and posterosuperior groups according to an imaginary radiological line extending from the most anterior floor of the orbit to the angle of the jaw. The TNM (tumour, node, mestastasis) classification is given in Table 19.1.

Basal cell carcinoma

Basal cell carcinoma of the nose

- Nose is most common site for BCC in the head and neck
- 30 times more common than squamous carcinoma
- Sixth to eighth decade; male:female 1:1

Although several histological types have been described, it is preferable to define them as either circumscribed or infiltrative. The clinical appearance can vary from small nodular growths to chronic ulcers or ulceronodular lesions. The border of an ulcer may be either rolled or flat. The apparent superficial limits may lead to an underestimation of the deep extent. Four out of 10 will recur and, although distant metastases are rare, recurrent morbidity and possible gross destruction of the face give high priority to successful first attempt therapy (see also Chapter 21).

Squamous carcinoma

Because the lateral wall of the nose, the maxillary antrum and the ethmoid sinuses are contiguous, it is usually impossible to say where a squamous carcinoma has begun. It is commonly accepted, however, that about 50% begin in the maxillary antrum. Almost every patient has signs of bony destruction when first seen because this is the only way that symptoms can occur. There is a male preponderence.

Squamous carcinoma of the nasal vestibule typically occurs in elderly men. In most cases the disease is localized (6% node positive). The nasal vestibule is rather exceptional, with a cutaneous surface functioning as a lin-

Table 19.1 T Classification and stage groupings of the paranasal sinuses

T	Primary tumour
Maxillary sinus	
T_1	Tumour limited to the antral mucosa with no erosion or destruction of bone
T_2	Tumour causing bone erosion or destruction, except for the posterior wall, including extension into hard palate and/or middle nasal meatus
T_3	Tumour invades any of the following: bone of posterior wall of maxillary sinus, subcutaneous tissues, skin of cheek, floor of medial wall of orbit
T_4	Tumour invades orbital contents beyond the floor or medial wall including apex and/or any of the following: cribriform plate, base of skull, nasopharynx, sphenoid sinus, frontal sinus
Ethmoid sinus	
*T_1	Tumour confined to ethmoid with or without bone erosion
*T_2	Tumour extends into nasal cavity
*T_3	Tumour extends to anterior orbit and/or maxillary sinus
*T_4	Tumour with intracranial extension, orbital extension including apex, involving sphenoid and/or frontal sinus and/or skin of nose

Stage groupings			
Stage 0	T_{is}	N_0	M_0
Stage I	T_1	N_0	M_0
Stage II	T_2	N_0	M_0
Stage III	T_1	N_1	M_0
	T_2	N_1	M_0
	T_3	N_0, N_1	M_0
*Stage IVA	T_4	N_0, N_1	M_0
	Any T	N_2	M_0
*Stage IVB	Any T	N_3	M_0
*Stage IVC	Any T	Any N	M_1

*New inclusion.

ing rather than a covering. The tendency for an indolent natural history is reflected in survival rates of 80%. It responds to both excision and radiotherapy and even some node-positive patients are long-term survivors.

Carcinoma of the columella, in contrast, is one of the most aggressive forms of nasal cancer (Mignogna *et al.*, 1995). Although most are squamous, basal cell lesions and melanomas are also described here. Recurrence rates are high and regrowths often cause bony destruction.

Direct spread of antroethmoid tumours

■ Antral to:
- nasal cavity
- ethmoid
- orbit via the inferior orbital fissure
- soft tissues of the cheek by erosion of the anterior wall
- palate or alveolar ridge through the dental foramina
- buccal sulcus
- infratemporal fossa
■ Ethmoid to:
- maxillary antrum
- orbit
- nose
- sphenoid by direct spread
- anterior fossa through the fovea or the cribriform plate

Dissemination of antroethmoid tumours

In 5% of patients with antroalveolar or antroethmoid tumours there is a lymphadenopathy at presentation. Not every node, however, contains tumour, because if the soft tissues of the face are affected, some may be inflammatory. If an ethmoidal tumour has metastasized to the neck nodes then the patient is incurable, but if tumour of the lower part of the maxillary antrum has metastasized then the patient has a small chance of cure.

One in three patients ultimately dies of metastases, the most common sites being the abdominal viscera, the lungs and the bones. As with other head and neck squamous carcinomas, the eventual cumulative rate of second primary tumour development is such that one patient in five will develop a second primary, usually in the bronchus.

Nasal neoplasms: immunohistochemistry

■ Melanoma: S-100; Vimentin; HMB-45
■ Esthesioneuroblastoma: sustentacular pattern S-100; neuroendocrine markers
■ Lymphoma: common leucocyte antigen
■ Muscle derived: muscle-pecific actin and desmin

Tumours of minor salivary glands

The adenoid cystic carcinoma and the mucoepidermoid carcinoma can occur in the nasal sinuses. Adenoid cystic carcinomas showing solid areas of malignant cells, rather than the classic Swiss-cheese pattern, are more malignant. Vascular invasion is more common, distant metastases are more frequent and death is more likely. Perineural invasion is said to occur and there is ample scope for this in the nasal sinuses via the infraorbital nerve, the maxillary nerve, the greater palatine nerve and the sphenopalatine foramen. They can also spread intracranially through the olfactory nerves and in the pterygoid space through the posterior dental nerves.

Sarcomas

Osteogenic sarcoma presents as an enlarging, firm mass that is rock hard on palpation. It is clearly seen radiologically. Surgical excision may be made difficult by extension to the skull base. The 5 year survival is in the range of 10–20%. Chondrosarcoma occurs in grades 1–3 pathologically. It is a very rare septal lesion and it can be difficult to distinguish the lowest grade from a chondroma. Pathological ring-form calcifications can produce a pathognomic appearance on computed tomography (CT). Magnetic resonance imaging (MRI) tends to produce a low-intensity image on T_1 weighting and a high-intensity image on T_2 weighting (Rassekh *et al.*, 1996). Soft-tissue sarcomas, particularly rhabdomyosarcoma, may occur in the sinonasal area, and are dealt with in Chapter 25. Malignant fibrous histiocytoma can arise in areas of previous bone disorders, such as Paget's disease and fibrous dysplasia. It has also been reported in patients who have undergone irradiation to the area. It presents as a gradually expanding mass that is hard on palpation and often difficult to differentiate from an osteogenic sarcoma. If it invades the skull base it becomes non-resectable.

Adenocarcinoma

These are uncommon tumours except in people working in the hardwood industry. They are also related to isopropyl alcohol and chrome inhalation. Inhaled dust particles will travel along the middle turbinate and larger particles will be deposited there, resulting in delayed mucociliary transport. Adenocarcinoma has the same bone-erosive properties as squamous carcinoma and presents in the same way. The metastatic rate to lymph nodes is identical. Histologically, adenocarcinomas are best classified into high grade and low grade.

High-grade adenocarcinoma has a bad prognosis, with 80% of patients ultimately dying of their disease, in contrast to low grade, which is eminently curable in at least 90% of patients (Cawte *et al.*, 1997). Low-grade lesions present in the sixth decade with nasal obstruction. Higher grade lesions present with more pain and deformity, as might be expected, and with a higher age and male preponderance (perhaps for occupational reasons).

Malignant melanoma

Malignant melanomas comprise about 1% of nasal and paranasal sinus cancers. Histologically, there is no relationship to Clark's skin classification. Origin from the sinus mucosa is uncommon. This is fortunate, because the survival of patients with melanoma of the sinuses is almost zero, whereas a reasonable response rate can be expected from treating nasal melanoma. Amelanotic melanomas quite frequently present as unilateral polyps, emphasizing the importance of sending all polypoidal material for pathological examination. The biological behaviour of nasal melanomas is totally unpredictable. Some can be removed never to reappear, while others progress relentlessly to widespread disseminated disease and death in a few months. Another group of melanomas responds to initial therapy and appears to be held in check by a competent immune system for many years until they also recur.

Sinonasal malignant melanoma

- Most commonly from septum/lateral nasal wall
- Slight male preponderance
- Peak age fifth to eighth decade
- More frequent in Orientals, notably Japanese
- 50% 3 year survival but an almost 0% 10 year survival line.
- Present as grey, blue or black polypoidal swellings
- Only 5% are secondary deposits from cutaneous lesions
- Regional satellites frequent
- Fewer than 40% will have a neck node
- Treatment in less fit patients should not be overzealous

The generally poor prognosis could, however, be due to a number of factors: non-specific symptoms, delay in diagnosis, older age group with ineffective immune systems, rich vascular and lymphatic system of mucosa, anatomical constraints of the primary site and possibly because it is histologically more aggressive. Discrete lesions should undergo wide local excision, usually via a lateral rhinotomy. If the peripheral margins are histologically clear, then a policy of wait and see should be adopted.

The less common sinus lesions tend to present late and excision thus requires radical surgery. This includes partial or total maxillectomy, with or without orbital exenteration if there is frank orbital involvement. In a frail, elderly patient, however, a simple debulking procedure via a lateral rhinotomy may be justified as palliation without unacceptable morbidity, because almost 85% relapse locally irrespective of treatment.

Elective radiation therapy (neck and/or primary site) improves the local–regional control rate but the impact on survival rate is not known. For patients wishing to avoid mutilating surgery there is a place for high-dose palliative radiotherapy, which also has a role in patients with symptomatic metastatic spread. Induced hyperthermia may enhance tumour response to radiation. Combination chemotherapy and immunotherapy have been used to treat mucosal melanomas. There are only a few studies suggesting some benefit, but there have been no randomized controlled trials (see also Chapter 25).

Esthesioneuroblastoma

This is also known as an olfactory neuroblastoma or neuroendocrine tumour, and until recently was rarely described. It resembles an anaplastic carcinoma and may remain undiagnosed unless the pathologist uses special tumour markers. The tumour arises in the upper part of the nasal cavity from stem cells of neural crest origin which differentiate into olfactory sensory cells. It is best regarded as one of the primitive neuroectodermal tumours. When the biopsy shows large nests of characteristic cells separated into compartments with rosette formation the histological diagnosis is easy, but sometimes the tissue provides only sheets of densely packed uniform round cells and it is these that are mistaken for undifferentiated carcinoma. Further clues to its nature include fibrillar intracellular background and marked microvascularity, with round or fusiform cells about the size of a lymphocyte.

Esthesioneuroblastoma

- Only 400 cases reported in the world literature
- Presents with nasal obstruction and a mass
- Differs from sympathetic neuroblastoma as all ages are affected
- Urinary vanillylmandelic acid and homovanillic acid, usually undetectable
- Two age peaks, around 20 and 50 years
- Term 'neuroendocrine tumour' proposed for those in the older age group
- 20 year old peak, less local recurrence, more metastasis
- 50 year old peak, more local recurrence, less metastasis

Esthesioneuroblastoma is a slow-growing tumour which may become very large and destructive and by its very nature must be regarded as involving the cribriform plate. A clinical staging has been proposed: group A tumours are confined to the nasal cavity, group B to the nasal cavity and one or more paranasal sinuses and group C tumours extend beyond these limits (Irish *et al.*, 1997). It is, however, difficult to estimate the spread of these tumours and to apply this system of staging.

Lymphoreticular neoplasms

Extramedullary plasmacytoma occurs usually in the head and neck. It is usually solitary and should be regarded as a tumour of well-differentiated B-lymphocytes. It replaces rather than invades tissue. Only 20% progress to generalized multiple myelomatosis.

Non-Hodgkin's lymphoma

Advances in immunocytochemical phenotyping and molecular genetics have resulted in the abolition of terms such as lethal midline granuloma or lymphomatoid granulomatosis (Cleary and Batsakis, 1994). Such terms originated because the lymphomatous infiltrate tends to be

mixed with an angiocentric alignment. Unlike Wegener's granuloma, however, although the local lesion can be very destructive, the patients are not ill and start with very mild symptoms. Most sinonasal T-cell lymphomas may be categorized as angiocentric immunoproliferative lesions.

In the West, sinonasal lymphomas are among the rarest (<0.5%) of the extranodal lymphomas, but in Asia they represent the second most frequent group, with a vast majority of T cell lesions (Liang *et al.*, 1995). In children also, extranodal lymphomas are more common overall (60% of non-Hodgkin's lymphoma) and those in the nose and oropharynx tend to have median age of only 5 years.

Nasal T-cell lymphoma

- Median age 50 years
- Male preponderance
- Worse prognosis than lymphoma in Waldeyer's ring
- Most have no other evidence of lymphoma
- Adverse prognostic factors
  - Asian patients, although even Western patients have only 50% survival
  - age > 60 years
  - advanced Ann Arbor stage
  - presence of B symptoms
- Express the T-cell markers CD2, CD45RO, CD43
- Associated with Epstein–Barr virus in all populations

B-cell lymphomas predominate in the paranasal sinuses and in Waldeyer's ring. The maxillary and ethmoid sinuses are most often involved and many patients have a long history.

Malignant neurogenous tumours

A number of different rare types of neural tumour are described involving the nose, including paraganglioma (Nguyen *et al.*, 1995) and schwannoma (Johnson *et al.*, 1996) (see Chapter 25).

Clinical features of sinonasal malignancy

History

- Antral
  - nasal obstruction
  - epistaxis
  - infraorbital anaesthesia
  - toothache
  - facial swelling
  - facial pain
  - trismus
- Ethmoid
  - nasal obstruction
  - epistaxis
  - proptosis or diplopia

Examine the patient with suspected sinus neoplasia for

- Fullness/numbness of the cheek
- Ptosis (Horner's syndrome).
- Proptosis and ophthalmoplegia (ophthalmologist)
- Evidence of tumour in the nose, nasopharynx, or mouth
- Loose teeth or ill-fitting dentures
- Persistent oroantral fistula
- Numbness of the hard palate (greater palatine nerve)
- Trismus
- Evidence of 9th and 10th cranial nerve palsies in the laryngopharynx
- Palpable disease on the hard palate, buccal sulcus or anterior antrum
- Lymphadenopathy

Investigations

Radiology

CT radiology is vital to define the site and extent of the disease in order to plan treatment. A CT of the upper neck and possibly a CT chest screen should be included in the protocol. Nearly every patient will show bone destruction. The critical areas are the cribriform plate, the fovea, the posterior wall of the maxillary sinus, the optic foramen, the medial orbit and the sphenoid sinus. This is best delineated with both coronal and axial scanning, the use of contrast and high-contrast bone algorithm images to depict questionable bone–tumour interfaces. None the less, spread may be overestimated by up to 30% because of surrounding oedema.

MR imaging has advantages over CT in this region for the following reasons.

- It is used to depict soft-tissue extension in the deep face, the intracranial compartment and the orbits.
- It is used in distinguishing tumour from sinusitis, which may require close correlation of T_1, T_2 and post contrast T_1 weighted images (Phillips, 1997).
- The T_1-weighted images of sinusitis show an isointense image, while T_2 and enhancement with T_1 show a high-intensity image (Stankewicz and Girgis, 1993).
- Tumours such as inverted papilloma will also be isointense on a T_1 image with contrast enhancement, but with T_2, tumours are isointense.

Laboratory investigations

If myeloma is suspected, plasma protein electrophoresis is performed and the urine examined for Bence Jones protein. If there is a watery nasal discharge, one should obtain a sample for β2-transferrin estimation to confirm whether it is cerebrospinal fluid (CSF). With olfactory neuroblastoma, it is important to remember that some tumours secrete catecholamines: a urine collection should be analysed before any general anaesthetic.

Biopsy

This is taken endoscopically. Any enlarged node in the neck should be aspirated for cytology or biopsied. A metastatic node may indicate that the patient is incurable; however, not every enlarged node is metastatic.

Treatment policy

Benign tumours

Osteomas of the frontal bone are removed using either a frontoethmoidectomy or preferably an osteoplastic frontal flap. Osteomas of the ethmoids are more difficult to treat and may cause blindness if treated inappropriately. They are best approached with a lateral rhinotomy or, if they are very close to the optic foramen, consideration should be given to a craniofacial resection.

Chondromas should be treated with wide local excision because of the aggressive, recurrent nature of these tumours. Ossifying fibromas and cementomas are easily shelled out and fibro-osseous dysplasia should be treated cosmetically by drilling away the excess tissue.

Intermediate tumours

Transitional cell papillomas tend to recur: after intranasal removal, the recurrence rate is 80%, after Caldwell–Luc 60% and after medial maxillectomy 30%. They are, therefore, best treated aggressively in the first instance with a lateral rhinotomy after the initial diagnostic polypectomy. The propensity to malignancy is not as frequent as was formerly thought, however, and several reports now describe successful endoscopic removal, although this is less successful for lesions with extensive antral disease. A technique is, however, described for transnasal endoscopic medial maxillectomy (Kamel, 1995). Endoscopic resection has the advantages of lack of external scar, shorter hospital stay, lower morbidity and less perioperative blood loss, and endoscopy is now vital in follow-up (Stanciewicz and Girgis, 1993). Endoscopic treatment of recurrences does not preclude later radical resection if required (Homer et al., 1997). Haemangiopericytomas are locally aggressive and should be widely excised, as should meningiomas.

Malignant tumours

- Surgery alone or in combination with radiotherapy is required in the majority of cases.
- Lymphomas are treated by grading and assessment of spread, and then by radiotherapy and chemotherapy (see Chapter 25). Midline reticuloses are treated with radiotherapy and perhaps immunosuppressive drugs such as azothioprine and steroids.
- Chemotherapy may be given as part of triple therapy, e.g. embryonal rhabdomyosarcoma, in combination with radiotherapy e.g. disseminated lymphoma, or for

palliation, e.g. poorly differentiated squamous cell carcinoma with disseminated disease.
■ Topical chemotherapy [5-fluorouracil (5-FU)] combined with repeated surgical debulking has been advocated for squamous cell carcinoma and adenocarcinoma in two centres but their results have not been replicated elsewhere.
■ Endoscopic resection may have a palliative role

Before treating any patient with a malignant sinus tumour it should be remembered that about half are incurable. This must not, however, lead to a policy of despair because if the tumour is not removed it will fungate into the mouth or orbit, causing a far worse deformity than any operation.

> *Causes of incurability*
>
> ■ Involvement of the nasopharynx and widespread intracranial and pterygoid involvement
> ■ Poor surgical risk
> ■ Distant metastases
> ■ Refusal to undergo surgery

Three out of 10 patients eventually lose their eye, a subject of much emotion. Too often the cure is compromised by leaving the eye, which is understandable as both surgeon and patient are loathe to sacrifice an eye that still functions normally. The dangers of keeping the eye, however, must be realized because the tumour will almost certainly recur and the eye will then be useless.

Involvement of the pterygoids is difficult to treat. Tumour here cannot be eradicated according to oncological principles. Attempts have been made to enlarge the surgical access to this area with infratemporal fossa approaches but it is still not an oncological operation. It is, however, better to make an attempt to clear the pterygoids rather than to leave the tumour to grow uncontrolled at this site.

Young people with undifferentiated tumours of the maxillary sinus are a special problem. If it is truly an undifferentiated carcinoma, then they are never cured by surgery and the treatment may be worse than the disease. They should, therefore, only be treated with radiotherapy. Before deciding on a treatment policy, the surgeon must to talk to the patient and the family. It is at times impossible to treat the nose or sinuses without severe disfigurement. This disfigurement may be coped with by the patient but if it is not, then the patient has not been helped. It is often impossible for the patient to perceive what he or she will look like after one of these operations or what it will entail. The surgeon, however, must do the utmost to ensure that informed consent has been given by the patient and family.

The surgeon then involves colleagues. It is important to give the prosthodontist at least 1 week to do any work necessary for the initial operation. The oncologist should meet the patient before the operation so that the transition to radiotherapy after surgery can be smooth. The patient should be examined by an ophthalmologist

to determine any clinical involvement of the orbit and, if a craniofacial operation is to be performed, then a neurosurgeon should at least be consulted.

There are now basically only three operations that are carried out for cancer of the maxillary and ethmoid sinuses: lateral rhinotomy, partial maxillectomy and craniofacial resection.

For squamous carcinoma, it is sometimes possible to perform a partial maxillectomy leaving the orbital-contents. It is never possible to do this for an adenocarcinoma because it involves the ethmoids. A squamous carcinoma involving the ethmoids should be subject to a craniofacial approach. The clearance margins should be somewhat wider for an adenocarcinoma. The periosteum of the orbit is frequently resistant to tumour growth and, although the patient should always give permission for an orbital exenteration before a craniofacial approach, it is sometimes possible to keep the orbit and merely remove the orbital periosteum in one area.

The treatment of malignant melanoma should be tailored to the tumour. If it lies discretely on a turbinate, a wide local excision should be performed and, if the periphery is clear of tumour, then a wait-and-see policy should be adopted. If it presents as polyps, a lateral rhinotomy should be the initial approach with permission to proceed to whatever resection seems appropriate in the light of the findings. If a decision is made to treat a patient with metastatic neck nodes, a radical neck dissection should be carried out, together with the primary excision, realizing that there is no possibility of an incontinuity resection. Several series report no long-term survivors from the disease (Gaze *et al.*, 1990; Spiro *et al.*, 1995).

The results of treatment of lymphoma of the nasal cavity using radiotherapy with or without chemotherapy in 21 patients showed a median survival of only 5.8 months and a 5 year survival of 24% (Yu *et al.*, 1997). Others quote 30–60% 5 year survival and Yu's group stresses the importance of adequate assessment to exclude infradiaphragmatic disease at the outset.

Esthesioneuroblastoma

Esthesioneuroblastoma is radiosensitive and adjuvant irradiation should be considered. There is some evidence that local control is considerably better following craniofacial resection, even if there is no obvious intracranial involvement.

Adjuvant therapy

Every patient who has a maxillectomy should have postoperative radiotherapy. If the eye has been preserved, appropriate steps should be taken to protect it. After 4 weeks, the cavity should be in good enough condition for the oncologist to apply a full dose to the area. The advantage of carrying out the operation first is that special attention can be given to areas where tumour clearance was minimal.

Chemotherapy has little place in the management of squamous or adenocarcinoma. It may be used for melanoma but its main place is in the management of lymphoma. The Japanese and the Dutch have described the use of 5-FU cream as an adjuvant therapy (Knegt *et al.*, 1985). They perform a debulking tumour operation and follow it by radiotherapy. The cavity is then packed with 5-FU on a weekly basis. Very careful debridement is carried out and packing the cavity is continued for several weeks.

Technique of nasal and sinus procedures

Operations on the skin around the nose

These are dealt with in Chapter 21.

Total rhinectomy

This operation is performed for squamous carcinoma that affects the skin of the external nose including the columella and the vestibule. The latter tumours may involve both the upper lip and the premaxilla. The excision to remove the nose involves taking as wide a margin as is possible to facilitate clearance. It is important to leave some or all of the nasal bones (if possible) both for contour, and to facilitate the placement of osseointegrated implants at the piriform aperture. These should be covered by a flap of unfolded external skin. The mucosa of the nose is stitched to the skin edges or alternatively a skin graft (split or full thickness) can be used. Occasionally, part of the internal lining of the nose (including the septum) is removed as well. The cavity is packed postoperatively using Whitehead's varnish. If the tumour involves either the upper lip and the premaxilla, then the resection includes these areas as well. The premaxilla reconstruction is with a prosthesis and the lip excision usually involves a two-thirds resection and reconstruction with bilateral pericular crescentic advancement. This is discussed in Chapter 15.

Lateral rhinotomy/medial maxillectomy

Anaesthesia

The patient should be anaesthetized with an oroendotracheal tube in a 15° head-up position. The eyes are protected during the operation by a temporary tarsorrhaphy and the wound area is infiltrated with 1% lignocaine with 1:200 000 adrenaline.

Incision

The incision, usually ascribed to Moure (who described it in 1902), was first described by Michaux in 1848 and begins midway between the medial canthus and the bridge of the nose, at the level of the upper border of the pupil; it then continues downwards in the nasomaxillary groove and curves medially below the lower ala to the midline at the columella; it does not routinely continue through the upper lip (Fig. 19.2) although it may be

extended to divide the lip, or superiorly on to the glabellar region if a craniofacial resection is planned.

Specific complications of lateral rhinotomy
■ Early complications
– haemorrhage
– blepharitis
– lid oedema
– wound infection
– cerebrospinal fluid leak
– meningitis
■ Late complications
– crusting: treated by frequent removal and saline/ bicarbonate douches
– epiphora: usually temporary as an effective dacrocystorhinostomy has been made
– diplopia eiplopia
– telecanthus
– cosmetic: alar lift, vestibular stenosis and webbing
– facial parasthesia
– frontonasal recess obstruction, with secondary mucocoele

The incision is made with a knife down to bone, and then the soft tissues are elevated from the anterior wall of the antrum laterally with a large periosteal elevator but, as far as possible, the periosteum remains attached to the nasal bones. The two flaps are held apart with a self-retaining retractor and/or a stay suture in the ala (Fig. 19.2). The periosteum is elevated, and if required the lacrimal sac displaced laterally. The medial canthal ligament may be partially detached and the anterior ethmoid vessels clipped.

An alternative incision that is becoming increasingly acceptable is the midfacial degloving approach. In the 15° head-up position, the buccogingival sulcus and nasal vestibules are infiltrated with 1% lignocaine with 1:200 000 adrenaline bilaterally, and bilateral temporary tarsorrhaphies are fashioned. An incision is made in the gingivolabial sulcus straight down to bone, linking the two maxillary tuberosities, and the soft tissues are elevated over the nasal spine from below (Fig. 19.3).

Then, bilateral intercartilaginous incisions are made, together with a full septal transfixion incision. The circumvestibular release is completed by using sharp dissection laterally and across the floor of the nose to link the lateral edge of the intercartilaginous incision with the base of the transfixion incision. Deepening the dissection

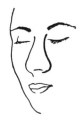

Figure 19.2 Moure's incision.

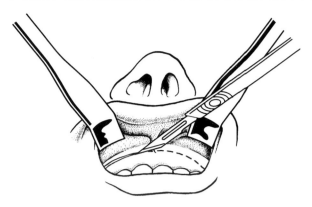

Figure 19.3 Bilateral sublabial incision elevated.

across the floor links the incisions to the buccogingival incision (see Fig. 19.4).

With good retraction, the facial tissues are elevated from the underlying bone to the frontoethmoid suture line in the midline (the infraorbital nerves more laterally). The lower lateral cartilages are elevated with the soft tissue, while the upper laterals are left attached to the piriform aperture. The access is good, a facial scar is avoided and healing is good. Early postoperative oedema is minimized by administering 40–125 mg of methyl prednisolone towards the end of the procedure, but patients should be warned of the specific complications. Vestibular stenosis is minimized by meticulous opposition of the skin edges with 4/0 catgut. A bipedicled flap of lateral nasal wall mucosa has been described to reduce further the risk of stenosis.

Complications of midfacial degloving

- Facial bruising
- Malar paraesthesiae
- Vestibular stenosis
- Crusting of the cavity
- Thickening of the glabella
- Telecanthus
- Heterotopia
- Nasal deformity (over-removal of the frontal process of the maxilla)

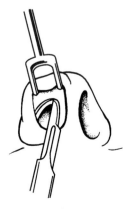

Figure 19.4 Nasal elements of the midfacial degloving incision.

Performance of the medial maxillectomy

The medial maxillectomy is an *en bloc* resection of the lateral nasal wall, including the bone at the lateral and suprolateral aspect of the piriform aperture, the medial 30% of the orbital floor and the orbital rim, together with the pars papyracea and the lacrimal fossa, which is described below (Schramm and Myers, 1978; Har-El and Lucente, 1996). An alternative is to preserve the inferomedial orbital rim and the walls of the piriform aperture, with either resection deep to this preserved frame of bone, or with its removal, replacement and miniplate fixation at the end of the procedure. The cosmetic advantages of these latter manoeuvres are doubtful.

Management of the nasolacrimal duct

Before the resection the surgeon must decide what to do with the nasolacrimal duct. It is often said that the most important thing is to identify and formally to transect it at the level of the orbital floor, but some authors describe either drilling it out or stenting it. A compromise is to transect the duct 10–15 mm distal to the periorbita, thereby freeing up the orifice of the canal and then inserting a pointed, e.g. no. 11, blade down the canal to transect it. The duct is then opened by two opposing 4 mm cuts and the edges are folded back on to the proximal duct or periorbita with 5/0 absorbable sutures (Har-El and Lucente, 1996). The lacrimal sac is dissected from the fossa and transected. This manoeuvre gives less postoperative epiphora than trying to probe or preserve the nasolacrimal duct, as it effectively fashions a large dacrocystorhinostomy.

Elevation and rotation of the nasal bone. The frontoethmoid suture, an important landmark that indicates the superior limit of resection, is identified. The anterior ethmoidal artery may be clipped at this point, but if possible the posterior ethmoidal artery is exposed and retained as a landmark. Before performing the excision osteotomies, rhinoplasty-type cuts are made to allow reflection and preservation of the nasal bone, thus minimizing postoperative deformity (Fig. 19.5). A low lateral osteotomy is followed by a superior one with a 2 mm

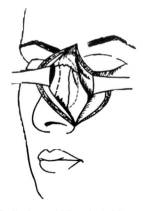

Figure 19.5 Preliminary 'rhinoplasty'-type osteotomies of the nasal bones.

chisel, 2 mm superior to the medial canthal ligament. The 2 mm chisel is also used to perform a perforating medial osteotomy with the aim of reflecting the nasal bone without detachment.

Creation of a defect in the anterior maxilla. It is helpful at this stage to perforate the anterior wall of the maxilla and enlarge the opening with Hajek's forceps. This manoeuvre in particular allows visualization of the posterior wall of the antrum when forming the definitive osteotomy cuts. In addition, the thick bone-nibbling forceps are the most efficient tool to divide the thick bone of the medial infraorbital rim, extending the access into the lacrimal fossa, but preserving the infraorbital nerve canal.

Removal of the specimen. Using a 9 mm osteotome, the surgeon makes a cut along the floor of the nose and maxillary antrum, extending back to the level of the posterior antral wall (region of the pterygoid plates, Fig. 19.6). The orbital contents are retracted laterally. A superior

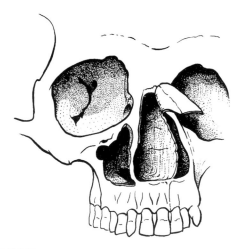

Figure 19.6 Access anterior antrostomy

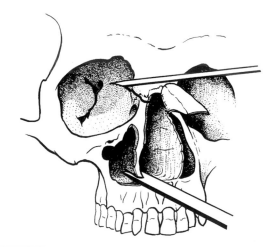

Figure 19.7 Superior and inferior resection osteotomies.

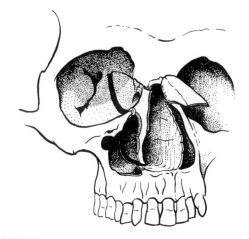

Figure 19.8 Intermediate osteotomy in medial orbit.

osteotomy cut is placed just below the frontoethmoid suture and extended to the region of the posterior ethmoidal artery (the optic nerve will be 6–10 mm posterior to this) (Figure 19.7). The osteotome may be used gently to lever the specimen on the frontal bone. Alternatively, the original nibbled cut in the medial infraorbital rim is now linked superomedially with the posterior end of the upper osteotomy (Fig. 19.8). The lacrimal sac is mobilized laterally.

Final mobilization of the specimen is as follows:

- introduce a 2 cm osteotome into the antrostomy, towards the medial posterior antral wall. This osteotome is elevated to the level of the upper cut and pushed medially
- remove and reintroduce the wide osteotome transnasally to the posterior choana, impact it on the anterior face of the sphenoid and push it laterally
- use heavy curved scissors, introduced first through the inferior cut, then the superior, flush with the anterior face of the sphenoid to divide the vertical posterior remaining attachments. The specimen is removed and haemostasis secured (clamping/cautery).

The sphenoid and remaining ethmoid cells are checked, if necessary with separate biopsies. Opening and suturing the lacrimal sac at this stage further reduces the risk of epiphora. Cannulation of the inferior lacrimal punctum will aid sac identification. The nose is packed with bismuth iodoform paraffin paste (BIPP) and the incisions closed with 3/0 chromic catgut and 5/0 Nurolon. Plaster of Paris tapes or splint will aid cosmetic recovery.

Maxillectomy

Preparation

The patient's face is prepared in the usual way but the eyebrows are not shaved because they would regrow in an irregular fashion. The patient is laid supine on the

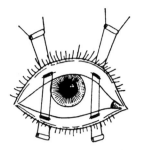

Figure 19.9 Temporary tarsorrhaphy.

table with the head extended. A temporary tarsorrhaphy (Fig. 19.9) is fashioned with 5/0 silk.

Two sutures are inserted, taking a bite of the lower lid and then a bite of the upper lid opposite to the initial stitch. Then the needle is threaded through a piece of thin red rubber catheter to stop the stitch cutting into the upper lid. The needle is next inserted into the upper lid, then the lower lid, passed through another red rubber catheter and tied. A tracheostomy (is required) is performed in the usual way and general anaesthesia continued via this route.

Incision

A Weber–Fergusson skin incision is marked out (Fig. 19.10), starting at the philtrum of the lip on the operative side and going up to the columella.

In some patients a complete Weber–Fergusson incision is not necessary so that part of the incision below the eye can be omitted (this in incision is called the Fergusson incision). Midfacial degloving is an alternative. The incision continues round the margin of the ala of the nose and up the lateral border of the nose to the medial corner of the eye, turning laterally in a rounded fashion to go 5 mm below the lid margin on the lower lid. If the surgeon goes too near the margin of the lower lid, the

patient may develop ectropion; too far away, he or she may develop lymphoedema. The incision is continued to just past the lateral canthus. If the eye is to be sacrificed, a circumferential incision is made through the conjunctiva, to preserve the lids.

Critical suture points are marked, taking great care to mark the vermilion border. An incision is made with a knife right down to the bone, taking the incision inside the mouth along the gingivobuccal sulcus as far back as the tuberosity of the maxilla, round the tuberosity and across just short of the midline at the junction of the hard and soft palates. It runs forward just lateral to the midline to the first incisior. (This part of the soft-tissue division may be done as a single step with the bony division.) The cheek flap including the buccinator muscle, is elevated with cutting diathermy but the orbicularis oculi muscle is left intact around the eye.

Excision

If the patient has upper teeth, the upper central incisor on the side of the operation is removed. With a knife, a stab wound is made into the nasopharynx at the junction of the hard and soft palate in the midline and a pair of right-angled forceps passed through this. A Gigli saw blade is passed through the nostril on the involved side, picked up with the forceps and brought out through the mouth. The hard palate is divided longitudinally through the floor of the nasal cavity, just lateral to the nasal septum, with the Gigli saw. Then an incision is made across the soft tissues of the posterior edge of the hard palate to the tuberosity of the maxilla, meeting the incision that was originally made in the gingivobuccal sulcus. This detaches the soft palate from the hard palate. With a Stryker saw or a fissure burr, the nasal process of the maxilla is divided, starting in the piriform aperture, and the cut continues just below the orbital rim around to the pterygomaxillary fissure (Fig. 19.11).

The lateral wall of the nose is mobilized by dividing between the superior and inferior turbinates using stout Mayo scissors. In order to gain access to the pterygoid space, the temporalis muscle is divided from its

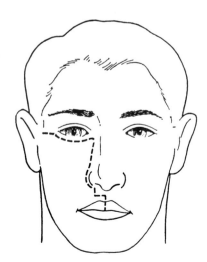

Figure 19.10 Weber–Fergusson incision.

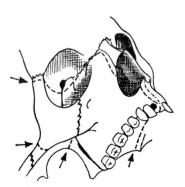

Figure 19.11 Maxillectomy: sites of division of bony struts.

attachment to the coronoid process of the mandible and the process at its origin transected from the ramus of the mandible. An osteotome is placed in the pterygomaxillary fissure and the pterygoids are divided from the maxilla, which can then be removed, cutting the soft-tissue attachments with Mayo scissors. Clearance of tumour is confirmed by taking a frozen section.

If the patient does not have dentures, the cavity is packed with BIPP and stay sutures are inserted from the palate remnant to the buccal mucosa to keep the pack in place. If he or she has an upper denture, or if a partial upper denture has been made prior to the operation, the pack can be kept in place with this.

Aftercare

- General care is given.
- The pack is removed in 10–14 days.
- A temporary denture is made by the prosthodontist from a provisional impression.
- The final prosthesis can be a one-piece or a two-piece model. With the latter then the obturator portion is kept in place either with a pivot fixation or with magnets. If it is a one-piece model, then the obturator portion should be hollow for lightness.

Complications

- General complications may occur.
- Notching of the lip is caused by an improper closure and atrophy of the orbicularis oris muscle. If it occurs then it can be corrected with a Z-plasty.
- If the obturator is too large it can create granulomas on originally bare areas in the cavity. These can look like recurrences and should always be removed for biopsy. If they are granulomas, then the obturator needs to be adjusted.

Reconstruction

In recent years a wide range of different methods of reconstruction of the considerable bony and soft tissue defect which results from maxillectomy have been described. Soft tissue free transfer may, for example, be used to reduce the size of the cavity, e.g. by rectus abdominis flap, to assist obturation. The flap may be raised with costal cartilages and these, with pedicled calvarial base, used to form a 'flying buttress' reconstruction (Kyutoku *et al.*, 1999). Rectus abdominis and latissimus dorsi flaps with attached ribs have also been used with a temporalis muscle transposition flap to animate the nasolabial fold and upper lip (Yoza *et al.*, 1997). Alternative methods include a fibula osseocutaneous flap with osseointegrated implants.

Craniofacial resection (Fig. 19.12)

The operation is performed in conjunction with a neurosurgeon.

Anaesthesia

It is important to maintain cerebral circulation and to cause shrinkage of the brain for easy manipulation. The

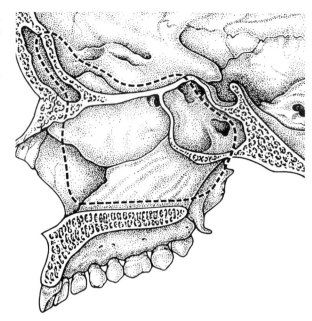

Figure 19.12 Area of sinus tissue usually removed in a craniofacial excision.

patient is given 200 ml of 20% mannitol in 20 min, and also 150 mg hydrocortisone. The arterial pressure is kept at normal or slightly elevated levels. Shrinkage of the brain is also assisted by deliberate hyperventilation.

Incision

The craniotomy can be performed from a bicoronal incision, which gives good access and allows the preparation of a good galeal flap for closure of the defect, but it tends to obstruct the facial incision and takes time to perform. Where the superior extent is limited, a midfacial degloving may be combined with a bicoronal flap, but access to the anterior ethmoid block may be more limited.

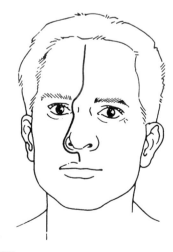

Figure 19.13 Incision for craniofacial resection: lateral rhinotomy incision combined with midline forehead incision.

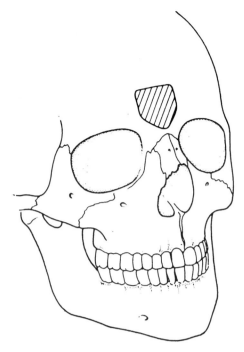

Figure 19.14 Shield-shaped access window cut in frontal bone.

The facial incision may be done with a lateral rhinotomy approach continued up through the medial canthus on to the forehead up to the hairline (Fig. 19.13). This allows retraction of the frontal bone. It is easier and quicker but it is more difficult to create a satisfactory galeal flap compared with the bicoronal incision. An alternative is to perform a cross-brow supraorbital incision, being careful to repair the wound so as to avoid interruption of the natural brow contour.

The Weber–Fergusson incision is required only if a complete maxillectomy is performed.

Craniotomy

Whichever incision is made, a shield-shaped segment is removed from the frontal bone (Fig. 19.14). Care is taken to make this segment come right down to the floor

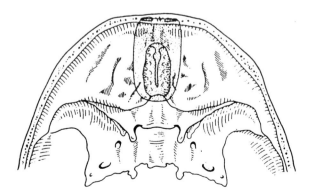

Figure 19.15 Superior view of anterior cranial fossa, showing extent of resection.

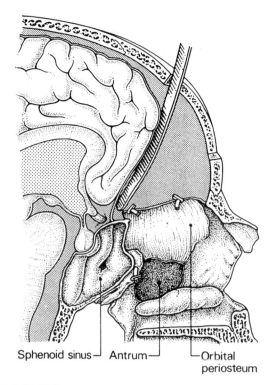

Sphenoid sinus — Antrum — Orbital periosteum

Figure 19.16 Frontal lobe retraction giving access to the fovea and cribriform plate.

of the anterior fossa so that one is not working over a ledge (Figs 19.14 and 19.15). Care is also taken not to cut the dura or to tear it, especially in older patients. It is better not to tear the sagittal sinus at this point or else the bleeding can be very troublesome. The dura is lifted off the cribriform plate and fovea back to the optic foramen, and the optic nerves can then be visualized (Fig. 19.16).

The frontal lobe is then retracted and operability assessed. An alternative craniotomy can be created low across the brow level and through the frontal sinus.

Further surgery is contraindicated if there is tumour extension

- into the frontal lobes
- beyond the posterior margin of the cribriform plate
- to involve both optic nerves
- laterally outside the boundaries of the fovea.

If the operation is to proceed then the maxilla is resected, in keeping with the extent of the tumour. It may be possible to retain the palate and even the orbital floor. The surgeon proceeds as described in the first part of the maxillectomy. With an osteotome, he or she cuts up to the frontonasal suture line and then along the frontoethmoidal suture. With a Gigli saw, the zygomatic arch is divided, as is the orbital floor through the inferior orbital fissure. The maxilla is disarticulated from the pterygoid plates or the pterygoid plates can be removed along with the maxilla.

Attention is then returned to the anterior fossa, and cuts are made through the fovea on each side and through the posterior part of the cribriform plate. Cutting through the anterior ethmoid cells allows the whole segment to be removed in a block.

Posterior extension makes *en bloc* resection difficult. Drilling away the posterior sinus wall exposes the greater palatine artery, which can be controlled with bipolar diathermy. Limited areas of pterygoid muscle involvement can be taken *en bloc*, but significant involvement may even require partial mandibulectomy (Donald, 1997). In addition, the posterior tumour margin may lie close to the internal carotid artery. Once the pterygoid muscles and plates have been cleared, the body of the sphenoid is well visualized. Tumours below the skull base may be approached via a lip split and mandibular swing. Alternatively, a transparotid approach to the infratemporal fossa may be extended superiorly, or a craniofacial disassembly and reconstruction of the facial skeleton performed (Nuss *et al.*, 1991).

Management of the eye

In recent years ocular preservation has been more and more successfully applied, even in cases of bony involvement. For low-grade tumours, e.g. fibrosarcoma, even areas of periorbital and orbital fat can be adequately resected and the rest of the ocular apparatus spared (Donald, 1997). If however, obvious extension through the periosteum is seen during the early part of the maxillectomy, then the eye is included in the resection at this point. If the periosteum is clear along the floor and the ethmoids, one should wait until the specimen has been removed and then take frozen sections from the posterior ethmoid in the area of the optic foramina. If these are clear, and if sufficient support remains laterally for the eye, then it can be preserved; but if the support of the eye is damaged, of if there is tumour in the posterior ethmoids, then the eye is removed at this point.

Closure

The dural defect is closed with the fascia lata graft using 5/0 Nurolon for the repair. The repair is strengthened by cutting a flap of frontalis and galeal aponeurosis, and slipping it under the dura in the anterior fossa. This can be further protected by putting in a cartilage graft from the nasal septum or a bone graft from the iliac crest. The facial wound is sutured meticulously or else there will be oedema around the inferior part of the orbital wound. A BIPP pack is put in place and the oral defect closed with either the patient's own denture or a specially made partial one.

Aftercare

- General care: supine bedrest is required for a few days following craniotomy.
- Antibiotics: because of the danger of meningitis and because the nasal cavity is connected to the anterior fossa, the patient is covered with an antibiotic mixture such as metronidazole (10 days) and co-amoxiclav (3 weeks).

- Neurological observations are made for at least 24 hours
- Anticonvulsants may be used for up to 1 year after the operation.
- Cerebrospinal fluid leak is expected. If the closure has been adequate there should not be a problem and it should seal quite quickly. If it does not, consideration has to be given to inserting a lumbar drain or even regrafting.

Complications of craniofacial resection

- Sudden death can occur if patients mobilize prematurely
- Persistent cerebrospinal fluid leak
- Meningitis
- Venous bleeding
- Convulsions

Radiotherapy techniques for tumours of the nasal cavity and sinuses

The techniques used by the oncologist for treatment of carcinoma of the nasal fossa, maxillary antrum and ethmoid sinuses are essentially the same whether the plan is to use radical radiotherapy alone, or to give preoperative or postoperative treatment. Initial surgery with planned postoperative radiotherapy is usually considered preferable to preoperative radiotherapy. For radiotherapy planning and treatment the patient lies supine, with the head fixed in a neutral position by an individually prepared beam-directing Perspex shell. The mouth is held open by a block to depress the tongue and lower lip which, by keeping them out of the treated volume, diminishes the intraoral acute mucosal reaction. The bite block has a central hole which allows the patient to breathe through the mouth during treatment.

The volume to be treated is determined on the basis of CT and MRI scans and clinical/or surgical assessment. It includes the primary site, areas of known tumour extension and also, because of the difficulties in accurate assessment, other routes of potential local spread. This entails treatment of a block of tissue containing the maxilla on the affected side, including the alveolus, the whole nasal cavity and ethmoid complex, the pterygopalatine fossa and often the orbit. In the unusual case where there is demonstrable nodal spread, the ipsilateral neck should also be irradiated.

Critical structures to be spared

- Contralateral eye
- Brainstem
- Upper cervical cord

Two fields are used for the treatment of antral tumours. The **anterior field** (Fig. 19.17) extends from its upper border at the superior margin of the orbit down to include the hard palate and alveolar ridge. Medially it extends across the midline to the opposite inner canthus, and its lateral border encompasses the gingivobuccal sulcus and

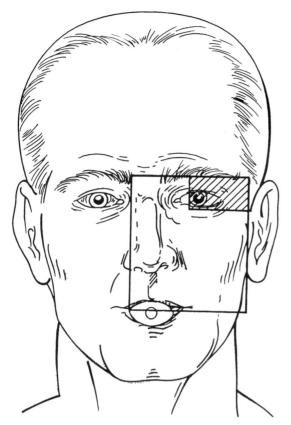

Figure 19.17 Anterior radiotherapy field for treatment of a carcinoma of the left maxillary antrum.

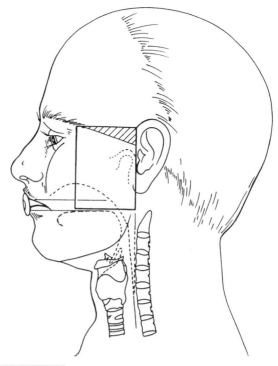

Figure 19.18 Lateral field for the irradiation of the antrum.

cheek. If there is no orbital involvement the ipsilateral cornea, lens and lacrimal gland should be shielded. If it is necessary to treat the orbit, the unpleasant acute corneal reaction can be minimized by cutting a hole in the shell and treating with the patient's eye open. If the soft tissues of the cheek are involved, wax bolus should be applied over this area of the shell to ensure that the skin receives an adequate dose, otherwise the shell may be cut out to minimize the acute skin reaction over the cheek.

The upper and lower limits of the **lateral field** (Fig. 19.18) match those of the anterior field. The lateral field extends posteriorly from the lateral orbital margin, that is behind the anterior chamber of the eye, to the anterior margin of the vertebral bodies, thus including the pterygopalatine fossa and lateral pharyngeal lymph nodes. The upper posterior corner of this field should be blocked, to shield the brainstem. The lateral field should be angled 5–10° posteriorly, to avoid irradiation of the contralateral eye. To be on the safe side, the dose received by the opposite eye should be checked by thermoluminescent dosimetry during the first one or two fractions.

A three–field technique may be preferred for the treatment of central tumours involving the nasal fossa and ethmoid sinuses, or if there is bilateral involvement of the maxillary antra. In this case two lateral opposed fields (wedged thick end anteriorly) and an unwedged anterior field are used. The anterior field may be shaped like an inverted T by blocking the orbits bilaterally if possible.

Megavoltage X-rays (4–6 MV) should be used. A variety of dose fractionation schedules is in current use, the most popular being 50–55 Gy in 20 fractions over 4 weeks or 60–65 Gy in 30–33 fractions over 6–6.5 weeks. For lymphoma, a lower dose of 40 Gy in 20 fractions over 4 weeks is usually adequate.

The principal acute side-effect is mucositis affecting the palate and upper alveolus on the treated side. Care should be taken to maintain oral hygiene and ensure that the patient receives adequate nourishment. Percutaneous gastrostomy (PEG) feeding may be necessary. In addition, the patient should be warned that he or she will lose the hair over the back of the head where the anterior beam exits.

A variety of intracavitary techniques has been described for postoperative irradiation or treatment of small local recurrences. A cast is made of the surgical defect in the maxilla. This is loaded with a suitable radionuclide and worn by the patient for a period calculated to give an appropriate dose. The principal limitation of this method is that there is a rapid fall-off of dose away from the surface of the mould, and so only the relatively superficial tissues are effectively treated.

Controversies in management

Is transitional cell papilloma a premalignant condition?

The problems of evaluating transitional cell papilloma arise from variations in the histology, the sample size and, most importantly, the source of the series. Most reports are from tertiary referral centres which see transitional cell papillomas that have become malignant. If the lesion does not show any focus of malignancy at the time of biopsy, then the chance of later development of a carcinoma is probably only about 1%.

What if the pathologist reports an undifferentiated carcinoma?

Undifferentiated carcinomas are rare. A similar histological picture is produced by lymphomas, amelanotic melanomas, olfactory neuroblastomas and rhabdomyosarcomas. If a report of undifferentiated carcinoma is received, the surgeon should ensure that the pathologist has used tumour markers to determine whether the epidermis really is the origin of the tumour. In this way some apparently untreatable tumours will become treatable.

What if the CT scan shows widespread infiltration of the tumour?

Blockage of the ostia will often lead to fluid accumulation in the sinuses and this cannot be differentiated from tumour by a coronal CT scan. Similarly, extension of tumours through the bony margins will cause surrounding oedema, which again is indistinguishable from tumour. Thus, a CT scan may overestimate tumour spread by as much as 30%. MRI is therefore useful in addition to CT in the staging of sinonasal tumours.

Is there a place for a radical maxillectomy with orbital exenteration instead of a craniofacial approach?

More control can be exerted over the management of the eye from above than from below. Coming from below to go to the posterior ethmoids is inherently a very dangerous procedure; with modern anaesthesia and postoperative care, there is very little morbidity in a craniofacial approach.

What does one do if a prosthodontist is not available?

This is a situation that still occurs in parts of the world. There is usually no problem with oral rehabilitation because there is always somebody in the district who can make an upper denture. At worst, a piece of gutta percha can be moulded into an obturator to sit on top of an ordinary denture. If no eye prosthesis is reconstructed, then the patient should wear a black patch over the eye or a pair of dark glasses.

Is it ever worthwhile rehabilitating the orbit with skin flaps?

A smaller cavity can be created by putting in a flap. A forehead or a sternomastoid flap or nowadays a free latissimus dorsi or radical free flap are commonly used. The latter is preferred since it is less bulky and thus facilitates the use of osseointegration and the subsequent fitting of a prothesis. A similar result, however, can be obtained by leaving the eyelids and suturing them together and grafting the underside. There is thus very little place for flap reconstruction of the orbit to make a prosthesis sit more comfortably.

Preoperative or postoperative radiotherapy?

A pragmatic policy is to use preoperative irradiation where there is doubt about the resectability of the tumour, surgery first for patients with clearly operable lesions and radical radiotherapy alone for patients whose general condition precludes major surgery.

Advantages of preoperative radiotherapy

- By shrinking the tumour, inoperable cancers may be rendered operable
- The magnitude of operation necessary may be reduced
- Reduces the chance that surgical manipulation may cause distant metastasis or local seeding, and is likely to be more effective without the hypoxia which may be caused by tissue disruption during surgery
- Avoids any treatment delay in therapy if wound healing is slow

Disadvantages of preoperative radiotherapy

- Surgical complications may be increased, either directly or through malnutrition
- Patient with a good initial response or unacceptable morbidity may then refuse surgery
- Tumour extent less well defined
- Wound healing may be impaired

Management of tumours of the septum and vestibule

Anterior nasal tumours present as small indolent ulcers. There is often a long diagnostic delay. The septum and the vestibule are lined by cartilage and thin squamous epithelium, and have a rich lymphatic drainage. Thus, 30% have invasion of cartilage and metastatic nodes. Thus a neck dissection may be required and the N_0 neck electively treated in high-risk cases. All histological types of tumour can occur in the area and there is no evidence as to what constitutes best treatment. Most series have been small, and there seems to be no difference in survival between primary surgery, primary radiotherapy or a combined treatment. The overall survival rate is between 20 and 30%. Surgical excision of the area presents a horrendous defect because it usually involves the upper lip. Resection usually involves total rhinectomy and excision of up to two-thirds of the upper lip. A forehead flap may be used if only soft-tissue replacement is required.

Otherwise, the basic reconstruction involves dental prosthetics and osseointegrated nasal replacement, and the lip reconstruction is performed with bilateral perialar crescentic advancement, supplement in rare circumstances by an Abbe flap from the lower lip.

Sinus tumours in children

Most sinus tumours in children are benign. Rhabdomyosarcomas are the most common malignant neoplasm. The former policy of triple therapy comprising wide excision, radiotherapy and chemotherapy has now been superseded. The paediatric oncologist often prefers initial surgery to be a confirmatory biopsy only. This is because surgery does not itself influence outcome, and extensive initial debulking makes it very difficult to assess subsequent clinical and radiological response to non-surgical modalities. Children with parameningeal tumours, e.g. sinonasal or nasopharyngeal rhabdomyosarcomas have a worse prognosis than children with rhabdomyosarcomas at non-parameningeal head and neck sites, e.g. the larynx or the floor of the mouth (see Chapter 25).

Prosthetic problems

Immediately after the excision a temporary obturator made of stent or gutta percha attached to a previously prepared upper denture is placed in the defect. The obturator material can be encouraged to stick to the upper denture by wires set in the upper surface of the denture. Grafting of the cavity is rarely necessary. The obturator should be left for 2 weeks and the denture and obturator should be removed under general anaesthesia. Care should be taken at this point not to split the lip if a Weber–Fergusson incision has been used. An impression is taken of the cavity and thereafter further fittings are conducted in the prosthodontist's clinic. The prosthodontist should try to create as large a prosthesis as possible to keep the facial contour, but small enough for the patient to be able to remove and clean it. The obturator should preferably be hollow for lightness. It can be fixed on to the denture by either studs or magnets or may form an integral part of it.

The eye presents greater difficulty to the prosthodontist. If the orbit is exenterated and no facial skin is removed then the lids are sewn together after excising the eyelashes and the undersurface grafted with a split-thickness skin graft. This creates a shallow depression over which the patient can wear a black patch. Alternatively, the prosthodontist can create a shallow prosthesis containing an artificial eye mounted on spectacle frames. If the eyelids are removed soft-tissue repair can be carried out using pedicled temporalis muscle and skin graft or free tissue transfer. The latter can employ a radial forearm flap with minimal bulk to allow subsequent osseointegration, but if this is not required, then a more bulky flap such as latissimus dorsi or rectus abdominis may be used. Recent advances with osseointegrated systems have considerably improved prosthetic attachments.

References and further reading

Acheson E. D., Cowdell R. H., Hadfield E. and Macbeth R. G. (1968) Nasal cancer in woodworkers in the furniture industry, *BMJ* ii: 587–96.

Atallah N. and Jay M. M. (1981) Osteomas of the paranasal sinuses, *J Laryngol Otol* 95: 291–304.

Baek C. H., Kim K. S. and Kang M. K. (1996) Primary mucosal melanoma of the nasal cavity, *Otolaryngol Head Neck Surg* 115: 582–3.

Billings K. R., Wang M. B., Sercarz J. A. and Fu Y. S. (1995) Clinical and pathologic distinction between primary and metastatic mucosal melanoma of the head and neck, *Otolaryngol Head Neck Surg* 112: 700–6.

Brandwein M. S., Rothstein A., Lawson W., Bodian C. and Urken M. L. (1997) Sinonasal melanoma. A clinicopathological study of 25 cases and literature meta-analysis, *Arch Otolaryngol Head Neck Surg* 123: 290–6.

Bilsky M. H., Kraus D. H., Strong E. W., Harrison L. B., Gutin P. H. and Shah J. P. (1997) Extended anterior craniofacial resection for intracranial extension of malignant tumours, *Am J Surg* 174: 565–8.

Catalano P. J., Brandwein M., Shah D. K., Urken M. L., Lawson W. and Biller H. F. (1996) Sinonasal hemangiopericytomas: a clinicopathologic and immunohistochemical study of seven cases, *Head Neck* 18: 42–53.

Cawte T., Taskin M., Kacker A. and Wahl S. (1997) Low-grade adenocarcinoma of nasal passages, *Otolaryngol Head Neck Surg* 117: 116–9.

Chiu N. T. and Weinstock M. A. (1996) Melanoma of oronasal mucosa. Population-based analysis of occurrence and mortality, *Arch Otolaryngol Head Neck Surg* 122: 985–8.

Cleary K. R. and Batsakis J. G. (1994) Pathology consultation. Sinonasal lymphomas, *Ann Otol Rhinol Laryngol* 103.

Comin C. E., Dini M. and Russo G. L. (1997) Pathology in focus. Oncocytoma of the nasal cavity: report of a case and review of the literature, *J Laryngol Otol* 111: 671–3.

Deitmer T. and Wiener C. (1996) Is there an occupational etiology of inverted papilloma of the nose and sinuses? *Acta Otolaryngol* 116: 762-5.

Edelstein D. R., Liberatore L., Bushkin S. and Han J. C. (1995) Applied anatomy of the posterior sinuses in relation to the optic nerve, trigeminal nerve and carotid artery, *Am J Rhinol* 9: 321–33.

Donald P. J. (1997) Management of sinus malignancy, *Curr Opin Otolaryngol Head Neck Surg* 5: 73–8.

Gaze M. N., Kerr G. R. and Smyth J. F. (1990) Mucosal melanomas of the head and neck: the Scottish experience, *Clin Oncol* 2: 277–83

Harbo G., Grau C., Bundgaard T., Overgaard M., Elbrond O., Sogaard H. and Overgaard J. (1997) Cancer of the nasal cavity and paranasal sinuses. A clinico-pathological study of 277 patients, *Acta Oncol* 36: 45–50.

Harrison D. F. N. (1984) Osseous and fibro-osseous conditions affecting the cranio-facial bones, *Ann Otol Rhinol Laryngol* 93: 199–203.

Har-El G. and Lucente F. E. (1996) Midfacial degloving approach to the nose, sinuses and skull base, *Am J Rhinol* 10: 17–22.

Hasegawa S. L., Mentzel T. and Fletcher C. D. M. (1997) Schwannomas of the sinonasal tract and nasopharynx, *Mod Path* 10: 777–84.

Homer J. J., Jones N. S. and Bradley P. J. (1997) The role of endoscopy in the management of nasal neoplasia, *Am J Rhinol* 11: 41–7.

Howard D. J. and Lund V. J. (1992) The midfacial degloving approach to sinonasal disease, *J Laryngol Otol* 106: 1059–62.

Irish J., Dasgupta R., Freeman J., Gullane P., Gentili F., Brown D. *et al.* (1997) Outcome and analysis of the surgical management of esthesioneuroblastoma, *J Otolaryngol* 26: 1.

Jakobsen M. H., Larsen S. K., Kirkegaard J. and Hansen H. S. (1997) Cancer of the nasal cavity and paranasal sinuses. Prognosis and outcome of treatment, *Acta Oncol* 36: 27–31.

Johnson P. J., Lydiatt D. D., Hollins R. R., Rydlund K. W. and Degenhardt J. A. (1996) Malignant nerve sheath tumour of the nasal septum, *Otolaryngol Head Neck Surg* 115: 132–4.

Kamel R. H. (1995) Intranasal endoscopic medial maxillectomy inverted papilloma, *Laryngoscope* 105: 847–53.

Kazaoka Y., Shinohara A., Yokou K. and Hasegawa T. (1999) Functional reconstruction after total maxillectomy using a fibula osteocutaneous flap with osseointegrated implants, *Plast Reconstr Surg* 103: 1244–6.

Kingdom T. T, Kaplan M. J. (1995) Mucosal melanoma of the nasal cavity and paranasal sinuses, *Head Neck* 17: 184–9.

Knegt P. P., de Jong PC, van Andel JG, de Boer MF, Eykenboom W. and van der Schans E. (1985) Carcinoma of the paranasal sinuses. Results of a prospective pilot study, *Cancer* 56: 57–62.

Kyutoku S., Tsuji H., Inone T., Kawakami, K., Han F. and Ogawa Y. (1999) Experience with the rectus abdominis myocutaneous flap with regularised hard tissue for immediate orbitofacial reconstruction, *Plast Reconstr Surg* 103: 395–402.

Liang R., Todd D., Chan T. K., Chiu E., Lie A., Kwong Y. L. *et al.* (1995) Treatment outcome and prognostic factors for primary nasal lymphoma, *J Clin Oncol* 13: 666–70.

Logsdon M. D., Ha C. S., Kavadi V. S., *et al.* (1997) Lymphoma of the nasal cavity and paranasal sinuses: improved outcome and altered prognostic factors with combined modality therapy, *Cancer* 80: 477–88.

Lund V. J., Howard D. J., Wei W. I. and Cheesman A. D. (1998) Craniofacial resection for tumours of the nasal cavity and paranasal sinuses – a 17 year experience, *Head Neck* 20: 97–105.

Martinez S. A. (1997) Low grade adenocarcinoma of nasal passages, *Otolaryngol Head Neck Surg* 117: 116–19.

Martinez S. A. (1996) Malignant nerve sheath tumour of the nasal septum, *Otolaryngol Head Neck Surg* 115: 132–4.

Manolidis S, and Donald P. J. (1997) Malignant mucosal melanoma of the head and neck: review of the literature and report of 14 patients, *Cancer* 80: 1373–86.

McCary W. S., Levine P. A. and Cantrell R. W. (1996) Preservation of the eye in the treatment of sinonasal malignant neoplasms with orbital involvement: a confirmation of the original treatise, *Arch Otolaryngol Head Neck Surg* 122: 657–9.

Michaels L. (1996) Benign mucosal tumours of the nose and paranasal sinuses, *Semin Diagnos Path* 13: 113–17.

Mignogna F. V. and Garay K. F. (1995) Surgical rescue of recurrent carcinoma of the nasal columella, *Am J Surg* 170: 453–6.

Nguyen Q. A., Gibbs P. M. and Rice D. H. (1995) Malignant nasal paraganglioma: a case report and review of literature, *Otolaryngol Head Neck Surg* 113: 157–61.

Nuss D. W., Janecka I. P. and Sen C. N. (1991) Craniofacial disassembly in the management of skull base tumours, *Otolaryngol Clin North Am* 24: 1465–97.

Ohngren L. G. (1933) Malignant tumours of the maxilloethmoidal region: a clinical study with special reference to the treatment with electrosurgery and irradiation, *Acta Otolaryngol* 19 (Suppl): 1–112.

Osguthorpe J. D. *Sinus neoplasia*, (1994) *Arch Otolaryngol Head Neck Surg* 120: 19–25.

Papadopoulos T., Rasiah K., Thompson J. F., Quinn M. J. and Crothy K. A. (1997) Melanoma of the nose, *Br J Surg* 84: 986–9.

Peralta E. A., Yarington C. T. Glenn M. G. (1998) Malignant melanoma of the head and neck: effect of treatment on survival, *Laryngoscope* 108: 220–3.

Phillips C. D. (1997) Current status and new developments in techniques for imaging the nose and sinuses, *Otolaryngol Clin North Am* 30: 371–87.

Rabosa E., Rosell G., Plaza G. and Martinez-Vidal A. (1997) Clinical records. Haemangioma of the maxillary sinus, *J Laryngol Otol* 111: 638–40.

Rassekh C. H., Nuss D. W., Kapadia S. B., Curtin H. D., Weissman J. L. and Janecka I. P. (1996) Chondrosacoma of the nasal septum: skull base imaging and clinicopathologic correlation, *Otolaryngol Head Neck Surg* 115: 29–37.

Ringertz N. (1938) Pathology of malignant tumors arising in the nasal and paranasal cavities and maxilla, *Acta Otolaryngol* 17 (suppl): 1–405.

Robinson C. F., Peterson M., Seiber W. K. *et al.* (1996) Mortality of Carpenter's Union members employed in the US construction or wood products industries, 1987–1990, *Am J Indust Med* 30: 674–94.

Schram V. L. and Myers E. N. (1978) Lateral rhinotomy, *Laryngoscope* 88: 1042–5.

Spiro J. D., Soo K. C. and Spiro R. H. (1995) Nonsquamous cell malignant neoplasms of the nasal cavities and paranasal sinuses, *Head Neck* 17: 114–18.

Stankiewicz J. A. and Girgis S. J. (1993) Endoscopic surgical treatment of nasal and paranasal sinus inverted papilloma, *Otolaryngol Head Neck Surg* 109: 988–95.

Taxy J. B. (1997) Squamous carcinoma of the nasal vestibute, *Am J Clin Pathol* 107: 698–703.

Trott M. S., Gewirtz A., Lavertu P., Wood B. G. and Sebek B. A. (1994) Sinonasal leiomyomas, *Otolaryngol Head Neck Surg* 111: 660–4.

Yoza S., Gunji H. and Ono I. (1997) Primary maxillary reconstruction after radical maxillectomy using a combined free flap and secondary dynamic suspension, *J Craniofacial Surg* 8: 65–73.

Yu K. H., Yu S. C., Teo P. M., Chan A. T., Yeo W. and Chow J. (1997) Nasal lymphoma: results of local radiotherapy with or without chemotherapy, *Head Neck*, 19: 251–9.

20 Tumours of the nasopharynx

'At what point then is the approach of danger to be expected?'
Abraham Lincoln, 1838

Surgical anatomy

The nasopharynx is a large space with rigid walls, approximately 4 cm high, 4 cm wide and 2 cm deep. The anterior wall is formed by the choana and nasal septum, the floor by the soft palate, and the lateral wall by the eustachian tubes and the fossae of Rosenmüller. The roof lies inferior to the body of the sphenoid and is occupied by the adenoids in the adolescent; it merges with the posterior wall of the pharynx. The eustachian tubes are triangular in shape, the anterior wall joining the soft palate and the posterior wall being large and prominent. As the posterior wall is mobile, it requires space and this is provided by the fossa of Rosenmüller. This is a lateral extension of the nasopharynx lying above and behind the medial end of the eustachian tube. By adult life it may be as deep as 1.5 cm and is cleft like. Its apex reaches the anterior margin of the carotid canal and its base opens into the nasopharynx at a point below the foramen lacerum medially. The inferior wall of the fossa is formed by a delicate mucosa covering the eustachian tube and levator palati muscle; the posterior wall is formed by the mucosa covering the dense pharyngobasilar fascia. The mandibular division of the fifth nerve lying in the parapharyngeal space is anterolateral to the apex of the fossa and is separated from it by fascia of the eustachian tube and the tensor palati muscle.

If a nasopharyngeal tumour penetrates the pharyngobasilar fascia, it invades the parapharyngeal space and can involve the foramen ovale, the foramen spinosum, the greater wing of the sphenoid and the retrostyloid compartment, which contains the carotid sheath, the last four cranial nerves and the cervical sympathetic trunk. This results in paralysis of the mandibular division of the trigeminal nerve, trismus, vocal cord paralysis, tongue paralysis, Horner's syndrome and, occasionally, pharyngeal and palatal paralysis. Anterior spread of tumour from the fossa of Rosenmüller blocks the eustachian tube, resulting in conductive deafness, but spread up the tube to the middle ear is extremely rare. Spread through the foramen lacerum and along the internal carotid artery causes paralysis of the motor nerves to the eye and the upper two divisions of the trigeminal nerve. The intimate relationship of the carotid artery in the fossa of Rosenmüller also explains the relatively frequent finding of radiological destruction of the greater wing of the sphenoid without invasion of the eustachian tube.

In infancy the nasopharyngeal epithelium is columnar ciliated but in adults most of the epithelium has undergone squamous metaplasia, leaving areas of columnar epithelium only in relation to the fossa of Rosenmüller.

There is abundant lymphoid stroma in the submucosa of the nasopharynx. The ease of access to rich lymphatic channels is probably responsible for the high incidence of cervical node metastasis in nasopharyngeal carcinoma. The first echelon of nodes is the lateral retropharyngeal group. The uppermost one is known as the node of Rouvière. These nodes lie deep in the upper neck and cannot be palpated. The nasopharynx is a midline structure and, therefore, it is not surprising to find a high rate of bilateral neck-node metastases.

Surgical pathology

Epidemiology

Nasopharyngeal cancer accounts for 18% of all malignant neoplasms in the Cantonese. It has a predilection for the Chinese who are natives of the Kwang Tung province. In Europe it forms less than 6% of all head and neck cancers but, in the Cantonese, it forms over 80%. In Singapore it is the second most common tumour: the normal Singaporean population distribution is 40% Chinese, 30% Malay, 28% Indian and 2% European, but the incidence of nasopharyngeal cancer is 87% Chinese, 10% Malay, 3% European and nil in the Indian population. In the Japanese, Korean and North Chinese the incidence is as low as in the UK or USA, but in Kenyans, Tunisians and Alaskans it is much higher than in non-mongoloid races. American-born, second-generation Chinese have a lower

Table 20.1 Incidence rates for nasopharyngeal carcinoma per 100 000 population

Region	Race	Male	Female
Hong Kong	All	28.5	11.2
Singapore	Chinese	18.1	7.4
USA, Hawaii	Chinese	8.9	3.7
USA, Hawaii	White	0.7	0.9
UK	All	0.2	0.1

IARC (1992).

risk of nasopharyngeal cancer than those born in China, suggesting that environmental as well as genetic ones factors important. Nonetheless, the risk is still eight times that of the resident non-Chinese population (Table 20.1).

Aetiology of nasopharyngeal carcinoma

■ Genetic factors
■ EBV infection
■ Dietary habits

The aetiology of the induction of nasopharyngeal cancer has been well explained. The three important factors are:

■ the Epstein–Barr virus (EBV), which acts as a carcinogen
■ a genetically determined susceptibility in the Cantonese
■ an environmental factor, which is thought to be the eating of salted preserved fish and a deficiency of vitamin C in young southern Chinese people.

In the Chinese the highest incidence is in the fourth decade of life; in the non-Chinese it is in the sixth decade. The male:female ratio in the Chinese is 3:1 and in the non-Chinese 2:1.

Environmental risk factors

In susceptible Chinese populations salted fish is one of the cheapest foods used to supplement rice and is probably eaten more often by the poorer segments of the population, in whom the disease is common. Chinese salted fish contains volatile nitrosamines which are potent carcinogens. Studies from Hong Kong have confirmed that feeding salted fish to babies during weaning was a major risk factor and experimental studies have shown that four out of 20 Wistar rats fed salted fish developed carcinoma in the nose and paranasal region. It has been suggested that over 90% of nasopharyngeal carcinomas occurring in young Hong Kong Chinese could be attributed to the consumption of Cantonese-style salted fish during childhood. More recent studies have shown that other preserved foods also function as independent risk factors, e.g. dried fish, salted duck eggs, salted mustard green and fermented soya bean paste. A diet rich in preserved foods is likely to be associated with a corresponding lack of fresh fruit and vegetables, and therefore be relatively deficient in vitamin C. The significance of environmental factors is supported by the epidemiological data, the occurrence of a plateau in the age incidence rate curve after the age of 40 years and the observation that, while the high risks for the indigenous Chinese population in the Far East have remained static for the last 50 years, the incidence for the disease in the second and third generations of Chinese people born in North America has shown a relative decline.

Immunology

Although nasopharyngeal carcinoma is an epithelial tumour which arises many years after the peak incidence of EBV infection, the lesion appears to be related to the virus as the patients have an antibody response to the viral capsid antigen (VCA), the early antigen (EA) and the nuclear antigen (EBNA). Furthermore, Epstein–Barr viral markers have been found in nasopharyngeal carcinoma cells. Only the undifferentiated or poorly differentiated forms of nasopharyngeal carcinoma are consistently associated with EBV. The fourth group of important Epstein–Barr-related antibody is antibody-dependent cellular cytotoxicity, which is known to be effective in the destruction of viral infected cells where the virus has induced the expression of membrane antigens. The titres of immunoglobulin G (IgG) and immunoglobulin A (IgA) to VCA and EA are useful diagnostic markers. Although the Ig levels are related to the tumour burden they are not particularly helpful in follow-up.

The IgA antibody to VCA can also be used to screen for the tumour in high-risk (Chinese) populations, or relatives of an index patient with a family history of nasopharyngeal cancer.

Genetic factors

Genetic factors play an important part in the aetiology of nasopharyngeal carcinoma. This is suggested by the high incidence in southern Chinese people and the frequency with which a positive family history can be elicited. None the less, it is currently impossible fully to disentangle genetic factors from environmental influences with any certainty. Despite the prevalence of the disease and the epidemiological data suggesting the importance of genetic factors in its causation, the cellular and molecular genetics of nasopharyngeal cancer have not been fully evaluated in the context of its epidemiology. Two areas have been examined in some detail: human leucocyte antigen (HLA) typing and chromosomal deletions and translocations which are related to oncogenes and tumour suppressor genes.

The major histocompatibility gene complex on the short arm of chromosome 6 has six loci: *HLA*-A, -B, -C, -DR, -DQ and -DS. There are many alleles for each locus and each determines a different antigen. Frequency of occurrence of these alleles varies among different ethnic groups. Despite the occurrence of more than 50 alleles at the HLA A and B loci, only a few are associated with nasopharyngeal carcinoma. HLA typing in Singapore Chinese patients has shown a higher prevalence of *HLA-A2, -BW6, -B17, -BW58, -DR3* and *-DR9*. Different HLA types are associated with different patterns of clinical behaviour in nasopharyngeal carcinoma, for example, *HLA-AW19–B17* is associated with short-term survival while *A2-BW46* is associated with intermediate-term survival. The occurrence of *A2* without *BW46* or *B17* is associated with long-term survival. The interpretation of these findings is not clear because there is a different distribution of HLA in different age groups but a relative risk from a particular HLA type can be calculated.

A numerical alteration in chromosome complement in human dermal fibroblast cultures – hyperdiploidy with a normal occurrence of tetraploidy – was found in almost half of a series of 39 cases of carcinoma of the nasopharynx. The same pattern has been reported to be associated with the *in vivo* expression of certain inheritable tumours and the average age of diagnosis was earlier in the group exhibiting the chromosomal abnormality. This has been taken to show a genetic predisposition for certain nasopharyngeal cancers. Deletions in chromosomal regions 3p14-21 and 9p21-22 (associated with a putative tumour suppressor gene) and translocations involving 5q have been identified. Amplification of p53 protein and Bcl2, C-myc and Ras oncogene products has been demonstrated.

Tumour types

Squamous cell carcinoma

Carcinoma constitutes 85% of all malignant tumours of the nasopharynx. Nasopharyngeal carcinoma is divided into three types in the World Health Organization (WHO) classification. All are regarded as varieties of squamous cell carcinoma. These three types are: (i) keratinizing squamous cell carcinoma which may be well, moderately or poorly differentiated; (ii) non-keratinizing carcinoma which is undifferentiated and although electron microscopy and immunohistochemistry show squamous origins, there are no light-microscopical features of this; and (iii) undifferentiated carcinoma of nasopharyngeal type. The nasopharyngeal carcinomas (formerly called transitional cell carcinoma and lymphoepithelioma or lymphoepithelial carcinoma) are now regarded as falling within the category of undifferentiated carcinoma of nasopharyngeal type. The lymphocytic infiltrate in undifferentated carcinoma can be predominant and lead to errors in diagnosis unless immunohistochemical techniques with lymphocyte markers and anticytokeratin antibodies are used to prevent confusion with lymphomas.

WHO classification of nasopharyngeal carcinoma

- Keratinizing squamous carcinoma
- Non-keratinizing carcinoma
- Undifferentiated carcinoma of nasopharyngeal type

While most classification systems attempt to categorize nasopharyngeal carcinomas into those arising from the vault and those arising from the lateral walls, it is usually impossible to say from where tumours arise. It is thought that most arise from the fossa of Rosenmüller but many will present with metastatic nodes before even declaring themselves in the nasopharynx. Almost half the patients will have metastatic nodes on first presentation. About one in three will have unilateral nodes and one in five bilateral nodes. The tumour spreads by direct infiltration into the basiocciput and the middle cranial fossa, eventually paralysing all cranial nerves from the third to the 12th. It can leave the nasopharynx by entering the orbit, the infratemporal fossa and the parapharyngeal space.

Other malignant tumours

The second most common adult tumour is lymphoma. In 95% of cases it is non-Hodgkin's lymphoma (NHL). Hodgkin's disease (HD) presenting in or involving the nasopharynx is very rare. One B-cell NHL variant is the plasmacytoma, which may be either solitary or part of a generalized multiple myelomatosis. Adenocarcinoma, adenoid cystic carcinoma and malignant melanoma may also rarely develop in the nasopharynx. In children, rhabdomyosarcoma is the most commonly encountered malignancy in the nasopharynx and accounts for 30% of all malignancies in this site in children. Rhabdomyosarcomas are classified as embryonal, alveolar, pleomorphic and botryoid. Histologically, the most common variety of rhabdomyosarcoma in the head and neck is the embryonal or botryoid embryonal form. Children with cancer should be referred to specialized paediatric oncology centres for further management.

Nasopharyngeal angiofibroma

This is a rare condition and very few clinicians have experience of it in depth. It seems to be more common in the Middle East and the Indian subcontinent than it is in Europe or the USA. Girls are very seldom affected and the mean age at diagnosis is around 14 years. It arises from the base of the medial pterygoid plate and the sphenopalatine foramen and thus is not truly nasopharyngeal. Secondary involvement of the nasopharynx occurs because of accessability of the site to additional vascular attachments, following pressure ulceration of the lining epithelium. The lesion consists of angiomatous tissue and a fibrous stroma; both the maturity and quantity of these components may vary within individual tumours. Some are thus angiofibromas and others are fibroangiomas. It is thought that spontaneous regression occurs with age but this is entirely unproven and open to much doubt. The tumours are histologically benign but expand to involve the ethmoids, the orbit and the skull base. The majority are operable but, with the passage of time and several recurrences, they can pass beyond the field of the surgeon, when treatment then becomes very difficult.

Investigations

History

Common presenting symptoms of nasopharyngeal carcinoma

- Nasal obstruction
- Cervical lymphadenopathy
- Conductive deafness
- Cranial nerve palsies

One in three patients with a carcinoma presents with nasal symptoms such as epistaxis or nasal obstruction, one in five with conductive deafness; one in five with lymph-node metastases; and one in 10 present with pain. The combination of conductive deafness, elevation and immobility of the homolateral soft palate together with pain in the side of the head (due to fifth cranial nerve involvement) represents symptoms of local invasion and is called Trotter's triad. The remainder presents with headache, diplopia, facial numbness, hypoaesthesia, trismus, ptosis and hoarseness. The average time between the appearance of the first symptom and first consultation is about 6 months. The patient's race is obviously very important and a Chinese person complaining of any of the above symptoms should be considered to have nasopharyngeal cancer until proven otherwise. A Caucasian over the age of 40 years complaining of unilateral conductive deafness, or with an enlarged cervical lymph node, should be regarded with a similarly high degree of suspicion. In patients with advanced nasopharyngeal tumours, endocrine changes such as Cushing's syndrome, dermatomyositis and pseudomyaesthenia gravis (Eaton–Lambert syndrome) have been reported.

Examination

The traditional use of a postnasal mirror alone to examine the nasopharynx must now be regarded as inadequate as it is impossible to visualize the whole area completely. Use of an endoscope is mandatory. Exophytic tumours are easily seen with a nasopharyngoscope or a postnasal mirror, but many tumours remain submucosal and may be missed. In large tumours the palate may be pushed down or even paralysed, as may the vocal cords. The tympanic membrane on one side may be indrawn and there may be evidence of serous otitis media. There may be ipsilateral tongue paralysis and eye tests may show diplopia or Horner's syndrome. If the tumour has spread into the parapharyngeal space, there may be trismus. With fifth nerve involvement there is often loss of facial, palatal or pharyngeal sensation. Seventy per cent of patients will have some degree of neck-node involvement, which can be either unilateral or bilateral enlargement, and this is very often the only presenting feature. Occasionally, an enlarged node of Rouvière can be seen as a bulge in the posterior pharyngeal wall.

A rhabdomyosarcoma presents with signs of a nasopharyngeal mass lesion, or of invasion into surrounding structures, in very much the same way as carcinoma and must, of course, be suspected if the patient is under the age of 12 years.

Similarly, angiofibroma occurs almost exclusively in boys around the age of puberty and should be suspected with someone at this age presenting with nasal symptoms. Angiofibromas are soft on palpation; fibroangiomas are often hard, tough and rubbery. There will not be any metastatic involvement, even though there is a large mass in the nasopharynx, and the patient will present with nasal symptoms or facial swelling.

Laboratory studies

A full blood count and erythrocyte sedimentation rate (ESR) are necessary, as repeated epistaxis may have caused anaemia and a high ESR may raise the possibility of a lymphoma. Routine blood biochemistry is also indicated.

Audiometry, including impedance tests, is carried out to test for eustachian tube function. Field tests and other specialized ophthalmic tests may also be required if there are visual symptoms or eye signs have been detected on examination.

Titres for EBV-related antigens may be ordered but are not regarded as essential. Patients with nasopharyngeal carcinoma have high titres of antibodies to Epstein–Barr viral capsid antigen and this increases with advancing clinical stage of the disease. Antibodies to the diffuse component of the EBV-induced early antigen are not usually demonstrable in stage I of the disease but, from stage II onwards, there is an increasingly high titre. VCA-specific IgA antibodies are invariably present in high-titre patients with nasopharyngeal cancer, and it has been suggested that the absence of these antibodies in a patient with clinical features suggestive of nasopharyngeal cancer may be used to exclude the diagnosis.

Imaging

Computed tomography (CT) is the investigation of choice. The widespread availability of high-quality CT imaging in the modern era means that the traditional evaluation of the extent of a nasopharyngeal tumour by plain X-rays and conventional tomograms of the skull base is now obsolete. With the ability to reconstruct coronal and axial views, the CT scan will define any evidence of destruction of pterygoid plates, foramen lacerum, foramen ovale, foramen spinosum or jugular foramen. Scans will give information about tumour extension into the ethmoid and sphenoid sinuses. They will also give further information about the presence of enlarged deep impalpable nodes in the retropharyngeal area and the rest of the neck.

Magnetic resonance imaging (MRI), with its superior density resolution, shows the tumour edge more clearly, and its vascular nature is demonstrated by negative signals from vessels within the tumour. MRI is also better at defining the extent of any intracranial extension. With gadolinium enhancement is possible to distinguish reliably trapped secretions within sinuses from tumour extension.

Distant metastases to bone, lung and liver are excluded using plain chest X-rays, skeletal scintigraphy and abdominal ultrasound. With modern spiral CT scanning, it is possible to extend the investigation from the skull base down to the abdomen to visualize any metastases in the lungs and liver as well as the primary tumour and nodal spread.

Angiography used to be the test of choice in the assessment of an angiofibroma. This is now only used when embolization is considered as a treatment modality. A CT scan will show erosion of the medial pterygoid plate, lateral extension into the infratemporal fossa and invasion of the middle fossa by way of the orbit or superior orbital fissure. It may show involvement of the sphenoid sinus in up to 70% of patients, of the infratemporal fossa in 60%, of the orbit in 30% and of the middle cranial fossa in 20%.

Biopsy

This should be conducted under general anaesthesia. If a mass is seen, then the palate can be held forward with two catheters, visualized with a postnasal mirror and biopsy performed transnasally with Tilley forceps. The biopsy may also be conducted under direct vision with a Yankauer's speculum, or under rigid endoscopic control.

Even when an obvious nasopharyngeal tumour is present, it is still advisable to perform a full examination

of the upper aerodigestive tract under anaesthesia to exclude any second primary tumours.

If no tumour is seen and the nasopharynx is being harvested by biopsy for the investigation of a metastatic node with no obvious primary, then it is probably best to use an adenoid curette to obtain as large a sample as possible from the nasopharynx. Isolated blind biopsies have a much lower harvest rate. If a nasopharyngeal angiofibroma is suspected, then a great deal of thought should go into whether or not to carry out a biopsy. It is usually preferable not to do a punch biopsy because of the uncontrollable bleeding that may result. Diagnosis in these cases is very often possible without a biopsy because of the clinical and radiological findings. Older subjects, in whom the diagnosis may be more in doubt, tend to have a more fibrous and less angiomatous lesion, making biopsy (with packing) acceptable.

Staging

Detailed and accurate staging is essential to determine the treatment policy and also to give an indication of prognosis. Over the years, various staging systems have been used. Earlier international classifications were flawed for several reasons. They divided the nasopharynx into often unidentifiable subsites and made an impractical distinction regarding the number of affected subsites. While recognizing the importance of bone erosion, they did not take into account cranial nerve palsies, which may occur

---

Table 20.2 TNM clinical classification for nasopharyngeal carcinoma

T: Primary tumour
T_X Primary tumour cannot be assessed
T_0 No evidence of primary tumour
T_{is} Carcinoma *in situ*
T_1 Tumour confined to nasopharynx*
T_2 Tumour extends to soft tissue of oropharynx and/or nasal fossa*
   T_{2a} without parapharyngeal extension*[†]
   T_{2b} with parapharyngeal extension*[†]
T_3 Tumour invades bony structures and/or paranasal sinuses*
T_4 Tumour with intracranial extension and/or involvement of cranial nerves, infratemporal fossa, hypopharynx or orbit*

N: Regional lymph nodes[‡]
N_X Regional lymph nodes cannot be assessed
N_0 No regional lymph-node metastasis*
N_1 Unilateral metastasis in lymph node(s), 6 cm or less in greatest dimension, above supraclavicular fossa*
N_2 Bilateral metastasis in lymph node(s), 6 cm or less in greatest dimension, above supraclavicular fossa*
N_3 Metastasis in lymph node(s)*
   (a) greater than 6 cm in dimension
   (b) in the supraclavicular fossa

M: Distant metastasis[†]
M_X Distant metastasis cannot be assessed
M_0 No distant metastasis
M_1 Distant metastasis

UICC (1997).
*New inclusion.
[†]Parapharyngeal extension denotes posterolateral infiltration of tumour beyond the pharyngobasilar fascia.
[‡]Midline nodes are considered ipsilateral nodes

Table 20.3 TNM stage* grouping for nasopharyngeal carcinoma

Stage 0	T_{is}	N_0	M_0
Stage I	T_1	N_0	M_0
Stage IIA	T_{2a}	N_0	M_0
Stage IIB	T_1	N_1	M_0
	T_{2a}	N_1	M_0
	T_{2b}	N_0	M_0
Stage III	T_1	N_2	M_0
	T_{2a}, T_{2b}	N_2	M_0
	T_3	N_0, N_1, N_2	M_0
Stage IVA	T_4	N_0, N_1, N_2	M_0
Stage IVB	Any T	N_3	M_0
Stage IVC	Any T	Any N	M_1

UICC (1997).
*New inclusion.

Table 20.4 Staging of nasopharyngeal angiofibroma

Stage I	Tumour confined to the nasopharynx
Stage II	Extension into the nasal cavity and/or sphenoid sinus
Stage III	Extension into antrum, ethmoid sinus, pterygomaxillary or infratemporal fossa, orbit, cheek or any combination
Stage IV	Intracranial extension

Chandler *et al.* (1984).

in the absence of bone erosion. In addition, the neck-node classification was geared towards a surgical approach, whereas a radiotherapeutic classification is more appropriate in this disease. Ho's classification, which has been in use for some time in the Far East, is more acceptable. The most recent TNM (tumour, node, metastasis) classification (fifth edition, 1997) is based on this (Tables 20.2–20.4).

The TNM classification for nasopharyngeal carcinoma is a pretreatment clinical system based on examination findings, endoscopy and biopsy, and imaging (cTNM). As primary radical surgery is not used, the postsurgical histopathological classification (pTNM) is irrelevant. For tumours which recur after a disease-free interval following initial treatment, restaging using the prefix r can be used, e.g. $rT_2N_0M_0$.

Treatment of nasopharyngeal carcinoma

Treatment policy for nasopharyngeal carcinoma at first presentation

The majority of patients are treated radically. Patients with distant metastases at presentation, however, and those medically unfit for treatment with curative intent, should receive palliative treatment and symptomatic care.

Radiation therapy is the primary treatment modality for nasopharyngeal carcinoma. The radiation field must be large, encompassing the nasopharynx, the base of the skull including the cranial foramina, the sphenoid sinus, the posterior ethmoid sinus, posterior orbit, posterior maxillary antrum and the posterior nasal cavity and, perhaps, the oropharynx and retropharyngeal nodes. Patients with clinically involved cervical nodes clearly need neck irradiation. The nasopharynx is a midline structure with bilateral lymphatic drainage, and so both sides of the neck should be treated even if only one side has detectable lymph-node enlargement. Patients without clinically involved cervical nodes should undergo elective irradiation of both sides of the neck to reduce the likelihood of subsequent nodal relapse because of the high incidence of clinically occult disease at presentation.

Chemotherapy, often with platinum-based combinations, is being used increasingly frequently in conjunction with radiotherapy for nasopharyngeal carcinoma. Early data suggested improved outcome for patients receiving chemoradiotherapy compared with historical controls treated with radiotherapy alone. Such comparisons are generally unreliable, but there are now limited data from randomized trials which support combined modality therapy. For example, a recently published US intergroup study (Al-Sarraf *et al.*, 1998) randomized 193 patients to either conventional radiotherapy or the same radiotherapy with three courses of concomitant cisplatin chemotherapy, followed by three additional courses of cisplatin and fluorouracil. The 3 year survival rate for the control (radiotherapy alone) group was 46%, compared with 76% for the experimental (chemoradiotherapy) group ($P < 0.001$).

Surgery has almost no place in the initial treatment of a patient with nasopharyngeal carcinoma.

Because of the large fields required, patients usually have bad side-effects from the irradiation, including anorexia, fatigue, mucositis and a persistent xerostomia. They may develop trismus secondary to irradiation of the mandibular joint. It is almost always possible to spare the lacrimal gland and eye, but if tumour extension makes this impossible, ocular complications such as keratoconjunctivitis may occur. The most severe complication formerly was transverse myelitis, but modern techniques now avoid this. Another potentially serious neurological complication is temporal lobe necrosis. Chemotherapy side-effects may include myelosuppression, ototoxicity and renal damage, depending on the schedule used.

Radiotherapy technique for nasopharyngeal carcinoma

The treatment volume includes the primary tumour, areas of actual or potential local spread, and the cervical lymph-node areas. Both sides of the neck are treated, even if enlarged nodes are palpable only on one side, because the nasopharynx is a midline structure with bilateral drainage. The neck nodes are always treated, even in those few patients without lymphadenopathy at presentation, because of the high incidence of subclinical disease. This large treatment volume by necessity includes the spinal cord, which is a dose-limiting structure. A two-phase technique is therefore used, enabling the dose to the cord to be kept within tolerance but still allowing adequate treatment of overt disease.

Radiotherapy technique for nasopharyngeal carcinoma

Target volume covers primary tumour and neck nodes bilaterally

- Phase I   *En bloc* treatment of nasopharynx and upper neck with parallel opposed lateral fields. Lower neck and supraclavicular fossae treated with anterior field
- Phase II   Reduced fields using electrons over posterior neck to keep spinal cord dose within tolerance

---

The patient is treated lying supine in an individually prepared Perspex shell, which extends from the level of the eyebrows to below the clavicles. The neck is extended to keep the anterior part of the oral cavity out of the field. The shell holds the patient immobile during treatment, and carries the marks indicating correct beam alignment and the position of the blocks used to shield critical structures.

For the first phase of treatment, the nasopharynx and upper neck are treated in continuity by large parallel opposed lateral fields. These extend from the level of the supraorbital ridge down to the shoulders. The anterior border is placed to include the upper neck, the oropharynx and the posterior parts of the nasal cavity and orbit within the treated volume. The posterior border encompasses the suboccipital area. The upper posterior corner is blocked to shield the brain, brainstem and optic chiasm. Care is taken, however, to ensure that this block does not impinge on the skull base, which needs to be treated, or on any intracranial extension of tumour. An additional block shields the eye and anterior orbit (Fig. 20.1). Sometimes an additional block may be needed to shield part of the mandible and oral mucosa.

The lower part of the neck cannot be treated satisfactorily with lateral fields because the shoulders get in the way, so an anterior field matched to the volume covered by the lateral fields is used. Care is taken to ensure that if possible the junction between the lateral and anterior fields is not through enlarged nodes. Blocks are used to shield the spinal cord and infraclavicular areas.

Simulator check films are retained as a permanent record of the intended treatment. At the start of treatment, verification films are taken on the radiotherapy machine to ensure that the actual set-up matches the intended set-up.

First-phase treatment is delivered with 4–6 MV photons from a linear accelerator, giving 40 Gy in 20

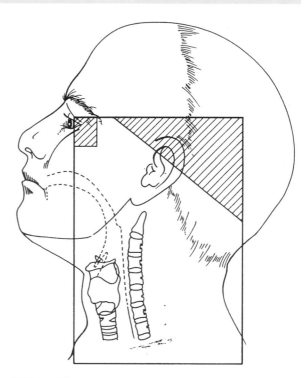

Figure 20.1 Radiotherapy field for the first phase of treatment of nasopharyngeal carcinoma.

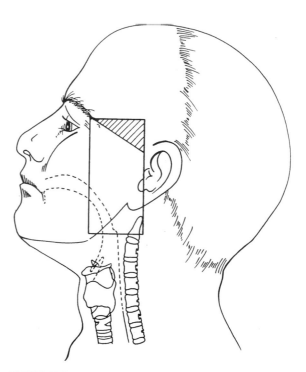

Figure 20.2 Smaller field covering only the nasopharynx for the second phase of treatment.

403

fractions over 4 weeks. During this time the patient is replanned for the second phase, which follows on immediately after the first. Two smaller lateral fields now cover the primary tumour in the nasopharynx, base of skull, parapharyngeal space, sphenoid and posterior ethmoid sinuses and any extension into the nasal cavity or oropharynx (Fig. 20.2). The posterior border is moved anteriorly, so that the lateral fields no longer cover the spinal cord. If there is gross disease in the nasal cavity or ethmoid sinuses, an anterior field may be added to give adequate coverage of this area without compromising the eyes or optic nerves. The use of a third field has the additional benefit of sparing the temporomandibular joints and lateral part of the temporal lobes. The neck is treated by a single anterior field which matches on to the lower side of the lateral fields. This field has a central block to shield the vulnerable cervical cord (Fig. 20.3). Any potential overlap between the upper lateral fields and the lower anterior field is blocked. The nodal areas overlying the spinal cord posterior to the upper lateral fields are treated with small electron beam fields. The limited penetration of electrons enables sparing of the spinal cord.

The principal phase II volume including the primary tumour and any palpable nodes receives a dose of 26 Gy in 13 fractions over 2.5 weeks, using 4–6 MV photons. The total dose in these areas is thus 66 Gy in 33 fractions over 6.5 weeks. Clinically uninvolved areas of the neck are adequately treated with a lower total dose of 50 Gy. Residual bulky node masses may receive a small additional boost with electrons, taking the total dose to 70 Gy.

As with other tumours such as supraglottic or piriform fossa carcinoma with extensive nodal disease, where irradiation of most of the neck is required, the principal acute side-effect is mucositis. As the parotid glands are included in the irradiated volume, xerostomia exacerbates this.

As it is easy for patients to stop eating and drinking almost completely, they must be kept under close surveillance, especially during the latter half of treatment. Appropriate analgesia, often with morphine, is necessary. The routine use of nutritional support via a percutaneous endoscopic gastrostomy (PEG) feeding tube has improved the comfort and outcome of patients receiving radiotherapy. Supplementary feeding via a PEG is more pleasant for the patient than nasogastric feeding. More important, however, is the fact that it allows continuation of the treatment as planned without interruptions or premature discontinuation. Even short gaps in treatment can reduce substantially the likelihood of cure.

Outcome following radiotherapy for nasopharyngeal carcinoma

The largest published series reporting the outcome of patients treated for nasopharyngeal carcinoma come, not surprisingly, from the Far East. Stage is the most important prognostic factor but it is difficult to give a meaningful overview of results stage by stage, as various staging systems have been used in different reports which are not strictly comparable and are different from those in use today. Nonetheless, one can expect approximate 5 year survival rates as set out below.

Approximate 5 year survival rates for nasopharyngeal carcinoma
■ Stage I 90%
■ Stage II 70%
■ Stage III 60%
■ Stage IV – without distant metastases 40%
– with distant metastases 0%

More recent reports indicate that outcome has improved in all stages. To some extent this may be an epiphenomenon related to stage migration due to the better imaging facilities now available. However, this is not the only explanation as overall results have also improved. For example, 10 year survival rates from series dating back to the 1960s and 1970s are in the region of 25–30%, whereas more recent series report 10 year survival rates in excess of 40%. There may be an element of earlier diagnosis and technically better treatment with radiotherapy.

Treatment of recurrent nasopharyngeal carcinoma

Recurrence of tumour in the nasopharynx has traditionally been treated with further radiotherapy but the incidence of severe complications is high. Intracavitary or intersitial brachytherapy may allow a high radiation dose to be delivered to tumour within the nasopharynx while sparing normal tissues which would be irradiated beyond tolerance limits by external beam treatment. Brachytherapy is of little value, however, when disease extends much beyond the nasopharynx.

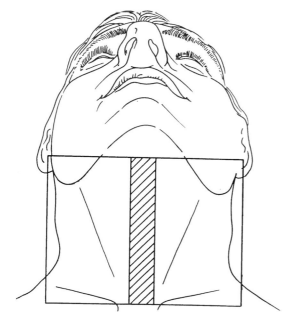

Figure 20.3 Split anterior neck field for nodal irradiation.

In the past, some radiotherapy failures arose because of a 'geographical miss' when it was not possible to image tumour extension so accurately, and others because of an inadequate dose being used when radiotherapy dose–response relationships were less well understood. In those circumstances, retreatment with radiotherapy not infrequently achieved the cure which was missed first time around. With current state-of-the-art imaging and modern radiotherapy techniques and schedules, the relapse rate is lower, but those tumours that do recur tend to be radioresistant and successful salvage treatment with radiotherapy is less likely.

Surgery has a limited place in recurrent disease. Occasionally, where there is certain control of the primary and there is persistent or recurrent neck disease, then a radical neck dissection may be performed. Regarding persistent or recurrent disease in the nasopharynx itself, laser excision of superficial disease has been described. As recurrence is usually invasive, often with bone destruction, its role is limited. For conventional surgery, various combined craniofacial procedures have been described to approach the midline compartment of the skull. The original description was by Derome, and involved a transbasal approach combined with a transoral approach. An alternative is the maxillary swing procedure, described below in the section on surgical approaches to the nasopharynx. Although these approaches are more useful for the excision of benign tumours, the occasional patient with an early recurrent (rT_1) cancer may be successfully salvaged. Facial disassembly and resection of recurrent nasopharyngeal carcinoma in carefully selected patients may have a greater chance of cure with less morbidity than reirradiation. Unfortunately, most recurrences spread laterally or superiorly and thus invalidate these procedures.

The results of chemotherapy for recurrent carcinoma of the nasopharynx are generally disappointing. Most cases which respond do so only for a short period. None the less, even a brief response may provide worthwhile palliation.

Treatment of other malignant tumour types

Lymphoma

Nasopharyngeal lymphoma requires individual assessment, staging and histological grading. Treatment should be undertaken by specialists in lymphoma management. With appropriate treatment, many patients are curable. Most patients will require chemotherapy, although in stage I disease radiotherapy alone may be appropriate and some patients will need combined modality therapy. Management of lymphoma is discussed in greater detail in Chapter 24.

Rhabdomyosarcoma

With modern treatment schedules, results of treatment for nasopharyngeal rhabdomyosarcoma are much better than before. Surgery is rarely indicated, other than for biopsy. The treatment is intensive multidrug chemotherapy with radiotherapy. Because of concern about the worse late effects of radiotherapy in younger children, those under the age of 3 years may be treated if possible by chemotherapy alone. Management of rhabdomyosarcoma is discussed in greater detail in Chapter 24.

Treatment of nasopharyngeal angiofibroma

Treatment policy

Nasopharyngeal angiofibromas should be treated surgically because if they are left alone, they expand into neighbouring cavities, notably the orbit, causing blindness. Radiotherapy has been used as a curative modality and also to reduce the vascularity of tumours before surgery. Its use as a curative modality, however, should be limited to inoperable cases because the patient is almost always a young boy and radiotherapy will produce, at best, retardation of facial growth and, at worse, tumour induction in later life.

Embolization is also enjoying increasing popularity as the skills of the radiologists improve. It requires considerable time and expertise to perform and, as well as being curative and preferable to the ligation of feeding vessels, it may actually produce an involution of the tumour. Even in skilled hands, embolization carries risks of morbidity and even mortality, and full information about the hazards involved must be given prior to seeking consent. Embolization is ideally performed by an expert neuroradiologist with neurosurgical back-up. Prior to the advent of embolisation, mortality related to haemorrhage from the surgical removal of large angiofibromas was appreciable. Embolization reduces the blood loss by over 50%: in one series mean blood loss fell from 1775 ml to only 675 ml.

If the tumours are confined to the nasopharynx with a small pedicle, then they are best approached and removed with a transpalatal approach. However, tumours that extend out of the nasopharynx into the posterior ethmoids and the infratemporal fossa should be removed via a lateral rhinotomy and a medial maxillectomy. This can be performed with a Moure's incision, and extended into a Fergusson incision or a Weber–Fergusson incision if infratemporal extension needs to be accessed. An alternative approach can be achieved by midfacial soft-tissue degloving, an approach to the medial maxilla and lateral nasal wall which leaves no facial scar.

Surgical technique for nasopharyngeal angiofibroma

Approaches to the nasopharynx

There are six approaches to the nasopharynx.

Surgical approaches to the nasopharynx

- Transoral
- Transpalatal
- Endoscopic transnasal
- Transmaxillary
- Transnasoantral
- Maxillary swing

Transoral. This is the approach used for nasopharyngeal biopsy, removal of adenoids and removal of nasopharyngeal cysts. The access is eased by anterior retraction of the palate and this is best done by passing rubber catheters through the nose and out of the mouth. This approach is of no value in the removal of angiofibroma.

Transpalatal. This is an approach that was formerly used for the removal of nasopharyngeal angiofibromas, but it is not as popular now as it once was. It gives better access to the anterior nasopharynx than the transoral route but provides inadequate access for the removal of an angiofibroma because there is poor access to the lateral nasopharynx, from which these angiofibromas arise. In addition, a palatal fistula may result in as many as 40% of patients.

If it is performed, then the best incision is one that is placed just inside the upper alveolus to provide a large palatal flap. The incision is made down to the bone with a knife and the soft tissues are elevated from the bone backwards to the posterior edge of the hard palate. The exposure is increased by extending the incision backwards into the soft palate and if necessary dividing the greater palatine vessels on one side. The bony hard palate is then removed as necessary, using a cutting burr and bone-nibbling forceps.

The closure of the palatal flap is with 2/0 silk. It is important that there is always bone underneath the incision line or else an oronasal fistula occurs. Since removal of the bony hard palate is always necessary in this approach, it is important to make the incision as far forward as possible.

Endoscopic transnasal. This may be used following embolization for disease confined to the nasopharynx with a very limited extension to the pterygomaxillary fossa and/or sphenoethmoid involvement. It may be used following a transantral maxillary artery ligation to enhance the effects of embolization. The pedicle may then be approached both laterally and medially, and ligaclips applied before the lesion is avulsed. The advantage over the formal lateral rhinotomy approach is that the only facial bone work is the anterior antrostomy to access the pterygomaxillary fissure, The disadvantage is that access is limited and visibility may be restricted. As with other transnasal approaches, the tumour must be delivered through the mouth.

Transmaxillary. The maxilla is approached with an alveolar degloving incision which runs from tuberosity to tuberosity. Once the maxilla is exposed, then Le Fort I osteotomies are carried out and the alveolus is fractured downwards. Occasionally, there can be troublesome bleeding from a torn maxillary artery which may be difficult to deal with via this approach. While it gives adequate access it may need intramaxillary fixation postoperatively (or at least titanium miniplates) and the osteotomy is contraindicated under the age of 12 years because of the risk to the canine dentition. This degree of tissue damage is not really acceptable for angiofibroma but has a place, for instance, in the removal of minor salivary gland lesions from the postnasal space.

Transnasoantral. This is now the preferred option now and there are two approaches to this. The first is a degloving incision which is similar to the incision used for the transmaxillary approach, together with intercartilaginous incisions and a transfixion incision of the nasal septum. The facial tissues can be elevated from both maxillae up to the frontoethmoid suture line. The inferior orbital rims can be easily identified on both sides and although there is quite a lot of facial swelling in the postoperative period, the technique avoids the creation of a facial scar.

The alternative approach is to use a Moure's incision and a lateral rhinotomy approach. This is more direct and gives slightly easier access, but it carries the complication of facial scarring.

Maxillary swing. The maxillary swing approach (Altemir, 1986; Wei *et al.*, 1991), requires exposure of the whole face except for the contralateral eye through a Weber–Fergusson incision, the horizontal limb of which is extended out to the zygoma. The vertical limb of the incision extends to the inner surface of the upper lip, along the hard palate between the two medial incisors. It then turns laterally at the junction of the hard and soft palates, to run behind the maxillary tuberosity. The soft tissues externally are left attached to the underlying maxilla except at a narrow strip of bone just adequate for an osteotomy below the infraorbital margin. Keeping the floor of the orbit intact, the maxillary tuberosity is separated from the pterygoid plates by the transoral insertion of a curved osteotome. The approach exposes the whole mucosal surface of the nasopharynx including the roof, posterior wall and lateral walls. Thus, an *en bloc* resection of a nasopharyngeal tumour with a cartilaginous portion of eustachian tube may be achieved. The internal carotid artery must be identified and preserved posterolateral to the eustachian tube. If required, needles and tubing for afterloading brachytherapy can be accurately placed during surgery. A further advantage is the relative ease of bone and soft-tissue reassembly.

Although Wei *et al.* (1995) reported on the use of their procedure in a further 18 patients, new procedures continue to be described to approach the nasopharynx. An example is the transcervicomandibulopalatal approach reported by Morton *et al.* (1996). The gradually increasing number of approaches reflects the inaccessibility of the area and the fact that no one method is entirely straightforward.

On occasion, the transpalatal, transmaxillary and maxillary swing approaches may require a temporary tracheostomy.

Removal of angiofibroma

Most angiofibromas are firm, and few are as vascular as expected. The vascularity of these tumours is now decreased by preoperative embolization 48 h before surgery. They extend into the nasal cavity, the infratemporal fossa, the ethmoids and the sphenoid. The tumour is approached by removing the medial wall of the maxilla and the ethmoids, and using blunt finger dissection round the side of the maxillary antrum into the infratemporal fossa. The tumour is freed from the nasopharynx and infratemporal fossa and pedicled on the pterygomaxillary fossa, from which it arises. With blunt dissection the two areas are joined and the tumour is removed. Any bleeding is controlled either directly or with a postnasal pack.

If a postnasal pack is inserted, then the patient needs to be covered with antibiotics. The incisions are closed with 3/0 chromic catgut or Vicryl to oral mucosa and 5/0 or 6/0 Ethilon to skin (if a skin incision has been used). The postnasal pack is removed after 48 h and it would be rare for any complications to develop after this period. In the degloving approach the facial swelling takes about a week to settle and intraoperative steroid administration may help to contain this. The circumalar incisions are meticulously closed using 4/0 chromic catgut to minimize the risk of vestibular stenosis.

Radiotherapy for juvenile angiofibroma

Surgery is the treatment of choice for these tumours, but for recurrent or inoperable cases, irradiation is a reasonable alternative, despite the slight risk of a subsequent radiation-induced malignancy. The tumour extent requires accurate delineation by CT scanning to enable the treated volume to be kept to a minimum. Lateral opposed portals or a three-field technique including an anterior field are suitable. A low dose of 30 Gy in 15 fractions over 3 weeks is adequate, but regression may be slow.

Recurrent angiofibroma

This can present a desperately difficult problem if it occurs after initial surgical removal. It is not so much of a problem after failed irradiation or embolization. It is said that fibroangiomas are more likely to recur than angiofibromas. These tumours do not have capsules and surgical removal may well leave tumour behind that hopefully will involute. If it does not, and if it regrows, then further surgery using, if necessary, a facial disassembly approach should be used. Stereotactic radiosurgery may be of value for small intracranial recurrences. The treatment of five patients with recurrent angiofibroma using doxorubicin and decarbazine has been described.

References and further reading

Al-Sarraf M., LeBlanc M., Giri P. G. S., Fu K. K., Cooper J., Vuong T. *et al.* (1998) Chemoradiotherapy versus radiotherapy in patients with advanced nasopharyngeal cancer: phase III randomised intergroup study 0099, *J Clin Oncol* **16**: 1310–17.

Altemir H. F. (1986) Transfacial access to the retromaxillary area, *J Maxillofac Surg* **14**: 165–70.

Chandler J. R., Goulding R., Moskowitz L. and Quencer R. M. (1984) Nasopharyngeal angiofibromas: staging and management, *Ann Otol Rhinol Laryngol* **93**: 322–9.

Cummings B. J., Blend R. and Keane T. (1984) Primary radiation therapy for juvenile nasopharyngeal angiofibroma, *Laryngoscope* **94**: 1599–605.

Fagan J. J., Snyderman C. H., Carrall R. J. and Janecka I. P. (1997) Nasopharyngeal angiofibromas: selecting a surgical approach, *Head Neck* **19**: 391–9.

Harrison D. F. N. (1987) The natural history, pathogenesis and treatment of juvenile angiofibroma, *Arch Otolaryngol Head Neck Surg* **113**: 936–42.

Howard D. J. and Lund V. J. (1992) The midfacial degloving approach to sinonasal disease, *J Laryngol Otol* **106**: 1059–62.

International Agency for Research on Cancer (1992) *Cancer Incidence in Five Continents* (D. M. Parkin, S. L. Whelan, J. Ferlay, L. Raymond and J. Young, Eds), IARC Scientific Publications, Lyon.

Lee A. W. M., Poon Y. F., Foo W., Law S. C. K., Cheung F. K., Chan, D. K. K. *et al.* (1992) Retrospective analysis of 5037 patients with nasopharyngeal carcinoma treated during 1976–1985. Overall survival and patterns of failure. *Int J Radiat Oncol Biol Phys* **23**: 261–70.

Morton R. P., Liavaag P. G., McLean M. and Freeman L. J. (1996) Transcervico-mandibulo-palatal approach for surgical salvage of recurrent nasopharyngeal cancer, *Head Neck* **18**: 352–8.

Poon Y. F. and Lau W. H. (1998) Current management of carcinoma of the nasopharynx, in *Current Radiation Oncology 3* (J. S. Tobias and P. R. M. Thomas, eds), Arnold, London, pp. 146–76.

Radkowski D., McGill T., Healy G. B., Ohlms L. and Jones D. J. (1996) Angiofibroma: changes in staging and treatment, *Arch Otolaryngol Head Neck Surg* **122**: 122–9.

Teo P., Kwan W. H., Yu P., Lee W. Y., Leung S. F. and Choi P. (1996) A retrospective study of the role of intracavitary brachytherapy and the prognostic factors determining local tumour control after primary radical radiotherapy in 903 non-disseminated nasopharyngeal carcinoma patients, *Clin Oncol* **8**: 160–6.

Teo P. M. L., Kwan W. H., Chan A. T. C., Lee W. Y., King W. W. K. and Mok C. U. (1998) How successful is high dose (≥ 60 Gy) reirradiation using mainly external beams in salvaging local failures of nasopharyngeal carcinoma? *Int J Radiat Oncol Biol Phys* **40**: 897–913.

Tseng H. Z. and Chao W. Y. (1997) Transnasal endoscopic approach for juvenile nasopharyngeal angiofibroma, *Am J Otolaryngol* **18**: 151–4.

UICC (1997) *TNM Classification of Malignant Tumours* (L. H. Sobin and C. H. Wittekind, eds), 5th edn, Wiley-Liss, New York.

Ungkanont K., Byers R. M., Weber R. S., Callender D. L., Wolf P. F., Goepfert H. (1996) Juvenile nasopharyngeal angiofibroma: an update of therapeutic management, *Head Neck* **18**: 60–6.

Wei W. I., Lam K. H. and Sham J. S. T. (1991) New approach to nasopharynx: the maxillary swing approach, *Head Neck* **13**: 200–7.

Wei W. I., Ho C. M., Yuen P. W., Fung C. F., Sham J. S. T. and Lam K. H. (1995) Maxillary swing approach for resection of tumours in and around the nasopharynx, *Arch Otolaryngol* **121**: 638–42.

21 Tumours of the skin and ear

'Rather a large scar than a small tombstone'
Sir Harold Gillies

SKIN CANCER

Introduction

Head and neck specialists may come across skin cancer in a number of ways. Some are primary referrals, others incidental findings, while a third category includes the tertiary referral of lesions affecting the ear, medial canthal region or nasolabial fold, columella or upper lip. Many will be best managed in collaboration with a dermatologist.

Principal skin cancers

- Basal cell carcinoma
- Squamous cell carcinoma
- Malignant melanoma

Epidemiology

Basal and squamous cell carcinoma comprise over 80% of skin cancers. These non-melanoma lesions now affect approximately 40 000 registered individuals in the UK annually, which is probably a gross underestimate of the true incidence. In a rural Irish survey, 10% of those over 75 years of age had had skin cancer. The ratios of skin cancer incidence are 30:4:1 basal:squamous:melanoma. In Caucasians the risk increases linearly towards the equator. In the USA, an estimated 2000 non-melanoma skin cancer-related deaths occur annually

Most skin cancer is caused by ultraviolet radiation, of which the UVB rays (290–320 nm) are the most dangerous. UVB may act as both an initiator and a promoter. The role of UVA (320–400 nm) is less clear. Some cutaneous chemical carcinogen risk factors are now of historic interest, but topical nitrogen mustard (used to treat T-cell lymphoma) increases the risk of non-melanoma skin cancer. The cancer risk in a benign pre-existing solar keratosis is only 0.1% per annum, whereas Bowen's disease (squamous carcinoma *in situ*) has a somewhat higher rate of malignant transformation.

In the autosomal recessive condition xeroderma pigmentosum patients are extremely sun sensitive, probably because they cannot repair DNA. The median age of onset of skin cancers is 8 years. Isoretinoin can prevent new tumour development. The effect of sunburn as an indicator of both sun exposure and sun sensitivity suggests a relationship between basal cell carcinoma and intense sun exposure, whereas squamous cell carcinoma may require prolonged exposure to sunlight (Zanetti *et al.*, 1996). Irritants that may cause squamous cell carcinoma include burns, hidradenitis suppurativa, lupus erythematosus and chronic ulcers (Marjolin's ulcer). Chronically immuno-suppressed patients, for example those with renal transplants, are at significantly increased risk of squamous skin cancer

---

Risk factors for development of non-melanoma skin cancer

- Red hair colour
- Fair hair
- Pale eye colour
- Lifetime sun exposure
- History of sunburns (BCC)
- Young age at first sunburn (BCC)
- Long-term immunosuppression
- Genetic risk factors (xeroderma pigmentosum)
- Chronic irritation: hand/neck (SCC)

BCC: basal cell carcinoma; SCC; squamous cell carcinoma.

Basal cell carcinoma

The most common skin tumour is basal cell carcinoma, and most are under 1 cm in diameter (Motley *et al.*, 1995). Exposure to sunlight is the main risk factor, but genetic factors also appear important: two thirds of lesions in one series showed loss of heterozygosity for chromosome 9q markers, irrespective of either biological characteristics and or exposure to sunlight (Gailani *et al.*, 1996). There are several high-risk sites where failure to eradicate the disease leads to aggressive recurrence: on the face the H-zone includes the cheek and nasolabial folds, medial canthus and preauricular region.

Basal cell carcinoma

- Up to 90% occur on the head and neck
- Rarely if ever metastasizes
- Peak age 60–65 years
- Variants include solid, cystic and pigmented
- Higher recurrence rates at medial canthus and nasolabial fold

---

Cutaneous squamous cell carcinoma

Squamous carcinoma of the skin is a malignant proliferation of epidermal keratinocytes. All have the capacity for metastatic spread, but those arising in keratoses on the dorsum of the hand are relatively indolent and late in metastasizing.

Cutaneous squamous cell carcinoma

- 70% on the head and neck
- Incidence appears to be increasing
- Peak age >70 years
- Clearest link to sun exposure of all skin cancers
- May have higher metastatic potential on the ear/upper lip

The TNM (tumour, node, mestastasis) staging and overall stage grouping for carcinoma of the skin (excluding the eyelid) is shown in Table 21.1.

Management of non-melanoma skin cancer

All suspicious skin lesions should be biopsied. It is important to exclude a diagnosis such as dermatitis artefacta which can mimic malignant disease (Fig. 21.1). Biopsy may be elliptical, incisional or punch. Elliptical excision is preferred by the pathologist and may be therapeutic if excision is used with an adequate margin in a small lesion. Many small lesions are managed by dermatologists, usually by excision, but also by curettage and cautery or liquid-nitrogen cryotherapy with a spray or probe, which is particularly useful for patients with multiple basal cell lesions.

Excision margins for non-melanoma skin cancer

For basal cell carcinoma under 1 cm, the resection margin should be at least 5 mm. Lesions > 1 cm should be excised with a 1 cm margin. All basal cell carcinomas recurrent after radiotherapy should have at least a 1 cm

Table 21.1 Carcinoma of the skin: TNM clinical classification

T: Primary tumour

T_X	Primary tumour cannot be assessed
T_0	No evidence of primary tumour
T_{is}	Carcinoma *in situ*
T_1	Tumour 2 cm or less in greatest dimension
T_2	Tumour more than 2 cm but not more than 5 cm in greatest dimension
T_3	Tumour more than 5 cm in greatest dimension
T_4	Tumour invades deep extradermal structures, i.e. cartilage, skeletal muscle, or bone

NB. In the case of multiple simultaneous tumours, the tumour with the highest T category is classified and the number of separate tumours is indicated in parentheses, e.g. $T_2(5)$

N: Regional lymph nodes

N_X	Regional lymph nodes cannot be assessed
N_0	No regional lymph-node metastasis
N_1	Regional lymph-node metastasis

M: Distant metastasis

M_X	Distant metastasis cannot be assessed
M_0	No distant metastasis
M_1	Distant metastasis

Overall stage grouping

Stage	T	N	M
Stage 0	T_{is}	N_0	M_0
Stage I	T_1	N_0	M_0
Stage II	T_2	N_0	M_0
	T_3	N_0	M_0
Stage III	T_4	N_0	M_0
	Any T	N_1	M_0
Stage IV	Any T	Any N	M_1

UICC (1997).

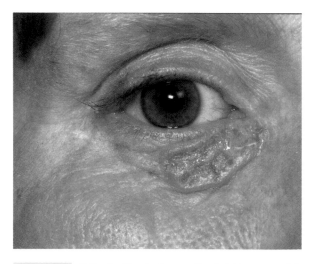

Figure 21.1 Patient with a lesion on the right lower eyelid. Malignancy was suspected but biopsy confirmed benign disease. The diagnosis was dermatitis artefacta secondary to eczema.

margin. The surgeon should consider using confirmatory frozen section with or without Moh's surgery. The margins for squamous cell carcinoma should be at least 1 cm. Radiorecurrences may require frozen section control and probably wider excision margins if possible.

Mohs micrographic surgery (Mohs, 1978) is especially useful to ensure complete excision of recurrent lesions, provided they can be readily identified on frozen section. The lesion is carefully marked before excision to allow orientation. An initial saucer-shaped excision of the area is stained and a deeper saucer is then removed. This too is then stained and orientated to assess residual tumour. Further deeper sections are taken as required, following the disease. Micrographic surgery is especially useful if the original anatomy has been distorted by previous therapy. Once histological clearance is confirmed, the area is either closed by a skin graft or left to granulate.

Radiotherapy is now used in under 10% of basal cell lesions in the UK. Rare aggressive lesions appear to be characterized by initial diameter >1 cm, more than two recurrences or extension into extracutaneous structures (Vico *et al.*, 1995).

Neck disease

You should consider elective neck imaging in high risk patients (e.g. ear, upper lip, T4 lesions and intermediate thickness melanoma). The type of elective neck dissection, if indicated, depends on both the site and pathology of the lesion. Palpable disease requires either modified radical or radical neck dissection and conservative parotidectomy (as required).

Cutaneous melanoma of the head and neck

Although classically associated with sun exposure, a number of factors have led recent authors to suggest the relationship is far from clear cut (Cascinelli *et al.*, 1995). The disease may also be related to human leucocyte antigen (HLA) linkage or to the *ras* oncogene.

Cutaneous melanoma

- Factors against simple link with sun exposure
  - in Europe, more common in the north
  - more common in covered areas of the body
  - outdoor workers less affected
  - more common in city than rural dwellers
- Unpredictable disease of increasing frequency
- Only 5% of skin carcinomas but 65% of skin cancer-related deaths
- 20% in the head and neck
- 1.5:1 male:female
- Variants
  - superficial spreading (most common)
  - lentigo maligna
  - acral lentiginous
  - mucosal lentiginous
  - nodular

The most common lesion is the superficial spreading, many of which appear to arise in association with a dysplastic naevus. Histology should be performed on paraffin sections if at all possible. Haematoxylin and eosin (H&E) staining may suffice, but diagnostic sensitivity is increased by immunohistochemical positivity to S-100 protein, vimentin or a number of monoclonal antibodies (e.g. HMB-45, MEL-1, NKI/3-C).

Histological prognostic parameters

The single best histological prognostic parameter is the histological thickness measured with an ocular micrometer. The risk of nodal metastasis in 5 years rises from 3% for lesions <0.76 mm though 15% for lesions between 1.5 and 4 mm thick, to 72% for those > 4 mm thick.

Histological prognostic parameters

Thickness	Inflammatory reation
Level	Mitotic rate
Histiotype	Cell type
Regression	Pigmentation
Ulceration	Vascular invasion
Growth pattern	Microscopic satellites

Clinical diagnosis rests on the ABCD Cascanelli criteria:

A: **asymmetry**, which is typical

B: **borders**, which are sharp and irregularly serrated, with the overall appearance of an island observed from an aircraft

C: **colour**, which is brownish, blackish or bluish, and unevenly distributed.

D: **diameter**, maximum is usually >7–9 mm.

The only additional test that may aid diagnosis is of cytology in ulcerated lesions.

The TNM staging and overall stage grouping for malignant melanoma of the skin is shown in Table 21.2.

Management of cutaneous melanoma

Wherever possible, the lesion should be excised with 1–2 mm clearance under local anaesthesia. This policy, contrary to some concerns, does not adversely affect prognosis provided that radical surgery is performed within 4 weeks of the excision biopsy. Incisional biopsy is not recommended except, for example, in removal of a large facial lesion where a disfiguring scar may result. The treatment of locoregional melanoma is surgical; disseminated disease is difficult to treat successfully with any modality.

The primary should be excised with a 1 cm margin for every 1 mm of thickness. A useful rule of thumb is to apply margins of 1 cm for a 1 mm lesion; 2 cm for an intermediate lesion and 3 cm for a thick lesion. Melanoma arising in a lentigo maligna should be treated as any other. In the node-positive neck if the primary is in the upper part of the face or temporal region an extended modified radical or radical neck dissection with conservative parotidectomy is recommended. Elective node dissection

Table 21.2   Malignant melanoma: TNM classification

T: Primary tumour
The extent of the tumour is classified after excision (pT classification)

pT: Primary tumour

pT_X	Primary tumour cannot be assessed
pT_0	No evidence of primary tumour
pT_{is}	Melanoma *in situ* (Clark level I) (atypical melanocytic hyperplasia, severe melanocytic dysplasia, not an invasive malignant lesion)
pT_1	Tumour 0.75 mm or less in thickness and invades the papillary dermis (Clark level II)
pT_2	Tumour more than 0.75 mm but no more than 1.5 mm in thickness and/or invades to the papillary–recticular dermal interface (Clark level III)
pT_3	Tumour more than 1.5 mm but no more than 4.0 mm in thickness and/or invades the reticular dermis (Clark level IV)
pT_{3a}	Tumour more than 1.5 mm but no more than 3.0 mm in thickness
pT_{3b}	Tumour more than 3.0 mm but no more than 4.0 mm in thickness
pT_4	Tumour more than 4.0 mm in thickness and/or invades subcutaneous tissue (Clark level V) and/or satellite(s) within 2 cm of the primary tumour
pT_{4a}	Tumour more than 4.0 mm in thickness and/or invades subcutaneous tissue
pT_{4b}	Satellite(s) within 2 cm of the primary tumour

NB. In case of discrepancy between tumour thickness and level, the pT category is based on the less favourable finding.

N: Regional lymph nodes

N_X	Regional lymph-nodes cannot be assessed
N_0	No regional lymph-node metastasis
N_1	Metastasis 3 m or less in greatest dimension in any regional lymph node(s)
N_2	Metastasis more than 3 cm in greatest dimension in any regional lymph node(s) and/or in-transit metastasis
	N_{2a} Metastasis more than 3 cm in greatest dimension in any regional lymph node(s)
	N_{2b} In-transit metastasis
	N_{2c} Both

NB. In-transit metastasis involves skin or subcutaneous tissue more than 2 cm from the primary tumour but not beyond the regional lymph nodes.

M: Distant metastasis

M_X	Distant metastasis cannot be assessed
M_0	No distant metastasis
M_1	Distant metastasis
	M_{1a} Metastasis in skin or subcutaneous tissue or lymph node(s) beyond the regional lymph nodes
	M_{1b} Visceral metastasis

Overall stage grouping

Stage 0	pT_{is}	N_0	M_0
Stage I	pT_1	N_0	M_0
	pT_2	N_0	M_0
Stage II	pT_3	N_0	M_0
Stage III	pT_4	N_0	M_0
	Any pT	N_1, N_2	M_0
Stage IV	Any pT	Any N	M_1

does not seem to improve survival. Of the chemotherapeutic agents, dacarbazine has a response rate of 15–25% as a single agent and most drug combinations do not achieve any additional benefit.

Operations for the removal of skin neoplasms

Most of the operations described here are for non-melanoma skin tumours. The nasal skin is fixed and inelastic, so that primary closure, after removal of tumours in this area, is often difficult. This means or full-thickness skin grafts or local flaps are usually required. Elsewhere in the face there is a much greater degree of laxity.

Lines of election for scars

Also known as the relaxed skin tension lines (RSTL), the most favourable lines for scars follow the wrinkles which form at right angles to the direction of contracture of the underlying muscles. Simple elliptical excision gives the best cosmetic result if in the axis of the RSTL. If dog ears develop at the outer ends, these can be excised after elevation and tension with a skin hook.

Primary closure

This may be the best option, particularly at certain sites such as the nasolabial crease. The tumour is excised in an ellipse and the incision continued down along the

(a)

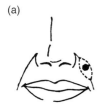

(b)

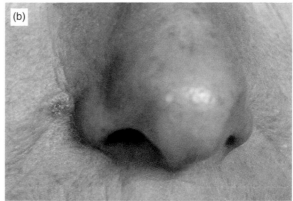

(c)

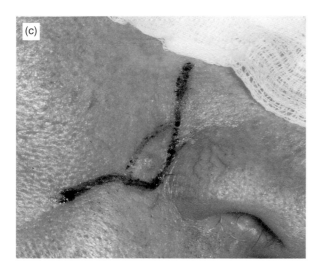

(d)

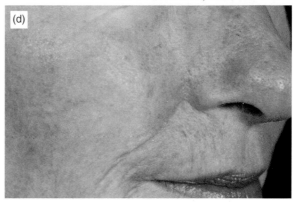

Figure 21.2 Excision of tumour of the nasolabial fold. (b) Basal cell carcinoma of the right nasolabial fold. (c) Treatment was with wide local excision and cheek advancement. (d) The final result.

nasolabial crease. The lateral side of the incision is widely undercut and moved medially for closure (Fig. 21.2). There may well be some tension and so the wound should be closed in two layers.

Some nasal bridge tumours may also be repaired by primary closure. The central bridge incision should be shaped like the head of an arrow (Fig. 21.3). By undercutting this almost down to the medial canthi on both sides it can be closed primarily without any tension or dog ears. Primary closure is often the method of choice in the older patient with greater skin laxity, but in the younger patient, or when primary closure is not possible, then either a full-thickness skin graft or a flap (i.e. glabellar) should be used (see later).

Split-thickness grafts

These still have a place for the coverage of large areas, e.g. the whole of the nose or the forehead. A thickly cut split skin graft usually gives a better result.

Full-thickness grafts

Full-thickness grafts include the epidermis and all layers of the dermis. The main head and neck donor sites are nasolabial, preauricular and postauricular, and lower neck (see Chapter 7). The nasolabial or preauricular grafts are best in older patients. The technique is especially useful

for the nose, because the colour match is so good. The graft should be designed to fit without tension, but also without skin overlap, which has an adverse effect on healing. A composite full-thickness graft incorporating cartilage to reconstruct the ala or lower lid can give excellent results. The graft should be only about 1.5 cm in diameter or less to ensure the best take rates.

Reasons for graft failure

■ Cross-infection
■ Cortical bone denuded of periosteum
■ Heavily contaminated or irradiated areas
■ Movement
■ Fluid collection deep to graft

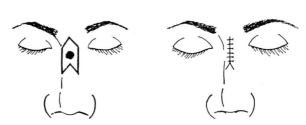

Figure 21.3 Excision of the tumour of the nasal bridge using primary closure.

A gauze or Jelonet template of the defect should therefore be fashioned and used in graft design. As little subcutaneous tissue as possible should be included. The graft should be supported by tie-over dressings. The donor site may be closed primarily.

Skin flaps

Flaps are of two types: those that work on the pivot principle, which are either rotation or transposition or sometimes a combination of both; and advancement flaps. See also Chapter 7, Reconstruction.

Pivot principle

Rotation flaps

Rotation flaps can be used to repair facial defects by conversion of the defect into a triangle, which is a segment of a circle. The flap is designed by extending the arc of the circle. The arc is about twice the sides of the triangle. The tension may be reduced either by lengthening the advancing edge by 1 cm or by a back-cut. Alternatively, a Burrow's triangle may be placed at any point on the arc of the circle.

Transposition flaps

Local flaps are best, as they have a good colour match and they contain adipose tissue, which may be required to supply missing thickness, e.g. in the nose. The pivot point of the flap is at its base at the incision point furthest from the defect. The tightest line will be from the pivot point to the opposite lower corner of the flap. The bilobed flap uses a smaller flap to fill the defect left by the larger. The first flap may be slightly smaller in diameter than the original defect, and the second is half the diameter of the first. The first flap is at 90° degrees to the long axis of the defect, while the second is at 180° to that axis. The technique is really a double transposition flap which masquerades as a rotation flap.

The Limburg flap is a rhomboid flap. All four sides of the excision must be of equal length, and the other two sides of the flap also of the same length. Most lesions can be converted to a rhomboid excision in such a way as to give eight possible rhomboid flap reconstructions, which gives the method a lot of flexibility and allows one to take account of the RSTL and adjacent structures.

Advancement flaps (listed below)

Methods of advancing facial skin to fill a defect

- Burrow's triangles
- V–Y advancement
- Pantographic expansion
- Transposition Z-plasty

Single advancement flaps

The excision of Burrow's triangles at the base of the flap extends the advancement of the flap without tension. A flap should not be used if there is any doubt about completeness of excision, or if a scar runs across its base. If an area is infected (e.g. post-trauma repair), it may be better to graft the area as the primary repair and use what may be the only suitable flap for reconstruction once the area is healthy. To increase coverage, at certain sites it is possible to use bilateral advancement flaps, each based on the principle of the single advancement flap. V–Y advancement, pantographic expansion and transposition Z-plasty are described in Chapter 7.

Anaesthesia for facial flaps

These operations may be performed under local anaesthesia, or with added infiltration of local anaesthetic (2% lignocaine and 1:80 000 adrenaline) if general anaesthesia is used. In the USA they are usually done using local anaesthetic only. When designing a flap for use with local anaesthesia, one must allow for the tissue swelling and oedema induced by the infiltration.

Preparation

The area should be carefully shaved and in men, rotation flaps should be planned so as not to transplant hair-bearing skin on to the nose. This applies especially when removing tumours from the area of the medial canthus, when no non-hair-bearing skin may be available in someone with bushy eyebrows, which meet in the midline.

The skin is cleaned with Cetavlon, as any solution containing spirit may be harmful to the eyes. It is also advisable to use Steridrapes. The eyes are protected by closing the lids with a piece of adhesive tape, but occasionally it may be necessary to perform a temporary tarsorrhaphy.

Technical considerations in facial flaps

- Outline flaps accurately with methylene blue before incising them
- Hold knife at right-angles to the skin edge: bevelling produces an ugly scar
- Use sharp pointed scissors to undermine
- Do not go too deep because branches of the facial nerve may be damaged
- Absolute haemostasis must be secured: use bipolar diathermy
- Tie any large vessels with 3/0 chromic catgut or Vicryl ties
- Use pressure with adrenaline swabs for the general ooze
- The flaps should move into position easily and the donor site should close easily; otherwise, more undermining is needed
- Use a drain only if necessary
- One-layer closure is now possible, e.g. 3/0 dermalene on a cutting needle
- Excise the inevitable dog ears only if the blood supply is not compromised
- 'Think big' in rotation flaps

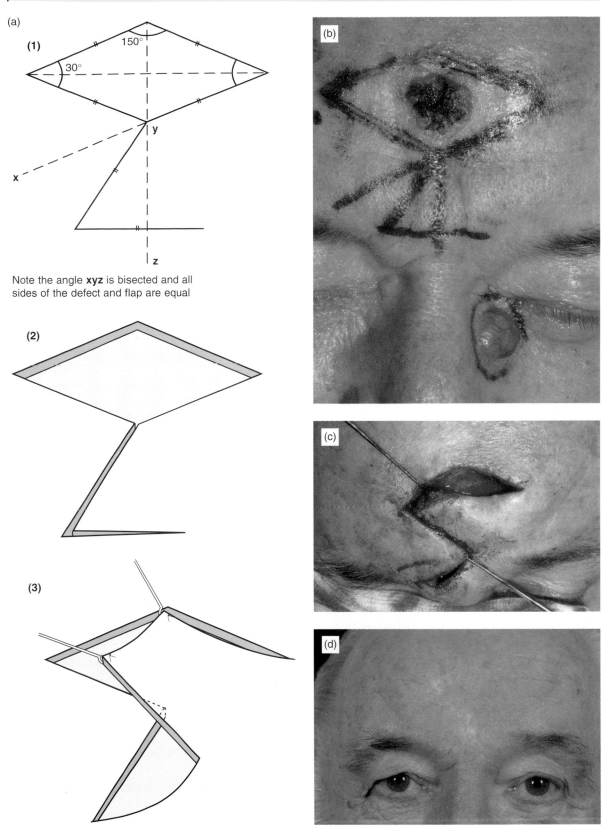

(a)

(1)

150°

30°

y

x

z

Note the angle **xyz** is bisected and all
sides of the defect and flap are equal

(2)

(3)

(b)

(c)

(d)

Figure 21.4 (a) Dimensions of the dufourmentel flap. (b, c) Patient with a basal cell carcinoma on the lower forehead
which is excised and repaired using the dufourmentel flap. The basal cell carcinoma on the left medial canthus has been
excised and repaired with a full-thickness skin graft. (d) The final result.

Aftercare

Once the wound is sutured, it may be left open or covered with a pressure dressing. The dressing is removed after 24 h and antibiotic cream can be applied to the edges of the wound if necessary. There is usually no need for drainage with small flaps and the stitches are removed in 5 days. Wound breakdown can occur as a result either of bleeding under the flap (which lifts it up), or too much tension due to insufficient undermining or a lack of tissue.

Specific sites

Specific sites for flap closure
▪ Temple, forehead and scalp
▪ Eyelids and medial canthus
▪ Nose
▪ Cheek
▪ Ear
▪ Neck

Temple, forehead and scalp

In the temple region there is often excess skin and lesions here can be dealt with by either excision with primary closure or a flap repair, usually a rhomboid transposition flap. Alternatively, V–Y advancement can be used. In the forehead, particularly in the midline, it is sometimes possible to achieve primary closure, but more often than not some form of reconstruction will be required. Lesions in the midline can be dealt with by triangular excision and bilateral advancement flaps or alternatively a dufour-

mentel flap from the forehead is possible (Fig. 21.4).

Larger lateral regions may be dealt with by rotational flaps. An alternative is split skin grafting to the forehead, which carries an associated morbidity. The scalp region has a rich blood supply but poor mobility and because of this many lesions require large rotational or transposition flaps and split skin grafting to the donor site. It is possible in some cases on the forehead and scalp to use tissue expansion.

For recurrent disease on the forehead after radiotherapy, the scalp can be advanced following excision to allow the bed to vascularize (the crane principle) before returning the hairline and split skin grafting the residual defect area (Fig. 21.5).

Eyelids and medial canthus

Many tumours in this area only affect the skin but have a high potential for recurrence. Because of this, the area is ideally suited (especially in the lower eyelid and medial canthal region) to wide excision and full-thickness skin graft repair. Otherwise, the medial canthus can be repaired laterally by a glabellar transposition flap (Figs 21.6 and 21.7).

For tumours on the eyelids the following factors should be noted.

▪ Tumours on the upper eyelid are uncommon. Many are superficial and can be resected and repaired with

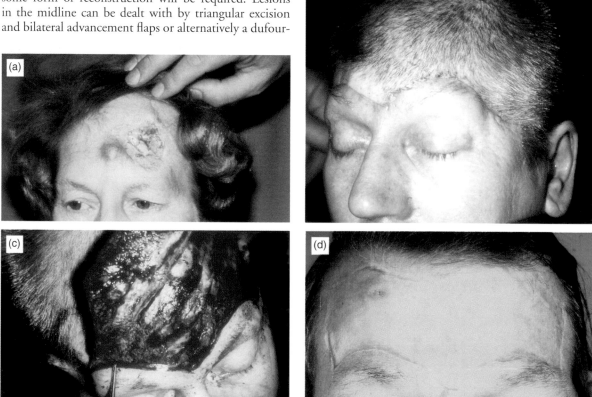

Figure 21.5 (a) Radiorecurrent basal cell carcinoma on the forehead. (b) The lesion is widely excised and initial repair completed with a 'bucket handle' scalp advancement flap. (c) The flap is returned 6 weeks later and (d) the vascularized bed covered with a thick split skin graft.

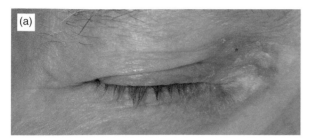

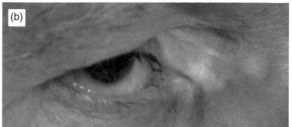

Figure 21.6 (a) Radiorecurrent basal cell carcinoma in the right medial canthus. (b)The lesion was treated by wide local excision and repair was with a full-thickness skin graft.

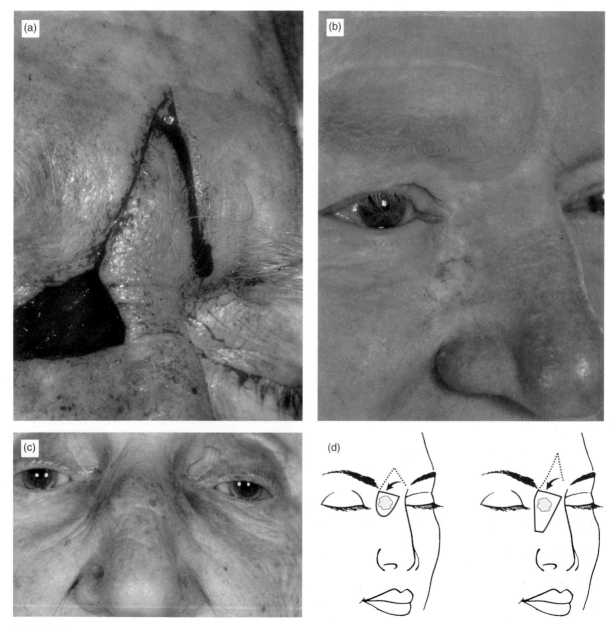

Figure 21.7 Basal cell carcinoma of the right medial canthus which has been (a) excised and (b) repaired with a glabellar transposition flap. (c) Larger lesions may be treated with an extended sliding glabellar flap . (d) Diagrams of these reconstructions.

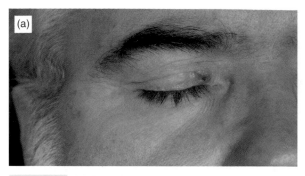
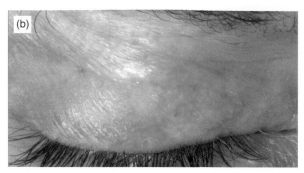

Figure 21.8 (a) Superficial basal cell carcinoma of the right upper eyelid. (b) Repair was with a full-thickness skin graft.

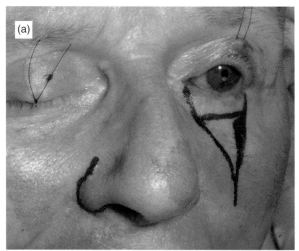

a full-thickness skin graft repair (Fig. 21.8), e.g. from the contralateral upper eyelid. Larger lesions that are full thickness require complicated reconstruction and the help of an oculoplastic surgeon is advisable since a lid switch flap from the lower eyelid may be required.

■ Superficial lower eyelid tumours can be resected and repaired using a full-thickness skin graft. Alternatively, a 'tripier' transposition flap from the upper eyelid may be used.

■ Up to one quarter of the lower eyelid may be resected and primary repair achieved.

■ Larger defects require more complicated reconstruction. Outside cover is provided by either Mustarde transposition flap with a Z-plasty or cervicofacial advancement for full lower eyelid reconstruction. Inside cover is provided by a chondromucosal graft (Fig. 21.9).

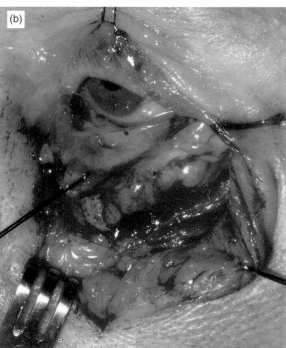
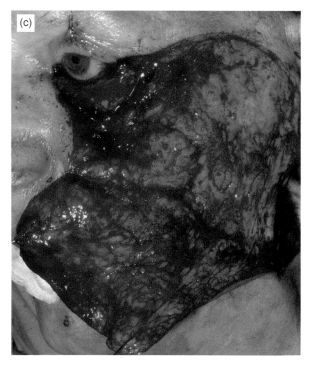

Figure 21.9 Full-thickness squamous cell carcinoma involving virtually the whole of the left lower eyelid. (b) The lesion was widely excised and the lateral canthal tendon divided. Repair was with a cervicofacial cheek advancement flap (c) and a chondromucosal graft was used for inside cover. (d)–(g) Continued opposite.

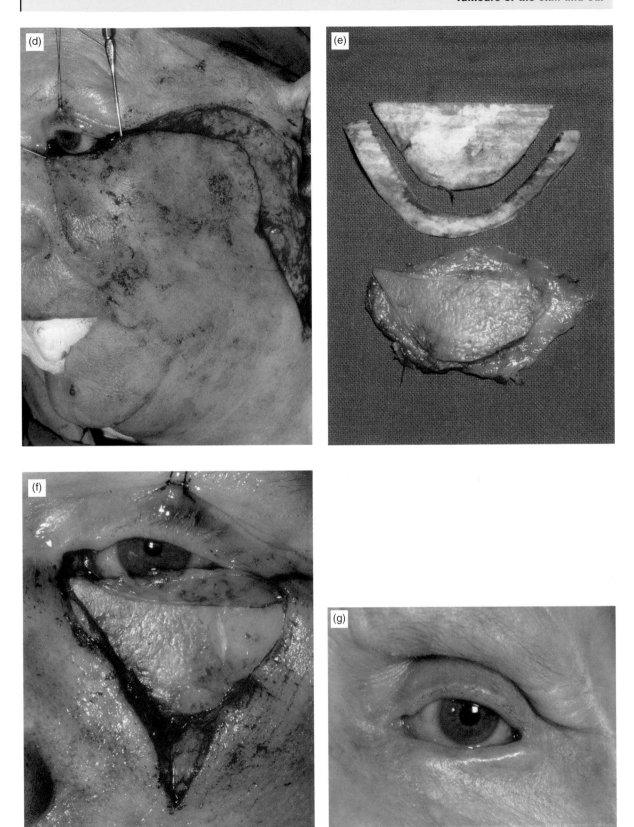

Figure 21.9 Full-thickness squamous cell carcinoma involving virtually the whole of the left lower eyelid. Repair was with a cervicofacial cheek advancement flap (d) and a chondromucosal graft was used for inside cover (e, f). Note the template for the chondromucosal graft in (e). (g) The final result.

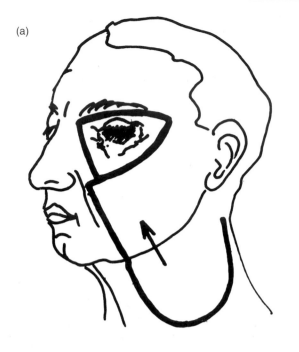
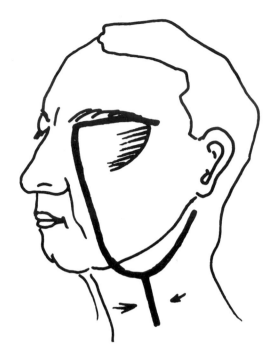

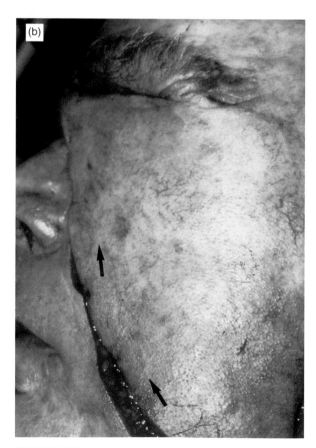
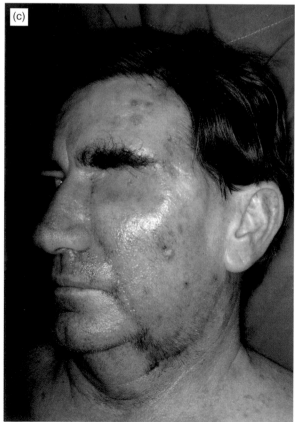

Figure 21.10   (a) Principles of the reverse cervicofacial cheek flap to close an orbital defect. (b) The movement of the flap; (c) the final result.

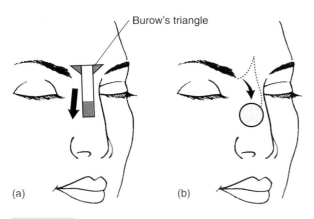

Burow's triangle

(a)   (b)

Figure 21.11 Principles of (a) the Rintala advancement flap and (b) the Reiger (bishop's mitre) rotation advancement flap.

■ Defects following orbital extenteration can be repaired (particularly in the elderly) with a reverse cervico-facial flap (Fig. 21.10). Otherwise, thin free flaps such as the radial forearm can be used to line the cavity and facilitate postoperative osseointegration.

Large lesions involving the lateral canthus can be repaired with a split transitional flap. Large medial canthal lesions can be repaired with a split finger medial forehead flap.

The nose. Apart from the smallest of lesions, primary closure is not usually possible on the nose owing to the sparsity of spare skin. However, the best way to repair the skin of the nose is with the skin of the nose. Mid-dorsum repair can be completed with either a full-thickness skin graft, the Rintala advancement or Reiger (bishop's mitre) rotation flaps (Figs 21.11 and 21.12). The lesions

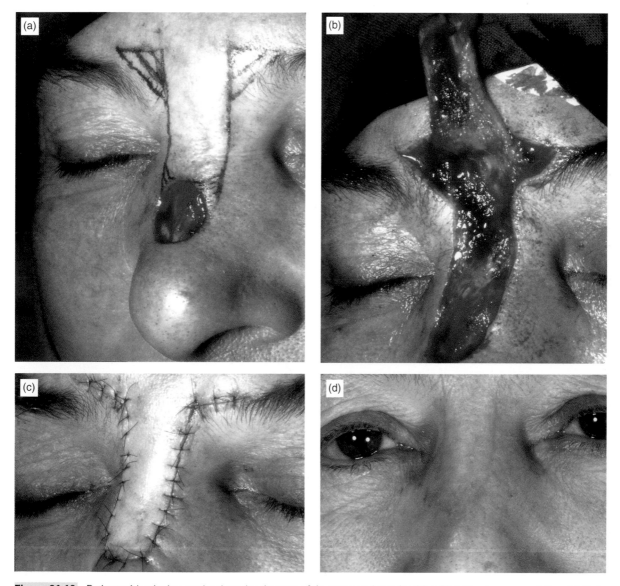

Figure 21.12 Patient with a lesion excised on the dorsum of the nose and repair with a Rintala advancement flap. (a) Note the marking of the Burow's triangles. (b, c) The flap is advanced down the nose. (d) The final result is shown.

(a)

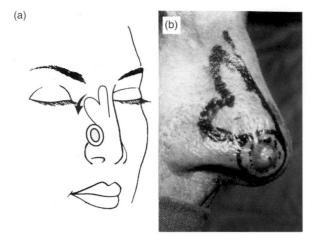

(b)

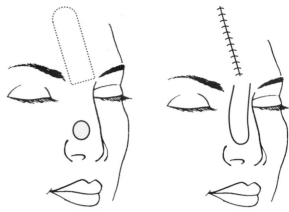

Figure 21.15 Repair of a full-thickness defect on the nose or alar rim. The flap is raised, sutured in and divided 3 weeks later. Larger defects on the nose may be resurfaced using the whole flap.

(c) (d)

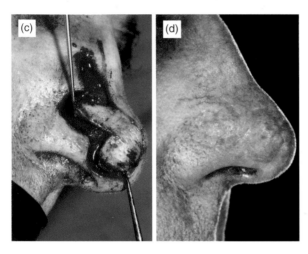

Figure 21.13 (a) Use of a bilobed flap on the nose. It is important to spend time accurately designing the flap. (b) Patient with a basal cell carcinoma on the lower lateral aspect of the nose. (c) The lesion is excised with a 6 mm margin, and repair was with a bilobed flap. (d) The final result.

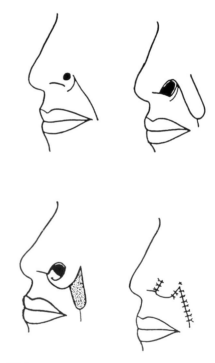

Figure 21.16 Creation of a new alar from a nasolabial transposition flap.

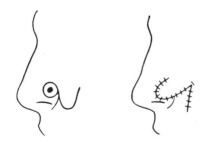

Figure 21.14 Excision of a tumour on the lower lateral surface of the nose. Repair was with a nasolabial transposition flap.

on the side of the nose can be repaired with full thickness skin grafts (and/or composite grafts), the bilobed flap (Fig. 21.13) or a transposition flap (including the rhomboid flap) from the nasolabial fold (Fig. 21.14). Alternatively, a forehead flap may be used (Fig. 21.15). The alar rim can be repaired with either a composite graft (small defects), a nasolabial flap (Fig. 21.16) or using

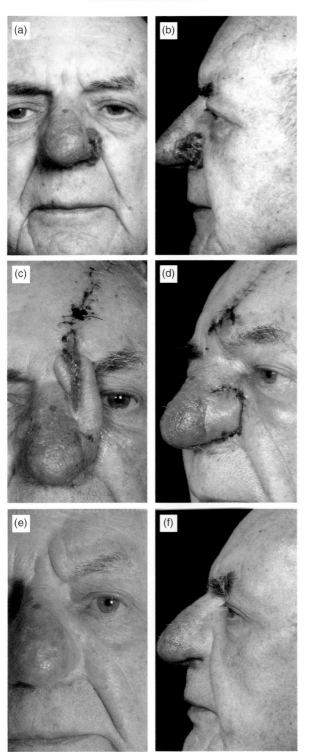

Figure 21.17 Use of a midline forehead flap to repair a defect in the left lower aspect of the nose and cheek. (a, b) A patient with a T$_4$ basal cell carcinoma of the lower aspect the nose and medial part of the cheek. (c) Wide excision was achieved, repair of the lateral side of the nose was with an infolded delayed forehead flap and the cheek was repaired using V–Y advancement. (d) The forehead flap was divided 3 weeks later. (e, f) The final result.

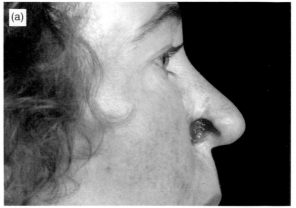

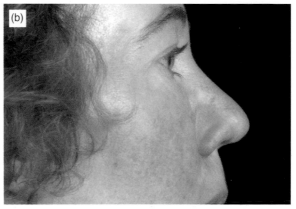

Figure 21.18 Patient with a multirecurrent basal cell carcinoma of the right alar base. (a) Treatment was with wide local resection and postoperative radiotherapy. (b) Reconstruction was with a prosthesis.

an infolded forehead flap as a staged procedure (Fig. 21.17). If there is any lack of local tissue or doubt about clearance, then a prosthesis may be more appropriate (Fig. 21.18). The nasal vestibule can be accessed by an external rhinoplasty approach and repaired with a full-thickness skin graft (Fig. 21.19). The columella is a difficult area to reconstruct. The usual method involves staged bilateral nasolabial flaps (Fig. 21.20).

Cheek

Because of the concave nature of the cheek and its large surface area, it is wise to think big and to repair small defects with large flaps that heal well. One should beware of using small rotational transposition flaps on the cheek because of subsequent problems with scarring. Lesions on the cheek are easily repaired using local skin, usually either in the form of a lateral cheek cervicofacial rotation flap (Figs 21.21 and 21.22) or as advancement, either as V–Y (Fig. 21.23) or pantographic expansion.

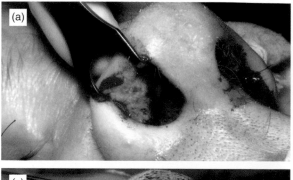

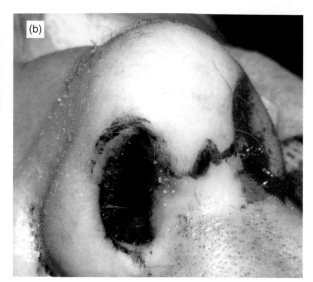

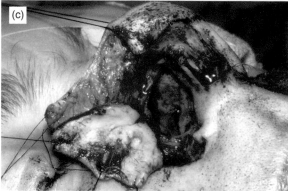

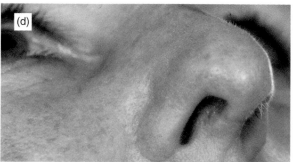

Figure 21.19 (a) Patient with a T$_1$ squamous cell carcinoma of the right nasal vestibule. (b, c) Treatment was with wide local excision using an external rhinoplasty approach. (d) The final result.

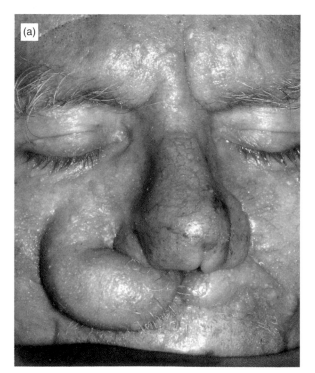

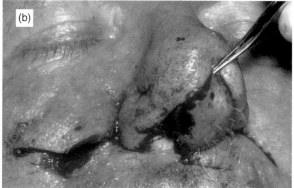

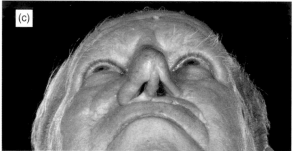

Figure 21.20 (a) Patient with a radiorecurrent basal cell carcinoma of the upper lip, columella and nasal tip treated by wide local resection and reconstruction with bilateral staged nasolabial flaps. (b) The flaps were divided and inset 3 weeks later. (c) The final result.

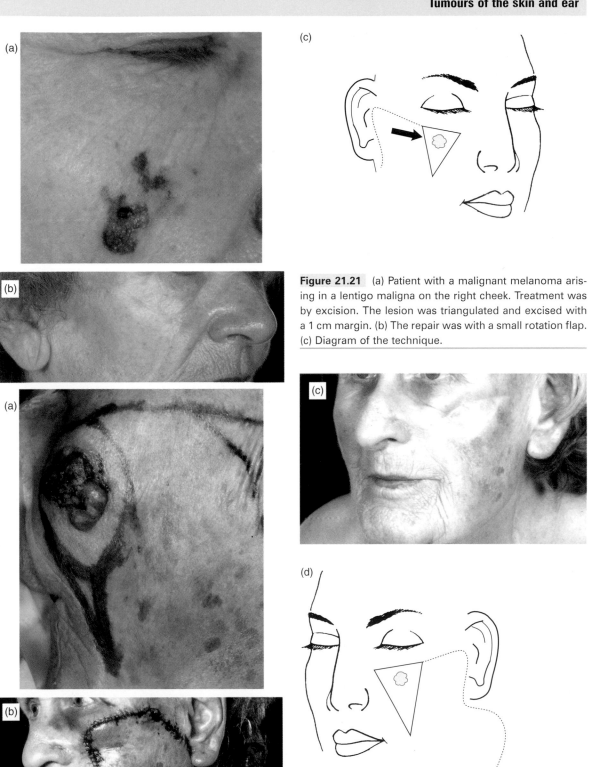

Figure 21.21 (a) Patient with a malignant melanoma arising in a lentigo maligna on the right cheek. Treatment was by excision. The lesion was triangulated and excised with a 1 cm margin. (b) The repair was with a small rotation flap. (c) Diagram of the technique.

Burow's triangle

Figure 21.22 (a) Patient with a T$_4$ squamous cell carcinoma on the left cheek. (b) Treatment was with wide local excision and repair with a large cheek cervicofacial advancement flap together with a Burow's triangle in the neck. (c) The final result. (d) Diagram of the technique.

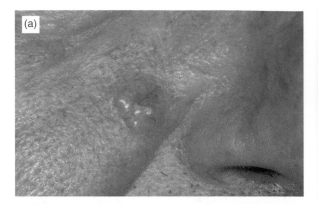

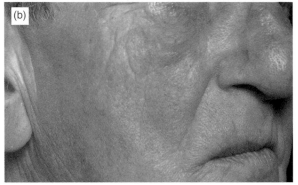

Figure 21.23 T$_2$ basal cell carcinoma right nasolabial fold. (b) Treatment was with excision and V-Y advancement.

External ear

Because of the complex major nature of the auricle, multiple curved surfaces and laxity of spare skin, the repair of local defects in the ear is fraught with difficulty. Small lesions on the extremity can be dealt with by wedge excision, but using this technique for larger defects leads to a 'telephone' deformity of the ear, so that either a star-shaped excision is usually necessary (Fig. 21.24) or the lesion can be excised as a rectangle with a Burow's triangle in the concha and repaired by advancement. Very small lesions in the concha that require any excision of skin and cartilage can be dealt with by a postauricular switch flap and primary closure of the donor site (Fig. 21.25).

Lesions in the external auditory meatus are difficult to deal with and unless a flap is introduced, some degree of stenosis inevitably occurs. Access is important and it is usually necessary to lift up the ear, widely resect the tumour under direct vision and introduce a postauricular transposition flap or cover to at least two-thirds of circumference with a skin split graft for the rest. The final result is usually excellent (Fig. 21.26). In contrast, larger lesions often require partial or total pinnectomy and prosthetic repair.

Postauricular lesions can be widely resected and repaired as for otoplasty (i.e. primary closure). Marginally more cartilage than skin is excised, in order to secure good skin apposition (Fig. 21.27). 4/0 monofilament

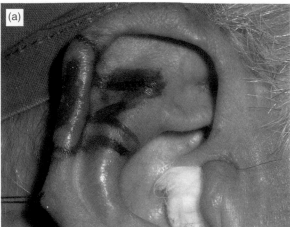

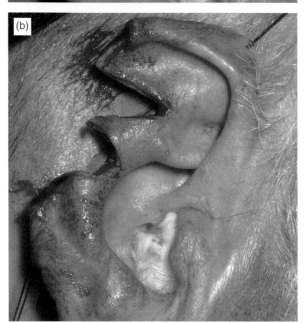

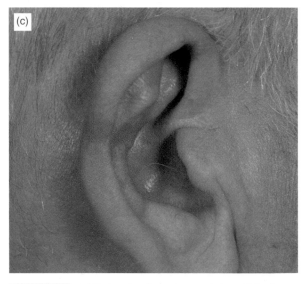

Figure 21.24 (a) T$_2$ basal cell carcinoma right auricle. Treatment was by (b) star-shaped excision and (c) primary repair.

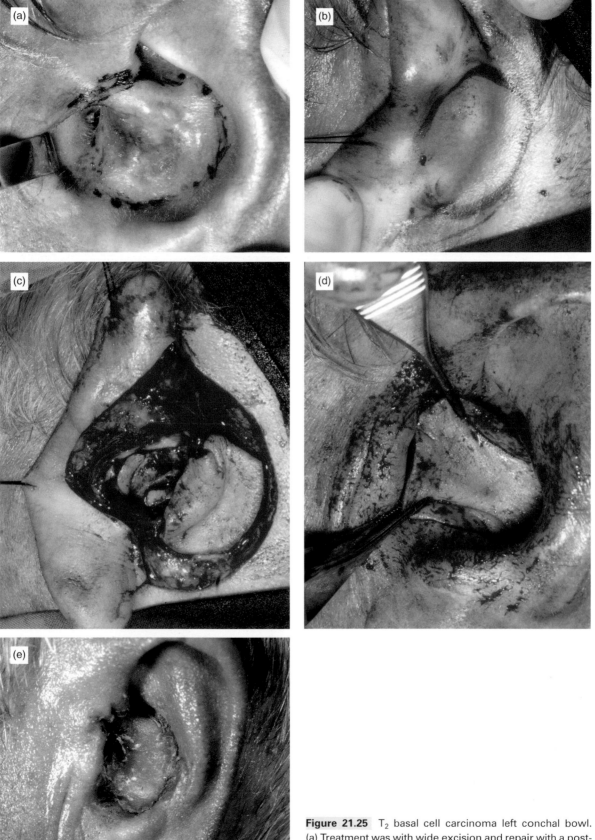

Figure 21.25 T$_2$ basal cell carcinoma left conchal bowl. (a) Treatment was with wide excision and repair with a post-auricular switch flap (b–d). The final result (e).

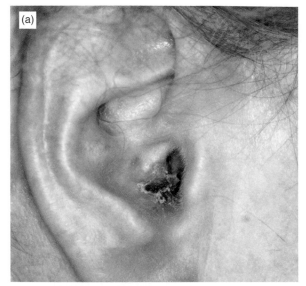

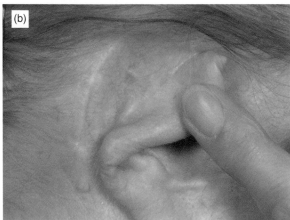

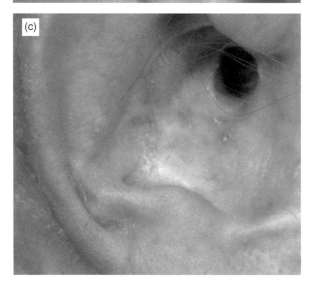

Figure 21.26 Radiorecurrent basal cell carcinoma right external auditory meatus. Treatment was with local excision (including the concha) and repair was with a postauricular transposition flap and additional split skin. (b) The donor site for the flap. (c) The final result.

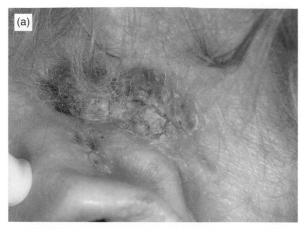

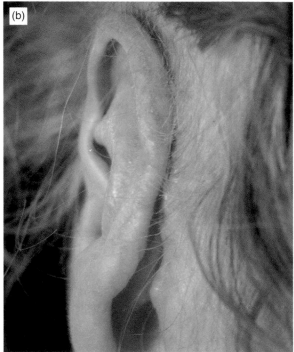

Figure 21.27 (a) T_4 basal cell carcinoma left postauricular region. (b) Treatment was by wide local excision and primary repair using the otoplasty technique.

non-absorbable suture is used to close the skin, but there is no need to use any suture in the cartilaginous layer.

Operations for partial full-thickness resection of small tumours with underlying cartilage require full-thickness skin grafting for repair:

- wedge resection with primary closure where two-thirds of the circumference of the pinna can be preserved (as already discussed)
- total pinnectomy with rotation scalp or lateral cervical flap or full-thickness skin graft repair and rehabilitation with a bone-anchored prosthesis as a

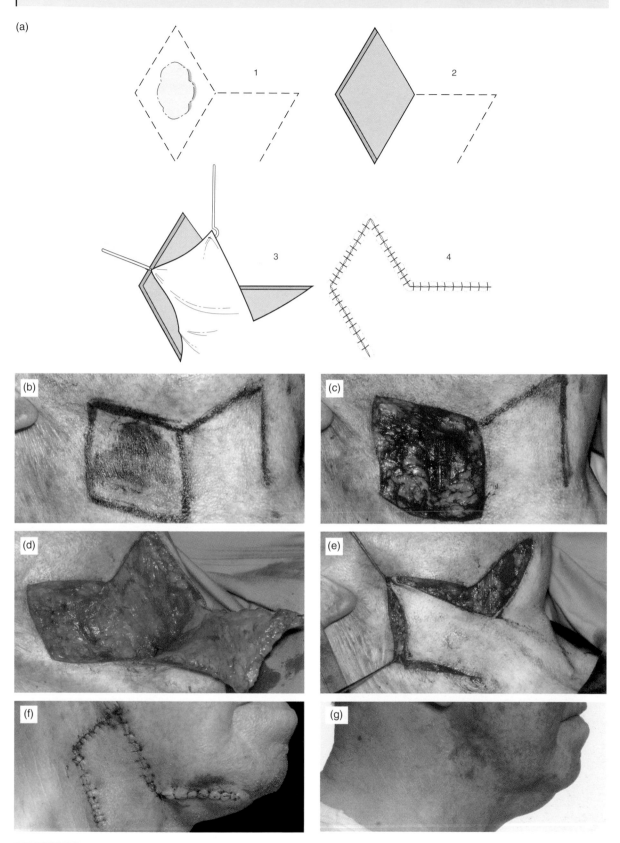

Figure 21.28 (a) Example of a named classic transposition flap: the Rhomboid or Limberg flap. (b) Patient with a lentigo maligna of the left upper neck. (c) The excision is marked as a rhomboid, the lesion is excised and (d) the flap raised and (e, f) transposed into the defect. (g) The final result.

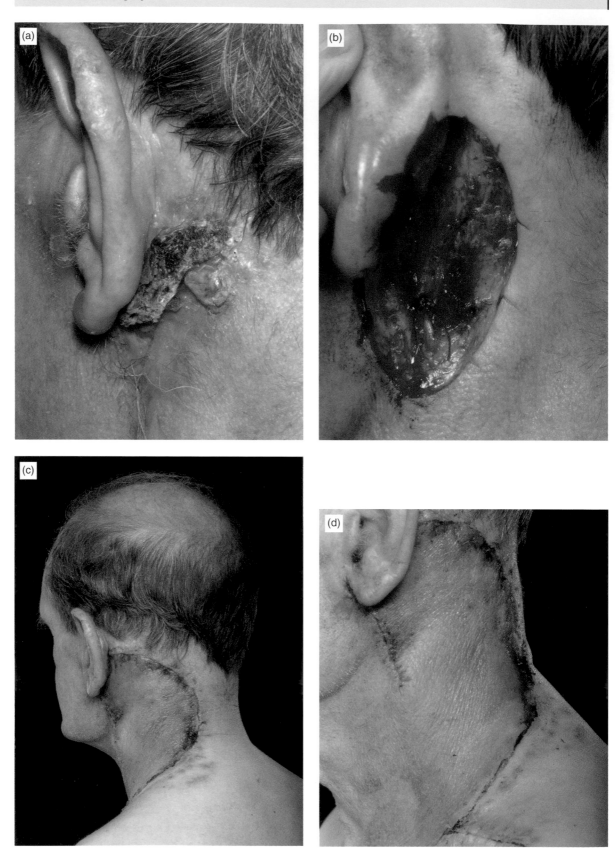

Figure 21.29 (a) Patient with a radiorecurrent basal cell carcinoma behind the left ear. (b) The tumour was widely resected using Moh's surgery; (c, d) repair was with a large cervical rotation flap.

secondary procedure. If the whole auricle is removed some skin is retained on the medial side of the auricle, attached to the skin behind the postaural crease. It can be used to close the defect. This is preferable to using split-thickness skin. In this case an osseointegrated artificial ear must be fitted.

The neck

Many lesions in the neck can be treated by excision and primary closure. Otherwise, local flap repair is usually possible using, for example, the rhomboid flap (Fig. 21.28) or a large rotation flap (Fig. 21.29).

Lips

Refer to Chapter 15, Tumours of the oral cavity and lip.

TUMOURS OF THE EAR

Surgical anatomy

Auricle

The skin of the lateral surface of the auricle is tightly bound down to the yellow elastic cartilaginous framework. The skin on the medial surface is much looser, owing to the subcutaneous layer. The skin immediately behind the postaural crease is free from large hair follicles and so is useful for full-thickness skin grafts. To remove a small tumour, a wedge of the helix of the auricle can be removed either for a composite graft or for tumour excision, with easy primary closure involving little alteration in the shape of the ear. (This has been discussed previously.) As the skin is so closely applied to the perichondrium, excision of part of the auricle requires a marginally greater removal of cartilage than skin, in order to secure an accurate repair. The superficial temporal artery sends a few branches to the lateral surface of the auricle, while the posterior auricular artery supplies the medial surface.

External auditory meatus

The external auditory canal can be subdivided into two parts:

- a cartilaginous portion: tumours arising here spread easily because the cartilaginous walls present little resistance; spread may be anteriorly into the parotid gland or posteriorly into the postauricular sulcus. The cartilage of the external auditory canal is an inward prolongation of the cartilage of the pinna, thus tumours spread readily in through this layer into the concha
- the bony portion: this is surrounded by dense bone, which provides an effective barrier to spread of the tumour that is then deflected along the canal into the middle ear.

Middle ear and mastoid

The middle ear and mastoid may be divided into two parts: petromastoid and tubotympanic. The petromastoid unit includes the tympanic cavity and the mastoid antrum.

Petromastoid tumours involve

- tympanic cavity only
- mastoid antrum only
- both the tympanic cavity and mastoid antrum
- both the tympanic cavity and external auditory canal
- Tubotympanic tumours arise
- in the middle ear and spread into the bony eustachian tube
- within the eustachian tube itself

Almost all carcinomas of the middle ear arise in patients with long-standing chronic otitis media, and usually following previous mastoidectomy. The markedly abnormal anatomy contributes largely to the poor prognosis in these patients. The labyrinth is remarkably resistant to tumour invasion. The bony portion of the eustachian tube ('protympanum') is anatomically part of the tympanic cavity. Tumour probably spreads within the surrounding fascial space rather than along the tube. Invasion of these fascial spaces gives the tumour access to the trigeminal or occulomotor nerves in the lateral wall of the cavernous sinus.

Routes of tumour spread

- **Medial:** the promontory of the middle ear is usually exposed with facial nerve exposure, or covered by only a thin layer of bone with facial paralysis. The tumour may spread into the petrous apex; the oval and round windows and the cells leading above, below and behind the labyrinth, with access to the petrous pyramid lying medial to the bend of the internal carotid artery.
- **Superior:** the tumour may spread through the thin tegmen tympani, in the presence or absence of a defect from previous surgery.
- **Inferior:** after mastoidectomy, the tumour has ready access to the base of the skull, particularly the jugular foramen, and this is one explanation for the paralysis of the lower cranial nerves. The same clinical picture follows metastasis to the node situated over the transverse process of the atlas in the lateral compartment of the retropharyngeal space.
- **Anterior:** the medial bony wall of the eustachian tube and the associated bony wall of the middle ear cavity are separated from the carotid canal by a thin layer of

bone, and this appears to be a frequent route of spread of tumours to the carotid canal.

- **Posterior:** spread may occur into the mastoid air cells, thence via the thin bony wall of the posterior group of air spaces into the internal auditory meatus.
- Local invasion: the tumour may invade of the remnants of the ossicles, the stapedius muscle and the facial canal.

Lymphatics of the external auditory meatus and auricle

There are three directions of lymph drainage:

- anteriorly to the parotid lymph glands, especially to the gland in front of the tragus
- inferiorly to the lymph glands that lie along the external jugular vein and those under the sternomastoid muscle
- posteriorly to the mastoid lymph nodes.

Lymphatics of the middle ear and mastoid

These are less well defined. Anatomically, the lymph vessels are arranged, like the blood vessels, in two sets on the medial and lateral surface of the tympanic membrane. Lymphatics from the tympanic cavity drain to retropharyngeal and parotid nodes. In carcinoma of the middle ear, however, the tympanic membrane has been destroyed. The lymphatic pathways in this situation have not been defined, but are probably sparse as lymphadenopathy is uncommon.

Pathology

The primary and secondary tumours of the ear are listed in Table 21.3

Only epithelial tumours of the external and middle ear will be discussed here. The mesodermal tumours, notably the glomus tumour, are now the province of the neuro-otologist (see Chapter 25), although some of the techniques described under petrosectomy may be applicable to this tumour.

The most common tumour of the auricle is carcinoma, which may be either squamous cell or basal cell, and their respective incidences vary from country to country. Both are more common in adult men and present as a warty lesion or an ulcer, usually on the helix. Biopsy is required to distinguish them from the benign tumours such as epithelioma adenoides cysticum, molluscum contagiosum and naevus. Basal cell tumours do not metastasize, but squamous cell tumours spread to involve the preauricular and postauricular nodes.

Tumours of the external auditory canal

Squamous carcinoma

Squamous carcinoma

- Constitutes about 90% of all malignant tumours
- Originates in any portion of the external auditory meatus, most often the bony canal
- Late extension along the perichondrium of the cartilaginous meatus
- Slow growing
- Tympanic membrane eventually weakens, and middle ear invasion with or without facial nerve paralysis develops
- Late invasion of the parotid gland anteriorly or the sternomastoid muscle posteriorly
- 20% have cervical lymphadenopathy
  - posterior canal wall: nodes overlying the insertion of the sternomastoid muscle
  - inferior canal wall: jugulodigastric lymph nodes (level III)
  - anterior canal wall: preauricular (parotid) lymph nodes

Adenocarcinoma

The glands of the external auditory meatus are typical apocrine sweat glands. Their secretion is a watery fluid devoid of lipids and they do not secrete the wax of the meatus, which is produced by sebaceous glands. Any tumours arising from these 'ceruminous' glands may all be described as a hidradenoma (ccruminoma):

- adenoma
- mucoepidermoid carcinoma
- adenoid cystic carcinoma
- adenocarcinoma.

These tumours present with canal blockage and share the following histological features:

- a two-layered epithelial structure, analogous to that of a normal sweat gland, consisting of an inner oxyphilic columnar layer and an outer myoepithelial layer
- a variable degree of interglandular stroma
- a papillary or cystic pattern.

An adenoma that is clearly benign requires local excision. For mucoepidermoid carcinoma wide excision of the entire external auditory canal, radical mastoidectomy, excision of the mandibular condyle and total parotidectomy with preservation of the facial nerve may be necessary.

Table 21.3   Primary and secondary tumours of the ear

Benign tumours	Malignant tumours
Primary	

Epithelial:
  Primary cholesteatoma (choristoma, adenoma)
	Epithelial:
	  Squamous carcinoma
	  Adenocarcinoma (hydradenocarcinoma)
	  Melanoma
	  Basal cell carcinoma
	  Sebaceous cell carcinoma

Mesenchymal:
  Jugulotympanic paraganglioma (glomus jugulare)
  Osteoma
  Haemangioma
  Neurogenic tumours
  Xanthoma
  Giant cell tumour
  Benign osteoblastoma
	Mesenchymal:
	  Sarcoma
	  Multiple myeloma
	  Haemangioendothelioma
	  Malignant xanthoma

Secondary	

Direct extension from:
  Nasopharynx
  External ear
  Parotid
  Meningioma
	Distant metastasis from:
	  Kidney
	  Lung
	  Prostate
	  Thyroid
	  Breast

Adenoid cystic carcinoma

- By far the most common ceruminous tumour
- Similar to same pathological type found elsewhere
- Painful
- Long natural history ranging from 10 to 30 years
- Death occurs from local invasion or distant metastases
- Radiotherapy can be valuable
- Treatment is extended radical mastoidectomy and total parotidectomy with excision of the external auditory canal and surrounding bone, part of the pinna, the mandibular condyle and any other involved surrounding structures

Adenocarcinoma

- Has a wide histological spectrum
- Basic pattern is that of two-layered eosinophilic glands
- Infiltrates widely into the middle ear and mastoid
- Is a very aggressive disease
- Often presents with facial paralysis
- Usually fatal within 4 years

Malignant melanoma is exceedingly rare; only one authentic tumour arising primarily in the meatus has been recorded. Basal cell carcinoma arising primarily in the external auditory meatus is rare. It tends to affect both genders equally and occurs in late middle life. Good survival results are obtained by sleeve resection.

Sebaceous cell carcinoma is extremely uncommon; fewer than 100 cases affecting any part of the body have been described. It can arise anywhere in the body, but most often in the head and neck, mainly on the concha and nose. Only one case has been reported affecting the ear.

Tumours of the middle ear

Choristoma is a mass of normal tissue at an abnormal site. Seven salivary gland choristomata of the middle ear have been reported, six of which were in females. All presented with deafness, usually lifelong, and many patients showed other anomalies of the middle ear, such as absence of the stapes and an abnormal course of the facial nerve. Attempts at removal are usually abandoned because of attachment to the facial nerve and because other middle ear structures cannot be identified.

Benign adenomata of the middle ear have recently been reported. Some previously reported series of middle ear adenocarcinomata may have included benign adenomata, which would explain the unusually good prognosis sometimes cited. Preoperative radiology shows a mass in the middle ear or mastoid, but no bone destruction.

Benign adenoma

- Male:female 1:1
- Peak age 40–50 years
- Main symptom is unilateral progressive deafness
- Principal clinical finding is a conductive hearing loss
- External canal is usually normal
- Tympanic membrane intact in 75%

Adenocarcinoma of the middle ear

- Extraordinarily rare in the middle ear, despite its glandular epithelium
- 13 cases reported in the literature
- Female predominance
- Median age of onset about 40 years
- Deafness, pain and facial paralysis
- Most treated by mastoidectomy followed by radiotherapy
- Six out of a series of eight patients were alive at 2 years

---

Squamous carcinoma

The petrous pyramid and especially the labyrinth resist tumour invasion. The path of least resistance is through the tegmen tympani into the middle cranial fossa. Dura provides a strong barrier. The cause of death is usually cachexia due to intolerable pain from cranial nerve involvement. Occasionally, invasion of the meninges leads to fatal intracranial complications; erosion of the jugular bulb or carotid artery may cause terminal haemorrhage.

Squamous carcinoma

- Comprises the vast majority of middle ear epithelial malignancies
- Causes extensive bony destruction
- Intracranial invasion is along nerves VII and VIII in the internal auditory canal, and also the petrosal nerve
- Temporomandibular joint and the parotid gland may be involved early
- IX to XII cranial nerve involvement indicates extension into the skull base and neck
- May also extend along the eustachian tube to the nasopharynx
- Lymphadenopathy in 10–15% at presentation; about 10% develop interval lymphadenopathy
- Rare distant metastases occur in liver, brain, lung and bones

---

Staging

Neither the International Union Against Cancer (UICC) nor the American Joint Committee (AJC) has developed a staging system for carcinoma of the ear. Some authors use the system shown in Table 21.4.

Epidemiology

Incidence

The incidence figures for the UK are available from 1967. The age-adjusted incidence (registration of new cases) rate

Table 21.4 Staging of carcinoma of the ear

T1	Tumour limited to the site of origin, no facial nerve paralysis and no bone destruction
T2	Tumour extending beyond the site of origin, indicated by facial paralysis or radiological evidence of bone destruction, but no extension beyond the organ of origin
T3	Clinical or radiological evidence of extension to surrounding structures (dura, base of the skull, parotid gland, temporomandibular joint, etc.)
T4	Patients with insufficient data for classification, including patients previously seen and treated elsewhere

remains steady at 1 per million per year for women and 0.8 per million per year for men. The male:female ratio is also therefore stable, at about 1:1.2.

Mortality

Mortality from cancer of the middle ear for the 10 year cohorts born around 1881–1921 reveals a marked gender difference. Each male cohort has experienced a lower age-specific mortality than the preceding cohort, while there has been no apparent change in the age-specific death rates for successive female cohorts. In men, the mortality decreases after 70–75 years of age, whereas the mortality continues to rise for women. The falling trend in mortality for men but not for women may be due to exposure to an occupational carcinogen, which was the cause of the relatively high incidence rate in men in the nineteenth century. In addition, many of these men were involved in the 1914–1918 war and it has been shown that mustard gas is associated with a higher risk of death from neoplasm of the respiratory tract (including the paranasal sinuses) than expected.

Aetiology of carcinoma

External auditory meatus
- Chronic inflammation
- Irradiation injury: repeated treatment of external otitis
- Speculative uninvestigated causes: carcinogens produced by indigenous microbial flora; production of carcinogens within cerumen
- Azoxymethane (a derivative of dimethylhydrazine) induces squamous cell carcinoma of the sebaceous glands of the ear in 15% of a treated population of experimental animals.

Middle ear
- Pre-existing chronic otitis media in up to 85%
- Irradiation-induced carcinomas are recorded.

Assessment

Clinical

A history of chronic otitis media suggests a tumour arising in the middle ear and absence of this history suggests origin in the external canal. Rarely, the history may also indicate aetiological factors such as previous irradiation. Most patients complain of discharge and deafness; vertigo is rare. Pain, particularly if deep and boring, indicates dural invasion.

Examination

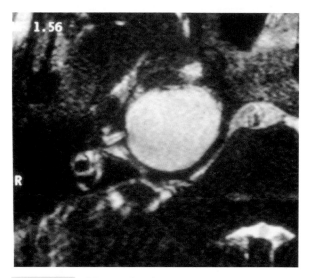

Figure 21.30 CT scan showing petrous tumour.

> ### Examination
>
> - Identify the extent of the tumour, and particularly assess curability
> - Facial paralysis
> - Trismus: invasion of the pterygoids or temporomandibular joint
> - Fullness of the parotid gland: spread through the cartilaginous meatus
> - Fullness of the infratemporal fossa
> - Perichondritis of the auricle
> - Lymphadenopathy, especially level II and preauricular/postauricular groups
> - Lower cranial nerve paresis: indicates extension of the tumour to the base of the skull

Confirmation of diagnosis

- Tumours of the pinna: incisional biopsy under local anaesthesia.
- Tumours of the ear canal and middle ear: punch biopsy under local or general anaesthesia.

Radiology

Computed tomographic (CT) scans usually show signs of chronic mastoid infection (Fig. 21.30). The avascular bone of the labyrinth resists carcinoma, and erosion of this area with direct invasion of the inner ear is a late radiological feature. Extension of the tumour anteriorly to penetrate the bony septum separating the middle ear cavity from the carotid artery is of great pathological importance. This is followed by spread around the artery and extension around the eustachian tube towards the postnasal space. Erosion of the carotid septum and the margins of the bony eustachian tube, and even-soft tissue extension of the tumour anteriorly, can be demonstrated by tomography and high-resolution CT scanning. Enlargement of the retropharyngeal lymph nodes may also be demonstrated by CT scan. Erosion may also be seen upwards through the tegmen tympani, backwards through the mastoid air cells and then through the thin plate of bone which forms the posterior wall of the pyramid and underlies the lateral sinus.

Once the tumour reaches the cranial cavity, the dura is infiltrated and this is rapidly followed by death. A carotid angiogram is thus of no value except to demonstrate a blocked lateral sinus.

- Retrograde jugular venography may be useful to assess the extent of the disease by demonstrating obstruction of the lateral sinus by tumour.
- The differential radiological diagnosis of squamous carcinoma of the middle ear includes tuberculosis otitis media, malignant otitis externa and glomus jugulare tumour.

Bone destruction medial to the sphenoid spine may be a contraindication to radical surgery.

Treatment policy

At least 10% of patients should not be offered any from of active treatment because the outlook is so gloomy due to extensive disease, poor general condition or distant metastases. The rest should be assessed for primary surgical treatment followed by postoperative radiotherapy. This is because:

- Reactions are lessened and the patients are made more comfortable.
- Higher doses can be given with less risk of complications.
- Five year survival is about 35%: external auditory meatus carcinoma results are about 10% better than those for tumours of the middle ear and mastoid.
- Surgery is usually of no value for primary recurrence after failed radiotherapy in middle ear tumours, but occasionally can be of value for non-squamous recurrences of external meatus lesions.

Carcinoma of the pinna

Primary surgical resection is the usual treatment, owing to the close proximity and possible involvement of cartilage. Superficial X-ray therapy is an alternative for some small tumours, but is contraindicated by:

- cartilage invasion
- fixation
- pain
- infection.

The extent of surgical resection depends on the size and histology of the tumour. Basal cell carcinoma requires a resection margin of 5–10 mm. Superficial lesions not invading cartilage may be excised with a disc of underlying cartilage. Deep lesions (invading cartilage) require full-thickness resection of the pinna.

Squamous carcinoma usually requires full-thickness resection. The margin for other non-skin sites is ideally 15–20 mm. This degree of clearance is usually neither feasible or necessary on the pinna.

Small tumours on the helix may be removed either in an ellipse- or a wedge-shaped excision larger ones require special techniques to reduce the cosmetic defect (see previously). After removal of tumours in the concha or antihelix, the resultant defect is impossible to close primarily and a postauricular flap is used. With larger tumours, involving removal of the whole or a large part of the auricle, there is no point in trying to rebuild the tissue and a prosthesis is the best replacement. If part of the ear is left then this can be used to hold the prosthesis. Larger defects are best repaired by an osseointegrated implant.

Tumours of, or invading the external auditory meatus, but not penetrating the middle ear

Surgical resection is the treatment of choice for all histologies. All cases should be treated by extended temporal bone resection. In exceptional cases (small tumours confined to the ear canal, basal cell carcinomas not invading deeply and the elderly and unfit) a lateral temporal bone resection may be used, with conservation of the facial nerve where possible. The petrosectomy cavity may be obliterated with a rotation, myocutaneous or free flap. Radical or modified radical neck dissection will be required in the presence of palpable or radiologically demonstrated cervical nodes.

Postoperative radiotherapy is indicated as soon as healing is complete.

- The temporal bone is one of the densest bones in the skull, and its invasion by tumour is inevitably associated with sepsis, which mitigates against the use of radiotherapy.
- It is very difficult to assess by clinical or radiological means the full extent of the petromastoid tumour. Preliminary surgical exploration is therefore necessary because this helps to remove necrotic or invaded bone and determine the extent of the tumour.

- The patient is usually made more comfortable by the operation and loses many of the symptoms.
- A cavity is provided for drainage and inspection.

Tumours of the parotid invading the facial nerve and temporal bone

The principles of treatment are:

- radical parotidectomy with sacrifice of the facial nerve, and frozen section histology on the proximal nerve stump. Where this is positive, the nerve should be resected proximally in its vertical mastoid portion with serial frozen sections until a clear margin of 10 mm is achieved. The head and ascending ramus of the mandible, and the pterygoid muscles, should be included in the radical resection
- lateral temporal bone resection combined with radical parotidectomy where the temporal bone is invaded
- primary facial reanimation by cable grafting using donor sensory nerve from a remote site
- postoperative radiotherapy as a routine
- secondary facial reanimation by appropriate techniques (e.g. gold weights, cross-facial anastomosis, free flap transfer with nerve anastomosis, faciohypoglossal anastomosis) where primary reanimation fails.

Carcinoma of the middle ear

Primary combined therapy is recommended since radiotherapy alone is not appropriate. These tumours are aggressive and carry a poor prognosis. Standard treatment is extended total petrosectomy with postoperative radiotherapy. The head and ascending ramus of the mandible should be excised, with parotidectomy and pterygoid muscle resection as necessary. Dural resection and repair may be required, with fascia lata grafts. Extensive tumours involving the temporal lobe are probably incurable, although occassional cure has been achieved with limited temporal lobe involvement. Involved brain should be removed with a margin of normal tissue. The pinna and surrounding skin are sacrificed. Postoperative radiotherapy is scheduled for 6 weeks following primary surgery.

Technique of petrosectomy

Preparation

- The postoperative facial paralysis and any nerve grafting proposed should be discussed. Facial function will not usually be better than a House Brackman grade 3 after a graft.
- The patient must be warned that he or she will be deaf after the operation, if not so already.
- Major vessels pass through the temporal bone and one must ensure adequate cross-match is obtained. The patient should be informed of the risk of haemorrhage. There may also be longer term sequelae in elderly subjects following surgery to the internal carotid artery.

Incision

The incision must encompass the entire ear, and in most cases the auricle will also be removed in continuity with the skin. The entire incision is shown in Fig. 21.31. The surgeon begins by marking the superior part 2 cm above the superior attachment of the auricle. This incision is used to expose the middle cranial fossa. A final check is made through the upper part of the incision as to the degree of dural involvement, to confirm the preoperative magnetic resonance imaging (MRI) and CT reports. The remaining part of the incision incorporates a standard parotidectomy incision. It starts at the upper level of the helix just in front of the auricle, dips down into the anterior incisura, gently curves under the lobe of the ear and continues down the neck to the level of the hyoid bone if the auricle is not to be removed. If a neck dissection is to be done the incision is continued to the point of the chin, and then a further incision is made in the lower part of the neck.

If the whole auricle is to be removed, the upper part of the incision continues round the ear to meet the original incision under the lobe of the ear. The facial and neck skin is elevated to expose the parotid gland. The tissues around the ear are elevated to expose as much mastoid bone as possible. The way in which this is done will depend on whether some auricle is to be kept or not. The anterior meatal wall must not be detached from the parotid or else a tumour-containing area will be entered. Early on, the internal jugular vein should be identified and ligated.

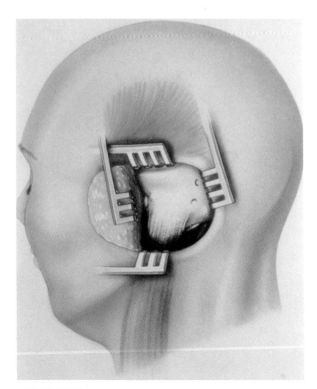

Figure 21.31 Extent of the incision for petrosectomy.

Excision

The skin incision above the auricle is continued straight down to the squamous temporal bone, and the soft tissues above and below are elevated. A cutting mastoid burr is used to cut through the squamous temporal bone over a distance of about 1 cm. Once the bone is opened, a Pennybacker retractor is introduced to open up the defect to allow wide exposure of the dura. The upper lateral venous sinus is identified and occluded. Then a blunt periosteal elevator is used to elevate the dura from the floor of the middle cranial fossa, provided that tumour has not penetrated the dura at this point. If it is invaded, it is possible to excise a small area, provided dural invasion does not extend medially to or beyond the apex of the petrous bone.

If the tumour is operable, the surgeon continues to remove the bone in an anterior direction using the Pennybacker's forceps, and divides the zygoma. The soft-tissue dissection is continued down the anterior border of the parotid gland, sacrificing the branches of the facial nerve. The dissection is continued deeply to the ascending ramus of the mandible. It is divided just below the notch to leave the temporomandibular joint which is left on the specimen.

The dissection continues posteriorly, first making the skin incision over the mastoid process. Again, the soft tissues are elevated off the bone and then the bone dissection continues using Pennybacker's forceps to expose the obliterated lateral sinus. The surgeon dissects forward through the floor of the middle ear so that the bone has now been divided on all sides. The specimen is now still attached by the firm bone of the petrous apex. This can be divided either by a cutting burr or with an osteoprobe. If an osteoprobe is used it is safer to use a curved pattern. The petrous apex can be cut through in one of these two ways and the specimen removed, if possible in one piece. Very often, however, the main specimen becomes detached before the hard bone of the petrous apex can be removed.

Repair

If the dura has been resected, it is repaired using a piece of fascia cut to the appropriate size and stitched in with 3/0 chromic catgut sutures. Small tears in the dura can be oversewn. The skin is repaired with a free flap; much the best is the rectus abdominis free flap, which is easy to harvest. It can be taken during the excision and it provides both muscle and skin. The muscle is very useful for filling the defect and sealing any small dural tears. The pectoralis major myocutaneous flap has the advantage of bulk but it may not always reach the upper limit of the defect. An alternative is the latissimus dorsi flap (pedicled or free). The facial nerve may be repaired by a cross-face nerve graft or a hypoglossal facial anastomosis. However, most patients have had enough after a petrosectomy and opt for accepting the defect.

The anterior scalp flap is now rarely used in the Western world, owing to the cosmetic defect. It may still have a place where resources are restricted.

Aftercare

- General care.
- Antibiotics: almost certainly the area was infected preoperatively so antibiotics are needed.
- Care of the eye: the eye should be monitored carefully; occasionally a lateral tarsorrhaphy is required.
- Cosmetic rehabilitation: if the patient is concerned about the paralysis of the corner of the mouth, it is possible to improve the position of the face at rest using a static fascia lata sling. The dynamic temporalis muscle sling tends to work less well. If the auricle has been removed it is possible to fit the patient with an artificial ear. The only exception to this may be in a woman with long straight hair.

Complications

- General complications.
- Intracranial complications. The main postoperative complications of this procedure relate to the cranial cavity. A cerebrospinal fluid leak is a distinct possibility, but usually closes spontaneously, particularly if a muscle-bearing free flap is used. Patients with cerebrospinal fluid leakage are particularly in need of antibiotic cover to reduce the chance of secondary meningitis. Re-exploration and repair are occasionally required.

Radiotherapy techniques

Carcinoma of the external auditory meatus and carcinoma of the middle ear and mastoid

One radiotherapeutic technique is used for carcinoma of the ear, whether it has arisen in the external auditory meatus, the middle ear cleft or mastoid air cells. The same technique is used for postoperative irradiation as for radical radiotherapy after only a biopsy. The treatment is planned and executed with the patient lying supine, immobilized in a Perspex beam-directing shell. The neck is well extended so that the treatment plane, which runs parallel to a line joining the top of the pinna to the floor of the orbit, is vertical. Clinical and radiological assessment defines the extent of disease to be treated, which as a minimum includes the petrous temporal bone, mastoid and adjacent lymph nodes. These are encompassed in a wedge-shaped volume, with its apex just anterior to the brainstem. The anterior border includes the preauricular lymph nodes and the posterior limit takes in the mastoid process. The upper margin runs along a line from the floor of the orbit to the top of the pinna. The lower margin includes the tip of the mastoid process and the submastoid lymph nodes (Fig. 21.32). This volume is designed to cover the tumour and possible extensions adequately, while sparing the eyes, brainstem and upper cervical cord from excessive dose. It is covered by anterior and posterior oblique fields, which are wedged to ensure dose homogeneity (Fig. 21.33). A dose of 66 Gy in 20–33 daily fractions over 4–6 weeks is given using megavoltage equipment.

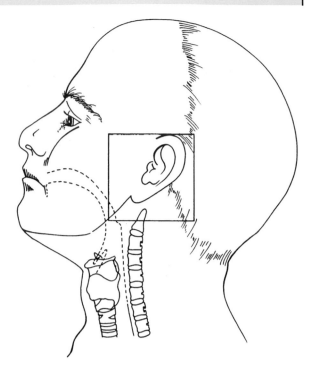

Figure 21.32 Volume to be irradiated in carcinoma of the middle ear and mastoid.

Carcinoma of the pinna

While small tumours of the helix may best be dealt with by surgery, small lesions at the entrance of the auditory canal and more extensive carcinomas can also be treated satisfactorily with electron beam therapy

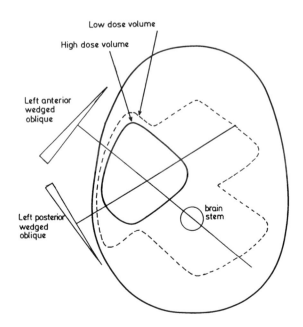

Figure 21.33 Plan of field arrangements for the irradiation of the middle ear and mastoid.

as an alternative to surgery to preserve the structure of the auricle. An appropriately shaped lead cut-out, allowing treatment of the tumour with a 1 cm margin, should be made. The external meatus should be plugged with wax to prevent deep penetration of the electrons through the air space. The surface of the tumour should be covered with an appropriate thickness of wax bolus, selected for the energy of electrons to be used, to give the required depth of penetration and a full surface dose. Using 10 MeV electrons, 45 Gy in 10 fractions over 2 weeks to 55 Gy in 20 fractions over 4 weeks should be given, depending on the size of the area treated.

Complications of radiotherapy

External auditory canal. Osteonecrosis of the bony portion of the canal is usually seen as an exposed area of bone that ultimately forms a scale-like sequestrum. It can be painful and tedious, but healing usually occurs. Sometimes, however, repair with a postaural flap may be required (Hill *et al.*, 1998). Stenosis can occur if radiation is given after a sleeve resection, or if local radium is inserted into the canal.

Middle ear and mastoid. Osteoradionecrosis usually means persistent disease unless the dosage given has been excessive.

Damage to the brain, brainstem or eyes. Damage to the eyes should be avoided, but it is impossible to irradiate the petrous temporal bone and much of the middle cranial fossa without irradiating cerebral tissue. Providing that large volumes of tissue are not irradiated to high doses the risk of damage seems to be small. Brain necrosis is more likely to follow radiotherapy in elderly patients whose vasculature is already the seat of arteriosclerotic changes.

The facial or auditory nerves in their extracranial course are never damaged by therapeutic radiation, and any impairment of their function is due either to involvement by cancer, or to a postoperative complication if radical surgery has been employed.

Conductive deafness after radiotherapy. This may occur in patients who have been successfully irradiated for carcinoma of the external auditory meatus. If the middle ear was normal to start with and the patient is free of recurrence, the possible causes include:

- thick mucus in the nasopharynx blocking the eustachian opening
- atresia of the eustachian orifice: this is rare and; results from necrosis of the eustachian cartilage, characterized by severe earache and trismus
- fibrosis of the fascial space surrounding the levator palati muscle.

The loss of conductive hearing following radical mastoidectomy for petromastoid carcinoma is not influ-

enced in any way by radiation. However, following irradiation to the petrous temporal bone, sometimes inner ear damage does occur which then can result in a degree of sensorineural hearing loss.

Radiotherapy technique for tumours of the skin

Basal cell carcinomas and the occasional squamous carcinoma which arise on the skin of the nose can usually be dealt with swiftly and effectively with radiotherapy. Because of their position, they tend to present early for treatment, although rarely one sees a patient with a very advanced tumour which has been neglected for years. The limited penetration of these tumours allows superficial X-rays (100 kV), which treat a depth of less than 1 cm, to be used in most cases. Larger tumours are better treated with electrons which have deeper, but still limited, penetration. For example, 10 MeV electrons will effectively treat a depth of 3 cm, but there is a rapid fall-off of dose beyond this.

The treated area:

- must be clearly defined
- will include the tumour with a margin of at least 5 mm all around.
- is demarcated by an appropriately sized lead cut-out to shield the surrounding skin
- if irregular, on an uneven contour such as the bridge of the nose, or adjacent, e.g. to the eye which needs to be meticulously shielded, requires an individually prepared lead cut-out. Otherwise, a standard one may be used.

The dose and fractionation prescribed depend principally on tumour size:

- <2–3 cm diameter: 35 Gy in five fractions over 1 week
- >2–3 cm diameter: 45 Gy in 10 fractions over 2 weeks
- frail, elderly patients may be given a single 20 Gy treatment, but the control rates and cosmetic results are less good
- consideration should be given to primary surgery for treatment of lesions involving the nasal cartilage, or which are bulky or deeply penetrating, for example at the columella. Otherwise, they require a higher radiotherapeutic dose: 55 Gy in 20 fractions over 4 weeks with electrons. Consideration should be given to primary surgery.

A skin reaction proceeding to moist desquamation will inevitably follow. This can be soothed with zinc and castor oil or 1% hydrocortisone cream. If the ala nasi is treated, there will also be a mucosal reaction within the vestibule. A fillet of lead inserted into the nasal cavity will prevent a reaction on the nasal septum. When the area is healed, the patient should be advised to avoid exposing it to direct sunshine, by either wearing a hat with a brim or using a sunblock cream. Late effects may include atrophy of the skin, depigmentation and the development of telangiectasia.

References and further reading

Cascinelli N., Clement C. and Belli F. (1995) Cutaneous melanoma, in *Oxford Textbook of Oncology* (M. Peckham, H. Pinned, U. Veronesi, Eds), Oxford University Press, pp. 902–28.

Gailani M. R., Lefell D. J., Ziegler A., Gross E. G., Brash D.E. and Bale A. E. (1996) Relationship between sunlight exposure and a key genetic alteration in basal cell carcinoma, *J Natl Cancer Inst* **88**: 349–54.

Gray D. T., Suman V. J., Su P. D., Clay R. P., Harmsen W. S. and Roenigk R. K. (1997) Trends in the population based incidence of squamous cell carcinoma of the skin first diagnosed between 1984 and 1992, *Arch Dermatol* **133**: 735–40.

Hill D. S., Gaze M. N. and Grant H. R. (1998) A simple reconstructive procedure for radiation-induced necrosis of the external auditory canal, *J. Laryngol Otol* **112**: 1142–6.

Kane W. J., Yugueros P., Clay R. P., and Woods J. E. (1997) *Treatment outcome* for *424* primary cases of clinical stage I cutaneous malignant melanoma of the head and neck, *Head and Neck* **19**: 457–65.

Moffat D. A., Grey P., Ballagh R. H. and Hardy D. G. (1997) Extended temporal bone resection for squamous cell carcinoma, *Otolaryngol Head Neck Surg* **116**: 617–23.

Mohs F. E. (1978) *Chemosurgery: Microscopically Controlled Surgery for Skin Cancer*, Charles C. Thomas, Springfield, IL.

Motley R. J., Gould D. J., Douglas W. S. and Simpson N. B. (1995) Treatment of basal cell carcinoma by dermatologists in the United Kingdom, *Br J Dermatol* **132**: 437–40.

Osguthorpe J. D., Abel C. G., Lang P. and Hochman M. (1997) Neurotropic cutaneous tumours of the head and neck, *Arch Otolaryngol Head Neck Surg* **123**: 871–6.

Papadopoulos T., Rasiah K., Thompson J. F., Quinn M. J. and Crotty K. A. (1997) Melanoma of the nose, *Br J Surg* **84**: 986–9.

Taxy J. B. (1997) Squamous carcinoma on the nasal vestibule. An analysis of five cases and literature review, *Am J Clin Pathol* **107**: 698–703.

Vico P., Fourez T., Nemec E., Andry G. and Deraemaeker R. (1995) Aggressive basal cell carcinoma of head and neck areas, *Eur J Surg Oncol* **21**: 490–7.

Zanetti R., Rosso S., Martinez C., Navarro C., Schraub S., Sancho-Garnier H. *et al.* (1996) The multicentre South European study *Helios* I : skin characteristics and sunburns in basal cell and squamous carcinomas of the skin, *Br J Cancer* **73**(11): 1440–6.

Tumours of major salivary glands

'Don't just do something ... stand there and think'
Ron Hoille

Introduction

The major salivary glands are common sources of benign pathology, both inflammatory and neoplastic. Salivary gland malignancy is rare and comprises a multiplicity of human types, reflecting the glands' heterogeneous cell populations. Both parotid and submandibular gland surgery may be complicated by neural damage. Thorough knowledge of surgical anatomy is imperative.

Surgical anatomy

There are four main salivary glands: two submandibular and two parotid glands. Multiple minor salivary glands occur elsewhere in the upper respiratory tract, especially in the hard palate and lateral pharyngeal wall. The removal of the major salivary glands is basically an anatomical dissection, so it is essential that any surgeon should know the anatomy of these regions intimately. The parotid gland is described as having a superficial and a deep lobe with an isthmus in between; these lobes are separated by the facial nerve, which runs through the gland. This is the case in the preserved cadaver, where the gland has been shrunk by formalin, but *in vivo* the gland should be regarded as a lump of bread dough poured over an egg whisk, the dough being the glandular tissue and the whisk the facial nerve. The facial nerve is surrounded by parotid tissue and intimately attached on all sides to glandular tissue.

The parotid gland extends from the zygoma superiorly to the oblique line of the sternomastoid inferiorly, and anteriorly to the midpoint of the masseter muscle. The duct runs over the anterior border of the masseter muscle to enter the mouth opposite the second molar tooth in the interdental line. The gland is covered by the investing fascia of the neck and there are six to eight lymph nodes outside this fascia and 10–12 lymph nodes embedded in the glandular tissue, largely in the superficial lobe. There are very few nodes in the deep lobe.

The deep 'lobe' of the parotid gland – the retromandibular portion – lies in the parapharyngeal space anterior to the carotid sheath and styloid process and posterior to the infratemporal fossa. Medially is the superior constrictor muscle separating it from the tonsil and oropharynx (Fig. 22.1). Tumours may extend deeply into the lateral parapharyngeal space either by passing through the narrow space between the mandible and stylomandibular ligament or by passing behind the ligament.

The facial nerve emerges from the stylomastoid foramen to enter the substance of the gland at its posteromedial surface. As the nerve exits from the stylomastoid foramen, it is surrounded by a thick layer of fascia, which is continuous with the periosteum of the skull base. It is, thus, very difficult to find the nerve at this point unless it is identified either distally or proximally within the mastoid process (Fig. 22.2).

Methods of facial nerve identification

- Tragal pointer
- Posterior belly of digastric
- Tympanomastoid suture
- Peripheral branches
- Mastoid process

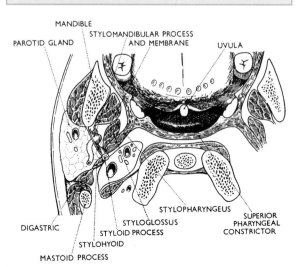

Figure 22.1 Transverse diagram of relations of the parotid gland.

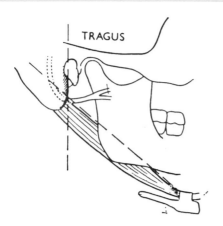

TRAGUS

Figure 22.2 Locating the facial nerve having traced the posterior belly digastric posteriorly. The nerve bisects the angle between the posterior belly of digastric and the tympanic plate.

The tragal cartilage ends on a point. The nerve is 1 cm deep and inferior to this, surrounded by a small aggregation of fat and overlain by a small blood vessel. If the posterior belly of the digastric muscle is followed up to the tympanic plate and the anterior mastoid process 5 mm below the bony meatal edge, the facial nerve may be found as it passes downwards, forwards and laterally, immediately above the upper border of the posterior belly of digastric, lateral and slightly posterior to the base of the styloid process. Alternatively, the anterior border of the mastoid process can be found and traced up to where it meets the vaginal process of the tympanic bone. The facial nerve bisects the angle between the two pieces of bone at the tympanomastoid suture.

Shortly after entering the substance of the parotid gland, the nerve divides into the two major trunks, the temporozygomatic and the cervicofacial. The branching of these nerves is rarely abnormal. In under 1% of cases, the nerve divides within the mastoid and exits as separate branches.

Many variations have been described based on the peripheral branching patterns. These may be summarized into five types, varying from no anastomoses between the five branches to multiple vertical anastomotic connections. The usual pattern is for terminal branches to go to the forehead, the eyebrow, the corner of the eye and lower eyelid from the temporozygomatic branch. The buccal branch can arise from either the upper division or the lower division of the nerve. This can give off vertical anastomotic branches to the temporozygomatic branch or the cervicofacial branch. It supplies the lower eyelid, the central portion of the face, the ala of the nose and the upper lip. The cervicofacial division divides into a mandibular branch to the upper lip, the corner of the mouth and the lower lip. The cervical branch supplies platysma and may be divided during a parotidectomy. This manoeuvre often causes abnormality of lip movement since platysma inserts into the angle of the mouth, and should thus be avoided if possible.

It is essential to know the surface markings of the peripheral divisions of the nerve, in case they have to be used to find the facial nerve in a retrograde manner. A safer way to find the nerve is to carry out a facial nerve decompression within the mastoid. The often-portrayed step of knocking the tip off the mastoid in order to find the facial nerve has more relationship to medical illustration than reality, because the nerve is surrounded by a mixture of fascia and periosteum and it is virtually impossible to find it safely with this manoeuvre.

The submandibular gland fills the major portion of the submandibular triangle. It has a superficial portion that lies on the mylohyoid muscle, bounded anteriorly by the belly of the digastric, and this curves around the posterior part of the mylohyoid muscle to lie on the hyoglossus muscle and thus terminate in a duct entering the floor of the mouth. On the fascia, superficial to the gland, runs the mandibular branch of the facial nerve; deep to the gland are the lingual nerve superiorly and the hypoglossal nerve inferiorly, both lying on the hyoglossus muscle. There are several lymph nodes on the surface of the submandibular gland: the two most important ones lie in front of and behind the facial artery at the edge of the mandible (close to the marginal mandibular branch of the facial nerve) and must be recognized and sampled during the treatment of mouth cancer. The paired sublingual glands lie just beneath the anterior floor of the mouth and are actually large collections of minor salivary glands. Secreted saliva enters the mouth through several short ducts.

The minor salivary glands are mucus-secreting glands, situated throughout the upper respiratory tract. There are about 250 glands on the hard palate, 100 on the soft palate and 10 on the uvula. Palatal glands are not found in the midline or anterior to a line between the first molar teeth, or on the gingiva. Other glands are found in the submucosa of the inner surface of the lips, around the opening of the parotid duct, in the mucous membrane of the cheek, in the floor of the mouth, in the palatoglossal folds, on the inferior surface of the tongue, and near the frenulum.

There are two main theories of salivary gland tumour origin. According to the bicellular theory of salivary tumorigenesis, the cells of the more proximal secretory ducts are thought to give rise to intercalated duct and myoepithelial cells. From these, glandular neoplasms originate, including the pleomorphic adenoma, oncocytoma, acinic cell carcinoma and adenoid cystic carcinoma. The excretory duct cell population is thought to give rise to epidermoid tumours, e.g. mucoepidermoid and squamous cell carcinomas. In the multicellular theory, each tumour type maps to a different cell type within the salivary gland unit: Warthin's and oncocytomas from the striated duct cells, acinic tumours from the acinar cells, mixed tumours from intercalated duct and myoepithelial cells, etc. This theory is supported by the observation that all salivary cell types retain mitotic potential.

More recently, however, the persistence of neuroectodermal antigens in both benign and malignant salivary tumour cell cultures has led to a single (neuroectodermal) stem cell theory of origin (Levine and Bradley, 1996). The rare lymphoepithelial carcinoma is associated, at least in Asian patients, with the Epstein–Barr virus, (EBV) which gains entry to cells via the surface C3d receptor, known to be present in salivary gland epithelium (Iezzoni et al., 1995). EBV has also been suggested to occur in association with Warthin's tumour, but the results of preliminary studies are conflicting.

Molecular biology

p53, DNA ploidy and chromosomal abnormalities

Studies using fluorescent in situ hybridization (FISH) to study a number of different salivary tumour types show that low-grade malignant tumours generally show small chromosomal gains or losses and are generally diploid or near diploid, whereas high-grade lesions showed marked polysomy and are DNA aneuploid. Clonal chromosomal abnormalities (usually gains rather than losses) are manifest in most DNA diploid and all DNA aneuploid malignant tumours. Benign tumours show more or less normal chromosomal patterns (El-Naggar et al., 1997).

About 20% of carcinomas are ex-pleomorphic adenomas, and 10% of pleomorphic adenomas have **polysomy of chromosome 17**. Chromosome 17 monosomy and polysomy have been related to p53 protein expression (often with *p53* gene deletion on FISH) in both tumour groups (Li et al., 1997). In adenoid cystic carcinoma, however, primary tumours have been shown to be negative for both p53 and WAF-1, whereas recurrent adenoid cystic lesions show frequent p53-positive cells and point mutations, suggesting that p53 alterations may be a later development in tumour progression (Papadaki et al., 1996).

c-erbB-2

The c-erbB-2 protein is a growth factor receptor encoded at a different region of the same chromosome (17) as the *p53* gene. Overexpression of both proteins is associated with neoplasia. In salivary glands, c-erbB-2 expression is associated with high-grade neoplasia but not those of myoepithelial cell origin (Rosa et al., 1997).

Ki-67

The Ki-67 nuclear antigen is used to estimate the growth fraction of tumours. A high level of expression in adenoid cystic carcinomas appears to be a very strong adverse prognostic indicator (Nordgard et al., 1997).

Hormonal receptors

There is some anecdotal evidence that salivary tumour such as adenoid cystic carcinoma may not only express sex hormone receptors (Jeannon et al., 1999) but may show clinical response to hormonal manipulation, e.g. by the antioestrogen tamoxifen.

Radiation-induced salivary gland tumours

A survey of 145 salivary gland tumours among atom bomb survivors (Saku et al., 1997) showed a disproportionate representation of both mucoepidermoid and Warthin's tumours at high radiation doses. Mortality from malignant tumours was inversely related to the radiation dose for that reason.

Benign tumours and non-neoplastic swellings

- Pleomorphic adenoma
- Warthin's tumour (adenolymphoma)
- Oncocytoma
- Vascular tumours
- Granulomatous diseases
  - Sarcoidosis
  - Tuberculosis
  - Actinomycosis
  - Cat scratch disease
- Cysts
- Benign tumours

Pleomorphic adenoma

- Male:female 1:1
- Average age at presentation 40 years
- 'Mixed cell tumour': arises from intercalated duct cells and myoepithelial cells
- Most common tumour of major salivary glands
- 90% of benign parotid tumours; 50% of all submandibular gland tumours
- A few bilateral tumours have been described

The tumour grows slowly with long quiescent periods and short periods of rapid growth. About one-quarter of patients with this tumour have vague local discomfort, but it is usually asymptomatic apart from the lump, and the facial nerve is never paralysed. Nearly all arise in the tail of the parotid gland, just anterior to the lobe of the ear. They can also occur in the retromandibular portion of the parotid gland, as either solitary deep-lobe tumours or dumb-bell tumours. They are very rare elsewhere in the parotid gland. On palpation, the tumour is usually smooth, superficial, round and mobile. The capsule of compressed normal parotid tissue varies in thickness and is lobulated because the tumour grows with pseudopodial extensions through this capsule.

The cut surface is usually greyish white but it may have blue tinges; there may also be secondary cyst formation and haemorrhage. One tumour in 10 is highly cellular and, although showing no sign of malignancy, such a tumour is more prone to recur. The tumour is highly implantable and the recurrence rate after primary surgery is about 5%. If simple enucleation is performed, however, the recurrence rate is between 20 and 30%.

Warthin's tumour

- Male:female 7:1
- 'Adenolymphoma'
- 6–8% of salivary tumours
- Arises in heterotopic parotid tissue occurring within parotid lymph nodes
- Average age at presentation 70 years
- 10% bilateral
- Usually fluctuant, slow-growing, smooth not bosselated, soft, compressible
- Usually in the parotid tail
- Never malignant
- Cystic ones contain mucoid fluid; solid lymphoid component
- Solid white areas are sometimes seen and these are due to lymphoid tissue

---

Oncocytoma

- Male:female 1: 1
- 1% of all salivary gland tumours
- Also known as an oxyphil cell adenoma
- Another adenoma; usually cystic
- Rare < 50 years
- Painless, slow-growing lump
- Arises from the striated duct cells
- Malignant variants are exceedingly rare

Vascular tumours

Haemangioma

- Over half of childhood salivary gland lesions
- Much more common in females than in males
- Usually diagnosed during the first year
- Soft, painless masses
- Parenchyma is replaced by vasoformative elements but normal glandular lobulation is maintained

---

The haemangioma may be capillary, cavernous, mixed or hypertrophic. About 50% of patients have a cutaneous haemangioma in the head and neck area. Spontaneous regression definitely occurs in some vascular tumours so that no treatment should be offered until the age of 10 or 12 years. Surgery should only be performed if the tumour is enlarging.

Lymphangiomas are usually present at birth and again are more common in girls than boys. The three types are simple lymphangioma, cavernous lymphangioma and cystic hygroma. The thin-walled lymph spaces invade the parotid and adjacent tissues and do not replace the glandular parenchyma like haemangiomas. The tumours are soft and fluctuant and usually transilluminate. If they cause disfigurement, they should be removed.

Granulomatous diseases

Sarcoidosis is usually bilateral and diffuse. A common presentation is, along with swelling of the parotid and lacrimal glands, chorioretinitis and progressive cranial nerve involvement, which is also known as Heerfordt's disease. Tuberculosis is rare but is a possible infection of the lymph nodes on or within the parotid gland. Actinomycosis can follow dental extraction or other oral trauma. Cat-scratch disease is passed from wild or domestic animals to humans by a scratch and is due to a Gram-negative bacillus.

Cysts

Simple **retention cysts** within the parotid tissue are rare, and one should suspect *Echinococcus* or a hydatid cyst, or human immunodeficiency virus (HIV)-related cysts. The most common cystic lesion is a Warthin's tumour and areas of pleomorphic adenoma may also be cystic (see above). Branchial cysts can occur within the lymph nodes in the gland and on the surface of the gland.

Lipomas can feel cystic. They usually lie lateral to the parotid gland but can extend anteriorly into the anterior compartment of the face. They must be differentiated from fatty infiltration, which is usually bilateral.

Benign lymphoepithelial lesion was described in 1952 by Godwin. It is a pathological process that arises in the intralobular ducts like a punctate parotitis. As the ducts dilate, their cells disrupt and epidermoid metaplasia begins. Lymphocytes aggregate around the ducts and the lumen becomes obliterated. It is probably part of a lymphoreticular proliferative disease; it is not yet clear whether a benign lymphoepithelial lesion evolves into malignancy or whether it is part of an immunological disorder that is going to become lymphoproliferative disease anyway. It is a lesion isolated to the parotid gland and shows none of the systemic manifestations of Sjögren's disease.

Sjögren's syndrome was first described in 1933 by Henrik Sjögren, a Stockholm ophthalmologist. It is a multisystem disease, involving almost every system in the body. It is classified into two forms. Primary Sjögren's disease (the sicca syndrome) consists of xerostomia and xerophthalmia without an associated connective tissue disease. Affected patients are often extremely upset by the dryness of the mouth and frequently show psychiatric disturbances. They seldom have salivary gland involvement and one in six will progress to lymphoma.

Secondary Sjögren's syndrome

- Triad of xerophthalmia, xerostomia and a connective tissue disorder
- Half of the patients have rheumatoid arthritis
- Also seen with systemic lupus erythematosus, scleroderma, polymyositis, primary biliary cirrhosis, autoimmune liver disease, chronic graft-versus-host disease
- 30% recurrent bouts of parotitis
- Small minority develops lymphoma

Malignant tumours

Tumours of the salivary glands are uncommon and together comprise less than 3% of all neoplasms of the head and neck. Most are benign, with the incidence of malignant tumours being approximately 1 per 100 000 of the population.

Prognostic factors in salivary gland malignancy

- Tumour histology
- Histological grade
- Anatomical site of origin
- Clinical stage
- Age
- Facial nerve paralysis
- Experience of the surgeon

The 'T' stage and overall stage grouping for salivary gland malignancies is shown in Table 22.1 and the World Health Organization (WHO) histological typing of these tumours is found in Appendix 1.

In patients with salivary gland carcinoma, survival depends on histological tumour type and grade, the anatomical site of origin and the clinical stage. In those patients with parotid gland cancers, male gender and age greater than 50 years also appear significantly to worsen the prognosis. Another important consideration is the experience of the surgeon. Further studies using multivariate analysis (Spiro, 1998) have concluded that clinical stage and the histological type together with the grade of the tumour are the only significant determinants of survival.

One in six parotid tumours is malignant, as are one in three submandibular tumours and one in two minor

---

Table 22.1 The 'T' and overall stage grouping of salivary gland malignancies

T_X	Primary tumour cannot be assessed
T_0	No evidence of primary tumour
T_{is}	Carcinoma *in situ*
T_1	Tumour 2 cm or less in greatest dimension without extraparenchymal extension*[†]
T_2	Tumour more than 2 cm but no more than 4 cm in greatest dimension without extraparenchymal extension*[†]
T_3	Tumour having extraparenchymal extension without seventh nerve involvement and/or more than 4 cm but no more than 6 cm in greatest dimension*[†]
T_4	Tumour invades base of skull, seventh nerve, and/or exceeds 6 cm in greatest diameter[†]

*Extraparenchymal extension is clinical or macroscopic evidence of invasion of skin, soft tissues, bones or nerve.
[†]New inclusion.
Microscopic evidence alone does not constitute extraparenchymal extension for classification purposes.

Stage grouping

Stage	T	N	M
Stage I	T_1	N_0	M_0
	T_2	N_0	M_0
Stage II	T_3	N_0	M_0
Stage III	T_1	N_1	M_0
	T_2	N_1	M_0
Stage IV	T_4	N_0	M_0
	T_3	N_1	M_0
	T_4	N_1	M_0
	Any T	N_2	M_0
	Any T	N_3	M_0
	Any T	Any N	M_1

UICC (1997).

salivary gland tumours. Malignant parotid tumours invade locally and usually extend into the retromandibular area of the parotid and the parapharyngeal space. They drain to the lymph nodes within the parapharyngeal space and to the deep jugular chain. They also metastasize to lymph nodes on the surface of the gland and to the prefacial and postfacial nodes. They will ultimately involve the temporomandibular joint and the external auditory meatus, and occasionally the petrous bone.

Salivary gland malignancy

- 12 per million of population
- 3% of head and neck malignant tumours.
- Male:female 1:1
- Usually present in the fifth decade
- Higher risk in Black populations, Eskimos, Scots and survivors from radiation exposure
- In parotid > 40% involve the lateral lobe only, 10% the deep lobe only, 27% will involve both lobes; 20% extend beyond the glandular tissue

---

Presentation with facial nerve paralysis in malignant tumours

Poorly differentiated carcinoma	23–26%
Adenoid cystic carcinoma	23–26%
Carcinoma ex-pleomorphic adenoma	9–14%
Mucoepidermoid carcinoma	8%
Acinic cell carcinoma	3%

Mucoepidermoid tumour

Mucoepidermoid tumour

- Male:female 1:1
- 4–9% of salivary tumours
- Major glands: > 90% arise in the parotid, 8% in the submandibular, 1% in the sublingual
- minor salivary glands: more common: 41% palate, 14% buccal, 9% tongue, 5% lip
- Most common salivary gland tumour in children
- Usually presents in the fifth decade
- Solid or cystic, usually not encapsulated
- 40% lymphadenopathy
- 40% 5 year survival if high grade

Several cell types are seen, including, epidermoid, columnar, clear and mucous. Pathologists have traditionally divided these tumours into low grade (well differentiated) and high grade (poorly differentiated). High-grade tumours comprise 10% of the total group and occur in older patients. However the value of grading is now disputed. They are commonly misdiagnosed as squamous carcinomas. A small proportion of the more common low-grade tumours will behave in the same aggressive manner but most behave like pleomorphic adenomas. The tumours are usually unencapsulated and show a reactive stroma.

Acinic cell tumour

Acinic cell tumour

- Male:female 1:1
- peak in fifth decade
- 2.5–4% of all parotid tumours
- Arises from the terminal tubular intercalated duct cells
- Sometimes bilateral
- Often encapsulated
- Second most common salivary tumour in children
- Most behave like pleomorphic adenomas
- Some have an aggressive malignant course
- Propensity for late recurrence, even 30 years after excision
- 5 year survival 90%; 20 year survival 50–60%.
- 10% of recurrences have regional lymphadenopathy, 15% have distant metastases

---

Adenoid cystic carcinoma

Adenoid cystic carcinoma

- Slightly more common in females than in males
- 40% of malignant tumours at all salivary sites.
- Four main pathological patterns: cribriform, tubuloglandular, solid cellular, cylindromatous
- Unencapsulated but appears circumscribed
- Most probable source: intercalcated ducts
- Median age at presentation in the sixth decade
- 25% parotid, 15% submandibular, 1% sublingual, 60% minor glands (70% oral)
- 8% lymphadenopathy at presentation, 7% late node appearance
- Moist and grey–pink on section, infiltrative growth pattern
- Marked tendency to invade nerves, with high frequency of pain

---

Only 15% will metastasize to lymph nodes, 8% at the time of presentation and 7% later. The hallmark, however, is the incidence of distant metastases in the lungs (40%), the brain (20%) and the bones (20%). Approximately 40% of patients will ultimately manifest distant metastases but the incidence of such metastases in patients dying of the disease approaches 70%.

Carcinoma ex-pleomorphic adenoma

Malignant mixed cell tumour

- Only 1% arise *ab initio*, the vast majority from a pre-existing pleomorphic adenoma
- Malignancy takes about 10 years to develop in an adenoma
- 1–5% of pleomorphic adenomas present for >10 years may become malignant
- May still be grossly encapsulated
- Suspicious features: pain, rapid growth spurt, excessive bosselation and infiltration at the periphery
- Metastases: regional lymph nodes in 25%, distant in 30%
- 5 year survival around 40%, 15 year survival 19%

Adenocarcinoma

This tumour comprises about 3% of parotid tumours and 10% of submandibular minor salivary gland tumours. The gender incidence is equal and it can occur at any age. It is one of the more common malignant salivary gland tumours seen in children. It may present as an asymptomatic mass or with typical malignant features. In the parotid, most occur in the deep lobe or extend beyond the gland when first seen. They are highly malignant with a high metastatic rate and the 5 year survival is only about 10%.

Squamous cell carcinoma

This is extremely rare in the parotid (1% of tumours) and is only slightly more common in the submandibular gland. Before arriving at a diagnosis of squamous cell carcinoma, the pathologist must exclude mucoepidermoid tumour or malignant pleomorphic adenoma. One must also rule out metastasis in the parotid lymph nodes from a neighbouring current or previously treated skin tumour, or from another head and neck primary site.

Squamous cell carcinoma

- Male:female 2:1
- Average age at presentation in the seventh decade
- Aggressive tumour
- No tendency to encapsulation
- Grows rapidly, causing pain, facial nerve paralysis, skin fixation and ulceration
- 50% metastatic neck nodes at presentation
- Very bad prognosis with any method of treatment

Lymphoepithelial carcinoma (undifferentiated carcinoma/malignant lymphoepithelial lesion)

This rare variant has been reported in major and minor salivary glands in fewer than 150 cases. It has a striking association with Asians, especially Inuit (Eskimos) and southern Chinese, in whom it seems to be associated with evidence of EBV (Iezzoni *et al.*, 1995; Sheen *et al.*, 1997).

Sarcomas

These are extremely rare but neurofibrosarcoma, rhabdomyosarcoma, histiocytoma and Kaposi's sarcoma have all been described. The management of sarcomas is outlined in Chapter 25.

Lymphomas

A lymphoma arising in an intraparotid lymph node may present initially as a parotid swelling. It is treated as any other lymphoma (see Chapter 25).

Metastatic tumours

The parotid gland has nodes within it and on the surface, so these can be the site of metastatic deposits. Eighty per cent of these are from skin of the face, temple or scalp, and they are usually melanoma or squamous carcinoma. The node metastases can be on the surface of the gland or in the deep portion of the stroma. They can also occur from infraclavicular sites.

Recurrent pleomorphic adenoma

This problem can be split into two categories. The first is where the recurrence can be expected after an inadequate lumpectomy for a pleomorphic adenoma. The second group is where the recurrence is unexpected after a superficial parotidectomy for pleomorphic adenoma. The possible causes of recurrence are bursting the capsule, carrying out an inadequate lumpectomy or the bursting of the capsule during manipulation, when the recurrence is frequently multiple. The problem of assessment, therefore, lies in knowing how far the tumour recurrence extends, and its relationship to facial nerve and skin, and being able to perform a total parotidectomy preserving as much facial nerve function as possible.

Investigations

History

Parotid tumours are usually unilateral, although Warthin's tumour can be bilateral. Pleomorphic adenomas almost always occur in the tail of the gland; if a tumour occurs in the body of the gland one should suspect that it is not a pleomorphic adenoma. Benign tumours grow slowly over a period of years, but malignant ones usually grow rapidly from the outset and the cardinal sign of malignancy is pain. They may also involve skin and/or the facial nerve. In inflammatory or calculus disease there is often marked fluctuation in the size of the glands, together with pain and tenderness. In these conditions, eating almost always causes an increase in pain and swelling.

Parotomegaly can occur with various endocrinopathies and systemic illnesses, so the patient should be asked about other conditions such as myxoedema, diabetes, Cushing's disease, cirrhosis, gout and alcoholism. Bulimia should be suspected in young girls with parotid enlargement. Certain drugs such as the contraceptive pill, thiouracil and coproxamol can also cause parotomegaly. One in three patients with Sjögren's syndrome will present with parotomegaly, and it is also seen in granulomas.

Examination conditions outside the parotid that mimic parotomegaly

- Hypertrophy of the masseter
- Dental cysts
- Branchial cysts
- Myxoma of the masseter
- Neuroma of the facial nerve
- Temporal artery aneurysm
- Mandibular tumours
- Mastoiditis
- Lymphadenitis of parotid nodes
- Sebaceous cysts

Having established that the swelling is truly salivary, the surgeon compares its margins with the anatomical limits of the gland. Inflammatory processes enlarge the whole gland, whereas neoplasia, at least in the early stages, presents as a discrete swelling within the gland.

Key points of physical examination of a major salivary gland

- Salivary or extraglandular?
- Whole gland swollen or a swelling within the gland?
- One gland is affected or multiple?
- Firm or cystic?
- Benign or malignant?
- Findings of bimanual palpation?
- Medial displacement of the pharynx?
- Can pus can be expressed from the duct?
- Is there associated lymphadenopathy?

One must establish if only one gland is affected or multiple glands are involved. Most tumours involve a single gland but sialectasis, benign lymphoepithelial

lesion, Sjögren's disease, calculus disease and the endocrine conditions mentioned above usually affect more than one gland.

The cardinal sign of malignancy is pain, and involvement of the skin or facial nerve is absolutely diagnostic of malignancy. In inflammatory disease, one must see whether any pus can be expressed from the duct: this may mean examining the oral cavity early on, when the gland is first palpated, and not as an afterthought, by which time no more pus may be expressible. The surgeon determines whether the tumour is firm or cystic. Pleomorphic adenomas may present in either way but a cystic feeling should make one consider a Warthin's tumour, a mucoepidermoid tumour or a parotid cyst.

Salivary glands should always be palpated bimanually. This is particularly important in the submandibular gland or if calculus disease is suspected. A pharyngeal extension of a deep-lobe tumour may be seen inside the pharynx.

Investigations of salivary gland disease

- Laboratory tests
- Radiology
- FNAC
- Open biopsy

Laboratory tests

The appropriate endocrine tests should be done to exclude diabetes, myxoedema or Cushing's disease. In Sjögren's syndrome, erythrocyte sedimentation rate, protein electrophoresis, antinuclear factor and rheumatoid factor are tested.

Radiology

- **Plain films.** Parotid stones are almost always radiolucent, while submandibular stones are nearly always radio-opaque. Intraoral films are especially useful in this latter condition. Plain films may also be useful in differentiating some of the extraparotid causes of parotomegaly. Chest X-ray is useful in suspected sarcoidosis or in malignant lesions such as adenoid cystic tumours.
- **Sialography.** This is the most useful radiological investigation in non-neoplastic salivary gland disease but is of little value in the investigation of mass lesions.
- **Ultrasonography.** This is useful in assessing the cystic nature of tumours. Retention cysts and true cysts of the parotid are sonolucent. Neoplasms appear as solid masses, except for Warthin's tumour. Malignant tumours have a low reflectivity, whereas mixed tumours show variable reflectivity.
- **Computed tomographic scanning.** This is the gold standard for investigation of parotid tumours. In the

work-up of a parotid tumour it is important to assess its extension in the deep lobe and its relation to the facial nerve. Computed tomographic (CT) scanning, combined with sialography, usually allows this differentiation.

■ **Magnetic resonance imaging.** In salivary glands, the contrast between tumour and the surrounding tissue is greater than with CT scanning but tissue detail is less well defined. Some radiologists attempt to distinguish benign from malignant lesions on magnetic resonance imaging (MRI).

Fine-needle aspiration cytology

In recent years, fine-needle aspiration cytology (FNAC) has become widely used in the diagnosis of salivary gland masses. The sensitivity and specificity in salivary gland diagnosis, however, depend on access to a cytopathologist who is both skilled and interested in the technique. If a tumour is obviously malignant and involving skin, then an incisional biopsy may be performed to establish the tumour type before removing it together with the area of the biopsy.

Open biopsy

■ **Discrete salivary gland mass.** On no account should this be subjected to incisional biopsy, unless there is clear clinical or cytological evidence of malignancy which cannot be conclusively categorized on cytological features. As there is a 90% chance that a single parotid mass is a pleomorphic adenoma, incisional biopsy as a primary investigation would cause tumour implantation.

■ **Diffuse enlargement of the salivary gland.** An incisional biopsy may be necessary, but this should usually be accompanied by a sublabial biopsy, to diagnose some of the granulomatous conditions, such as Sjögren's syndrome.

Treatment policy

The main problem with simple parotid masses is that a fairly major operation is performed without a diagnosis being known. In 90% of cases, the clinical diagnosis is correct and a suspected simple tumour turns out to be a simple tumour. Occasionally, however, a malignant tumour may present as an isolated mass without pain, facial nerve or skin involvement. The diagnosis may be suspected during surgery but usually becomes apparent only when the pathology report is received.

In the case of a simple mass suspected of being a pleomorphic adenoma, a superficial parotid lobectomy is performed. Enucleation must never be performed. Even though it could be done quite safely for a Warthin's tumour or an oncocytoma, the diagnosis is not known at this point in the operation, and a frozen section is not acceptable because of the danger of implanting a pleomorphic adenoma as well as the unreliability of frozen-section pathological diagnosis.

When some authors write about enucleation, they mean that they find the nerve and dissect the lower division, thus carrying out a lumpectomy with a cuff of healthy tissue around it usually with microscopic assessment of the dissection margins. This is an acceptable method of treating small pleomorphic adenomas and does not need to be followed with irradiation. When embarking on a superficial lobectomy, one must be prepared to carry out a total parotidectomy if it is indicated, and thus be able to complete a total parotidectomy, preserving the facial nerve. Total conservative parotidectomy with preservation of the facial nerve may be indicated for larger tumours (>4 cm) in any case.

If, during the operation, the appearance of the tumour is such as to suggest malignancy, then a frozen section must be performed. If, at this point, it appears impossible to resect the tumour without damage to, or resection of, the facial nerve, then the wound must be closed and the changed situation discussed with the patient. In most cases, it is possible to dissect the tumour off the nerve. Furthermore, although nerve resection may increase disease-free survival, there is relatively little, if any, convincing evidence that this is associated with an improved prognosis. If, after the operation, the pathologist reports an intermediate grade of tumour or even a small adenoid cystic or malignant mixed-cell tumour, then the wound should be reopened, a total conservative parotidectomy carried out, and postoperative irradiation considered.

Factors influencing treatment policy in suspected parotid malignancy

■ Age
■ Metastatic spread: nodal and distant
■ Facial nerve involvement
■ Mandibular involvement
■ Temporal bone involvement
■ Skin involvement
■ Trismus
■ Tumour site
■ Tumour size, stage and grade

The operation may vary from a total conservative parotidectomy with preservation of all or part of the nerve to a total radical parotidectomy, hemimandibulectomy, facial nerve sacrifice, petrosectomy, radical neck dissection and excision of skin in the area with subsequent reconstruction. Complete surgical excision is usually adequate for low-grade carcinomas while postoperative radiotherapy will usually be required for high-grade malignancy. Other indications for postoperative radiotherapy include high stage, if the adequacy of resection is in doubt or the tumour has ominous pathological features. A suggested grading system for salivary gland carcinomas is shown in the box below.

Guide to grading of salivary carcinomas

- Acinic cell carcinoma – Low grade
- Mucoepidermoid carcinoma – High/Low grade
- Adenoic cystic carcinoma – High/Low grade
- Polymorphous low-grade adenocarcinoma (terminal duct adenocarcinoma) – Low grade
- Epithelial–myoepithelial carcinoma – Low grade
- Basal cell adenocarcinoma – Low grade
- Sebaceous carcinoma – Low grade
- Papillary cystadenocarcinoma – Low grade
- Mucinous adenocarcinoma – Low grade
- Oncocytic carcinoma – High grade
- Salivary duct carcinoma – High grade
- Adenocarcinoma – High or Low grade
- Malignant myoepithelioma (myoepithelial carcinoma) – Low grade
- Squamous cell carcinoma – High grade
- Small cell carcinoma – High grade
- Undifferentiated carcinoma – High grade
- Other carcinomas

Those in both the low- and high-grade groups represent a spectrum of diseases where an intermediate grade is possible. Each case should be treated on its merits.

While radical surgery if possible is the treatment of choice, a significant proportion of patients have disease which is inoperable either by virtue of disease extent, or because of their age and general condition. In such cases primary radical irradiation after biopsy should be considered.

With recurrent pleomorphic adenoma, the aim of treatment is to carry out a total parotidectomy with preservation of as much facial nerve function as possible. Identification of the facial nerve is difficult in this instance because of scar tissue and the use of a stimulator is to be recommended. Finding the facial nerve using the peripheral branches is also very useful in this situation. Once the facial nerve is identified, a total conservative parotidectomy may be attempted. It is usually possible, however, to keep a large number of the branches of the facial nerve intact, thus leaving the patient with useful nerve function. Otherwise, any severed branches should be grafted.

For adenoid cystic carcinoma, there is an approximately 30% overall 10 year survival and 25% disease-free survival (Sur *et al.*, 1997). Survival was found in Sur's series of 50 patients not to relate to age, site, type of salivary gland involved, stage, node positivity or neural invasion. The extent of surgical resection had a significant impact on disease-free interval but, because of the slow-growing nature of adenoid cystic tumours, not on overall survival. There was a small but insignificant advantage in Sur's series of postoperative radiotherapy to patients who had microscopic residual disease following surgery.

A larger series of adenoid cystic carcinomas involving 198 patients with known or suspected microscopic residual disease after surgery at the MD Anderson hospital

(Garden, 1995) showed very good local control from post-operative radiotherapy. The authors concluded that the 86% 10 year local control was related to the use of post-operative irradiation. Perineural invasion was an adverse prognostic factor only if a major (named) nerve was involved. Distant metastases developed in 37% of this cohort.

Tumours in the submandibular gland are less common and are relatively simple to deal with. Those that are considered benign can be removed with a wide-field suprahyoid submandibular gland resection. Those that are considered to be malignant must be taken as floor-of-the-mouth tumours and the gland removed together with selective, modified radical or radical neck dissection as appropriate. Involvement of surrounding structures may mean resection of the lingual nerve, the floor of the mouth or occasionally the mandible.

Technique of salivary gland operations

Superficial parotidectomy

Preparation and anaesthetic

The anaesthetic tube is taped to the opposite corner of the mouth, taking care not to distort the outline of the mouth. Before the operation the anaesthetist should be asked not to use relaxant drugs which prevent facial nerve stimulation.

The patient is placed with a 15° head-up tilt to reduce venous congestion. A sandbag is placed under the ipsilateral shoulder and the head turned away from the surgeon. The contralateral eyelids are taped closed. The skin of one side of the face and neck is prepared from the midline to the clavicle, and from 2.5 cm behind the mastoid process down to the shoulder. It is important to expose the whole of the side of the face as the head drape is put on. It is important that the preparation includes the external meatus and a piece of sterile cotton wool is inserted to stop it filling with blood clot. A large steridrape is applied to the exposed face and also used to reinforce the fixation of the head drapes.

Incision

The beginner may find it helpful to mark out on the skin not only the surface contour of the tumour but also the angle of the mandible and the level of the greater horn of the hyoid, before marking the incision (Fig. 22.3). It begins near the upper part of the auricle, curves downwards into the tragal notch to avoid a scar contracture, continues downwards to the lobe of the ear, then curves backwards at almost a right angle to the tip of the mastoid process, and finally curves gently downwards towards the hyoid bone in a skin crease (cervicomastofacial).

The incision extends down to the parotid fascia and, in the neck, through platysma to but not through the deep cervical fascia covering the sternomastoid muscle. It is often difficult to find the right plane over the gland where is no platysma. The skin flaps are elevated forwards

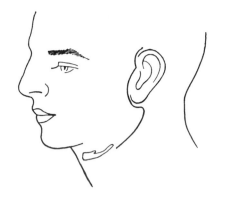

Figure 22.3 Parotidectomy incision.

to the edge of the masseter muscle. The golden rule is: 'under the platysma in the neck, over the platysma in the face'.

The great auricular nerve runs obliquely upwards and forwards at the junction of the upper and middle thirds of the sternomastoid muscle. It must not be divided indiscriminately as it is a useful graft if the facial nerve must be resected (as long as it is well away from tumour). It is, however, impossible to remove the gland without dividing the great auricular nerve and this should be done as near the gland as possible, preserving its two terminal branches. The flap is elevated and turned forwards, and moist swabs are placed on top of it. Very little posterior dissection is necessary, but the lobe of the ear should be freed and stitched to the upper drape.

The technique of parotidectomy via a rhytidectomy incision has slowly gained popularity, especially in North America, over the last 30 years. The preauricular component is similar to the conventional incision, but begins on the anterior margin of the helix. Inferiorly, instead of curving down into the neck, the wound continues as a postauricular incision which extends straight back for 4 cm into the hairline at the level of the external auditory canal (Murthy *et al.*, 1997). The approach may be suitable for some small, benign tumours.

Mobilization of the posterior surface

The key to this part of the operation is the cartilaginous external auditory meatus. The gland is separated from this until the whole of the cartilaginous meatus is free. The best approach is to start at the upper end of the parotid gland and separate this with scissors; this is quite safe as the facial nerve lies very much deeper than the cartilaginous meatus. Keeping directly on the perichondrium; this avoids shredding the gland and injuring the nerve. Pledgets on the end of artery forceps are also helpful in creating relatively bloodless dissection. The surgeon continues to elevate the gland off the cartilage right down to its lower border where it lies on the sternomastoid. With a knife the gland is elevated off the sternomastoid until the anterior border of the muscle is seen. This is retracted and the posterior belly of the digastric muscle and the

stylohyoid muscle are identified, and traced back to the mastoid process. Preserving the posterior facial vein for as long as possible will minimize passive congestive bleeding.

Exposure of the facial nerve

The use of a nerve stimulator is most important at this point and it should be noted in the operative record. The methods to identify the nerve are described above (surgical anatomy). In some circumstances other methods must be used. If the tumour is very large and overlies the previous approaches, or if the gland has been operated on before, then it may be necessary to approach the nerve by finding the buccal branch (which supplies the upper lip). It runs parallel to and 1 cm below the arch of the zygoma as it runs towards the corner of the mouth. It is possible to find it at the anterior part of the gland and trace it backwards to the main trunk. Retrograde dissection places the branch followed at risk. Thus, it is better to use the buccal branch than the mandibular, the paralysis of which leads to an ugly cosmetic deformity.

The gland is held forwards with a malleable retractor, and the nerve located by opening up an artery forceps parallel to the nerve using the above landmarks (Fig. 22.4). During the early stages of the dissection numerous fine strands appear running in the direction of the facial nerve. Most beginners are worried that these are the nerve, but they do not respond to stimulation and when the nerve is finally seen deep in the wound it is instantly recognizable as a thick, white cord, 2 or 3 mm wide. Final confirmation of nerve identification is made by stimulating it. From now on, only bipolar diathermy is used.

Before operating on a parotid gland the surgeon should be thoroughly conversant with all possible anomalies of the facial nerve. It may be pushed deep, inferiorly, or superiorly by a tumour. It may also divide within the stylomastoid foramen, where it appears as five separate branches. The forceps are inserted along the nerve sheath and spread to make a tunnel. Cutting along this with scissors, the cut ends of the gland are grasped with artery forceps to retract them and stop the bleeding (Fig. 22.5). Repeating these four steps, **insert, spread, lift, cut,** one can tunnel along each branch consecutively, starting at the top and working downwards and, by cutting the piece of parotid that lies between two branches (Fig. 22.6), peel the parotid out from above downwards. Try, if possible, to preserve the vertically disposed anastomotic filaments that join the nerves. Always test each piece of tissue with the stimulator before cutting it.

As the gland is dissected and lifted downwards, the duct is located about its midportion, divided, and ligated with 3/0 Vicryl or silk. When the gland is finally removed the facial nerve should be seen fully dissected out. All of the terminal branches, the major bifurcations and the main trunk should be stimulated. If one part of the nerve does not respond to stimulation, then that part should be examined closely to make sure

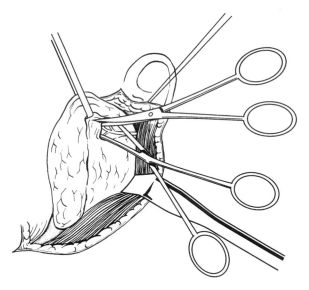

Figure 22.4 Use of 'baby' mosquito forceps to expose and protect the facial nerve while the tunnel is cut with dissecting scissors.

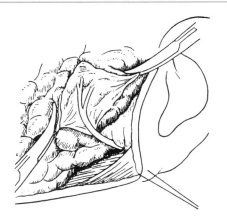

Figure 22.5 The cut edges of the tunnel are held apart by artery forceps.

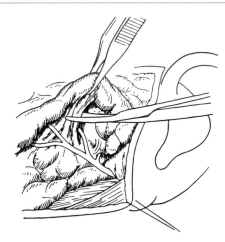

Figure 22.6 Once the tunnel has been completed along two adjacent nerve branches, the intervening bridge of parotid tissue is divided to allow the gland to be pulled inferiorly.

that there is no break in continuity of the nerve. Occasionally, interruption of conduction of a nerve may be caused by a haematoma in the medial surface of the perineural sheath. The only way to recognize this is with a stimulator.

Particular care should be taken when following the inferior branches. Not only can these be very fine, but they are also much more mobile than the branches of the upper division, which tend to remain applied to the deep lobe and are thus less likely to be drawn up inadvertently into the field of dissection.

Closure

When the parotid gland has been removed, the wound is washed with saline and all bleeding points secured. The nerve is stimulated to confirm its function and a note made in the operative record of its function at the end of the procedure. One 12 FG suction drain is put in place and brought out posteriorly under the hairline. If it is brought out in the neck an ugly puncture mark will be visible, which is undesirable, especially in women. The skin is closed in two layers. In the upper part of the wound, the deeper layer may be a dermal suture using 4/0 Vicryl. This may even allow the skin to be closed with steristrips, avoiding suture marks. Otherwise, nothing thicker than 5/0 should be used in the face. The cervical part of the wound is usually closed with 3/0 chromic catgut or 4/0 Vicryl to platysma and the subcutaneous tissues, and either 4/0 or 5/0 Prolene or Ethilon (without tension), or clips to the skin. When inserting the subcutaneous sutures it is easy to pucker the skin underneath the ear lobe, since as it is both thin and often redundant after the removal of an underlying swelling in the tail of the gland. Extra care is therefore needed at this point. Occasional patients with additional risk factors for postoperative haemorrhage may benefit from the application of a pressure dressing for 24 h. In the absence of wound complications, any skin sutures should be left in for only 3–5 days to minimize scarring.

Total conservative parotidectomy

Indications for total conservative parotidectomy

- Benign neoplasms of the deep lobe
- Recurrent pleomorphic adenoma
- Certain malignant tumours
- Recurrent severe suppurative parotitis secondary to calculi/ductal stenosis
- First-arch branchial abnormality

When the superficial parotidectomy has been completed, the superficial lobe is usually left pedicled inferiorly between the cervical and mandibular branches of the facial nerve (Fig. 22.7). Sometimes the specimen is pedicled between the upper and lower divisions, depending on the configuration of the relevant pathology.

Under certain circumstances it can be acceptable to mobilize the deep lobe as a separate specimen. It is necessary to use fine scissors and a nerve hook to elevate the facial nerve. The posterior facial vein and external carotid artery are ligated inferiorly.

The deep lobe can be mobilized from the styloid process, the ascending ramus of the mandible and the temporomandibular joint using small scissors or a pledget. At the upper part of the dissection the upper end of the posterior facial vein, as well as the superficial temporal and maxillary terminal branches of the external carotid artery, need to be ligated. A segment of the external carotid artery is therefore removed on the deep lobe to allow its final mobilization. Very occasionally it can be spared. The complications of this operation are similar to those of superficial parotidectomy but with a somewhat higher incidence of temporary and permanent facial weakness.

Total radical parotidectomy

The skin incision is as for superficial parotidectomy but with upward extension in the temporal hairline and lower extension in a neck crease, as required. An extension inferiorly may be necessary to carry out neck dissection. A total parotidectomy is performed with sacrifice of the facial nerve. The nerve should only be removed when macroscopic invasion by tumour is confirmed. Access to the nerve to facilitate preservation can be improved by mastoid exploration and/or neck dissection. Clearance of tumour within the nerve should be confirmed by frozen section in cases of adenoid cystic carcinoma. The distal branches of the facial nerve are marked with silk, and primary cable grafting is performed using branches of the cervical plexus or the sural nerve. Freeze–thawed muscle is an acceptable alternative.

Postoperative care

A tarsorrhaphy will probably be required if the whole nerve is sacrificed. In cases of complete facial paralysis, where nerve grafting is not performed or is unsuccessful, facial slings, pedicled muscle transposition or, very rarely, free muscle transfer may be required.

Extended radical parotidectomy

Radical parotidectomy may be extended to include contiguous structures such as the ascending ramus of the mandible (and occasionally the temporomandibular joint), the zygomatic arch, the temporalis and sternomastoid muscle (anterior part), as well as the lower part of the medial pterygoid muscle, the bony and cartilaginous meatus and the mastoid process. This operation is usually carried out in conjunction with a radical neck dissection.

Skin may be involved and can be included when total conservative parotidectomy is carried out for recurrent benign and low-grade malignant tumours. Most cases can be reconstructed by shaping the excision as an ellipse which follows the incision and then performing a mini-

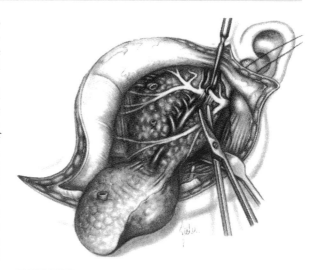

Figure 22.7 Superficial lobe pedicled between the cervical and mandibular branches of the facial nerve prior to deep lobe dissection on total conservative parotidectomy.

facelift. Larger defects can be filled using pedicled muscle-only or myocutaneous flaps (pectoralis major or latissimus dorsi) or free tissue transfer (latissimus dorsi or rectus abdominis).

Neck dissection

Elective neck dissection for the N_0 neck may be indicated in high-grade mucoepidermoid and squamous cell carcinoma (SCC), as well as adenocarcinomas of the parotid gland. In such cases, all five levels should be dissected (in theory, a modified radical neck dissection type 3). However, since the operation is usually performed with a parotidectomy (extended neck dissection), removal of the sternomastoid muscle facilitates identification of the facial nerve, so that speed and ease of operation often dictate that it is more convenient to carry out a modified radical neck dissection type 1. This operation can also be performed when access is required for the reconstruction of defects which require pedicled myocutaneous pectoralis major or latissimus dorsi flaps.

With low-grade tumours, neck-node sampling can be carried out in level I with frozen-section control. Positive disease facilitates proceeding to neck dissection, as described above. Palpable nodes should be treated by modified radical or radical neck dissection.

Complications

Specific complications of parotidectomy
■ Facial nerve injury
■ Frey's syndrome
■ Numbness of the ear
■ Salivary fistula
■ Xerostomia

The steps to avoid **nerve injury** have been pointed out in the description of the operative technique. If a division of the nerve is transected, it can be repaired with 6/0 Ethilon; 7/0 or 8/0 may be required for the branches. The operating microscope is essential in this technique. When stitching the nerve it is important to stitch nerve sheath edge to nerve sheath edge, and not to evert the nerve or buckle it. Epineurium and perineurium should be carefully opposed. It is possible to put two stitches in the sheath of each branch, and four to five sutures may be placed in the main trunk. If a haematoma is found in the perineural sheath, it is slit open with a sickle knife and the haematoma evacuated.

If the main trunk of the nerve is transected and re-anastomosed, then there is no point in looking for any recovery of movement in under 6 months. The maximum improvement will occur at about 10–12 months. If the nerve is intact on stimulation at the end of the operation as described but weakness of part of the face is seen on the day after operation, then the patient can be reassured that movement should usually return. The quickest part of the face to recover normal function is the middle portion as there is a rich neural anastomosis to this area.

Frey's syndrome (gustatory hyperhidrosis of the cheek) was described by Duphenix in 1757, following lacerations around the parotid gland. Lucia Frey, a French neurologist, implicated the auriculotemporal nerve in her much later classic account (1923) of a Polish cavalry officer with an infected parotid wound. (Sood *et al.*, 1998). This syndrome consists of painful sweating around the ear when the patient eats. It occurs in up to 50% of parotidectomies, if the appropriate enquiries are made, but about 10% of patients will volunteer symptoms of the syndrome. Gustatory sweating can be demonstrated in about 90% of patients. The onset is usually within 6 weeks to 3 months of the operation. Only 10–15% of sufferers will require further treatment.

The **auriculotemporal nerve** provides both parasympathetic innervation to the parotid gland and sympathetic innervation to sweat glands and subcutaneous blood vessels. The neurotransmitter for both fibres is acetylcholine. It is therefore postulated that Frey's syndrome is due to regrowth of the secretomotor parasympathetic fibres into the distal cut ends of the sympathetic fibres in the skin. As both fibres share the same neurotransmitter, whenever the patient eats, the reflex for salivation occurs, the skin blood vessels dilate and the sweat glands secrete. The delay in onset is thought to match the time taken for regeneration.

Most patients will require only reassurance that this is a well-recognized development which will resolve spontaneously in the vast majority. In those rare cases where it is needed, conservative therapy with anti-perspirant may be tolerated by the patient and buy time for the surgeon: aluminium chloride hexahydrate is said to be the most effective. Topical anticholinergics such as glycopyrolate reduce both gustatory sweating and flushing. The use of topical anticholinergics is contraindicated in glaucoma, obstructive uropathy, diabetes and a number of other general medical conditions, as a proportion is absorbed systemically. An alternative is botulinum toxin A, which interferes with exocytosis of synaptic vesicles at cholinergic nerve endings. Because of the young age of most patients, radiotherapy is now very rarely used in the treatment of Frey's syndrome.

Surgical treatment is directed at interrupting the autonomic nerve supply. This can be done most easily by performing a tympanic neurectomy. This is carried out via a tympanotomy; the fibres of Jacobsen's nerve on the promontory are identified as they run vertically across the promontory anterior to the round window and divided. (In 20% of patients the nerve may lie in a bony canal.) Early results of the procedure are very variable. If a sufficient segment is excised, regrowth is said not to occur, but some authors also report recurrence at 12 months. The range of alternative procedures which have been described for the treatment of Frey's syndrome over the years (section of the auriculotemporal nerve, interposition of fascia lata or fat between the secretomotor fibres and the skin, stellate ganglion blockade and intracranial neurolysis of the glossopharyngeal nerve) emphasizes the lack of established benefit from any intervention.

A number of modifications to parotidectomy have been developed in order to reduce the incidence of Frey's syndrome, including the elevation of a superficial musculoaponeurotic system (SMAS) flap or a sternomastoid flap as an interposition to prevent aberrant autonomic reinnervaton of the skin. The latter also has some cosmetic advantage, as it reduces the postoperative soft-tissue defect. The former may become more popular if parotidectomy via a rhytidectomy incision grows in popularity.

Numbness of the ear always follows parotidectomy because the great auricular nerve needs to be cut. Recovery of sensation may slowly take place over the next year.

It is surprising that **salivary fistula** does not occur after every superficial parotidectomy as the bare surface of the deep lobe is left exposed. This happens rarely after a superficial parotidectomy, however, and if it does occur it always ceases spontaneously with time and pressure dressings.

Removal of a superficial lobe only removes 30% of the saliva-producing tissue, so **xerostomia** is almost unknown after superficial parotidectomy.

Removal of a submandibular gland

The patient lies supine on the table, with the head turned to the opposite side and slightly extended. An area bounded by the mouth, the mastoid process, the clavicle and the midline is prepared. Towels are positioned so that the angle of the mouth can be seen; it is helpful to use a steridrape to cover the field.

An incision 10 cm long is made, 2.5 cm below the mandible, in a skin crease, and curved slightly upwards anteriorly. The incision is taken through the platysma and flaps are elevated superiorly to the rim of the mandible and inferiorly to just below the hyoid bone, keeping the platysma in the skin flap. This plane may be obscured after sialadenitis.

The mandibular branch of the facial nerve comes into the neck one finger's breadth in front of the angle of the mandible and crosses the facial vessels. It then loops upwards after a variable distance towards the corner of the mouth. The best way to preserve the nerve is to incise through the fascia of the gland at the level of the hyoid bone and reflect a flap upwards in the plane between the fascia and the surface of the gland. In this way the nerve need never be identified but will never be transected. If a facial nerve stimulator is available, then identification of the nerve is very much easier and it can be dissected upwards with accuracy. When the fascial cuff is developed and dissected upwards it is stitched to the upper flap, with care taken not to include the nerve in the tie (Fig. 22.8). Only bipolar diathermy should be used in the upper part of the flap.

The next step is mobilization of the gland. The surgeon starts by identifying the facial vessels as they cross the mandible, one finger's breadth in front of the angle of the jaw. They are identified and tied separately with 3/0 silk. Because the fascial cuff has been elevated off the gland the dissection of the upper border of the gland from the mandible is an easy matter and only a few small vessels need be cauterized.

Separating the anterior part of the gland from the fat in the submental region can be tedious because of multiple small vessels, but a good plane is easily obtained with a knife. The hyoid bone is followed posteriorly and the lower part of the gland elevated. The next step is to free the part of the gland that curves back over the mylohyoid muscle. This part of the gland can usually be pushed backwards off the mylohyoid muscle but this manoeuvre often has to be aided with the use of a knife until the free edge of the mylohyoid muscle is seen. The anterior part of the gland is grasped with Allis forceps and held upwards and outwards, and the facial artery and vein entering the lower part of the gland are identified, transected and ligated separately. It is often advisable to transfix the facial artery proximally. Next, the posterior border of the mylohyoid muscle is retracted anteriorly to show the submandibular duct. This pulls the lingual nerve down in a U-shaped curve (Fig. 22.9) and it can be freed with a knife.

This often causes troublesome bleeding from small veins in the area. These must be identified accurately and on no account should blind attempts be made to secure haemostasis as this will almost invariably result in damage to the lingual nerve. Very often, pressure will stop the bleeding in this area. Before the submandibular duct is tied, the hypoglossal nerve is identified as it lies below the duct; then the duct is clamped, cut and ligated. The gland can then be removed and final haemostasis secured. A suction drain is put in place and the skin closed with 3/0 chronic catgut.

Complications of the removal of the submandibular gland

- Injury to marginal mandibular branch of VII
- Lingual nerve injury (and chorda tympani syndrome)
- Hypoglossal nerve injury

The nerve most at risk is the mandibular branch of the facial nerve and steps to avoid this have been mentioned previously. Injury has been reported in 11–36% as a temporary phenomenon and in 7% as permanent (Milton *et al.*, 1986). If it occurs it gives rather an ugly cosmetic deformity and is not really an acceptable complication for a benign condition.

Lingual nerve injury can also be avoided but it may occur in as many as 3–5% of patients if blind attempts at haemostasis are made after freeing the lingual nerve. There is little that can be done if this occurs. The same applies to any injury to the hypoglossal nerve, although this is very rare.

In the chorda tympani syndrome, there is misdirected autonomic reinnervation of the overlying skin, analogous to Frey's syndrome.

Radiotherapy technique

Parotid gland

Whilst radium needle implantation was once popular, especially for postenucleation treatment of pleomorphic

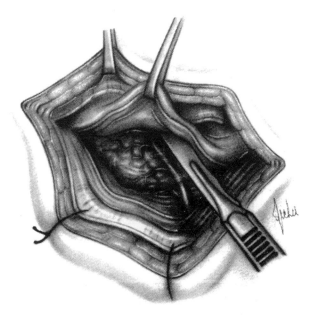

Figure 22.8 Protection of the mandibular branch of the facial nerve by developing a fascial cuff.

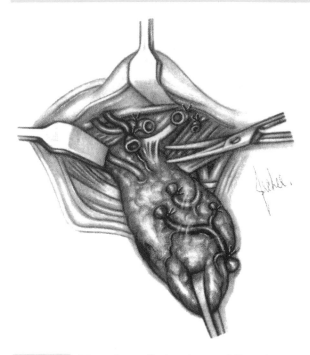

Figure 22.9 The submandibular duct and lingual nerve are visualized by anterior retraction of the mylohyoid muscle.

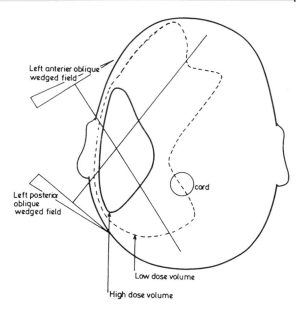

Figure 22.10 Plan of radiotherapy field arrangement for irradiation of the parotid gland.

adenomas, external beam therapy with 4–6 MV X-rays is now most often used. This enables the homogeneous treatment of the large block of tissue at risk. The technique is essentially the same for radical irradiation of an inoperable tumour as it is for postoperative radiotherapy. The wedge-shaped volume (Fig. 22.10) extends from the top of the zygoma superiorly, down to the hyoid bone, and from the anterior border of masseter to the mastoid. Medially it extends to the midline. It thus includes the entire parotid bed, the parotid duct, the parapharyngeal space and adjacent and upper deep cervical lymph nodes, as well as covering the surgical scar. The upper limit may need to be extended if there is base-of-skull invasion, or any likelihood of spread of an adenoid cystic carcinoma along the facial nerve into the skull. If there is established lymph-node involvement or if, as in the case of squamous or undifferentiated tumours, there is a significant risk of occult nodal disease, the ipsilateral lower neck should also be irradiated. The patient is immobilized in a beam-directing shell lying supine with the neck extended. This position enables the upper border of the volume to lie vertically along the orbital floor (Fig. 22.11), ensuring that the posterior oblique beam does not exit through the contralateral eye. It is also easier with the patient in this position to ensure that the cervical spinal cord lies outside the high-dose volume than it is if the head is turned to one side.

The volume to be treated is covered with a pair of appropriately wedged lateral oblique fields, one anterior and one posterior. If the lower neck is to be treated, a single anterior field can be used, the upper border of which is carefully matched on to the lower border of the wedged pair. Where there is skin involvement by tumour, 0.5 cm

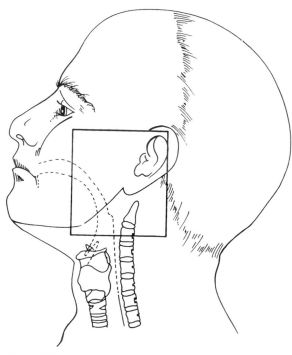

Figure 22.11 Volume to be irradiated in parotid tumours.

of wax bolus is applied to the shell to circumvent the skin-sparing effect of megavoltage irradiation. If not, the shell can be cut out to minimize the cutaneous reaction. A dose of 55 Gy in 20 fractions over 4 weeks or its equivalent should be used. For the postoperative treatment of pleomorphic adenomas, a direct electron field is a good alternative to a wedged pair arrangement of photon beams.

Submandibular gland

The radiotherapy technique used here is essentially the same as that used for floor-of-mouth tumours (Chapter 15).

References and further reading

El-Naggar A. K., Dinh M., Tucker S. L., Gillenwater A., Luna M. A. and Batsaki J. G. (1997) Chromosomal and DNA ploidy characterisation of salivary gland neoplasms by combined FISH and flow cytometry, *Hum Pathol* 28: 881–6.

Armstrong J. G., Harrison L. B., Spiro R. H., Fass D. E., Strong E. W. and Fuks Z. Y. (1990) Malignant tumors of the major salivary gland origin, *Arch Otolaryngol Head Neck Surg* 116: 290–3.

Cajulis R. S. (1997) Fine needle aspiration biopsy of salivary glands. A five year experience with emphasis on diagnostic pitfalls, *Acta Cytologica* 41: 1412–20.

Christallini E. G. (1997) Fine needle aspiration biopsy of salivary gland 1985–1995, *Acta Cytol* 41: 1421–5.

El-Naggar A. K., Dinh M., Tucker S. L., Gillenwater A., Luna H. A. and Batsakis J. G. (1997) Chromosomal and DNA ploidy characterization of salivary gland neoplasms by combined FISH and flow cytometry. *Hum Pathol* 28: 881–886.

Frankenthaler R. A. (1991) Prognostic variables in parotid gland cancer, *Arch Otolaryngol Head Neck Surg* 117: 1251–6.

Garden A. S. (1995) The influence of positive margins and nerve invasion in adenoid cystic carcinoma of the head and neck treated with surgery and radiation, *Int J Radiat Oncol Biol Phys* 32: 619–26.

Harrison L. B., Armstrong J. G., Spiro R. H., Fass D. E. and Strong E. W. (1990) Postoperative radiation therapy for major salivary gland malignancies, *J Surg Oncol* 45: 52–5.

Iezzoni J. C., Gaffey M. J. and Weiss L. M. (1995) The role of Epstein–Barr virus in lymphoepithelioma-like carcinomas, *Am J Clin Pathol* 103: 308–15.

Jeannon J. P., Soames J. V., Bell H. and Wilson J. A. (1999) *Clin Otolaryngol*, Immunohistochemical detection of oestrogen and progesterone receptors in salivary tumours, *Clin Otolaryngol* 24, 52–4.

Kane W. S. (1991) Primary parotid malignancies, *Arch Otolaryngol Head Neck Surg* 117: 307–15.

Kaplan M. J. and Johns M. E. (1993) Malignant neoplasms of the salivary glands, in *Otolaryngology Head and Neck Surgery*, Vol. 2, 2nd edn, Mosby Year Book, St Louis, MO.

Levin R. J. and Bradley M. K. (1996) Neuroectodermal antigens persist in benign and malignant salivary gland tumour cultures, *Arch Otolaryngol Head Neck Surg* 122: 551–8.

Li X., Tsuji T., Wen S., Mimura Y., Sasaki K. and Shinozaki F. (1997) Detection of numeric abnormalities of chromosome 17 and p53 deletions by fluorescence in situ hybridization in pleomorphic adenoma. *Cancer* 79: 2314–9.

Milton C. M., Thomas B. M. and Bickerton R. C. (1986) Morbidity study of submandibular gland excision, *Ann R Coll Surg Eng* 68: 148–50.

Murthy P., Hussain A. and McLay K. A. (1997) Parotidectomy through a rhytidectomy incision, *Clin Oncol* 22: 206–8.

Nordgard S., Franzen G., Boysen M. and Halvorsen T. B. (1997) Ki-67 as a prognostic marker in adenoid cystic carcinoma assessed with the monoclonal antibody MIBI in paraffin sections, *Laryngoscope* 107: 531–6.

Papadaki H., Finkelstein S. D., Kounelis S. *et al.* (1996) The role of p53 mutation and protein expression in primary and recurrent adenoid cystic carcinoma, *Hum Pathol* 27: 567–72.

Renehan A., Gleave E. N., Hancock B. D. *et al.* (1996) Long term follow up of over 1000 patients with salivary gland tumours treated in a single centre, *Br J Surg* 83: 1750–4.

Rosa C. J., Felix A., Fonseca I. and Soares J. (1997) Immuno-expression of c-erbB-2 and p53 in benign and malignant salivary neoplasms with myoepithelial differentiation, *J Clin Pathol* 50: 661–3.

Saku T., Hayashi Y., Takahara O. *et al.* (1997) Salivary gland tumours among atomic bomb survivors, 1950–1987, *Cancer* 79: 1465–75.

Seifert G. (1991) In collaboration with pathologists in 6 countries, *World Health Organisation (WHO) International Histological Classification of tumours*, 2nd edn, Springer, London.

Shadaba A., Gaze M. N., Grant H. R. (1997) The response of adenoid cystic carcinoma to tamoxifen, *J Laryngol Otol* 111: 1186–89.

Sheen T. S. Tsai C., Ko J. Y. *et al.* (1997) Undifferentiated carcinoma of the major salivary glands, *Cancer* 80: 357–63.

Spiro R. H. and Huvos A. G. (1992) Stage means more than grade in adenoid cystic carcinoma, *Am J Surg* 164: 623–8.

Smith W. P., Markus A. F. and Peters W. J. N. (1993) Submandibular gland surgery: an audit of clinical findings, pathology and postoperative morbidity. *Ann Roy Coll Surg Eng* 75: 164–7.

Sood S., Quraishi M. S. and Bradley P. J. (1998) Frey's syndrome and parotid surgery, *Clin Oncol* 23: 291–301.

Spiro R. H., Hajdu S. I. and Strong E. W. (1976) Tumors of the submaxillary gland, *Am J Surg* 132: 463–8.

Spiro J. D. and Spiro R. H. (1994) Submandibular gland tumors, in *The Neck, Diagnosis and Surgery* (W. W. Shockley and H. C. Pillsbury, eds), Mosby, St Louis, MO, pp. 295–306.

Spiro R. H. (1998) Management of malignant tumours of the salivary glands, *Oncology* 12: 671–83.

Suen J. Y. and Snyderman N. L. (1993) Benign neoplasms of the salivary glands, in *Otolaryngology Head and Neck Surgery*, Vol. 2, 2nd edn, Mosby Year Book, St Louis, MO.

Sur R. K., Donde B., Levin V. *et al.* (1997) Adenoid cystic carcinoma of the salivary glands; a review of 10 years, *Laryngoscope* 107: 1276–80.

Weber R. S., Byers R. M., Petit B. *et al.* (1990) Submandibular gland tumors, adverse histologic factors and therapeutic implications, *Arch Otolaryngol Head Neck Surg* 116: 1055–60.

Wilson J. A., McIntyre A., Haacke P. and Maran A. G. D. (1987) Fine needle aspiration biopsy and the otolaryngologist, *J Laryngol Otol* **101**: 595–600.

Wilson J. A. (1991) Excision of the submandibular gland, *Curr Pract Surg* **3**: 34–7.

UICC (1997) *TNM Classification of Malignant Tumours (UICC)* (L. H. Sobin and C. H. Wittekind, eds), 5th edn, Wiley-Liss, New York.

Xinwel L., Tatsuo T., Shumin W. *et al.* (1997) Detection of numeric abnormalities of chromosome 17 and p53 deletions by fluorescence *in situ* hybridization in pleomorphic adenomas and carcinomas in pleomorphic adenoma, *Cancer* **79**: 2314–9.

Appendix 22.1: The World Health Organization's histological classification of salivary gland tumours (1991)

1 Adenomas
1.1 Pleomorphic adenoma
1.2 Myoepitheloma (myoepithelial adenoma)
1.3 Basal cell adenoma
1.4 Warthin's tumour (adenolymphoma)
1.5 Oncocytoma (oncocytic adenoma)
1.6 Canalicular adenoma
1.7 Sebaceous adenoma
1.8 Ductal papilloma
   1.8.1 Inverted ductal papilloma
   1.8.2 Intraductal papilloma
   1.8.3 Sialadenoma papilliferum
1.9 Cystadenoma
   1.9.1 Papillary cystadenoma
   1.9.2 Mucinous cystadenoma

2 Carcinomas
2.1 Acinic cell carcinoma
2.2 Mucoepidermoid carcinoma
2.3 Adenoid cystic carcinoma
2.4 Polymorphous low-grade adenocarcinoma (terminal duct adenocarcinoma)
2.5 Epithelial–myoepithelial carcinoma
2.6 Basal cell adenocarcinoma
2.7 Sebaceous carcinoma
2.8 Papillary cystadenocarcinoma
2.9 Mucinous adenocarcinoma
2.10 Oncocytic carcinoma
2.11 Salivary duct carcinoma
2.12 Adenocarcinoma
2.13 Malignant myoepithelioma (myoepithelial carcinoma)
2.15 Squamous cell carcinoma
2.16 Small cell carcinoma
2.17 Undifferentiated carcinoma
2.18 Other carcinomas

3 Non-epithelial tumours

4 Malignant lymphomas

5 Secondary tumours

6 Unclassified tumours

7 Tumour-like lesions
7.1 Sialadenitis
7.2 Oncocytosis
7.3 Necrotizing sialometaplasia (salivary gland infarction)
7.4 Benign lymphoepithelial lesion
7.5 Salivary gland cysts
7.6 Chronic sclerosing sialdenitis of submandibular gland (Kuttner tumour)
7.7 Cystic lymphoid hyperplasia in patients with acquired immunodeficiency syndrome.

23 Tumours of the thyroid and parathyroid glands

'Diagnosis precedes treatment'
Russell John Howard, 1875–1942

THYROID GLAND

Introduction

The management of thyroid tumours represents a small but significant workload for the modern head and neck oncologist. In the UK, it is estimated that approximately 8% of the population have nodular thyroid disease and, of these, a significant proportion are solitary. Thyroid nodules are more common in women and increase in frequency with age. While thyroid nodules are common, thyroid cancer is uncommon and the most common way for it to present is as a solitary thyroid nodule. The fundamental and crucial question which faces the surgeon is how to detect the 10% of solitary thyroid nodules with cancer so that safe and effective surgery can be offered to those who require it. **Fine-needle aspiration cytology** (FNAC) is now the cornerstone of investigation for many of these patients and evaluation and subsequent treatment usually involve assessment by a multidisciplinary team fully conversant in all aspects of thyroid cancer therapy. This usually means a head and neck surgeon, a clinical oncologist and an endocrinologist working together in a combined thyroid clinic. In many cases combined treatment is highly effective and this results in an excellent prognosis for the majority of patients.

A similar approach to patients with primary hyperparathyroidism resulting from either an adenoma or multiple gland hyperplasia means that excellent results can be obtained if patients are treated by a dedicated team involving an endocrinologist and a specialist surgeon.

Surgical anatomy

The morbidity created by a poorly performed thyroid gland operation can exceed the morbidity caused by leaving some thyroid lesions alone. Therefore, it is vital to know the important points of thyroid surgical anatomy and pathology as well as the natural history of thyroid disease.

The thyroid gland is made up of two lateral lobes which extend from the sides of the thyroid cartilage to the sixth tracheal ring. These are joined together by the isthmus which overlies the second to fourth tracheal rings. In addition, there is sometimes a pyramidal lobe which projects up from the isthmus, usually on the left-hand side. The gland is enclosed in pretracheal fascia, covered by the strap muscles and overlapped by the sternomastoid muscles. The anterior jugular veins cross over the isthmus. On the deep aspect of the gland lie the larynx and the trachea, with the pharynx and the oesophagus behind and the carotid sheath laterally.

On either side, two important nerves, the external branch of the superior laryngeal nerve and the recurrent laryngeal nerve, lie in close proximity to the gland and its blood supply.

The external branch of the superior laryngeal nerve lies deep to the upper pole of the gland as it passes to the cricothyroid muscle in the sternothyrolaryngeal (Joll's) triangle. This is formed laterally by the upper pole of the gland and the vessels, superiorly by the attachment of the strap muscles and deep investing layer of fascia to the thyroid and medially by the midline (Fig. 23.1). Its floor is cricothyroid, its contents are usually the external laryngeal nerve running on cricothyroid and its roof is the strap

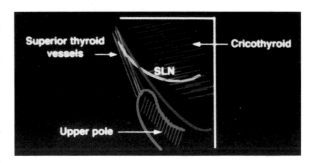

Figure 23.1 Relationships of the sternothyrolaryngeal (Joll's) triangle showing the external branch of the superior laryngeal nerve (SLN) running on cricothyroid.

muscles. In about 15% of cases, the external laryngeal nerve runs with the superior thyroid vessels and leaves them close to the gland. It is therefore, important to attempt to identify and preserve the nerve wherever possible. The superior thyroid artery and vein, which run down to the upper pole from the external carotid artery and internal jugular vein, are in close proximity to this nerve, which can therefore be damaged if the vessels are ligated too high. The effect of sectioning of the external branch of superior laryngeal nerve is that the patient's vocal range is then limited but, unless he or she is a singer, this deficit is unlikely to be noticed.

Blood vessels of the thyroid gland

Arterial supply
- Superior thyroid artery
- Inferior thyroid artery
- Thyroid ima artery (inconstant)

Venous drainage
- Superior thyroid vein
- Middle thyroid vein
- Inferior thyroid veins

The recurrent laryngeal nerves (Fig. 23.2) run in the tracheo-oesophageal groove and can be in front of, pass through or behind the inferior thyroid arteries. This relationship was used in the past as a method to identify the nerve but is not usually relied on nowadays. The inferior thyroid arteries arise from the thyrocervical trunks, branches of the first part of the subclavian artery,

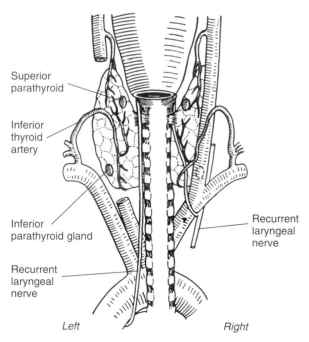

Superior parathyroid

Inferior thyroid artery

Inferior parathyroid gland

Recurrent laryngeal nerve

Recurrent laryngeal nerve

Left   *Right*

Figure 23.2 Posterior relations of the thyroid gland showing the inferior thyroid arteries, the recurrent laryngeal nerves and the usual position of the parathyroid glands.

and pierce the prevertebral fascia medial to the carotid sheath to enter the posterior part of the gland. Before any branch of the inferior thyroid artery is divided, it is necessary to identify the recurrent laryngeal nerve on each side as the anatomy can be variable. The best way to identify the nerve is to look for it low down in the tracheo-oesophageal groove where it forms one of the sides of Beahr's triangle (Fig. 23.3), the other two sides being formed by the common carotid and inferior thyroid arteries. The nerves may occasionally lie lateral to the tracheo-oesophageal groove and can then pass under, over or between the branches of the inferior thyroid artery. At the level of the upper two or three tracheal rings, the recurrent laryngeal nerves are closely applied to the posterior surface of the thyroid gland and may penetrate it in the region of Berry's ligament (which represents a posterior condensation of pretracheal fascia where the gland is tethered to the trachea). They usually divide into anterior and posterior branches before entering the larynx. On the right side it is important to remember that in approximately 2% of cases, the nerve may be non-recurrent and is then found in the paracarotid tunnel where it runs with the inferior thyroid vessels en route to the larynx. There may be extralaryngeal divisions as far as 3–4 cm below the inferior border of the cricoid. Additional blood supply sometimes comes from an inconstant vessel, the thyroidea ima artery which, when present, arises from either the aortic arch or the innominate artery.

Venous drainage is to the internal jugular vein via the superior thyroid vein, which drains the upper pole, and the middle thyroid vein, which drains from the lateral side of the gland. In addition, there are often multiple inferior thyroid veins which drain the lower pole to the brachiocephalic veins.

The superior pair of parathyroid glands (Figs 23.2 and 23.3) is usually in or near the capsule of the upper third of the thyroid gland, where they lie posteriorly at the level of the cricoid cartilage cephalic to the inferior thyroid artery. The lower pair is much less posteriorly placed on the lower poles, where they lie caudal to the branches of the inferior thyroid artery. Parathyroid tissue can, however, occur anywhere in the neck (see section on parathyroid surgery).

The lymphatic drainage of the thyroid is shown in the box below.

Lymphatic drainage of the thyroid gland

Major
- Middle jugular nodes – Level III
- Lower jugular nodes – Level IV
- Posterior triangle nodes – Level V

Lesser
- Pretracheal and paratracheal nodes – Level VI
- Superior mediastinal nodes – Level VII

The major lymphatic drainage is to the middle and lower deep jugular nodes (levels III and IV) and to the nodes in the posterior triangle (level V). Some lymphatics drain

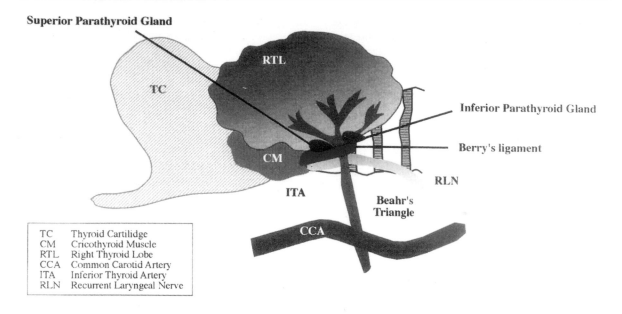

Superior Parathyroid Gland

RTL

TC

Inferior Parathyroid Gland

Berry's ligament

CM

RLN

ITA

Beahr's
Triangle

CCA

TC	Thyroid Cartilidge
CM	Cricothyroid Muscle
RTL	Right Thyroid Lobe
CCA	Common Carotid Artery
ITA	Inferior Thyroid Artery
RLN	Recurrent Laryngeal Nerve

Diagram to show the relationships of the Recurrent Laryngeal Nerve

*Note: The RLN may pass in front, behind or between the branches of the ITA.
Such relationships should not be relied upon when searching for the nerve.*

Figure 23.3 Usual position of the recurrent laryngeal nerve. It lies in the tracheo-oesophageal grove and forms the third side of Beahr's triangle. The other two sides of the triangle are formed by the inferior thyroid artery and the common carotid artery. Note the usual position of the parathyroids.

to the pre- and paratracheal nodes in the anterior compartment (level VI) and thence to the mediastinal nodes (level VII).

Surgical pathology

Incidence

Carcinoma of the thyroid gland is uncommon, but there is a wide geographical variation in its incidence. In the UK the annual incidence is about between two and three per 100 000 of the population and this results in about 1000 new cases per year. In Switzerland, where goitre is very common because of the diminished iodine intake, the mortality rate from cancer of the thyroid is approximately 10 times that in England and Wales. There is a female preponderance of approximately 3:1. Although thyroid cancer can occur at almost any age, the majority of patients, especially those with follicular, medullary and anaplastic cancers, are elderly. In adolescents and young adults, thyroid cancer is predominantly of the well-differentiated papillary type.

Aetiology

Several factors are now known to be of importance in the causation of thyroid cancer.

People living in areas where the natural diet is deficient in iodine may have difficulty in producing adequate amounts of the iodine-containing thyroid hormones thyroxine (T_4) and tri-iodothyronine (T_3). As a result, they may either become overtly hypothyroid or at least develop compensated hypothyroidism. In both cases there will be an increased secretion of thyroid-stimulating hormone (TSH) by the anterior pituitary gland. This can lead to enlargement of the gland and endemic goitre, and prolonged TSH stimulation may be a factor in causing the abnormal gland to undergo malignant change. Now that the relationship between iodine deficiency, endemic goitre and thyroid cancer is understood, it should be possible to reduce the incidence with the use of dietary iodine supplementation. The cancers arising in these nodular parenchymatous goitres are most often follicular in type. Conversely, in Iceland, where the intake of iodine is high, thyroid carcinoma is usually of papillary type.

The presence of a solitary thyroid nodule is also a risk factor for malignancy (Fig. 23.4). The incidence of malignancy within a clinically apparent solitary thyroid nodule is approximately 10%. On investigation, many apparently solitary nodules will be shown to be part of a multinodular goitre. If imaging investigations show the nodule to be truly solitary, then the likelihood of it being malignant increases to about 20%.

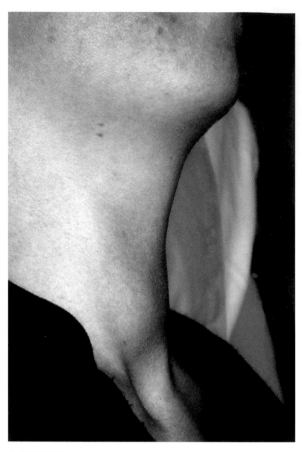

Figure 23.4 Right-sided solitary thyroid nodule in a young female patient. The risk of malignancy is approximately 10%.

A nodule is more likely to be malignant if:

- There is a past history of ionizing radiation
- It occurs in a patient with a family history of thyroid cancer
- There is a history of previous thyroid cancer
- It is enlarging (particularly on suppressive doses of thyroxine)
- The nodule develops in a person under 14 or over 65 years of age
- The patient is male

Another well-recognized aetiological factor in thyroid carcinoma is ionizing radiation. Between 1920 and 1940, young patients were treated by radiation to cause involution of the thymus, or of the tonsils and adenoids, to treat adolescent acne, to treat tuberculous cervical adenitis, to control unwanted facial hair, and as a valid therapy for other malignancies. The association of irradiation with the subsequent development of thyroid cancer has been well documented over the past 30 years. One investigation found 8.3 cases of thyroid cancer per 1000 irradiated patients after a follow-up of 20 years. This exceeded the spontaneous rate by 100 times. The high-dose group had a rate 300 times that expected, and it was calculated that the mortality from thyroid cancer due to irradiation would be 38–52 cases per million persons exposed per cGy of thyroid dose per year. The latent period before cancers occur is often 10–15 years and the peak incidence is 20–30 years after exposure. It has also been found that about 60% of the radiation-created tumours are multifocal and 25% are node positive. However, nodules are common after ionizing radiation and occur in up to 30–40% of patients and of these, approximately 60% are benign. Because of this, it is reasonable to perform FNAC as an initial investigation rather than proceed to surgery in every case. Many of the cancers which occur following irradiation are papillary adenocarcinomas. Following the nuclear disaster at Chernobyl in the former USSR, there has been a recognized significant increase in differentiated thyroid cancers in children from the surrounding areas.

Genetic predisposition is also an important aetiological factor. There appears to be a definite tendency for hyperthyroidism, goitre and thyroid carcinoma to occur in members of the same family. Medullary carcinoma of the thyroid often has a genetic basis. It may occur in patients who have other synchronous or metachronous endocrine neoplasia. This is found in several variants of the multiple endocrine neoplasia (MEN) syndrome. MEN type IIA was described by Sipple in 1961 and sometimes bears his name. It is inherited as an autosomal dominant condition with complete penetrance but variable expressivity. In this syndrome, medullary thyroid carcinoma occurs in association with phaeochromocytoma and hyperparathyroidism. Medullary cancer develops in all affected family members and is usually detectable by the second decade of life, although a palpable thyroid nodule may not become evident until the age of 40 years. In patients with known familial disease, the genetic mutation on the RET proto-oncogene should be sought. If present, it should be looked for in all first-degree relatives who wish to be tested. Children can be tested at any time after birth. Healthy family members found to have the mutation should be considered for prophylactic total thyroidectomy after screening to exclude a phaeochromocytoma. MEN type IIB is characterized by a more aggressive medullary thyroid cancer, phaeochromocytoma, a Marfanoid appearance with multiple mucosal neuromas affecting the lips, tongue and oropharynx and ganglioneuromas of the gastrointestinal tract. In addition, an autosomal dominant familial variety of indolent medullary thyroid cancer with a good prognosis, not associated with other tumours (familial non-MEN MTC), is recognized.

Predisposing factors for thyroid malignancy

- Prolonged stimulation by elevated TSH
- Solitary thyroid nodule
- Ionizing radiation
- Genetic factors
- Chronic lymphocytic thyroiditis

Thyroid lymphoma most often occurs against a background of autoimmune lymphocytic **thyroiditis** (Hashimoto's disease).

Histopathological types of thyroid tumour

Tumours affecting the thyroid gland are usually either benign or malignant tumours arising from within the thyroid gland itself. Much less commonly, the thyroid may be involved by direct spread of cancers from adjacent organs such as the larynx, hypopharynx and cervical oesophagus. Very rarely haematogenous metastases from cancers arising at other sites are found (Table 23.1).

Benign enlargement of the thyroid gland is common. Colloid and adenomatous goitres, characterized by multiple nodules of varying size and consistency, are the types most often encountered. The nodules are demarcated but not encapsulated. Many have a gelatinous consistency with areas of degeneration or calcification. Microscopically, they contain nodules of various sizes with flattened follicular epithelium. A variant of adenomatous goitre is the adenomatous nodule which is a solitary dominant mass that mimics adenoma. They may be difficult to distinguish on cytology from a true adenoma.

The adenoma is the most common benign thyroid neoplasm. This usually presents as a solitary thyroid nodule or as a dominant nodule in a multinodular gland. Adenomas are most common in middle-aged females, are not premalignant and rarely become toxic, but may function and become autonomous. Grossly, they are distinguished from goitrous nodules by their capsule. Microscopic patterns include follicular, microfollicular, Hürthle cell and embryonal. Malignancy cannot usually be excluded by cytological or microscopic patterns, but

is diagnosed by capsular or vascular invasion. Rarely, papillary adenomas have been reported, but they are probably all low-grade papillary carcinomas. Teratomas occur exclusively in infants. They too are rare and invariably benign.

Malignant tumours of the thyroid gland can originate from any of the cellular components of the gland: follicular and parafollicular cells, lymphoid cells and stromal cells. The vast majority, however, arise from follicular cells, and other types are rare. Follicular cell neoplasms can be classified into three major categories: papillary, follicular and anaplastic (undifferentiated). The only known neoplasm of parafollicular cell origin is the medullary carcinoma. Malignant lymphomas are uncommon, usually arising within a lymphocytic thyroiditis, and sarcomas are very rare. Only a few cases of squamous cell carcinoma of the thyroid have been described. Much more common is direct spread by continuity and contiguity from carcinomas of either the larynx or postcricoid region.

The World Health Organization (WHO) classification of thyroid tumours is shown in Appendix 23.1.

Papillary adenocarcinoma

Papillary adenocarcinoma accounts for 80% of all cases of thyroid malignancy. It occurs in all age groups and is virtually the only thyroid cancer of children. Its most frequent age incidence, however, is from 40 to 49 years. Typically, papillary adenocarcinoma presents as a nodule in the thyroid. Macroscopically, it is a firm and unencapsulated tumour which is sharply circumscribed by the surrounding normal thyroid tissue. It is multicentric in 80% of cases and frequently involves both lobes.

Papillary thyroid cancer is referred to as minimal (or microcarcinoma) when it is less than 1.0 cm in diameter. The occult sclerosing carcinoma appears as an irregular white scar within a normal or goitrous gland. Such lesions are often incidental findings at sonography, following surgery for benign disease and at autopsy. Minimal and occult tumours are of interest because their incidence far exceeds that of papillary cancers greater than 1.0 cm in diameter, and the prognosis for patients with small tumours is so good that a conservative approach may be justified. Intrathyroidal tumours measure greater than 1.0 cm but are confined to the gland, whereas extrathyroidal tumours extend outside the capsule of the gland to involve the soft tissues of the neck or the regional lymph nodes.

Table 23.1 Classification of thyroid tumours

Benign	Malignant
	Primary
Follicular cell adenoma	Papillary carcinoma (80%)
	Pure papillary
Hürthle cell adenoma	Mixed papillary-follicular
	Follicular variant
Teratoma	
	Follicular carcinoma (10%)
	Hürthle cell carcinoma
	Medullary carcinoma (5%)
	Anaplastic carcinoma
	Lymphoma
	Sarcoma
	Squamous cell carcinoma
	Secondary
	Kidney, lung, colon and breast

Extent of papillary thyroid cancers

- Minimal (or microcarcinoma): <1.0 cm
- Intrathyroidal: >1.0 cm
- Extrathyroidal: beyond gland capsule and/or lymph-node metastases

Histologically, these cancers are divided into pure papillary, mixed papillary–follicular and the follicular variant of papillary carcinoma. The mixed pattern is most common, with pure papillary the rarest. The papillary component is characterized by a fibrous stalk with a periphery of follicular epithelium. Laminated calcifications called psammoma bodies are often found in the stalk region. The nuclei often appear clear and are described as ground-glass or orphan Annie nuclei. The biological behaviour and prognosis are the same for all three.

Papillary carcinoma

- Histological variants include:
  - Pure papillary carcinoma
  - Mixed papillary–follicular carcinoma
  - Follicular variant of papillary carcinoma
- Is associated with a high incidence (60%) of enlarged cervical lymph nodes in levels III–VII
- The primary tumour may be impalpable and, therefore, often presents with lymph node enlargement
- One in five patients has pulmonary metastases at presentation
- Bone metastases are substantially less common
- In the older age groups, the tumour tends to behave in a more aggressive fashion and may invade the larynx and trachea
- The 10 year survival from minimal, occult or intrathyroid papillary carcinoma is over 90% but when it is extrathyroidal, the 10 year survival falls to 60%

Follicular adenocarcinoma

Follicular adenocarcinoma occurs in the older age groups, being most common between 50 and 59 years, and seldom being seen under the age of 30. It is substantially less common than papillary cancer, accounting for only 10–20% of all cases of thyroid malignancy. The incidence appears to be decreasing in endemic goitre areas where iodine intake has been increased. Follicular carcinoma most commonly presents as a solitary thyroid nodule, either as a new problem or less frequently as an obviously malignant change in a thyroid swelling that may have been present for many years. Alternatively, follicular cancers may present with symptoms or signs of metastasis. Bone or lung involvement is found in 20–30%, but lymph-node involvement (about 10%) is less common than is the case with papillary cancer.

Typically, follicular cancer has a well-defined capsule and cases can be divided into two subgroups depending on whether the capsule has been breached or not. Histologically, it is a carcinoma composed of follicles with no papillary structures. The nuclei are non-vesicular and psammoma bodies are not seen. Although follicular neoplasms can be identified on FNAC, it is generally not possible to distinguish an adenoma from a carcinoma. Surgery, most often lobectomy, is usually required to provide tissue for histological examination to show whether a follicular neoplasm is benign or malignant. Histological features of malignancy include vascular and capsular invasion.

Hürthle cell tumours

The Hürthle cell, also known as the eosinophilic cell, oncocyte or oxyphilic cell, was first described by the German histologist Hürthle in 1894. It is a round cell with eosinophilic, finely granular cytoplasm which is indicative of abundant mitochondria. It is derived from follicular epithelium and possesses a limited ability to produce thyroglobulin, although it does not usually concentrate iodine well. The true nature of the cell is unclear, but it may represent a degenerative or metaplastic phenomenon. Hürthle cells are found in nodular goitres, chronic lymphocytic thyroiditis, diffuse toxic goitre, postradiation and postchemotherapy, as part of the ageing process as well as in Hürthle cell adenomas and carcinomas.

Hürthle cell tumours are extremely uncommon. Histological distinction between benign and malignant tumours is difficult and controversial. Malignant tumours display capsular and vascular invasion and may invade surrounding thyroid tissue and extrathyroid structures. Lymph-node metastases are common. Benign tumours display none of these features. Errors in the past and an association between increasing tumour size and malignancy have led some authors to recommend total thyroidectomy for all Hürthle cell tumours more than 2 cm in size.

Medullary thyroid carcinoma

Medullary carcinoma accounts for about 5% of all cases of thyroid malignancy. It may occur as part of the MEN syndrome (see above), as familial non-MEN disease or be sporadic. In patients with MEN it is frequently bilateral (90%) and multifocal. In sporadic cases, medullary carcinoma is likely to be unifocal. The cervical node metastasis varies from 25 to 50%. Medullary cancers arise from the parafollicular or C cells. Parafollicular cells secrete calcitonin which is therefore a valuable tumour marker.

Medullary carcinoma of the thyroid

- MEN IIA
- MEN IIB
- Familial non-MEN
- Sporadic

Macroscopically, the tumour is grey or white with a gritty texture and areas of haemorrhage, necrosis, fibrosis and calcification. Histologically, it consists of uniform spindle-shaped cells within a variable fibrous stroma which may contain amyloid.

Lymphoma

Primary thyroid lymphomas are uncommon, accounting for fewer than 5% of all cases of lymphoma. They usually present as a rapidly increasing swelling of the neck in an elderly woman. This clinical presentation can be very similar to that of anaplastic thyroid carcinoma and so histological confirmation of the diagnosis is necessary. On purely morphological grounds lymphoma can sometimes resemble anaplastic carcinoma, so appropriate immuno-cytochemistry is essential to distinguish these two diseases. Accurate diagnosis is important as the treatment of the two conditions is different, and the response to treatment and prognosis of lymphoma is very much better than that of anaplastic cancer.

Grossly, most thyroid lymphomas appear as large grey fleshy masses, often extending outside the capsule. Infiltration of the residual thyroid tissue may be seen. Lymphoma usually arises on a background of chronic autoimmune thyroiditis and the non-tumour thyroid tissue may show the gross appearance of lymphocytic thyroiditis. Histologically, the majority of lymphomas are high-grade B-cell non-Hodgkin's lymphoma. Very rarely, low-grade mucoid-associated lymphoid tissue (MALT) lymphomas may be encountered. Most often, primary thyroid lymphomas are localized stage I or II disease. Occasionally, the thyroid may be involved in patients with widespread systemic lymphoma.

Anaplastic cancers

Anaplastic tumours are more common in the elderly and in women, and many of them are superimposed on a long-standing enlargement of the thyroid gland, which then begins to increase in size rapidly, associated with pain referred to the ear and hoarseness. They are aggressively malignant and have a high metastatic potential. They rapidly invade surrounding structures, such as the larynx, pharynx and oesophagus, and carry a uniformly bad prognosis. Treatment is often ineffective and the over-whelming majority of patients are dead within 1 year of presentation.

Histologically, anaplastic or undifferentiated thyroid cancers have no characteristic architecture and bear no resemblance to normal thyroid cells. Traditionally, they have been divided into two categories depending on the predominant cell morphology: the uncommon small cell carcinoma and the spindle and giant cell carcinoma. In the more common latter category there exists a wide variety of histological patterns. The differential diagnosis includes lymphoma, sarcoma, spindle cell medullary cancer and metastatic cancer. If metastatic neoplasms from other sites involve the thyroid, the most common sources are the kidney and the breast.

Clinical assessment

History

The majority of patients with thyroid tumours will present with a solitary thyroid nodule. The patient's age is a critical factor in determining the likelihood of a solitary nodule being malignant. A solitary thyroid nodule in a patient under 30 years old has a 10–20% chance of malignancy and the risk is even higher in ath very young and

elderly. Of those that are malignant, up to 80% may have cervical lymph-node micrometastases. The risk lessens in middle age, and increases again after the age of 50–60 years when, in elderly males, the likelihood of a solitary thyroid mass being malignant is doubled (20–40%). The incidence of anaplastic thyroid cancer increases after the age of 50–60 years.

Twenty per cent of patients will present with palpable neck-node metastases. One in five will have hoarseness or symptoms of airway or oesophageal compression. Pain, often referred to the ear, is a less common feature. Rapid growth of a mass, and unilateral vocal cord paralysis are less common and more ominous signs. It is important to establish any history of radiation in childhood or a family history of thyroid disease.

Presenting symptoms of thyroid tumours

- Solitary thyroid nodule
- Cervical lymphadenopathy
- Rapidly enlarging goitre
- Pain in the neck
- Stridor due to tracheal compression
- Dysphagia due to oesophageal compression
- Hoarseness due to vocal cord palsy
- Metastases

Examination

The thyroid gland is examined, looking particularly for hardness. The surgeon notes whether any swelling is mobile and goes up and down when the patient swallows, and tries to get below the swelling in the midline. If there is a retrosternal prolongation of the tumour, the patient's neck is extended to see whether the tumour comes up into the neck. Cysts feel as if they are full of fluid, colloid nodules feel doughy, and papillary and medullary cancers frequently feel like hard rubber nodules. Anaplastic tumours are hard, fixed and craggy, and lymphomas are frequently diffuse.

The neck and axillae are palpated carefully for lymph nodes and finally, the pharynx, larynx (and upper trachea if indicated) are examined by direct fibre-optic endoscopy to look for vocal cord paralysis or invasion by tumour.

Radiology

Chest X-ray may show tracheal deviation, mediastinal extension or lymphadenopathy, pulmonary metastases and comorbidity. Soft-tissue X-rays of the neck and thoracic inlet may also show deviation and compression of the trachea (although flow-loop studies have been shown to be more accurate than plain films) and finely stippled areas due to calcification in psammoma bodies are seen in papillary thyroid cancer. The appearance of a rim or eggshell calcification suggests a benign lesion. Bilateral calcification at the upper lateral portion of the gland suggests medullary carcinoma, whereas heavy irregular calcification suggests a multinodular goitre.

Ultrasound is helpful in measuring tumour size, diagnosing multinodular goitres and excluding contralateral disease. Ultrasonography can also be used to evaluate complex cysts and can distinguish purely cystic nodules from complex cysts with a solid component but is unable to reliably distinguish benign from malignant disease. Only rarely is a cystic nodule associated with a thyroid cancer. The resolution of ultrasound is good, and it can detect cysts as small as 1 mm and solid lesions as small as 3 mm in diameter. Psammoma bodies may again be demonstrated.

Scintigraphy, which has been available for longer than both magnetic resonance imaging (MRI) and computed tomography (CT), has traditionally been regarded as the gold standard for investigation of the solitary thyroid nodule. However, it is poorly specific and sensitive in the diagnosis of thyroid cancer. Iodine-123 (^{123}I) is probably the optimal radionuclide for thyroid imaging because of its physical properties but, as it is cyclotron generated, cost and availability limit its use. The very short half-life radionuclide technetium-99m (^{99m}Tc), in the chemical form of pertechnetate (TcO$_4^-$), is therefore usually used for thyroid imaging because it is trapped by the thyroid gland in a similar manner to the iodide ion, it is cheap and readily available, and the radiation dose is low. Pertechnetate uptake does not always match the physiological uptake of iodide, however, since its uptake is low (0.4–4%), leading to a high background activity. Nonetheless, with careful attention to scanning technique, the majority of nodules greater than 5 mm in diameter can be visualized on scintigraphy. False-negative results are often associated with smaller lesions in the isthmus, but these are usually easy to palpate and therefore do not cause a significant problem.

More than 90% of lesions identified will not concentrate the radionuclide ('cold' nodules). These clinically solitary non-functional nodules may be an adenoma, a carcinoma, a cyst, a dominant nodule in a non-palpable multinodular goitre or one of a variety of other rare entities. The likelihood of malignancy in a cold nodule is about 20% (Fig. 23.5a). If a cyst has been excluded on ultrasound, then the likelihood of a semisolid or solid cold nodule being malignant rises to about 50% (Fig. 23.5b).

Truly functioning nodules (i.e. 'hot' nodules) using ^{123}I are unlikely to be malignant. Sometimes confusion occurs when lesions are said to be 'warm' on scintigraphy. This is usually a false-positive result because of the vascularity of the lesion, or because the lesion is overlapped by normal functioning thyroid tissue. It may be helpful in such circumstances to perform a repeat scan after 12 h. If the lesion is still 'hot' then malignancy is very unlikely.

A diagnostic strategy for the solitary or dominant thyroid nodule is shown in Fig. 23.6. Other radiopharmaceuticals can be used in the investigation and treatment of thyroid tumours. ^{123}I-MIBG (metaiodobenzylguanidine) is taken up by tumours of neural crest origin such as phaeochromocytoma and some cases of medullary thyroid cancer. It is therefore useful in imaging suspected cases of MEN. Gallium scanning with ^{67}Ga citrate can be useful in detecting lymphoma, and may be used in patients with longstanding Hashimoto's thyroiditis who develop a solitary nodule. ^{131}I radioiodine is used following surgery for well-differentiated cancers of follicular cell origin to ablate the residual normal thyroid tissue, and to search for and treat metastatic disease.

Computed tomography of the neck and thorax is of help in assessing the extent and relationship of larger thyroid tumours, particularly involvement of the larynx,

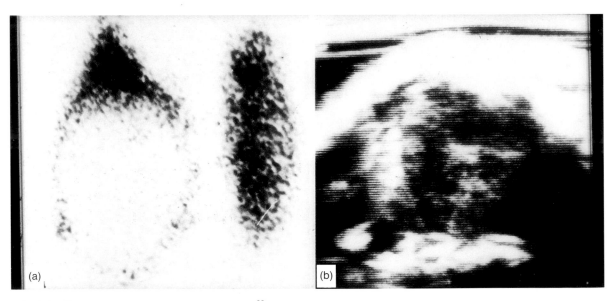

Figure 23.5 (a) Right-sided 'cold' nodule on ^{99m}Tc scintigraphy. The risk of malignancy is approximately 20%. (b) Solitary thyroid nodule which was 'cold' on scintigraphy and semisolid on ultrasound. The risk of malignancy is now approximately 50%.

A DIAGNOSTIC STRATEGY TO EVALUATE THE "SOLITARY" OR "DOMINANT" THYROID NODULE

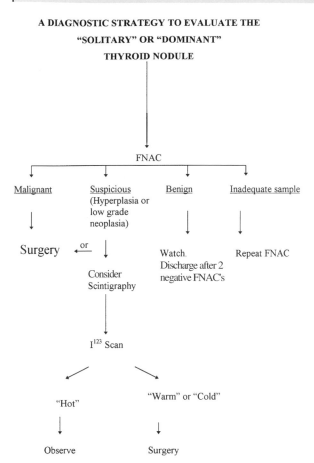

FNAC

- Malignant
  - ↓
  - Surgery ←─ or ─┐
- Suspicious (Hyperplasia or low grade neoplasia)
  - ↓
  - Consider Scintigraphy
    - ↓
    - I¹²³ Scan
      - ↙ "Hot" ↘ "Warm" or "Cold"
      - ↓ Observe   ↓ Surgery
- Benign
  - ↓
  - Watch. Discharge after 2 negative FNAC's
- Inadequate sample
  - ↓
  - Repeat FNAC

Figure 23.6 Diagnostic strategy for the evaluation of a 'solitary' or 'dominant' thyroid nodule.

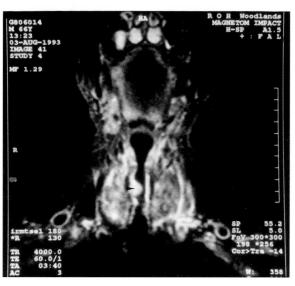

Figure 23.7 Coronal MRI scan showing follicular carcinoma invading the right trachea (arrow). The disease was localized above the suprasternal notch and treatment was with total thyroidectomy, extended total laryngectomy and upper tracheal resection facilitated by manubrial split and subsequent primary pharyngeal repair.

trachea, pharynx oesophagus and major vessels (Fig. 23.7). It is also used to demonstrate nodal deposits in the neck and mediastinum, direct retrosternal extension and pulmonary metastases. Abdominal CT is also used for lymphoma staging and when a phaeochromocytoma is suspected.

Magnetic resonance imaging allows multiplanar image aquisition (Figs 23.8 and 23.9) and has good inherent soft-tissue contrast. It also allows possible vessel involvement to be assessed with MR angiography (Fig. 23.10) Additional advantages over CT include the fact that iodine-containing contrast is not required and there is no radiation exposure. Both MRI and CT may be difficult investigations for patients with a compromised airway for whom lying flat is uncomfortable.

Laboratory investigations

All patients should have baseline thyroid function tests (TSH, and free T4 with free T3 as appropriate). Suppression of TSH is a common and non-specific finding in subjects with goitre. Overt thyroid dysfunction, indicated by raised serum concentrations of free T4 and T3 or biochemical hypothyroidism, is frequently associated

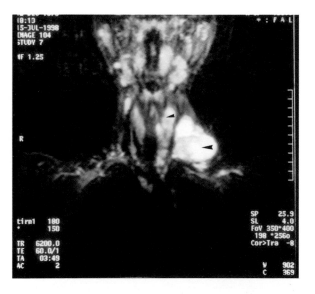

Figure 23.8 Coronal MRI showing extensive papillary carcinoma of the thyroid gland. Significant primary disease is seen in the left lobe of the gland (small arrow) as well as in level VI and levels III, IV and V (large arrow). Treatment was with total thyroidectomy, left modified radical neck dissection and subsequent radioiodine ablation.

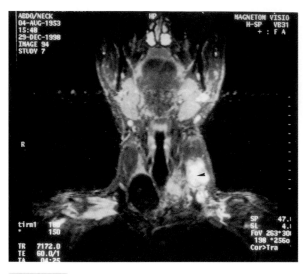

Figure 23.9 Coronal MRI showing extensive medullary carcinoma of the thyroid gland. Primary disease is seen in the right lobe of the gland with metastatic disease on the right in level II and on the left in levels III, IV and V extending into VII (arrow). Treatment was with total thyroidectomy, bilateral neck dissection with mediastinal exploration and postoperative radiotherapy. Disease involved the lower end of the left internal jugular vein at its junction with the subclavian.

with thyroid enlargment and such patients do not generally require further investigation in terms of the nature of their thyroid enlargement. Assessment of thyroid antibody status is not mandatory but may assist in the diagnosis of chronic lymphocytic thyroiditis, predict postoperative hypothroidism and help in the interpretation of both thyroid function and serum thyroglobulin measurements. Preoperative measurement of thyroglobulin is not helpful. If medullary carcinoma is suspected, the serum calcium and calcitonin is measured.

Cytology

The interpretation of fine needle aspirates by an experienced cytopathologist has had a major impact in the management of thyroid disease. It has reduced the need for imaging and surgery, and increased the yield of cancers in patients who have an operation. FNAC is safe, cheap and reliable, although it is not possible to distinguish between benign and malignant follicular neoplasms on cytology alone. This technique is described in Chapter 2. FNAC should be undertaken with caution to exclude a malignancy in patients with a history of radiation exposure, because a cancer may be present in up to 40%, is often multifocal and can easily be missed by aspiration cytology. Sometimes a cutting needle-core biopsy is appropriate to make the diagnosis but often a thyroid lobectomy will be performed as an excision biopsy to obtain material for histological purposes if a preoperative diagnosis cannot reliably be made on FNAC and imaging criteria.

Excision biopsy of a small, lateralized tumour usually entails ipsilateral lobectomy with removal of the isthmus and a small portion of the contralateral lobe. Partial lobectomy or lumpectomy is unacceptable because this is associated with a higher recurrence rate and poorer survival if the diagnosis is cancer. Removal of the isthmus prevents an unsightly bulge developing as a result of compensatory hypertrophy. For small nodules of the isthmus,

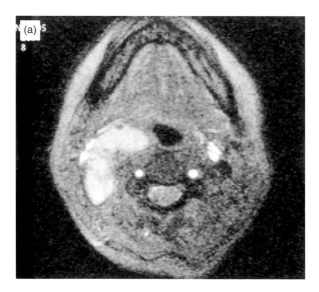
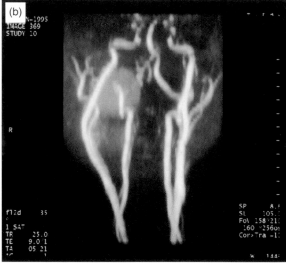

Figure 23.10 Patient with recurrent papillary carcinoma of the thyroid gland presenting 18 years later following partial thyroidectomy and limited neck clearance. (a) A right parapharyngeal mass was noted presenting in the oropharynx and (b) on MR angiography is seen extending to the skull base and displacing the right internal carotid artery laterally. No evidence of vessel wall involvement was noted. Treatment was with completion thyroidectomy, removal of the parapharyngeal mass and subsequent radioiodine ablation. The patient remains alive and well.

Table 23.2 Prognostic factors associated with thyroid cancer

Patient factors	Tumour factors	Management factors
Age	Tumour size	Delay in therapy
Sex	Tumour histology	Extent of surgery
	Nodal metastases (in elderly patients)	Experience of the surgeon
	Local invasion	Thyroid hormone therapy
	Distant metastases	Treatment with postoperative radioiodine

Table 23.3 TNM classification for carcinoma of the thyroid gland

T: Primary tumour

T_X	Primary tumour cannot be assessed
T_0	No evidence of primary tumour
T_1	Tumour 1 cm or less in greatest dimension, limited to the thyroid
T_2	Tumour more than 1 cm but no more than 4 cm in greatest dimension, limited to the thyroid
T_3	Tumour more than 4 cm in greatest dimension, limited to the thyroid
T_4	Tumour of any size extending beyond the thyroid capsule

NB. All categories may be subdivided: (a) solitary tumour; (b) multifocal tumour (the largest determines the classification)

N: Regional lymph nodes
The regional lymph nodes are the cervical and upper mediastinal nodes

N_X	Regional lymph nodes cannot be assessed
N_0	No regional lymph-node metastasis
N_1	Regional lymph-node metastasis
N_{1a}	Metastasis in ipsilateral cervical lymph node(s)
N_{1b}	Metastasis in bilateral, midline or contralateral cervical or mediastinal lymph node(s)

M: Distant metastasis

M_X	Distant metastasis cannot be assessed
M_0	No distant metastasis
M_1	Distant metastasis

pTNM pathological classification
The pT, pN and pM categories correspond to the T, N and M categories.

*pN_0 Histological examination of a selective neck dissection will ordinarily include six or more lymph nodes.

*New inclusion.

removal of the central portion of the gland with a margin of at least 1 cm is adequate. A patient undergoing surgery to obtain tissue for the histological diagnosis of an undiagnosed nodule must be made aware that the planned operation is a diagnostic one, and that further surgery may be necessary if malignancy is confirmed.

Prognostic factors

There are a number of **prognostic factors** associated with differentiated (papillary, papillary–follicular and follicular) thyroid cancer and these can be divided into **patient, tumour** and **management** factors. They are listed in Table 23.2.

Patients aged under 45 years have a better prognosis than older patients and women do better than men. There is a linear relationship between tumour size and prognosis and the grade of tumour is important. The tall cell variant of papillary carcinoma is particularly aggressive, as are follicular tumours which exhibit marked invasion. Local and distant spread are significant prognostic factors, as are the extent of surgery, the experience of the surgeon and whether or not the patient received postoperative radioiodine following near-total or total thyroidectomy.

For **medullary thyroid cancer**, the important prognostic factors are TNM stage, whether or not there has been previous surgery and what the pre- and postoperative calcitonin levels were.

Staging

The most widely used staging classification is the *TNM Classification of Malignant Tumours* (5th edn, 1997). The classification applies only to carcinomas and is based on some of the prognostic factors listed above. There should be histological confirmation of the disease and division of cases by histological type. The TNM (tumour, node, metastasis) classification for carcinoma of the thyroid gland is set out in Table 23.3. Separate stage groupings are recommended for papillary and follicular, medullary and undifferentiated carcinomas (Table 23.4).

Treatment policy

The treatment of thyroid malignancy is multidisciplinary in nature, involving five distinct and complementary modalities. Selection of the most appropriate combination depends on both the tumour pathology and extent of disease. It should usually be possible to have a definitive diagnosis on the basis of cytology and imaging before any major surgery is undertaken.

Treatment modalities for thyroid malignancy

- Surgery
- Radioactive iodine
- External beam radiotherapy
- Thyroxine therapy
- Chemotherapy

Papillary adenocarcinoma

The extent of surgery in the management of early papillary cancers is controversial. Some will advocate total thyroidectomy, others a more conservative approach.

Table 23.4 Stage grouping for carcinoma of the thyroid gland

Papillary or follicular	<45 years			≥45 years		
Stage I	Any T	Any N	M_0	T_1	N_0	M_0
Stage II	Any T	Any N	M_1	T_2	N_0	M_0
				T_3	N_0	M_0
Stage III				T_4	N_0	M_0
				Any T	N_1	M_0
Stage IV				Any T	Any N	M_1
Medullary						
Stage I	T_1	N_0	M_0			
Stage II	T_2	N_0	M_0			
	T_3	N_0	M_0			
	T_4	N_0	M_0			
Stage III	Any T	N_1	M_0			
Stage IV	Any T	Any N	M_1			
Undifferentiated						
Stage IV (all cases are stage IV)	Any T	Any N	Any M			

There is little disagreement about surgery for more advanced tumours. A patient with papillary adenocarcinoma with a large mass in one lobe of the thyroid associated with metastatic lymph nodes in the neck requires a total thyroidectomy and neck dissection.

The advantages of limited surgery in carefully selected patients with early cancers are fewer surgical complications, the prognosis is excellent and if recurrence occurs further treatment is still likely to be curative. Advocates of more extensive initial surgery argue that multicentric foci of cancer are present in 80% of patients and consequently local control rates are better if total thyroidectomy is performed, complications are no greater if the operation is undertaken by a skilled and experienced surgeon and the very small risk of an anaplastic transformation supervening is eliminated by total surgery. In addition, the use of radioactive iodine is only advisable after total thyroidectomy, and serum thyroglobulin levels are a more sensitive marker for recurrence if all normal thyroid tissue is removed. Finally, it should not be forgotten that to reoperate on the thyroid is technically more difficult than to perform an adequate operation the first time around, when fewer complications are likely to result.

Selection of a treatment policy by allocation into risk groups depending on gender, age, stage, and histology (GASH) seems reasonable (Table 23.5). Use of such a policy assumes that patients have had optimal preoperative imaging to give an accurate estimate of tumour size, identify multicentricity and define local, nodal or distant spread, and that a cytological diagnosis has been made preoperatively wherever possible. A suggested treatment strategy for differentiated (papillary and follicular) thyroid cancer is shown in Fig. 23.11.

Table 23.5 Risk* stratification treatment based on the TNM classification

Age
Gender
Tumour size
Tumour histology
Nodal and distant metastases

*Gender included.

Low-risk patient with low-risk tumour = lobectomy

Low-risk patient with high-risk tumour = lobectomy or total thyroidectomy

High-risk patient with low-risk tumour = lobectomy or total thyroidectomy

High-risk patient with high-risk tumour = total thyroidectomy

■ = intermediate group.

Low-risk patients include females under the age of 45.

High-risk patients include all males, and females over 45.

Low-risk patients include papillarycarcinomas less than 1 cm in size, and minimally invasive follicular carcinomas less that 1 cm in size.

High-risk tumours include papillary and follicular carcinomas greater than 1 cm in size. Also included is any tumour associated with significant multifocality, local or distant spread.

Patients under **16** with a diagnosis of cancer should be regarded as **high risk** and, are usually best treated aggressively.

Figure 23.11 Surgical treatment of differentiated thyroid cancer.

Solitary papillary thyroid cancers which are less than 1.0 cm (pT_1) and surrounded by an adequate cuff of normal thyroid tissue, in the absence of cervical or distant metastases, can be safely treated by unilateral lobectomy, TSH suppression with Thyroxine and thyroglobulin surveillance. Similarly tumours in the isthmus can be treated by an isthmusectomy and a 1 cm margin.

Low-risk patients, that is females under 45 years of age with solitary, non-metastatic tumours greater than 1 cm but less than 3 cm in diameter (small $pT_2N_0M_0$ tumours) can also probably be safely treated with lobectomy, TSH suppression with thyroxine and measurement of the serum thyroglobulin. In men, and women with larger tumours the risk of recurrence is higher. Many such patients should have total thyroidectomy, postoperative radioiodine ablation of residual normal thyroid tissue, TSH suppression with thyroxine and measurement of the serum thyroglobulin.

All patients with tumours greater than 4 cm (PT_3) and those with tumours of any size in which there is significant multifocal disease, extracapsular spread, lymph-node metastases or distant metastases should have a total thyroidectomy, selective neck dissection as required to clear disease, radioiodine, TSH suppression with thyroxine and measurement of the serum thyroglobulin.

The routine use of frozen section during surgery for differentiated thyroid cancer is not usually of value. However, it can be useful in resolving management issues when the diagnosis is in doubt either at the primary site or in the neck.

So, for many patients, total thyroidectomy with parathyroid preservation is the operation of choice. If there is concern regarding the morbidity resulting from a truly total thyroidectomy, a near-total thyroidectomy can be performed in the absence of contralateral disease. In this procedure a sliver of the contralateral lobe, including one parathyroid, is preserved. The remnant of normal thyroid tissue can then be ablated with radioiodine.

The extent of nodal surgery depends on the extent of lymphatic involvement. The lymphatics of the thyroid gland drain to nodes in the tracheo-oesophageal groove, to mediastinal (particularly thymic) nodes, to the prelaryngeal nodes and to the jugular chain; some of the lymphatic trunks also pass through the wall of the trachea. From this it is obvious that a true radical neck dissection for a thyroid cancer, with all its draining nodes, would be a massive and mutilating bilateral procedure. What is therefore practised instead is removal of all enlarged nodes, including where necessary those in the mediastinum, without attempting a full clearance of uninvolved nodes in the neck, or sacrificing the sternomastoid muscle, jugular vein or accessory nerve unless absolutely necessary. In the clinically N_0 neck, level VI should be routinely dissected and levels II–V and VII palpated at the time of surgery. Suspicious nodes can be subjected to frozen section and, if involved, a selective neck dissection (at least levels II–IV) should be performed.

Clinically palpable disease in levels II–V indicates at least a selective neck dissection involving these levels and depending on the size and extent of the disease, a modified radical, radical or extended radical neck dissection may be required. The aim of the combined total thyroidectomy and limited lymphadenectomy is to remove all macroscopic malignancy.

When a multinodular goitre is removed by either lobectomy or thyroidectomy and an unsuspected occult papillary thyroid carcinoma is discovered, as long as excision margins are complete, then future treatment involves TSH suppression with thyroxine and measurement of the serum thyroglobulin. If there is any question about incomplete clearance, multifocality or a follicular element to the tumour then completion thyroidectomy and radioiodine are necessary.

If papillary thyroid cancer is discovered in a thyroglossal duct cyst, and if excision is complete (Sistrunk's operation), there are no cervical metastases and the thyroid gland is normal on palpation and imaging, treatment is with TSH suppression with thyroxine and measurement of the serum thyroglobulin. If there is any suspicion of disease in the gland itself, particularly in a young person, total thyroidectomy should be performed and future treatment guided by the histopathological findings.

Following total thyroidectomy, radioiodine ablation of the residual normal thyroid tissue with 3 GBq of ^{131}I can be performed in the immediate postoperative period, before thyroid hormone replacement has been started. If there is any delay before radioiodine can be administered, liothyronine can be used as thyroid hormone replacement and stopped 10 days before radioiodine is given. Radioiodine ablation of normal thyroid function is performed whether or not the tumour concentrates iodine. In fact, most papillary carcinomas have a follicular component and about 80% of well-differentiated carcinomas of follicular cell origin – not just follicular carcinoma – accumulate iodine adequately for imaging and therapy. Scanning with radioiodine, 200 MBq of ^{131}I, to confirm ablation of the thyroid remnant and to demonstrate functioning residual disease or metastases is undertaken at 3 months, by which time the initial treatment should have abolished residual normal tissue. Earlier assessment is not possible, as the avidity of tumour for iodine is always considerably less than that of normal thyroid tissue. If any uptake is demonstrated, a therapy dose, 5.5 GBq of ^{131}I, is given. This is repeated every 3–6 months until all tumour is eradicated or the disease progresses.

Postoperative external beam radiotherapy should be considered if the operative clearance was dubious or macroscopically incomplete, or if there was extensive nodal involvement.

After this combined primary treatment with optimal surgery and radioiodine or external irradiation, the patient should be placed on a dose of thyroxine, adequate to suppress TSH levels fully (usually 200 µg daily). Thereafter, patients should be followed up regularly. As the disease may recur after decades of inactivity, surveillance should probably be for life. Thyroglobulin assay has now replaced routine radioiodine scanning, although of course this is indicated if thyroglobulin levels rise.

Follicular adenocarcinoma

The management of follicular adenocarcinoma is very similar to that of papillary tumours. The mainstay of treatment is surgery. Small tumours less than 1 cm diameter (pT_1) with minimal invasion may safely be managed by lobectomy alone (Fig. 23.11), followed by TSH supression with thyroxine and measurement of the serum thyroglobulin. For the more advanced tumours, surgery usually entails a total thyroidectomy, although some patients in the intermediate group with tumours less than 3 cm with minimal invasion (as for papillary cancer) may be treated conservatively with hemithyroidectomy. Each case should be judged on its merits. The neck and mediastinum are managed as described for papillary carcinoma. Subsequently ablation of any thyroid remnants is performed, followed in 3 months by screening for residual disease in the neck or distant metastases.

Haematogenous spread is more common with follicular than with papillary carcinoma. The most frequently affected sites are lung and bone. In contrast to squamous carcinoma of the head and neck, and indeed most other solid tumours, distant dissemination is not a death sentence. About half of those receiving radioiodine for pulmonary deposits alone will survive for 10 or 15 years. The prognosis is, however, much worse for those with osseous disease, and in patients whose tumours fail to concentrate iodine. With follicular tumours, adequate iodine uptake is less likely in the elderly and in those with less well-differentiated tumours. Following initial treatment, suppressive T_4 replacement and regular surveillance with thyroglobulin measurement are indicated, as in the case of papillary carcinoma. Hürthle cell cancers should be managed as follicular cancers.

Medullary carcinoma

The principal treatment advised for the patient with medullary carcinoma is **surgery**. This should be **radical** and entails total thyroidectomy and removal of any enlarged lymph-node masses. There is no role for elective neck surgery. Palpable disease requires modified radical or radical neck dissection. The operation is extended into the superior mediastinum if necessary. If an unexpected diagnosis of medullary carcinoma is made following lobectomy, lymph-node biopsy or other incomplete surgery, reoperation is required to remove all possible remaining disease. As these tumours arise from the parafollicular cells, it is not surprising that they do not accumulate radioiodine.

Postoperative radiotherapy is indicated if there is any suggestion of macroscopic residual disease in the neck and/or multiple large nodal metastases with extracapsular extension. Patients with disease considered inoperable either due to the advanced nature of the primary tumour or nodal disease, or because of serious intercurrent illness, should be considered for radiotherapy. Although the aim of this is principally palliative, a full radical treatment course is required and cure may be anticipated in a proportion. Although medullary carcinoma is more chemoresponsive than carcinoma of follicular cell

origin, and some patients have benefited from palliative chemotherapy, there is no regimen that can be considered as routine for patients with this disease. Because of its significant toxicity and limited efficacy, cytotoxic drug treatment should only be considered for patients with distressing symptoms refractory to other treatments. A proportion of medullary thyroid cancers take up MIBG and ^{131}I-MIBG therapy is a possible treatment for recurrent or metastatic disease.

Genetic studies and screening for familial medullary carcinoma

In excess of 90% of patients with any form of familial medullary thyroid carcinoma (MTC) have been shown to have a mutation of the RET proto-oncogene. Moreover, 98% of cases of MEN2A have mutations in one of just six codons. These plus mutation in an additional two condons have been found in isolated familial MTC while just one single different mutation has been found in 95% of all cases of MEN2B. Such a restricted range of mutations means that selective analysis of the RET gene is a very feasible and useful technique.

It is important to differentiate MTC which is truly sporadic from the apparently sporadic case which in fact is an index case of a familial form of the disease. The finding of multiple foci of tumours together with definite 'C' cell hyperplasia virtually guarantees the diagnosis of familial disease although their absence does not exclude it. A family history of any of the tumours associated with MEN2 should raise suspicion.

In likely sporadic cases, family screening should not be undertaken initially and the emphasis should be on increasing the certainty that the case is sporadic. If the clinical information is insufficient to be conclusive, a limited analysis of the RET proto-oncogene should be undertaken looking for the common mutations. If this examination is normal, this will reduce the likelihood of familial MEN2A or familial MTC to less than 0.5%.

If a genetic abnormality is found, then this should be used to screen other family member. Patients with likely MEN2B should also have their RET proto-oncogene analysed expecting to find an abnormality which can be used to screen offspring.

Stimulated calcitonin measurements which previously were the mainstay of diagnosing the disease have been almost completely replaced by genetic testing. They should only be considered where there is very strong suspicion of familial disease and a normal genetic analysis in the affected case.

It is strongly advised that family screening and genetic counselling is done by, or in close association with, a clinical genetics department so that everyone is aware of the implications of the tests **before** they are undertaken.

Thyroid lymphoma

If the clinical condition at presentation permits, patients with thyroid lymphoma should be fully staged prior to treatment. The system is the same as for extranodal lymphoma at other sites. That is, patients with disease confined to the thyroid comprise stage I, those also with nodal disease in the neck or mediastinum are in stage II and those with subdiaphragmatic nodal disease fall into stage III. Evidence of extranodal involvement in organs other than the thyroid, such as the liver, gut or bone marrow indicates stage IV disease.

Although no surgery other than biopsy is usually considered to be necessary for lymphoma at other sites, surgical removal of bulky disease has been shown to improve both local control and survival in patients with thyroid lymphoma. Thyroidectomy is therefore sometimes indicated (but not usually feasible), so that radiotherapy remains the principal treatment for this condition. While radiotherapy may produce a very dramatic resolution of the tumour mass, treatment must continue until the end of the prescribed course to ensure sustained local control. Patients with high-grade histology and more advanced disease should, in addition, receive appropriate chemotherapy, if permitted by their general condition.

Investigations for thyroid lymphoma

- Thyroid function tests
- Thyroid antibodies
- FNAC and open biopsy (or tru-cut)
- Whole body CT
- Bone marrow and trephine
- Lactate dehydrogenase (LDH)
- ESR

Anaplastic tumours

A biopsy is mandatory to confirm that a patient suspected to have an anaplastic carcinoma **does not have lymphoma** which may be curable. Sometimes the isthmus will need to be divided and a tracheostomy performed if there is airway obstruction. Apart from this surgery and radioiodine have no part to play in the management of anaplastic carcinoma. Regression may be achieved by radical radiotherapy, but early recurrence is the rule, leading almost inevitably to **death within 6–12 months**. Historical reports of cure following radiotherapy were probably due to lymphoma being misdiagnosed as anaplastic cancer in the days before immunocytochemistry was routinely available. Attempts to improve the dismal prognosis in this disease with chemotherapy have been disappointing and none is recommended. In some patients the disease may be so advanced at presentation that, once the diagnosis is confirmed, no active treatment is the kindest policy.

Investigations for anaplastic thyroid cancer

- Thyroid function tests
- Thyroid antibodies
- FNAC and open biopsy (or tru-cut)
- Neck and chest CT (or chest X-ray)

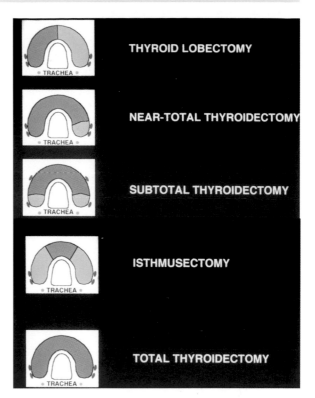

THYROID LOBECTOMY

NEAR-TOTAL THYROIDECTOMY

SUBTOTAL THYROIDECTOMY

ISTHMUSECTOMY

TOTAL THYROIDECTOMY

Figure 23.12 Various operations that can be performed on the thyroid.

Technique of operations on the thyroid gland

Several surgical procedures have been used in the treatment of thyroid tumours and their indications have been discussed. The following definitions are proposed (Fig. 23.12).

- **Lumpectomy:** removal of the nodule alone with minimal surrounding thyroid tissue
- **Partial thyroidectomy:** removal of the nodule with a larger margin of surrounding thyroid tissue
- **Total lobectomy or hemithyroidectomy:** complete removal of one thyroid lobe and the isthmus
- **Subtotal thyroidectomy:** bilateral removal of more than one half of the thyroid gland on each side plus the isthmus
- **Near-total thyroidectomy:** total lobectomy and isthmusectomy with removal of more than 90% of the contralateral lobe
- **Total thyroidectomy:** removal of both thyroid lobes and the isthmus
- **Completion thyroidectomy:** a subsequent procedure to convert a lesser operation into a near-total or total thyroidectomy

---

In general, the **minimum** operation which should be done for a suspected or confirmed cancer is a **total** lobectomy. Subsequent surgery may be a **completion thyroidectomy**. Often, if cancer is confirmed, a **near-total thyroidectomy** will be performed as the initial operation.

Lobectomy

Incision. The patient is positioned with the neck extended and a sandbag under the shoulders. The neck is prepared and drape the neck in the usual way. A collar incision is marked out in a skin crease approximately 2 cm above the suprasternal notch. One must never cut without making a mark as this can easily lead to an asymmetrical scar. The surgeon cuts through skin and platysma, and with traction on the flaps elevates them down to the sternum and up to the upper edge of the thyroid cartilage. The flaps are then retracted using a Joll's thyroid retractor.

Gland mobilization. Standing on the contralateral side, the surgeon divides the deep investing layer of fascia in the midline and mobilizes the gland from the strap muscles. The anterior jugular veins may need dividing. For larger swellings and malignant tumours which invade the strap muscles, these structures may have to be divided and/or resected. As their nerve supply (ansa cervicalis) enters low down, they should be divided high. Next, the middle thyroid vein is identified and ligated (Fig. 23.13). The paracarotid tunnel is accessed, the carotid artery retracted laterally and the thyroid retracted medially to identify the posterior capsule of the gland and Beahr's triangle (Fig. 23.3). The next step is to identify and preserve the recurrent laryngeal nerve and the parathyroid glands.

Identification of the recurrent laryngeal nerve. One of the crucial steps in a thyroid lobectomy is preservation of the recurrent laryngeal nerve: it is first identified and then its safety ensured (Figs 23.3 and 23.14). The nerve is located **low** in the neck where it lies in the **tracheo-oesophageal groove** and forms the third side of **Beahr's triangle**. On the **left** side, the nerve hugs the groove and is angled at 45° as it exits the chest. On the right side, since the nerve does not enter the chest, it is 45° to the

midline as well as 45° laterally. This means that it may be more **superficial** and hence encountered earlier than on the **left**. Before entering the larynx, the nerve may divide into two or three branches which should be identified and preserved. Magnification with loupes may help. One of these branches is usually a sensory branch (the loop of Galen). If the nerve cannot be identified, it may be non-recurrent. This occurs in 1–2% of cases on the right side. The nerve is located running with the inferior thyroid vessels and is preserved in the conventional manner. It is a good idea to practise recognition of the recurrent laryngeal nerve during total laryngectomy when it does not matter whether it is cut.

Localization and preservation of the parathyroid glands. The surgical anatomy of the parathyroid glands, together with localization for preservation, are discussed later (see section on parathyroid surgery). When the parathyroids have been identified and their blood supply has been preserved, they are peeled down off the gland with the pretracheal fascia (Fig. 23.15). Devascularized parathyroids should be transplanted.

Mobilization of the upper and lower poles. Once the recurrent laryngeal nerve has been identified, the gland should be mobilized top and bottom. The upper pole is mobilized (Fig. 23.16) and retracted laterally, and the superior thyroid vessels are ligated separately close to the gland. The external branch of the superior laryngeal nerve should be preserved as it runs in Joll's triangle, medial to the upper pole vessels, where it lies on cricothyroid and its identification at this point can be enhanced by the use of a nerve stimulator. The lower pole is mobilized by dividing the inferior thyroid vessels. The recurrent laryngeal nerve can be inadvertently damaged during division of either the upper or lower poles. Because of this, it must always be identified early in the operation.

Removal of the gland. The recurrent laryngeal nerve is traced upwards by lifting the gland off it and peeling down the pretracheal fascia together with the parathyroid glands.

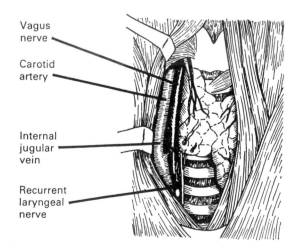

Figure 23.13   Division of the middle thyroid vein.

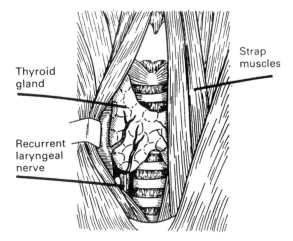

Figure 23.14   Exposure of the recurrent laryngeal nerve.

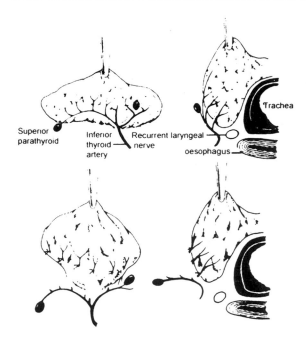

Figure 23.15 Thyroidectomy technique with extracapsular dissection for parathyroid preservation.

Without lifting or squeezing the nerve, the surgeon dissects all tissues off it, leaving it undisturbed in its bed if possible. Bipolar diathermy is perfectly acceptable to use near the nerve; otherwise, all bleeding points are tied using small mosquito forceps and fine ties, being careful never to catch the nerve in a tie.

Now that the gland is mobilized, the whole lobe can be swung medially. The inferior thyroid artery is preserved, together with its branches to the parathyroids. The pericapsular branches are ligated. At this point the gland

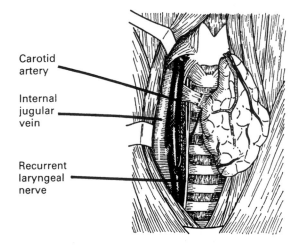

Figure 23.16 Superior thyroid pedicle is divided and following division of the lower pole vessels, the gland is rotated medially to allow the division of Berry's ligament by sharp dissection (as shown), which allows removal of the lobe of the gland with preservation of the recurrent laryngeal nerve.

is attached to the trachea by a condensation of fascia called Berry's ligament. This is divided by sharp dissection (Fig. 23.16) to allow the lobe to be removed together with the isthmus to prevent an unsightly bump occuring after surgery due to hypertrophy of the gland in the midline.

Then, the jugular lymphatic chain is palpated, and any suspicious nodes are removed and sent for frozen section. The anaesthetist may perform a valsalva manoeuvre on the patient to help to identify any potential sources of bleeding. Particular attention is paid to the inferior thyroid veins and the area in the apex of the triangle formed by the recurrent laryngeal nerve where it enters the larynx and the side wall of the trachea. Branches of the inferior thyroid artery that come from below the recurrent laryngeal nerve at this point can be particularly troublesome, particularly if a small remnant of thyroid tissue has been left behind at Berry's ligament (which is often the case).

Finally, a suction drain is placed in the wound, and both the thyroid bed and the superficial space are drained. The wound is closed in two layers using either clips or a subcutaneous suture. At the end of the operation, the anaesthetist should check vocal-cord mobility.

Total thyroidectomy for cancer

This operation is in essence a bilateral lobectomy. The following points are important when performing the operation for malignancy.

- **Incision** is the same as for a lobectomy except that it may need extending to facilitate a neck dissection or mediastinal exploration.
- **Access** is facilated by dividing the strap muscles, which often need resecting if involved by tumour or a completion thyroidectomy with level VI dissection is being performed.
- Both recurrent laryngeal nerves should be identified and preserved if possible
- The surgeon should **operate** on the non-involved side first.
- One must not be afraid to **resect** an involved nerve.
- The parathyroids must be **preserved** wherever possible. It is usually possible to keep two glands, particularly when operating on a non-involved contralateral lobe where a small sliver of thyroid can be left (near-total thyroidectomy) to maintain an intact blood supply.
- **Mediastinal access** may be required to identify the nerves low down, facilitate neck dissection by allowing inferior access to the internal jugular vein at its junction with the subclavian, and finally to allow mediastinal dissection.
- The operation includes a **level VI dissection**. Any further neck disease is treated on its merits.
- Extension of disease into the **larynx** may be shaved off if clearance is judged satisfactory. Since the spread of disease into the larynx is often posteriorly in the region of the ligament of Berry, partial laryngectomy is not feasible so that an extended laryngectomy may be required.
- If a small amount of pharyngeal muscle is involved, this can be locally resected. Extensive pharyngeal

involvement requires pharyngolaryngectomy and free jejunal transfer (or gastric transposition if the former is unavailable).

■ Involvement of the trachea is not uncommon. Disease on the surface can usually be shaved off but invasive disease requires resection. If it is localized, then wedge resection may be possible. For anterior disease, another option is to simply insert a tracheostomy tube and allow healing by decannulation. This is the favoured option if the airway is compromised. More extensive disease requires a sleeve resection. Up to 4 cm of trachea can be resected with primary anastomosis following suprahyoid release and mobilization of the trachea down to the carina. The technique of tracheal anastomosis is discussed in Chapter 10.

■ Major vessel involvement is rare in patients with thyroid cancer but is a major concern in those with extensive disease. The internal jugular vein is the most commonly involved vessel and can be resected in the conventional way. Differentiated thyroid cancer often extends into major arteries in the neck and mediastinum but rarely invades the vessel wall. The disease can usually be dissected from the artery wall. Any concern regarding involvement is an indication for assessment with imaging. Magnetic resonance (MR) angiography can be particularly helpful (Fig. 23.10). In patients with medullary thyroid cancer, the disease may invade major vessels so imaging is mandatory in the presence of extensive disease.

Aftercare

■ General care
■ In the immediate postoperative period, one should watch for bleeding and airway embarrassment
■ The full blood count and serum calcium are checked on the morning after surgery.
■ Following thyroid lobectomy, there is no need to commence thyroxine replacement unless the patient develops hypothyroidism. Thyroid function tests are performed in clinic at 6 weeks following surgery. Clinicians should note that TSH measurements at this time may be misleading when diagnosing the need for long-term thyroxine replacement therapy. A final decision is best left until 3–6 months following surgery. Patients are more likely to require treatment if the thyroid antibodies are positive.
■ Following thyroid lobectomy for malignancy, patients are commenced on suppressive doses of thyroxine. After total thyroidectomy for malignancy, T_4 is commenced immediately unless radioiodine ablation is planned within the next 4 weeks, when the patient can go on to liothyronine (T_3). This is discussed in the next section.

Complications

■ General complications.
■ **Respiratory obstruction.** This should not occur after a lobectomy, but may occur after a total thyroidectomy if there was tracheal compression before operation or if both recurrent laryngeal nerves have been exposed.

■ **Bleeding.** Two common sites of bleeding after thyroidectomy are the inferior thyroid veins and the branches of the inferior thyroid artery in the vicinity of the recurrent laryngeal nerve. The danger is pressure on the exposed trachea, resulting in respiratory obstruction. If this happens, the wound can be opened in the ward and the patient returned to theatre. Any bleeding points in the vicinity of the recurrent laryngeal nerve should be clamped and tied carefully using mosquito forceps and fine ties or bipolar diathermy.

■ **Hypoparathyroidism**: immediate or delayed. This should be looked for by serum calcium estimation, in the immediate period after operation and at intervals of 6 months. If it occurs treatment is with calcium replacement and vitamin D supplements. This is discussed in Chapter 6.

■ Following neck dissection for disease low in the neck, the thoracic duct is particularly at risk and care should be taken to identify this structure and its tributaries at the time of surgery, so as to avoid any potential disasters in the early postoperative period.

Radiotherapy techniques

Radioiodine treatment

The protocol to be followed for both ablation of residual normal thyroid tissue and treatment of functioning local residual disease or distant metastases is the same. The patient should be admitted to a hospital and accommodated in a single room equipped, for radiation protection purposes, with private toilet facilities or a commode. The patient should have been warned to avoid iodine-containing foods over the previous 3 weeks and should not have had any recent radiological investigations such as intravenous urography which use iodine-containing contrast media. As most patients with thyroid cancer are women, many of child-bearing age, the possibility of pregnancy must be excluded before radioiodine therapy is given. Lactating mothers must stop breastfeeding their infants. The patient should either not have commenced or have stopped thyroid hormone replacement in time to allow endogenous TSH levels to rise and stimulate uptake of iodine. This is 4 weeks for thyroxine or 10 days for liothyronine. The TSH level should be measured before radioiodine therapy.

The isotope of iodine used for therapy is ^{131}I, given as a drink or capsule of sodium iodide. The dose prescribed is 3 GBq for ablation of a small thyroid remnant or 5.5 GBq (150 mCi) for treatment of tumour. The whole-body effective half-life of this radionuclide is considerably shorter than its physical half-life of 8 days, as the variable biological half-life is often less than 1 day. In contrast, such is the avidity of differentiated thyroid carcinoma for iodine that the effective half-life in tumour, although again variable, is at least 3 days. The significance of this is that scanning 3 or 4 days after administration of a therapy dose allows imaging of the tumour after the whole-body radioiodine level has become negligible. Accumulation of radioiodine occurs not only in the thyroid gland and carcinoma, but also in the bladder and salivary glands. In order to minimize the radiation dose to pelvic organs and prevent sialitis or xerostomia, the patient should drink plenty to establish a diuresis and suck lemon sweets to stimulate salivation. The patient is discharged home when the measured whole-body radioactivity has fallen to the permissible level of 30 MBq if travelling home by private car or, if going by bus or train, to 15 MBq. When the need for further ^{131}I therapy or diagnostic scanning is anticipated, suppressive thyroid hormone replacement should be with liothyronine, 20 μg three times daily, rather than with thyroxine, as its half-life is considerably shorter, enabling a more rapid rise in TSH levels after its withdrawal. It is necessary to stop liothyronine replacement about 10 days prior to radioiodine administration in order to allow TSH levels to rise adequately. A protocol

for the administration of radioactive iodine following total thyroidectomy is shown in Fig. 23.17.

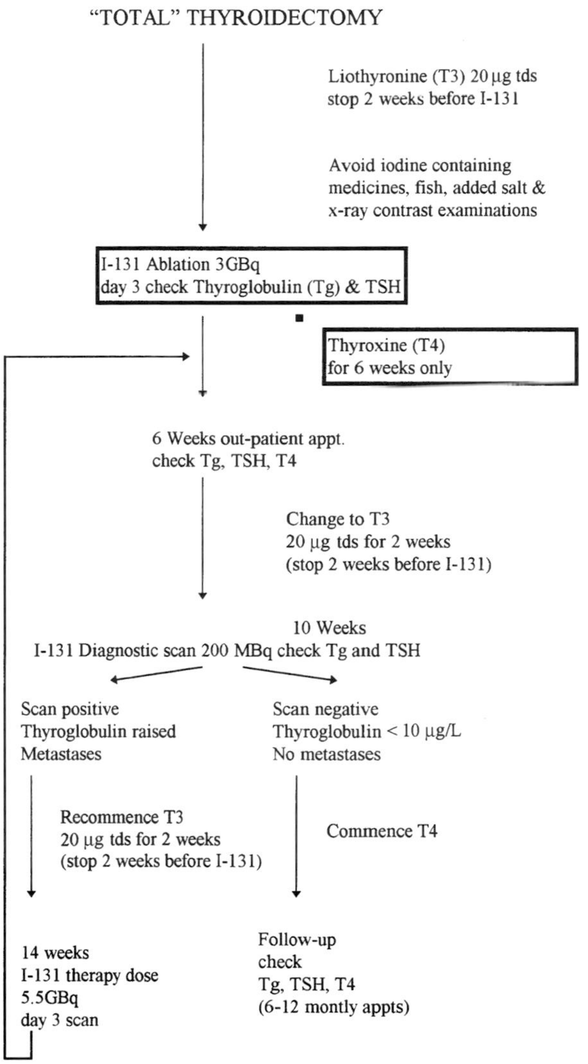

External beam radiotherapy

The planning of radiotherapy for thyroid carcinoma is complicated by various factors. First, a large volume must be covered to encompass both the primary tumour and draining nodal areas. Secondly, the body contour changes rapidly in both the sagittal and coronal planes. In addition, the spinal cord lies just behind the target volume. Great care must be taken to ensure that the radiation dose received by this critical structure is kept within its tolerance, while an adequate radiation dose must be delivered to the tumour. For simulation and treatment the patient lies supine, with the cervical spine as straight as possible, immobilized in a shell. This covers the whole neck and upper chest, extending from the base of the skull, down to nipple level. The central axis of the treatment beam is angled so that it is perpendicular to the spinal cord. To enable accurate dosimetry, at least three contours are taken (Fig. 23.18), parallel to the central axis, on which the position of the tumour, cord and air gaps can be marked. The advent of CT planning has made this process much easier and more accurate.

The volume to be treated depends on the tumour type and extent of disease. For treatment of differentiated carcinoma of follicular cell origin following optimal surgery without bulky nodal disease, the treatment volume can be limited to the tumour bed and adjacent nodal areas bilaterally. The upper and lower margins of the volume are the hyoid bone and the suprasternal notch. When there has been extensive nodal disease, the volume must be extended posteriorly to include all cervical nodes and also inferiorly to the carina to include the superior mediastinum.

Similarly, in the case of anaplastic and medullary carcinoma, a large volume must also be treated. In addition, treatment of the medial supraclavicular fossa nodes is also recommended in these histological types if there was bulky central disease. In cases of lymphoma yet more generous fields are used, with the upper limit at

"TOTAL" THYROIDECTOMY

Liothyronine (T3) 20 μg tds
stop 2 weeks before I-131

Avoid iodine containing
medicines, fish, added salt &
x-ray contrast examinations

I-131 Ablation 3GBq
day 3 check Thyroglobulin (Tg) & TSH

Thyroxine (T4)
for 6 weeks only

6 Weeks out-patient appt.
check Tg, TSH, T4

Change to T3
20 μg tds for 2 weeks
(stop 2 weeks before I-131)

10 Weeks
I-131 Diagnostic scan 200 MBq check Tg and TSH

Scan positive
Thyroglobulin raised
Metastases

Scan negative
Thyroglobulin < 10 μg/L
No metastases

Recommence T3
20 μg tds for 2 weeks
(stop 2 weeks before I-131)

Commence T4

14 weeks
I-131 therapy dose
5.5GBq
day 3 scan

Follow-up
check
Tg, TSH, T4
(6-12 montly appts)

Figure 23.17 Protocol for the administration of radioactive iodine following total thyroidectomy.

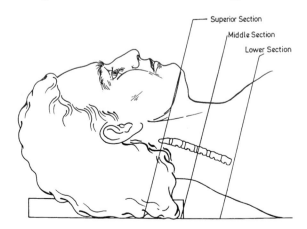

Figure 23.18 Levels at which contours are taken for radiotherapy planning purposes.

both superior and inferior glands is from the inferior thyroid artery and in a third of these cases, there is also a significant supply to the glands through the thyroid capsule. In the remainder, both glands are supplied either by an anastomotic arch from the superior and inferior thyroid vessels or by the superior thyroid artery alone.

The superior glands are more constant in their location and usually lie near the cricothyroid joint close to the recurrent laryngeal nerve, cephalic to the inferior thyroid artery (Fig. 23.3), which is probably the best initial marker to locate the glands. The inferior glands are often more variable in their location, being caudal to where the recurrent laryngeal nerve and the inferior thyroid artery cross at the apex of Beahr's triangle. In half of the cases, the inferior parathyroid glands are found in and around the lower pole of thyroid gland and a quarter may be close to, or within residual thymus tissue. As a general rule, parathyroid glands are located symmetrically on either side of the neck and this is often helpful when looking for a missing gland. Most people have four parathyroids, but approximately 10% have more than 4 glands, while only 3% have fewer than four glands. A healthy parathyroid usually measures on average just under 1 cm^3 and is usually oval, varying in colour from light yellow in older patients to a reddish brownish colour in younger ones. The fat content increases with age. It is useful to remember that in normal saline, fat floats and parathyroid tissue sinks.

Parathyroid hormone

Parathyroid hormone (PTH) is a single straight-chain peptide containing 84 amino acids which is measured by highly sensitive radioimmunoassay. It influences calcium metabolism by having a direct effect on bone and kidney.

Actions of parathyroid hormone

- Increases osteolytic activity of osteocytes and osteoclasts
- Increases bone remodelling
- Increases tubular reabsorption of calcium
- Increases phosphate excretion
- Increases the production of 1,25-dihydroxycholecalciferol (the active metabolite of vitamin D)
- Facilitates the uptake of calcium from the kidney, bone and intestine

Primary hyperparathyroidism

Clinical features

This disease has a wide clinical spectrum and affects many organ systems. Although the classic presentation of 'stones, bones, moans and abdominal groans' is often quoted, many patients have mild symptoms or are asymptomatic. Its frequency increases with age and it is more common in females.

Features of hyperparathyroidism

- Renal stones (25%)
- Urinary frequency, nocturia and polyuria
- Nephrocalcinosis, nephrolithiasis and progressive renal failure
- General malaise
- Painful bones due to generalized bone dimineralization and rarely osteitis fibrosis cystica, historically the main presentation (Von Recklinghausen's disease of bone)
- Chondrocalcinosis and joint effusions
- Gout and pseudogout
- Psychiatric symptoms, often mild, including depression, impaired concentration or memory loss. Becoming more common in the elderly

Rarely in some patients, hypercalcaemic crisis can occur when the serum calcium rises in excess of 3 mmol/l. This is a medical emergency and is recognized by increasing weakness, nausea, vomiting and anorexia with drowsiness and confusion. Untreated, it can lead to oliguric renal failure with cardiac arrhythmia and sudden death. It is managed by normal saline infusion, a frusemide diuresis and attention to any electrolyte imbalance. Any further treatment addresses the cause.

Pathology

The majority of cases of primary hyperparathyroidism (80%) are due to a single adenoma. In approximately 15% of cases, the disease is due to multiple gland hyperplasia and double adenomas account for about 2–5% of cases. Parathyroid carcinoma is extremely rare and accounts for less than 1% of patients with primary hyperparathyroidism.

Diagnostic assessment and evaluation

The diagnosis of primary hyperparathyroidism can be accurately made in the presence of an elevated serum calcium and parathormone level on the background of normal renal function. A number of clinical conditions can cause hypercalcaemia in the presence of a normal parathormone level.

Hypercalcaemia with normal parathormone level

- Malignancy with bony metastases
- Malignancy with parathyroid hormone-related peptide production
- Granulomatous diseases such as sarcoidosis
- Vitamin D intoxication
- Milk alkali syndrome
- Thyrotoxicosis
- Phaeochromocytoma
- Prolonged immobilization

A positive family history of hypercalcaemia should raise the suspicion of hereditary hyperparathyroidism and the MEN syndrome. Familial hyperparathyroidism is commonly an autosomal dominant disorder when all of the parathyroid glands are hyperplastic. Rarely it may occur in a recessive form with only one hyperplastic parathyroid gland. When presented with a patient with familial hyperparathyroidism, other endocrine neoplasms (especially a phaeochromocytoma) associated with MEN syndrome need to be excluded, as does familial hypocalciuric hypercalcaemia.

MEN type I syndrome, hyperparathyroidism is present along with either islet cell tumours of the pancreas (75%) or pituitary tumours (60%). In the MEN type IIA syndrome, patients present with medullary thyroid carcinoma and C cell hyperplasia and 50% of patients have a phaeochromocytoma. Hyperparathyroidism occurs in about 40% of patients. In the MEN IIB syndrome, patients have those features described in the MEN type I syndrome along with a more characteristic appearance which includes a Marfanoid habitus and submucosal neuromas.

In the MEN type I syndrome, there is a high recurrence rate of almost 50% of hyperparathyroidism following either subtotal parathyroidectomy or total parathyroidectomy with autotransplantation. Because of this, the treatment of choice is usually total parathyroidectomy with autotransplantation in the forearm so that further surgical access to parathyroid tissue is easily achieved via the arm. In patients with the MEN type II syndrome, the hypercalcaemia is usually much milder and regularly controlled by subtotal parathyroidectomy, but when all of the parathyroid glands are grossly enlarged and the serum calcium level is grossly elevated, then total parathyroidectomy with autotransplantation is justified.

Surgical indications

The majority of patients with primary hyperparathyroidism is treated by surgical exploration of the neck (Fig. 23.21). In the presence of symptomatic disease and a serum calcium level above 2.6 mmol/l then surgery provides expected cure rates around 95% or greater. In those patients with asymptomatic disease and only mildly elevated serum calcium levels then a conservative approach may be undertaken as long as vigilant medical follow-up is available, although nowadays many would suggest that even asymptomatic patients are best treated surgically, especially patients under 50 years old.

Preoperative imaging studies

Imaging studies are unnecessary prior to first explorations. In those patients who have had failed initial surgical explorations and still remain hypercalcaemic, a preoperative imaging study may be valuable to help to locate the site of the adenoma. Such techniques include ^{99m}Tc Sestamibi radionuclide imaging and/or ultrasound, CT and MRI scanning. All of these techniques have significant false-positive and false-negative rates with subsequent overall accuracy rates of between 60 and 90% in most series. They may be of help but at present there remains no significant evidence that the use of preoperative imaging can help in any way to decrease surgical

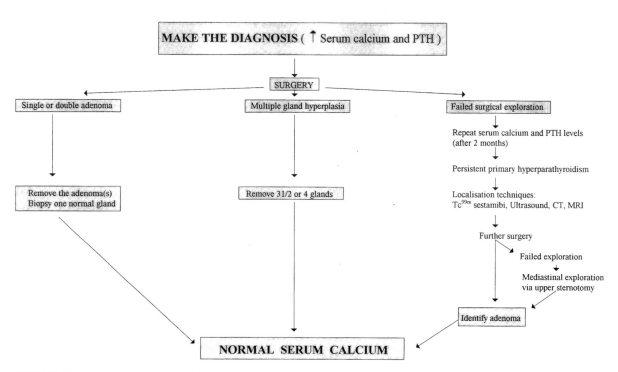

Figure 23.21 Surgical treatment of primary hyperparathyroidism.

costs, lessen surgical complications, shorten the operating time or prevent inevitable surgical failure in some cases. Ultimately, these failures may require selective venous sampling.

Technique of parathyroidectomy

In this operation, attention should be paid to meticulous technique, adequate exposure and secure haemostasis. Any blood staining of the tissues can lead to difficulty with parathyroid identification. Some surgeons use Methylene Blue intravenously 40 min before surgical exploration to assist with parathyroid identification. Owing to the high blood flow of the glands, they selectively concentrate the dye and stand out against the surrounding tissues. The timing of the infusion is crucial.

Key steps in parathyroidectomy

- The incision is as per thyroidectomy.
- The skin flaps are elevated.
- The investing fascia is divided in the midline, the strap muscle retracted and the thyroid gland capsule exposed posteriorly.
- The middle thyroid vein is ligated.
- The paracarotid tunnel is accessed.
- The periglandular tissue in Beahr's triangle is identified to allow excellent exposure of the entire posterior thyroid capsule (Fig. 23.3).
- The superior parathyroid gland is identified first and the surgeon checks whether its blood supply is coming from the inferior or superior thyroid artery.
- The majority of superior glands (80%) will be located in a 2 cm area approximately 1 cm above the intersection of the recurrent laryngeal nerve and the inferior thyroid artery at the apex of Beahr's triangle. The surgeon checks that they are not adherent to, or partially concealed in, the connective tissue adjacent to the thyroid capsule, or indeed embedded within the thyroid gland. It may be necessary to divide the superior thyroid vessels to locate the superior parathyroid gland.
- The majority of the inferior glands will be located in a pericapsular or capsular location below the inferior thyroid artery on the inferior, lateral or posterior surface of the thyroid and closely attached to the capsule of the gland (Fig. 23.22). In about a quarter of patients, they will be intimately associated with the thymus gland.
- Since most parathyroid glands are symmetric, both sides should be explored and carefully evaluated before considering further exploration of any ectopic sites.
- The most common ectopic location sites for a missing superior gland are in the retro- oesophageal and retropharyngeal areas.
- The most common ectopic location for a missing inferior gland is within the superior mediastinum. Often it is within a thymus remnant, which can usually be delivered into the neck so that sternotomy is rarely required.

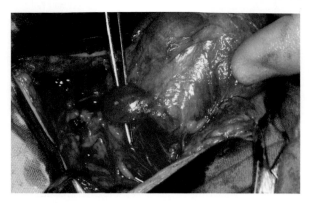

Figure 23.22 Lower pole parathyroid adenoma identified at surgery (courtesy of Mr A. Ready).

- When searching for an ectopic gland, the following areas should therefore, be assessed in order of preference:

  1. retro-oesophageal, and retropharyngeal area (superior glands);
  2. superior mediastinum (inferior glands): after clearing the inferior poles of the thyroid gland, most ectopic glands in the thymus can be removed via transcervical thymectomy and care is taken to dissect the paratracheal tissues and preserve both recurrent laryngeal nerves;
  3. thyroid lobectomy;
  4. exploration of the carotid sheath from the bifurcation to the superior mediastinum;
  5. upper sternal split and mediastinal exploration (very rarely).

Biopsy of parathyroid glands

During parathyroid surgery, it is essential to confirm the presence of normal, healthy parathyroid glands to exclude the possibility of four-gland hyperplasia. This is done by taking a biopsy of the antihilar surface and submitting the tissue to frozen section.

Parathyroid carcinoma

- Occurs in about 1% of patients with primary hyperparathyroidism.
- High serum calcium levels (3.0 mmol/l or above).
- Grossly elevated serum parathormone levels (at least four times normal).
- Greyish-white, firm tumours which invade locally by continuity and contiguity.
- Lymph-node metastases occur in approximately 30% of cases; treatment is by wide local excision including ipsilateral thyroid lobectomy and regional lymph nodes.
- Postoperative radiotherapy is indicated if resection margins are involved.

- Chemotherapy is ineffective
- 5 year survival is 50%.
- Distant metastases may occur in liver, bone and lung.
- Death is usually due to the metabolic consequences of gross hypercalcaemia.
- Most are a surprise, being diagnosed at surgical exploration or on histology.

Postoperative course following parathyroidectomy

The majority of patients has a normal serum calcium within 48 h following surgery. In some cases, particularly when the preoperative serum calcium was grossly elevated, there may be temporary postoperative hypocalcaemia which is treated in the conventional manner with oral or occasionally intravenous calcium supplements. Longer term vitamin D is sometimes required.

Treatment of persistent and recurrent hyperparathyroidism following failed surgical exploration

The problems of persistent and recurrent hyperparathyroidism present significant challenges to the surgeon since treatment is associated with lower success rates and a recognized increase in complications. Whilst a few failures will be due to misdiagnosis, the majority relate to the initial operation and who performed it, and the surgeon's failure to detect an ectopic adenoma, supernumerary gland or multiglandular hyperplasia. Often, these failures are the result of inexperienced surgeons missing glands that are not actually ectopic.

Before any further surgery is performed the following points should be noted.

- The diagnosis must be confirmed by raised serum calcium and PTH.
- Possible risks and benefit are assessed. If a patient is asymptomatic, conservative treatment may be considered.
- An experienced parathyroid surgeon should be involved.
- All previous operation notes are reviewed to establish whether all common sites for parathyroid location were explored, was part of the thyroid explored or removed, were healthy glands identified, what technique was used to do this and were any clips or sutures left in the neck as markers.
- All previous histology is reviewed.
- Recurrence can be due to implantation. Therefore, it is important not to fracture any glands during initial exploration.
- Appropriate localization studies are arranged to assist in accurate preoperative diagnosis. Radionuclide scanning with ^{99m}Tc Sestamibi imaging and ultrasonography is usually the first-choice investigation, with MRI and CT being reserved for possible mediastinal ectopic adenomas.

- The state of the vocal cords is evaluated.
- The majority of missing glands are located within the neck. Meticulous neck re-exploration is performed and all likely sites are explored using a systematic approach. A lateral strap muscle approach, anterior to sternomastoid, is recommended to avoid midline adhesions and facilitate preservation of the recurrent laryngeal nerves.
- Failure to identify diseased parathyroid tissue in the neck and thyroid means that mediastinal exploration should be performed. This is only usually indicated in the minority of cases (less than 1%).
- Most mediastinal parathyroid glands are intrathymic or at the level of the innominate vein. Other locations include the aortic arch near the origin of the great vessels, the pulmonary hila, the pericardium, the tracheal carina and the aortopulmonary window.

Parathyroid autotransplantation and cryopreservation

Fresh parathyroid glands, when autotransplanted, are estimated to function in up to 90% of patients. The site of autotransplantation is usually the forearm. It is also possible to cryopreserve functioning parathyroid tissue and this may function when autotransplanted in approximately 60% of cases. Following the discovery of a missing parathyroid gland or ectopic adenoma, when this is the only known functioning parathyroid tissue remaining in the patient, some parathyroid tissue should be transplanted in the forearm and if possible a portion cryopreserved.

Autotransplants can be monitored by measuring serum parathormone levels in blood samples taken from each arm. Transplant function can, therefore, be subsequently adjusted by the addition or removal of further cryopreserved tissue.

Secondary hyperparathyroidism and chronic renal failure

Secondary hyperparathyroidism develops in most, if not all patients with chronic renal failure. This is a normal response of the parathyroids trying to maintain the serum calcium. The stimulus for increased PTH reduction is chronic hypocalcaemia and hyperphosphataemia. The effects of this have already been described. Some patients with longstanding chronic renal failure develop persisting or worsening hyperparathyroidism following successful renal transplantation. This is called tertiary hyperparathyroidism.

In those patients with secondary hyperparathyroidism and chronic renal failure where symptoms cannot be controlled medically and where parathyroid hormone is significantly raised, parathyroidectomy is indicated. Many of the troublesome symptoms of this condition, including bone pain, pruritis and mental function, improve after surgery.

Subtotal parathyroidectomy may be performed since it preserves access sites in the forearm which are important in renal transplantation patients. However, total parathyroidectomy with autotransplantation and cryopreservation (and later control with alfacalcidol) is as effective, especially in non-compliant patients with secondary hyperparathyroidism.

The surgical approach has already been described and in view of the metabolic problems that many of these patients have, quite profound postoperative hypocalcaemia often develops. This should be managed aggressively along with the other associated electrolyte problems.

References

Black E. G., Sheppard M. C. and Hoffenberg R. (1987) Serial serum thyroglobulin measurements in the management of differentiated thyroid carcinoma, *Clin Endocrinol* 27: 115–20.

Brierley J. D., Panzarella T., Tsang R. W., Gospodarowicz M. K. and O'Sullivan B (1997) A comparison of different staging systems. Predicatibiltiy of patient outcome. Thyroid carcinoma as an example, *Cancer* 79: 2414–23.

Byar D. P., Green S. B. and Dor P., *et al.* (1979) A prognostic index for thyroid carcinoma. A study of the EORTC thyroid cancer cooperative group, *Eur J Cancer* 15: 1033–41.

Cady B. and Rossi R. (1988) An expanded view of risk-group definition in differentiated thyroid carcinoma, *Surgery* 104: 947–53.

Cernea C. R., Ferraz A. R. and Furlari J., *et al.* (1992) Identification of the external branch of the superior laryngeal nerve during thyroidectomy. *Am J Surg* 164: 634–9.

Chow E., Tsang R. W., Brierley J. D. and Filice S. (1998) Parathyroid carcinoma – The Princess Margaret Hospital Experience, *Int J Radiat Oncol Biol Phys*, 41: 569–72.

Clark O. H. (1985) Hyperparathyroidism, in *Endocrine Surgery of the Thyroid and Parathyroid Glands* (O. H. Clark, ed.), Mosby, St Louis, MO.

Eisle D. (1993) Complications of thyroid surgery, in *Complications in head and neck surgery* (D. Eisle, ed.), Vol. 47, Mosley Press, St Louis, MO, pp. 423–36.

Eisle D. W. and Goldstone A. C. (1991) Electrophysiologic identification and preservation of the superior laryngeal nerve during thyroid surgery, *Laryngoscope* 101: 313–15.

Ellenhorn J. D. I., Shah J. P. and Brennan M. F. (1993) Impact of therapeutic regional lymph node dissection for medullary carcinoma of the thyroid gland, *Surgery* 114: 1078–82.

Franklyn J., Daykin J., Young J., Oates G. D. and Sheppard M. (1993) Fine needle aspiration cytology in diffuse or multinodular goitre compared with solitary thyroid nodules, *Br Med J* 307: 240.

Gittoes N. J. K., Miller M. R., Daykin J., Sheppard M. C. and Franklyn J. A. (1994) Upper airways obstruction in 153 consecutive patients presenting with thyroid enlargement, *Br Med J* 312: 484.

Harada T., Shimaoka K., Mimura T. and Ito K. (1987) Current treatment of Graves' disease, *Surg Clin North Am* 67: 29–314.

Harness J. K., Lit Fung M. D., Thompson N. W., Burney R. E. and McLeod M. K. (1986) Total thyroidectomy: complications and technique, *World Surg* 10: 781–6.

Hay I. D., Bergstralh E. J., Goellner J. R., Ebersold J. R. and Grant C. S. (1993) Predicting outcome in papillary thyroid carcinoma: development of a reliable prognostic scoring system in a cohort of 1779 patients surgically treated at one institution during 1940 through 1989, *Surgery* 114: 1050–8.

Hay I. D., Grant C. S., Taylor W. F. and McConahey W. M. (1987) Ipsilateral lobectomy versus bilateral lobar resection in papillary thyroid carcinoma: a retrospective analysis of surgical outcome using a novel prognostic scoring system, *Surgery* 102: 1088–95.

Hay I. D., Grant C. S., Taylor W. F. and McConahey W. M. (1987) Ipsilateral lobectomy versus bilateral lobar resection in papillary thyroid carcinoma: a retrospective analysis of surgical outcome using a novel prognostic scoring system, *Surgery* 102: 1088–95.

Jossart G. G. and Clark O. H. (1994) Well differentiated thyroid cancer, *Curr Prob in Surg* 31: 936–1011.

Kark A. E., Kissin M. W., Auerbach R. and Meikle M. (1984) Voice changes after thyroidectomy: role of the external laryngeal nerve, *Br Med J* 289: 1412–15.

Kumar H., Daykin J., Holder R., Watkinson J. C. Sheppard M. C. and Franklyn J. A. (1999) Gender, clinical findings and serum thyroidtropin measurements in the prediction of thyroid neoplasia in 1005 patients presenting with thyroid enlargement and investigated by fine needle aspiration cytology, *Thyroid* 11: 1105–9.

Lynn J. and Bloom S. (eds) (1996) *Heinemann Surgical Endocrinology*, Butterworth Heinemann, Oxford.

Mazzaferri E. L. (1993) Management of solitary thyroid nodule (Editorial) *New Eng J Med* 328: 553–9.

Mazzaferri E. L. (1999) An overview of the management of papillary and follicular thyroid carcinoma, *Thyroid* 9: 421–7.

Mazzaferri E. L. and Jhiang S. M. (1994) Long term impact of initial surgical and medical therapy on papillary and follicular thyroid cancer, *Am J Med* 97: 418–28.

Moley J. F., Wells S. A., Dilley W. G. and Tissell L. E. (1993) Reoperation for recurrent of persistent medullary thyroid cancer. *Surgery* 114: 1090–1096.

Moosa M. and Mazzaferri E.L. (1998) Management of thyroid neoplasms, in *Otolaryngology, Head and Neck Surgery* (C. W. Cummings, J. M. Fredrickson, L. A. Harker, C. J. Krause, M. A. Richardson and D. E. Schuller, eds), Mosby, St Louis, MO, pp. 2480–518.

Ponder B. (1990) Multiple endocrine neoplasia type 2: the search for the gene continues, *Br Med J* 300: 484–5.

Shah J. P., Loree T. R., Dharker D. *et al* (1992) Prognostic factors in differentiated carcinoma of the thyroid gland, *Am J Surg* 164: 658–61.

Shah J. P, Loree, T. R., Dharker D. and Strong E. W. (1993) Lobectomy versus total thyroidectomy for differentiated carcinoma of the thyroid: a matched-pair analysis, *Am J Surg* 166: 331–4.

Shah, J. (1996) Thyroid and parathyroids, in *Head and Neck Surgery*, 2nd edn), Mosby Wolfe, New York, 10: 393–240.

Shah J. P, Loree T. R. and Dharker D., *et al.* (1992) Prognostic factors in differentiated carcinoma of the thyroid gland, *Am J Surg* 164: 658–61.

Shaha A. R., Loree T. R. and Shah J. P. (1994) Intermediate risk group and differentiated carcinoma of the thyroid, *Surgery* 116: 1036–41.

Summers G. W. (1998) Surgical management of parathyroid disorders, in *Otolaryngology and Head and Neck Surgery*, 3rd edn, Vol. 3 (C. W. Cummings, J. M. Fredrickson L. A. Harker, C. J. Krause, M. A. Richardson and D. E. Schuller, eds), Mosby, St Louis, MO, Chapter 131, pp. 2519–29.

Thompson N. W., Eckhauser F. and Harness J. (1982) Anatomy of primary hyperparathyroidism, *Surgery* **92**: 814–21.

Tunbridge W. M. G., Evered D. C. and Hall R., *et al* (1977) The spectrum of thyroid disease in a community: The Whickham Survey, *Clin Endocrinol* **7**: 481–93.

UICC (International Union against Cancer) (1997) *TNM Classification of Malignant Tumours* (L. H. Sobin and C. H. Wittekind, eds), 5th edn, Wiley-Liss, New York.

Walsh R., Watkinson J. C. and Franklyn J. (1999) The management of the solitary thyroid nodule (A review), *Clinical Otolarynology* **27**: 388–97.

Watkinson J. C. (1998) Tumours of the thyroid gland, in *Diseases of the Head and Neck, Nose and Throat* (A. S. Jones, D. E. Phillips and F. J. M. Hilgers, eds), Arnold, London, pp. 347–70.

Appendix 23.1: the WHO classification of thyroid tumours.

World Health Organization revised histologic classification of thyroid tumours

I. Epithelial tumours
A. *Benign*
 1. Follicular adenoma
  (a) Architectural patterns
   (i) Normocollicular (simple)
   (ii) Macrofollicular (colloid)
   (iii) Microfollicular (fetal)
   (iv) Trabecular and solid (embryonal)
   (v) Atypical
  (b) Cytologic patterns
   (i) Oxyphilic cell type
   (ii) Clear cell type
   (iii) Mucin-producing cell type
   (iv) Signet-ring cell type
   (v) Atypical
 2. Others
  (a) Salivary gland-type tumours
  (b) Adenolipomas
  (c) Hyalinizing trabecular tumours

B. *Malignant*
 1. Follicular carcinoma
  (a) Degree of invasiveness
   (i) Minimally invasive (encapsulated)
   (ii) Widely invasive
  (b) Variants
   (i) Oxyphilic (Hürthle) cell type
   (ii) Clear cell type
 2. Papillary carcinoma
  (a) Variants
   (i) Papillary microcarcinoma
   (ii) Encapsulated variant
   (iii) Follicular variant
   (iv) Diffuse sclerosing variant
   (v) Oxyphilic (Hürthle) cell type
 3. Medullary thyroid cancer
  (a) Variant
   (i) Mixed medullary-follicular carcinoma
 4. Undifferentiated (anaplastic) carcinoma
 5. Other carcinomas
  (a) Mucinous carcinoma
  (b) Squamous cell carcinoma
  (c) Mucoepidermoid carcinoma

II. Nonepithelial tumours

III. Malignant lymphomas

IV. Miscellaneous tumours
 1. Parathyroid tumours
 2. Paragangliomas
 3. Spindle cell tumours with mucous cysts
 4. Teratomas

V. Secondary tumours

VI. Unclassified tumours

VII. Tumour-like lesions
 1. Hyperplastic goitres
 2. Thyroid cysts
 3. Solid cell nests
 4. Ectopic thyroid tissue
 5. Chronic thyroiditis
 6. Riedel's thyroiditis
 7. Amyloid goitre

24 Conservation surgery

'Less can mean more'
Ron Spiro, 1993

Introduction

The traditional approach to surgical treatment of head and neck cancer unlikely to respond well to radiotherapy has been one of radical resection. More often than not, this approach involved significant loss of function and marked deformity of both tumour and donor sites. Moreover, despite improved techniques for cancer resection and reconstruction during the 1980s and the 1990s, surgery has not been instrumental in improving survival figures for head and neck cancer as a whole. However, trying to demonstrate any benefit in terms of survival by a change in surgical practice will always be difficult, if not impossible, because of the low volume of head and neck cancer within the spectrum of malignant disease. However, bearing in mind what progressive radiotherapy and chemotherapy schedules have achieved in containment of locoregional disease, the concept of 'conservation' surgery offers a further treatment option to the patient with malignant disease of the head and neck (Sheppard *et al.*, 1998).

What is conservation surgery?

The idea of conservation surgery is probably as old as that of radical surgery. It is taken to mean different things by different clinicians, however, which may have some bearing on its scarcity within clinical practice, certainly within the UK. It is far more prevalent in other parts of Europe and North America, where financial factors and treatment availability may play a part. Conservation surgery for head and neck cancer is defined as 'a surgical procedure which when combined with radio- and/or chemotherapy aims to effect the same cure as radical surgery, but with preservation of both structure and function'. In other words, conservative surgery can result in cure, through the added benefits of advances in other treatment modalities – a fact which has been ignored in the past.

Conservation surgery: the considerations

■ The tumour
■ The patient
■ The operation
■ The view of the oncology team – medical and ancillary

The tumour

In general, the larger the tumour, the more likely it is to be inoperable or need a major resection. Estimation of tumour size and operability is now greatly improved by radiology (Chapter 3). When trying to preserve structure and function, it is vital to have radiological staging of the tumour to supplement the clinical information to determine whether conservation is feasible in the first instance. The only exceptions are some cases of malignant disease of the neck – selective neck dissection would be considered depending on the site of the tumour, so that, for example an elective supra-omohyoid neck dissection should be considered in tumours of the oral cavity. Imaging also allows operative techniques to be modified to spare at least part of an organ or structure, e.g. sparing of the outer cortex of the mandible. Conservative surgery is rarely used in radiorecurrent malignancy. The only possible exception to this is the T_1 glottic carcinoma which has recurred after radiotherapy, but the decision to preserve the larynx in this case is not to be undertaken lightly.

The patient

■ Both surgeon and oncologist must talk to the patient and explain all of the possible (multimodality) treatment options.
■ The patient must appreciate that certain conservative procedures may be more demanding for them, e.g. it may be more difficult to recover from a supraglottic laryngectomy than total excision.

- Commonsense must prevail. One has to determine what the patient has in the first place to preserve. There is no rationale for performing a supraglottic laryngectomy in an elderly patient with poststroke dysphagia.

The team required for conservation therapy

- Oncologists – to determine tumour suitability for conservation surgery
- surgeons
- expert radiologists
- dedicated nurses
- speech therapists
- nutrition teams.

Conservation surgery: structure and function

Conservation procedures are most commonly applied in the neck and the larynx. From the patient's point of view, the latter has the greater impact for obvious reasons. Operative details will be dealt with elsewhere, but this section will outline options available to the oncology team and the patient.

> ### Sites of conservation surgery
>
> - Neck
> - Larynx
> - Pharynx
> - Parotid
> - Thyroid
> - Sinuses

Neck

The treatment of malignant neck disease is performed either on an elective basis for certain tumours with N_0 disease, or when metastases are already evident. There is no prospective evidence that elective neck dissection improves survival. Elective treatment of the neck may improve regional control if the likelihood of metastasis is greater than 20%.

> ### Tumours with >20% risk of occult metastasis
>
> - Oral cavity
> - Oropharynx (tonsil and tongue base)
> - Hypopharynx (piriform fossa)
> - Supraglottic larynx

Nowadays, rather than the N_0 neck in all of these situations having to be treated by radical or modified radical neck dissection, there is a wealth of modifications based on the documented pattern of disease spread within the lymphatic groups of the neck, so that structures and thereby function may be preserved.

Classification of conservative neck dissection and guidelines for their usage

Comprehensive neck dissections include the radical neck dissection and three modifications, but always refers to a procedure in which all of groups I–V are removed.

Modified radical neck dissection. This operation is based on the work of Suarez, Bocca and Pignataro which indicated that the *en bloc* removal of the cervical lymphatics can be accomplished by stripping the fascia from the sternomastoid and internal jugular vein. No lymphatic communication was ever noted between these structures and the cervical lymphatics. These studies point out that both the spinal accessory and the hypoglossal nerve do not follow the aponeurotic compartments, but rather run across them; however, their conclusion was that if the tumour did not directly involve the nerves, they could be spared.

From the above information and a desire to minimize the shoulder dysfunction associated with spinal accessory nerve sacrifice came the development of the modified radical neck dissection.

> ### Type I modified radical neck dissection
>
> - Removes the same lymphatics as the radical neck dissection
> - Spinal accessory nerve is spared
> - Used less commonly in the N_0 neck
> - Reasonable for N^+ disease involving the sternomastoid or internal jugular vein without the spinal accessory nerve

In a recent study by Anderson, radical neck dissection was compared with type I modified radical neck dissection. Neither survival nor tumour control in the neck was affected by preservation of the spinal accessory nerve. The pattern of failure was the same for the two different procedures; the nerve preservation did not predispose to recurrence in that area.

> ### Type II modified radical neck dissection
>
> - Removes the same lymphatics as the radical neck dissection
> - Spinal accessory nerve and internal jugular vein are spared
> - Similarly indicated in N^+ necks with involvement of the sternomastoid, but without involvement of the nerve and vein

> ### Type III modified radical neck dissection (comprehensive 'functional' neck dissection)
>
> - Removes the same lymphatics as the radical neck dissection
> - Spinal accessory nerve, sternomastoid and internal jugular vein are spared
> - The indications are controversial

In Europe, type III modified radical neck dissection is popular in the treatment of hypopharyngeal and laryngeal tumours with N_0 necks. Molinari *et al.* propose this procedure for N_1 necks when the involved nodes are mobile and no greater than 2.5–3 cm. Bocca proposes this operation for any neck that has indications for a radical neck dissection as long as the nodes are not fixed. The results from Byer's study demonstrate recurrence rates similar to those associated with radical neck dissection.

Selective neck dissection. This type of dissection arose from the work of Shah *et al.*, who identified the pathways of lymphatic spread in the head and neck. Only those regions with high risk for metastasis are removed. This is a subject of great controversy but some surgeons feel that in necks with limited disease (N_1), these procedures provide the same therapeutic value as their more radical counterparts. Recent work by Byers indicates that patients undergoing selective neck dissection with mobile N_1 disease in the first echelon of lymphatic drainage have similar recurrence rates to those having a radical neck dissection. Another recent investigation by Kowalski (1993) recommends selective neck dissection for oral cavity cancers with positive nodes at level I. Sobol's prospective study indicates that (i) by 16 weeks, patients performed significantly better than those who had radical neck dissection, and (ii) supraomohyoid neck dissection allows a quicker return to normal function than modified radical dissection, especially in the first year.

Selective neck dissection

■ Provides the same staging information as radical neck dissection
■ Prognosis and the necessity of radiotherapy can be assessed
■ Manipulation of the spinal accessory nerve is minimized
■ Short-term shoulder morbidity

The following types of selective neck dissection may be undertaken.

In supraomohyoid neck dissection, levels I, II and III are removed, sparing the sternomastoid, internal jugular vein and the accessory nerve. It is indicated in the treatment of oral cavity lesions.

In lateral neck dissection, levels II, III and IV are removed, sparing the sternomastoid, internal jugular vein and the accessory nerve. This is indicated in tumours of the larynx, oropharynx and hypopharynx when the neck is N_0, although some advocate this approach with the N_1 neck with nodes limited to level II.

In posterolateral neck dissection, levels II, III, IV and V are removed, sparing the sternomastoid, internal jugular vein and the accessory nerve. It is useful in the treatment of skin tumours with metastatic potential located in the posterior scalp or neck such as melanomas, squamous cell carcinomas and Merkel cell carcinomas.

Larynx

The most common carcinoma arising within the head and neck has been the subject of some controversy over the last 30 years regarding the place of conservation surgery. There still remains, however, a great division in terms of treatment strategy, between North America, Australia and southern Europe, where partial laryngeal surgery is not unusual, and the UK, where it is the exception rather than the rule. There are various reasons for this: pathological, financial and political. For example, the UK has a better developed radiotherapy service nation-wide than some other parts of Europe. Australia also has a well-developed radiotherapy service, but with very variable ease of access because of the population distribution. Even areas with readily available good radiotherapy, however, may opt for conservation surgery. Why, therefore, should conservation surgery be considered for laryngeal cancer at all, especially for a T_3 and T_4 lesion which may, depending on its anatomical site, do poorly with primary radiotherapy, leaving total laryngectomy as the only salvage option? Certainly in these cases, therefore, conservative surgery could be applicable in order to retain the voice. However, partial laryngeal surgery can also be used in the earliest stages of laryngeal cancer, with radiotherapy for recurrence and salvage surgery held in reserve.

Options

Having decided that conservation surgery in the larynx might be worth considering, the surgical alternatives available for this particular area of the head and neck are legion. The following range of operations reflects the varying tumour biology of laryngeal subsites

---

■ Transoral laser resection
  – partial epiglottectomy
  – partial cordectomy
■ Partial laryngectomy
  – supraglottic laryngectomy
  – vertical hemi laryngectomy
  – supracricoid laryngectomy (or subtotal laryngectomy)
■ Near-total laryngectomy

Supraglottis

The CO_2 laser has been used in the supraglottic area (e.g. for T_1 suprahyoid epiglottic carcinoma) since introduced by Strong, Jako and Vaughan at Boston University in 1969. It was commonly used. Originally, the excision of larger tumours was to allow stabilization of the airway by epiglottectomy, resection of one aryepiglottic fold and in some cases resection of the ventricular fold, which was well tolerated. The key to successful transoral supraglottic laryngeal resection is good visualization. This became easier with the invention of the adjustable laryngoscope which allowed a full view of the supraglottis (Lindholm). The rationale in this approach was that removal of all endoscopically detectable cancer should increase the effectiveness of definitive radiation therapy. In addition, the laser reduces some of the problems of radiation therapy such as oedema.

If the pre-epiglottic space is not grossly invaded and if the tumour has not extended into the anterior commissure at the level of the vocal cord, the transoral supraglottic resection is both safe and effective. Where there is grossly invaded pre-epiglottic space, therapy entails an open procedure. Tracheostomy is rarely necessary for patients with T_1–T_3 tumour transoral resection since the airways are usually significantly improved. The most significant postoperative problem is aspiration. Nonetheless, patients tend to swallow better and leave the hospital earlier following laser therapy than open resection.

For the larger supraglottic lesion thought unsuitable for transoral laser resection, the next option is supraglottic laryngectomy.

Structures removed in supraglottic laryngectomy

- Epiglottis
- False vocal cords
- Aryepiglottic folds
- Arytenoid cartilages
- Ventricle
- Upper one third of the thyroid cartilage
- Thyrohyoid membrane.

The true vocal cords and arytenoids are retained for vocalization and deglutition. The oncological basis for this procedure invokes the resistance to spread of the fibroelastic membranes within the larynx (the conus elasticus, the quadrangular membrane, the thyrohyoid membrane and the hyoepiglottic ligament). However, a recent study by Weinstein et al. (1995) disputed the resistance to spread of the supraglottic region into the glottis.

Indications for supraglottic laryngectomy

- T_2 carcinomas limited to the supraglottis
- Acutely traumatized supraglottis
- Delayed strictures after infection or injury

Contraindications to supraglottic laryngectomy

- Tumour extension onto the cricoid cartilage
- Bilateral arytenoid involvement
- Arytenoid fixation
- Extension on to the glottis or the presence of impaired vocal-cord mobility
- Thyroid cartilage invasion
- Involvement of the apex of the piriform sinus or postcricoid region
- Involvement of the base of the tongue >1 cm posterior to the circumvallate papillae
- Decreased pulmonary reserve

Supraglottic laryngectomees have problems with aspiration, dysphagia and delayed decannulation. The surgeon should be aware of two critical factors in the recovery of swallowing, which are good airway closure at the laryngeal inlet, the space between arytenoids and base of tongue, and movement of the tongue base to make complete contact with the posterior pharyngeal wall. Local control rates of up to 97% have been obtained from supraglottic laryngectomy. There appears no survival benefit from the routine addition of postoperative radiation. Several studies confirm surgical local control rates for T_1, T_2 and T_3 supraglottic carcinoma of 90–100% (against reported radiation control rates of 60%). Such reports seem optimistic, given the relatively greater surgical failure rate after total laryngectomy.

Supracricoid laryngectomy (subtotal laryngectomy)

Supraglottic carcinomas that are unsuitable for horizontal supraglottic laryngectomy can be resected with the partial horizontal supracricoid laryngectomy with reconstruction by cricohyoidopexy. This procedure results in the complete removal of the paraglottic and pre-epiglottic spaces in continuity with the thyroid and epiglottic cartilages. Maintenance of the cricoid cartilage allows for early decannulation, and the preservation of a mobile arytenoid cartilage results in physiological speech and swallowing. The sensory and motor innervation to remaining laryngeal structures is maintained by sparing both the recurrent and superior laryngeal nerves bilaterally. Laryngeal sphincter function is achieved by active opposition of the arytenoid cartilages with the base of the tongue forming a transverse neoglottic opening.

Possible indications for supracricoid laryngectomy

- T_1 and supraglottic lesions with ventricle extension
- T_2 of infrahyoid epiglottis or posterior one-third of the false cord
- Supraglottic lesions extending to glottis or anterior commissure, with or without vocal cord mobility
- T_3 transglottic carcinoma with limitation of the vocal cord
- Selective T_4 lesions invading thyroid cartilage

Exclusion criteria for supracricoid laryngectomy

- Bulky pre-epiglottic space involvement
- Gross thyroid cartilage destruction
- Interarytenoid or bilateral arytenoid involvement
- Fixed arytenoid
- Subglottic extension > 1 cm anteriorly or > 0.5 cm posteriorly
- Inadequate pulmonary reserve

Reported 3 year survival following supracricoid laryngectomy is up to 80%. The functional results obtained by Lacourreye et al. (1990) showed that all patients were decannulated (average 7 days). Normal deglutition was achieved by 74.6% of their patients. Physiological phonation was achieved by all patients within 2 months. The vocal quality was harsh but allowed normal social interactions.

In conclusion, the supraglottic and supracricoid laryngectomy are oncologically sound procedures with an extremely high local control rate. The tumours in general have a high propensity to regional and distal metastasis which decreases long-term survival. The surgical procedures appear more effective than radiation therapy for local control and overall survival. From the patient's perspective, the lack of a permanent stoma with the associated symptom of tracheal mucus production offers a clear advantage over total laryngectomy.

Glottis

Like the supraglottis, malignant lesions of the glottis are treatable with transoral laser resection. There is as yet no evidence that radiotherapy confers survival advantage over laser ablation for a T_1 'mid-cord' glottic carcinoma. After laser surgery, radiotherapy remains as a second-line option should further recurrence occur. There are no adequate prospective data comparing voice-quality outcomes after the two modalities. The application of laser surgery is more straightforward in the glottis than the subglottis, where tumours present later.

Contraindications to glottic laser resection

- Tumours larger than T_{1a}
- Anterior or posterior commissure involvement
- Involvement of the laryngeal ventricle

More extensive resections can be carried out by performing a laser cordectomy or cordectomy by a laryngofissure approach, but voice outcomes may be less favourable than with vertical hemilaryngectomy.

Vertical hemilaryngectomy is increasing in popularity for glottic tumours unsutable for transoral resection.

Indications for vertical hemilaryngectomy in glottic cancer

- Larger glottic tumour extending along the length of one cord, even to the anterior commissure
- T_2 lesions with supraglottic, but not subglottic, involvement
- Ipsilateral arytenoid tumour free (better functional outcome)

Contraindications to hemilaryngectomy

- Anterior commissure cartilage involvement: careful imaging is essential
- Preoperative swallowing problems
- Poor pulmonary reserve

The temporary tracheostomy is closed at 7–10 days. Hemilaryngectomy demands a high degree of motivation from both the patient and the speech therapist and would be unsuitable for some patients. In extended vertical hemilaryngectomy one half of the larynx is completely resected together with two-thirds of the remain-ing hemilarynx, leaving an uninvolved arytenoid on the other side. This effectively removes both paraglottic spaces. The remaining mucosa is tubed leaving the correctly selected and well-motivated patient able to phonate without aspirating. Although considered acceptable by some, for T_3 tumours of the glottis, it has never had widespread acceptance because of doubts concerning its oncological efficacy. Recent results suggest, however, that it is as effective as other treatment modalities, with the advantage of voice preservation. Nonetheless, the patient has a permanent tracheostomy and voice outcomes are no better than those with a good voice prosthesis following a total laryngectomy.

Subglottis

The subglottis is the least suitable region for laryngeal conservation surgery. Lesions quickly invade the perichondrium of the thyroid and cricoid cartilages, and at least 20% of patients have lymph-node metastases at presentation, often in the form of occult paratracheal spread.

Conservation surgery and laryngeal radiorecurrence

The standard approach to laryngeal radiorecurrence is salvage total laryngectomy. There can be difficulties in operating in the region of irradiated cartilage, but there are indications for conservation hemilaryngectomy.

Requirements for salvage conservation surgery

- Recurrence on the suprahyoid epiglottis: supracricoid laryngectomy/subtotal laryngectomy
- Recurrence at the site of a previous T_{1a} glottic carcinoma: vertical hemilaryngectomy
- Recurrence is small, ideally no larger than the primary tumour
- The original surgical/oncology team reviews the patient
- Resection margins are clear of tumour at the time of surgery
- Consent is obtained for a total laryngectomy should conservation prove impossible

---

Hypopharynx

When a patient presents with a carcinoma in the hypopharynx, the likelihood is that the larynx will be removed as part of curative surgical therapy. Conservative surgery in this anatomical region poses a major problem and is the exception rather than the rule, mainly as a result of the extent of the tumour at first presentation. The most common tumour is that of the piriform fossa (about 60%). Even smaller piriform fossa tumours can involve the larynx and in one patient in four, the thyroid gland is invaded by larger tumours. The same problems apply to postcricoid carcinomas which, like oesophageal tumours, also have a risk of submucosal spread. In the USA it is more common to find a small piriform fossa carcinoma than, for example, in the UK.

As a consequence, piriform fossa lesions are at times removed by extended supraglottic laryngectomy, but this would not meet with universal approval on either side of the Atlantic.

The hypopharyngeal tumour that may be considered more suitable for conservation surgery is that on the posterior wall. However, this is the least common, making up only approximately 5% of all cases.

Favourable features for conservation surgery of posterior pharyngeal wall tumours

- Usually exophytic rather than infiltrative
- Do not tend to invade the anterior larynx
- Lower limit is just above the arytenoid cartilage

If there is no extension below the arytenoid cartilage into the cervical oesophagus or laterally into the piriform sinus, then resection via a lateral pharyngotomy is a viable proposition so the larynx might be preserved. It cannot be emphasized enough, however, that because of the nature of hypopharyngeal carcinomas, a meticulous assessment of the tumour is mandatory.

Oropharyngeal, floor of mouth cancer and the mandible

Limited intraoral excision of oropharyngeal tumours is generally condemned. For some T_1 and T_2 tonsil and soft palate carcinomas, however, wide excision of the primary lesion with a simultaneous or staged discontinuous neck dissection has its proponents. Only if the resection does not compromise oral, palatal or nasopharyngeal function is this considered conservative surgery. Traditionally, removal of a portion of the mandible with the primary lesion was considered necessary for surgical access. However, malignant cells are not found in the periosteal lymphatics unless the gross tumour lesions are in direct contact with the mandibular mucoperiosteum. For lesions lying close to but not directly involving the lingual surface of the mandible, partial marginal mandibular resections may be considered, preserving mandibular continuity. Plain radiographs, isotope bone scans, computed tomographic (CT) and magnetic resonance imaging (MRI) scans are available to determine bone involvement, but the most accurate method seems to be direct intraoperative inspection. If the periosteum strips cleanly, then invasion of the bone is unlikely. Conservation mandible surgery is not feasible if the patient has radiorecurrent disease since radiotherapy alters the natural history of tumour spread within the bone

In cancer of the floor of the mouth, mandibular involvement also necessitates surgical treatment. Involvement of the periosteum or very superficial cortical erosion can be treated with marginal mandibulectomy. Advanced cortical involvement or marrow involvement requires segmental mandibulectomy. The inferior alveolar nerve should always be sampled at the resection margin in mandibulectomies to rule perineural spread. The edentulous mandible is more susceptible to invasion.

Parotid tumours and the facial nerve

A treatment protocol from the University of Virginia summarizes well the type of resection necessary in malignant parotid tumours with conservation of the facial nerve where possible. This is advantageous from the patient's point of view, but commonsense must prevail when dealing with more aggressive and larger tumours as illustrated by these guidelines, which are based on the factors which influence survival. Patients are categorized into the following four groups.

Group 1: T_1 and T_2N_0 low-grade malignancies (low-grade mucoepidermoid and acinic cell). Excision of tumour with a cuff of normal tissue is recommended.

- total parotidectomy
- regional lymph nodes are evaluated at operation
- VII is preserved.

Group 2: T_1N_0 (<2 cm diameter), T_2N_0 (>2 cm, <4 cm) high-grade malignancies (adenocarcinoma, malignant mixed, undifferentiated and squamous) and T_3N_0 (>4 cm, <6 cm) low-grade malignancies:

- total parotidectomy with excision of digastric nodes
- preservation of facial nerve: involved VII is resected back to clear margins on frozen section and immediately grafted
- wide-field radiotherapy to include the upper-echelon nodes.

Group 3: T_3N_0 or any N^+ high-grade cancers and recurrent cancers:

- radical parotidectomy with sacrifice of facial nerve and modified neck dissection if N_0
- radical neck dissection is recommended for N^+ necks
- if VII is involved into the mastoid, it is followed until negative margins are obtained
- primary nerve grafting is recommended
- wide-field postoperative radiotherapy, from skull base to clavicle.

Group 4: all T_4 (> 6 cm) tumours:

- radical parotidectomy and neck dissection
- may resect masseter muscle, buccal fat pad, skin, mandible, ear canal, mastoid, or other involved structures
- VII nerve may be grafted
- postoperative radiotherapy is routine.

Facial nerve conservation is mandatory in benign tumours such as pleomorphic adenomas, even in deep lobe tumours. The only exception is recurrent pleomorphic adenoma, where owing to technical difficulties, the nerve may have to sacrificed.

Conservative thyroid surgery

When considering thyroidectomy in malignant disease, three factors related to conservation are considered:

- the recurrent laryngeal nerves
- the parathyroid glands
- invasion of other local structures, e.g. the larynx.

Based primarily on stage, sex and the behaviour of the histological variants, it is possible to formulate operative plans with conservation of the aforementioned structures in mind. Low-risk patients with low-risk tumours can safely be treated with hemithyroidectomy, TSH suppression with thyroxine and serial measurements of serum thyroglobulin. The remainder are usually best treated by near-total or total thyroidectomy, postoperative radio-iodine ablation, TSH suppression with thyroxane and serial measurements of sodium thyroglobulin.

Papillary and mixed papillary/follicular carcinoma

■ Comprise > 80% of tumours
■ Peak onset third and fourth decades
■ Female:male 3:1
■ Prognosis is directly related to size of the tumour (<1 cm)
■ Tumours that invade or extend beyond the thyroid capsule have a worse prognosis
■ Low incidence of distant metastasis, related to the lack of early vascular invasion

---

Arguments for conservative surgical therapy

■ Low rate of clinical tumour recurrence (5–24%)
■ Hypoparathyroidism in up to 40% in patients undergoing total thyroidectomy
■ Increased risk of recurrent laryngeal nerve injury in total thyroidectomy

---

Arguments for total thyroidectomy

■ Tumour foci in up to 88% of contralateral lobes and in cervical lymph nodes
■ Several large studies with <3% incidence of recurrent nerve injury and permanent hypoparathyroidism
■ With adjuvant radioiodine therapy and thyroid suppression, gives a significantly lower recurrence rate and mortality if tumour >1 cm
■ Desirable to reduce the amount of normal gland tissue that will take up radioiodine

---

Papillary carcinomas

Indications for hemithyroidectomy and isthmusthectomy

■ Well circumscribed
■ Isolated with no evidence of cervical metastases
■ Less than 1 cm
■ Young (20–40 years old) female patient with no history of radiation exposure

---

All others should be treated with a near-total or total thyroidectomy, central neck dissection and ipsilateral selective neck dissection of at least levels II–V as required. Iodine-131 may be taken up well by papillary/follicular thyroid carcinoma and should be used postoperatively.

Follicular carcinomas

Follicular carcinoma

■ Comprises about 15% of all thyroid carcinomas
■ More malignant than papillary carcinoma but lymphadenopathy rarer (8–13%)
■ Occurs in a slightly older age group than papillary, less common in children
■ Only rarely complicates radiation exposure
■ Mortality related to degree of vascular invasion
■ Patients > 40 years have more aggressive disease which concentrates iodine less well
■ Vascular invasion and distant metastasis common to lung, bone, brain, liver, bladder and skin

---

Conservative surgical therapy is similar to papillary carcinoma. Those patients listed below can safely be treated by hemithyroidectomy, TSH suppression with thyroxane and serial measurements of serum thyroglobulin.

■ minimally invasive tumours 1 cm diameter
■ age < 40 years old and female.

The rest should undergo near-total or total thyroidectomy and central neck dissection (with neck ipsilateral selective neck dissection for involved nodes). Postoperative therapy with ^{131}I at 6 weeks and thyroxine suppression therapy are as for papillary carcinoma.

Hürthle carcinomas

Hürthle cell variant of follicular carcinoma

■ Variant of follicular carcinoma: defined by the presence of oxyphilic cells
■ Occurs in an even older age group (mean age 55 years)
■ Coexistent well-differentiated carcinoma in 40% of patients
■ Previous radiation therapy in 7–39% of patients
■ Less favourable prognosis
■ Lymph-node involvement in up to 50% of patients
■ No iodine uptake
■ Prognosis variable

In the absence of invasion of the capsule, lymph nodes, distant metastases or vascular invasion the lesion is considered benign. Serial section of the lesion is required to confirm that simple hemithyroidectomy and isthmusthectomy with central neck dissection is adequate. The remaining lobe must be examined carefully for coexistent disease at the time of initial surgery. All other lesions should be treated with near-total or total thyroidectomy and central neck dissection as described above.

Surgical management of laryngotracheal invasion: to conserve or not?

Thyroid carcinoma that invades the airway can in most instances be treated with partial laryngectomy or partial tracheal resection. Full-thickness cartilage resection is usually necessary even when there is no evidence of intraluminal involvement. Partial laryngectomy is not usually an option, owing to the different invasion patterns of thyroid cancer from endolaryngeal squamous cancer. Total laryngectomy and circumferential tracheal resection may be required in patients with extensive disease. Addition of a laryngeal drop will be required if more than 4 cm is resected. Following resection of a shorter segment, primary closure may be possible. The relatively benign nature of well-differentiated thyroid cancer has led some to believe that it is better to leave some local disease than to remove local vital structures. Patients who eventually die of thyroid cancer, however, most often do so as a result of local recurrence with invasion of vital structures. Thus, conservative surgery may not be the best option and should only be considered if imaging and operative findings are favourable.

Tumours of the sinuses: conservative approaches

> **Management challenges in malignant tumours of the paranasal sinuses**
>
> ■ 50% will be incurable
> ■ Wide range of histological variants
> ■ More likely to present in the younger patient
> ■ Severe disfigurement of the midface or the eye can be a distinct possibility

Three operations dominate current surgical approaches

■ lateral rhinotomy
■ partial maxillectomy
■ anterior craniofacial resection.

For squamous cell carcinoma within the maxilla, it is possible to perform a partial maxillectomy preserve both the orbital floor and orbit. However, in adenocarcinoma this often not possible because of ethmoid involvement. A squamous or adenocarcinoma of the ethmoids should be resected by an anterior craniofacial approach. This need not mean loss of an eye, as the orbital periosteum is frequently resistant to tumour invasion and although it is wise to have consent for orbital exenteration, it is sometimes possible to spare the orbit and resect orbital periosteum in one area. Whenever orbital preservation is a distinct possibility, it is important to remember that far more control is achieved via a craniofacial approach rather than coming from below via a radical maxillectomy.

Slightly more favourable in terms of structure conservation is malignant melanoma, as resection can often be tailored to the tumour. If it occurs discretely on an inferior turbinate then wide local excision is perfectly reasonable. Even if more extensive, perhaps as a polypoid mass, then a lateral rhinotomy with good resection margins can suffice. This is really the only malignant tumour occurring within the nose and paranasal sinuses where a 'wait and see' policy following relatively limited surgery is an option.

References and further reading

Andersen P. E., Shah J. P., Cambronero E. and Spiro R. H. (1994) The role of comprehensive neck dissection with preservation of the spinal accessory nerve in the clinically positive neck, *Am J Surg* **168**: 499–502.

Beckhardt R. N., Murray J. G., Ford C. N., *et al.* (1994) Factors influencing functional outcome in supraglottic laryngectomy, *Head Neck* **16**: 232–9.

Bocca E., Pignataro O., Oldini C. and Cappa C. (1984) Functional neck dissection: an evaluation and review of 843 cases, *Laryngoscope* **94**: 942–5.

Byers R. M., Wolf P. F. and Ballantyne A. J. (1988) Rationale for elective modified neck, *Head Neck Surg* **10**: 160–7.

Chevalier D. and Piquet J. J. (1994) Subtotal laryngectomy with cricohyoidopexy for supraglottic carcinoma a review of 61 cases, *Am J Surg* **168**: 472–3.

Don D. (1995) Evaluation of cervical lymph node metastases in squamous cell carcinoma of the head and neck, *Laryngoscope* **105**: 669–774.

Eckel H. E., Volling P., Pototschnig C., Zorowka P. and Thumfart W. (1995) Transoral laser resection with staged discontinuous neck dissection for oral cavity and oropharynx squamous cell carcinoma, *Laryngoscope* **105**: 53–60.

Henick D. (1995) Supraomohyoid neck dissection as a staging procedure for squamous cell carcinomas of the oral cavity and oropharynx, *Head Neck* **17**: 119–123.

Hilgers F. J., Ackerstaff A. H., Aaronson N. K., Schouwenburg P. F. and Van Zandwijk N. (1990) Physical and psychosocial consequences of total laryngectomy, *Clin Otolaryngol* **15**: 421–5.

Kashima H. K. (1993) *Postoperative Dysphagia. Complications in Head and Neck Surgery* (Eisele, D. W. ed.), Mosby, St Louis, MO, pp. 157–63.

Kitahara S., Inouye T., Tanabe T., Haniu Y. and Widick M. H. (1994) Reconstruction of the hypopharynx using hemilarynx for localized pyriform sinus cancer, *Laryngoscope* **104**: 1401–3.

Kligerman J., Lima R. A., Soares J. R., Prado L., Dias F. L., Freitas E. Q. and Olivatto L. O. (1994) Supraomohyoid neck dissection in the treatment of T_1/T_2 squamous cell carcinoma of the oral cavity, *Am J Surg* **168**: 391–394.

Kowalski L., Magrin J., Waksman G., Santog F. and Lopes H. E. (1993) Supraomohyoid neck dissection in the treatment of head and neck tumours, *Arch Otolaryngol Head Neck Surg* **119**: 958–963.

Krespi Y. P. and Levine T. M. (1991) Tumours of the nose and paranasal sinuses, in *Otolaryngology* (M. M. Paprella *et al.*, eds), W.B. Saunders, Philadelphia, PA.

Laccourreye H., Laccourreye O., Weinstein G., Menard M. and Brasnu D. (1990) Supracricoid laryngectomy with cricohyoidopexy: a partial laryngeal procedure for glottic carcinoma, *Ann Otol Rhinol Laryngol* **99**: 421–6.

Laccourreye O., Merite-Drancy A., Brasnu D., Chabardes E., Cauchois R., Menard M. and Laccourreye H. (1993) Supracricoid hemilaryngopharyngectomy in selected piriform sinus carcinoma staged as T_2, *Laryngoscope* **103**: 1373–9.

Larson D. L. and Sanger J. R. (1995) Management of the mandible in oral cancer, *Semin Surg Oncol* **11**: 190–9.

Logemann J. A., Gibbons P., Rademaker A. W., *et al.* (1994) Mechanisms of recovery of swallow after supraglottic laryngectomy, *J Speech Hear Res* **37**: 965–74.

McGuirt W., Johnson J. T., Myers E. N. Rothfield R. and Wagner R. (1995) Floor of mouth carcinoma, the management of the clinically negative neck, *Arch Otolaryngol Head Neck Surg* 121: 278–82.

Molinari R., Cantu G., Chiesa F. and Grandi C. (1980) Retrospective comparison of conservative and radical neck dissection is laryngeal cancer, *Ann Otol Rhinol Laryngol* 89: 578–81.

Nakatsuka T., Harii K., Ueda K., Ebihara S., Asai M., Hirano K., *et al.* (1997) Preservation of the larynx after resection of a carcinoma of the posterior wall of the hypopharynx: versatility of a free flap patch graft, *Head Neck* 19: 137 42.

Nibu K., Kamata S., Kawabata K., Nakamizo M., Niguri T. and Hoki K. (1997) Partial laryngectomy in the treatment of radiation-failure of early glottic carcinom, *Head Neck* 19: 116–20.

Norris C. M., Busse P. M. and Clark J. R. (1993) Evolving role of surgery after induction chemotherapy and primary site radiation in head and neck cancer, *Semin Surg Oncol* 9: 3–13.

Pruyn J. F., De Jong P. C., Bosman L. J., Van Poppel J. W., Van Den Borne H. W., Ryckman R. M. and De Meij K. (1986) Psychosocial aspects of head and neck cancer – a review of the literature, *Clin Otolaryngol* 11: 469–74.

Ramadan H. H. and Allen G. C. (1993) The influence of elective neck dissection on neck relapse in N_0 supraglottic carcinoma, *Am J Otolaryngol* 14: 278–281.

Shah J. P. and Andersen P. E. (1994) The impact of nodal metastasis on modifications of neck dissection, *Ann Surg Oncol* 1: 521–32.

Shah J. P,. Candela F. C. and Poddar A. K. (1990) Patterns of cervical lymph node metastasis from squamous carcinomas of the oral cavity, *Cancer* 66: 109–13

Shah J. P., Loree T. R., Dharker D. and Strong E. W. (1993) Lobectomy versus total thyroidectomy for differentiated of the thyroid: a matched-pair analysis, *Am J Surg* 166: 331–5.

Sheppard I. J., Watkinson J. C. and Glaholm J. (1998) Conservation surgery in head and neck cancer (editorial), *Clin Otolaryngol* 23: 385–7.

Spiro R. H. (1991) Diagnosis and pitfalls in the treatment of parotid tumours, *Semin Surg Oncol* 7: 20–4.

Spiro R. H., Strong E. W. and Shah J. P. (1994) Classification of neck dissection: variations on a new theme, *Am J Surg* 168: 415–8.

Spiro R. H., Morgan G. J., Strong E. W. and Shah J. P. (1996) Supraomohyoid neck dissection, *Am J Surg* 172: 650–3.

Sobol S., Jensen C. and Sawycr W. P. (1985) Objcctive comparision of physical dysfunction after neck dissection, *Am J Surg* 150: 503–9.

Stern S. J. (1993). Orbital preservation in maxillectomy, *Otolaryngol Head Neck Surg* 109: 111–15.

Suarez C., Rodrigus J. P. and Herranez J. (1995) Supraglottic laryngectomy with or without postoperative radiotherapy in supraglottic carcinoma. *Ann Otol Rhinol Laryngol* 104: 3858–63.

Urba S. and Wolf G. T. (1991) Organ preservation in multimodality therapy of head and neck cancer, *Hematol Oncol Clin North Am* 5: 713–24.

Vijay S. D., Bahri H. and Stone P. C. (1972) Preepiglottic space, *Arch Otolaryngol* 95: 130–3.

Weinstein G. S., Laccourreye O. and Brasnu D. (1995) Reconsidering a paradigm: the spread of supraglottic carcinoma to the glottis, *Laryngoscope* 105: 1129–33.

Weiss M. (1994) Use of decision analysis planning a management strategy for the stage N_0 neck, *Arch Otolaryngol Head Neck Surg* 120: 699.

Zeitels S. M. and Kirchner J. A. (1995) Hyoepiglottic ligament in supraglottic cancer, *Ann Otol Rhinol Laryngol* 104: 770–5.

25 Rare tumours

'With April's firstborn flowers, and all things rare
That heaven's air in this huge rondure hems'
William Shakespeare, Sonnet XXI

Introduction

The majority of cancers which arise in the head and neck region are squamous carcinomas of the upper aerodigestive tract. These have been covered in Chapter 1, and the various chapters relating to each anatomical site. A significant minority, however, are of different types. Some are site specific, such as the various carcinomas of the thyroid gland which have been dealt with in Chapter 23. Some are tissue specific, such as salivary gland cancers. Although these may also occur in minor salivary glands which are widely distributed throughout the mucosa of the upper aerodigestive tract, they are included with tumours of the major salivary glands in Chapter 22.

Other tumours which are not exclusively in the province of the head and neck surgeon, and can occur in many other parts of the body, are described in this chapter. They include the various types of lymphoma and sarcoma, melanoma, neurogenic tumours and malignancies related to the acquired immunodeficiency syndrome (AIDS). When they present with head and neck symptoms and signs, the head and neck surgeon plays a pivotal role in obtaining tissue for diagnosis. Treatment, however, is often based on non-surgical modalities and may not be affected by the primary site of the tumour, and it is therefore essential to involve relevant colleagues at an early stage in each patient's management.

Rare tumours

- Lymphoid malignancy
  - Hodgkin's disease
  - non-Hodgkin's lymphoma
- Sarcomas
  - bone
  - soft tissue
- Mucosal malignant melanoma
- Neurogenic tumours
- AIDS-related cancer

Lymphoid malignancy

Hodgkin's disease

Epidemiology

The London physician, pathologist and Quaker philanthropist Thomas Hodgkin described six patients with lymphadenopathy in 1832. Three of these cases have more recently been proven to be due to the disease which now bears his name. Hodgkin's disease can occur at any age, although it is rare in children under 5 years of age. There is a rising incidence in older adolescents and younger adults, with a peak between the ages of 20 and 30 years. After that it becomes less common, although the incidence rates rise again in old age. Males are more commonly affected than females.

The cause is not known, but several epidemiological features suggest a complex interaction between genetic and environmental factors. In less developed countries such as Columbia and Nigeria, the peak incidence occurs at a younger age than in, for example, Denmark and New Zealand. Hodgkin's disease is not common in Japan, but is more common in ethnic Japanese who have emigrated to the USA. Occasionally, familial or social clustering is seen. Hodgkin's disease is also more common in higher socioeconomic groups. Cases are more likely than controls to have evidence of Epstein–Barr virus (EBV) infection and malignant cells have been shown to contain EBV DNA. Nonetheless, an association does not prove causality and furthermore not every case shows EBV infection.

Histopathology

In Hodgkin's disease, the typical lymph-node architecture is effaced by a mixture comprising predominantly normal cells and a lesser proportion of abnormal lymphoid cells. The normal (reactive) cell population includes lymphocytes, histiocytes, eosinophils and plasma cells. The malignant population comprises the classical multinucleate cells first recognized by Sternberg of Vienna in 1898, and Reed of Baltimore in 1902, called

Reed–Sternberg cells, and their mononuclear variant, called the Hodgkin cell. The appearance of Reed–Sternberg cells is characteristic: they are large with an eosinophilic cytoplasm, and they contain usually two, but sometimes four or more, mirror-image lobulated nuclei with a darkly staining nuclear membrane, pale chromatin and a prominent eosinophilic nucleolus. There is often an element of fibrosis within the abnormal gland.

For more than 30 years, Hodgkin's disease has been subdivided in the Rye Classification according to the predominant cell types and the presence or absence of fibrosis. There is an association between the histological type of the disease and the clinical presentation (age and stage) and outcome. Categorization of an individual case therefore appears to be of importance prognostically, but it is rare for the histological type to influence therapeutic choices, and histological subtype may be of less relevance once age and stage are taken into account.

Rye Classification of Hodgkin's disease

- ■ Lymphocyte predominant (rare)
  - Nodular subtype
  - Diffuse subtype
- ■ Nodular sclerosing (most common)
  - Type 1
  - Type 2
- ■ Mixed cellularity (less common)
- ■ Lymphocyte depleted (rare)

Lymphocyte-predominant Hodgkin's disease is not common. As its name suggests, the predominant cell type is the lymphocyte, and sometimes the histiocyte. Plasma cells, eosinophils and Reed–Sternberg cells are very sparse. It tends to be associated with early stage disease and a very good prognosis. Recent immunohistochemical studies have shown important differences between this type of Hodgkin's disease and the more common nodular sclerosing and mixed cellularity variants, suggesting that it is more closely related to some types of non-Hodgkin's lymphoma (NHL) than classical Hodgkin's disease. The nodular subtype can be associated with a chronic relapsing course similar to low-grade follicular NHL and can occasionally transform into high-grade B-cell NHL.

Nodular sclerosing Hodgkin's disease is the most common type. Microscopically, it is characterized by variable amounts of fibrous tissue bands which divide up the lymph node into nodules containing the malignant and reactive cells. Young female patients with large mediastinal masses are usually of this type. Nodular sclerosing Hodgkin's disease may be subdivided into two subtypes on the basis of the cellular infiltrate. Type 1 disease has many lymphocytes and is associated with a relatively favourable prognosis. Type 2 has fewer lymphocytes and a larger proportion of pleomorphic Reed–Sternberg and Hodgkin's cells, and is associated with a worse outcome.

Mixed cellularity Hodgkin's disease contains significant numbers of Reed–Sternberg and Hodgkin's cells set in a mixed background of eosinophils, lymphocytes, histio-

cytes and plasma cells without fibrous banding. Patients with mixed cellularity disease are more likely to have infradiaphragmatic disease spread and a correspondingly poor prognosis.

In lymphocyte-depleted Hodgkin's disease, which fortunately accounts for only about 5% of cases, Reed–Sternberg cells are predominant and there is little by way of a reactive infiltrate. Areas of necrosis may be present. Diffuse fibrosis may occur, but collagen banding is not seen. Lymphocyte-depleted disease is more commonly seen in the elderly and is more likely to be associated with extralymphatic spread.

Clinical presentation

The majority of patients present with painless enlarged lymph nodes, most commonly in the neck. The size of the nodes may wax and wane over a period of months before the diagnosis is made. Mediastinal lymph nodes are commonly involved and the presentation may be with superior vena cava obstruction. Infradiaphragmatic lymph-node involvement is less common. While involvement of the para-aortic nodes is not infrequently found by staging investigations, an inguinal presentation is rare.

Approximate frequency of lymph-node involvement in Hodgkin's disease

- ■ Cervical 70%
- ■ Mediastinal nodes 50%
- ■ Axillary nodes 30%
- ■ Para-aortic nodes 30%
- ■ Inguinal nodes 10%

Involvement of extranodal lymphatic tissue is well recognized. The spleen is most commonly affected. Involvement of Waldeyer's ring is, however, unusual. It is much less common in Hodgkin's disease than in NHL. Occasionally, however, one encounters a patient with Hodgkin's disease who has undergone either a tonsillectomy or adenoidectomy without histological analysis of the resected tissue a few months prior to the diagnosis being made. Involvement of non-lymphoid tissue such as liver, bone or bone marrow is recognized as being of importance, but is unusual at presentation.

Approximate frequency of non-lymph node involvement in Hodgkin's disease

- ■ Spleen 30%
- ■ Liver 5%
- ■ Bone marrow 5%
- ■ Waldeyer's ring 1–2%

Systemic symptoms are reported in up to one-third of patients. These include the so-called B symptoms of weight loss, fever and night sweats which affect the staging classification. Other symptoms such as pruritis and the rarely encountered but classical phenomenon of pain after drinking alcohol are not regarded as B symptoms.

Breathlessness may occur for various reasons including pleural or pericardial effusion, and anaemia may be due to bone-marrow infiltration or a Coombs-positive autoimmune process.

Staging

Nowadays, clinical staging is usually all that is required in Hodgkin's disease. The anatomical extent of the disease, as determined by clinical examination and imaging, is allocated a number from I to IV (Table 25.1). The investigations necessary include plain chest radiography, computed tomography (CT) of the neck, thorax, abdomen and pelvis and abdominal ultrasound examination. Other investigations such as a bone scan may be called for by symptoms such as pain. Bone-marrow aspirate and trephine is no longer routinely performed in early stage disease, but may be indicated if there are B symptoms, anaemia or a markedly raised erythrocyte sedimentation rate (ESR), for example.

The stage number is given a suffix A or B depending whether or not constitutional symptoms of fever, night sweats or weight loss are present (B) or absent (A).

B symptoms in Hodgkin's disease

- Fever
- Weight loss
- Night sweats

Previously, when imaging techniques were much less sophisticated than at present, clinical staging was less reliable. When radiotherapy was the principal curative treatment, it was essential to know the precise extent of disease. Pathological staging was therefore usually undertaken in patients with supradiaphragmatic clinical stage I or II disease. In this process, the patient was subjected to a laparotomy at which many lymph nodes were sampled for histology, the spleen was removed and the liver was biopsied. In this way about a quarter of patients with unselected clinical stage IA or IIA disease, and about a half of patients with unselected stage IB or IIB disease were found to have more advanced disease than was previously thought. Nowadays staging laparotomy is essentially obsolete.

Adverse prognostic factors in Hodgkin's disease

- B symptoms
- Bulky disease, e.g. large mediastinal masses
- Involvement of many lymph-node groups
- Unfavourable histology
- Old age

Principally, the likelihood of cure in unselected clinically staged patients is the same as for comparable populations who have been pathologically staged. This is because it is now possible to select out those clinically staged patients who have a significant likelihood of having more extensive disease. The adverse prognostic factors include B symptoms, large mediastinal masses, involvement of many lymph-node groups, unfavourable histology and old age. In these patients, chemotherapy should be the principal treatment and the precise anatomical extent of disease is irrelevant. Radiotherapy can be reserved as the principal treatment for patients with localized, biologically favourable disease. If they relapse because of undetected intra-abdominal disease, salvage chemotherapy offers a high likelihood of cure.

In addition, laparotomy has its own acute morbidity and, rarely, mortality. Splenectomy leads to long-term immunodeficiency, particularly with regard to fulminant septicaemia caused by encapsulated bacteria such as *Pneumococcus* and *Meningococcus* which can be rapidly fatal. Patients who have undergone splenectomy therefore require lifelong penicillin prophylaxis and regular immunization against pneumococcal infection.

Table 25.1 Ann Arbor staging classification

Stage	Definition
I	Involvement of a single extranodal site (I_E) or a single lymph-node region (for example cervical, axillary, inguinal, mediastinal, hilar) or lymphoid structure such as spleen, thymus or Waldeyer's ring
II	Involvement of two or more lymph-node regions or lymph-node structures on the same side of the diaphragm or localized involvement of an extranodal organ or site and of one or more lymph node regions on the same side of the diaphragm (II_E)
III	Involvement of lymph-node regions or lymph-node structures on both sides of the diaphragm
IV	Diffuse or disseminated involvement of one or more extranodal organs or tissues with or without associated lymph-node involvement
A or B	The suffix A is used in the absence of, and the suffix B is used in the presence of, any of the following three constitutional symptoms: • Otherwise unexplained weight loss of more than 10% over the previous 6 months • The presence of an otherwise unexplained persistent or recurrent, fluctuating fever (>38°C) during the previous month • Recurrent drenching night sweats during the previous month

Treatment

The initial treatment choices in Hodgkin's disease lie between radiotherapy and chemotherapy or combined modality treatment. There are few hard and fast rules, and various alternative strategies are acceptable and produce good results. Surgery, while obviously essential for obtaining tissue for diagnosis, is never used in the treatment of Hodgkin's disease.

For adult patients with localized (clinial stage I or II) disease without adverse features such as B symptoms, unfavourable histology or a bulky mediastinal mass radiotherapy alone is usually the treatment of choice. This may be wide-field treatment, encompassing not only known sites of disease but also adjacent nodal groups which are not clinically involved, but could harbour occult foci of disease. Most commonly for supradiaphragmatic disease this would involve radiotherapy to the 'mantle' field. This encompasses glands in the neck, mediastinum and axillae, shielding out the oral cavity, larynx shoulders and lungs. Mantle radiotherapy is not suitable for those rare patients with involvement of Waldeyer's ring, because of the xerostomia which would be produced by the inevitable coincidental irradiation of the salivary glands. Nor is mantle radiotherapy suitable for patients with bulky mediastinal disease, as the volume of lung tissue which would be encompassed is too great. For those few patients with infradiaphragmatic presentations, an 'inverted Y' field is used, covering the para-aortic, iliac and inguinal node regions. For patients with favourable prognosis stage I disease, such as a 25-year-old woman with type 1 nodular sclerosing Hodgkin's disease confined to a single small node in the mid or upper neck, involved field radiotherapy, covering only the node group known to be affected, is good treatment associated with less morbidity.

When radiotherapy is used for Hodgkin's disease, a 4 week course delivering 35–45 Gy is usually adequate, as the disease is substantially more radiosensitive than squamous cancer.

Patients with stage III or IV disease, and patients with earlier stage disease and unfavourable features will receive initial combination chemotherapy. Advanced Hodgkin's disease was one of the first disseminated cancers to be recognized as chemocurable when the MOPP regimen comprising mustine, vincristine, procarbazine and prednisolone was introduced into clinical practice over 30 years ago. Since then, many chemotherapy schedules have been evaluated. Some, such as LOPP (chlorambucil, vincristine, procarbazine and prednisolone), MVPP (mustine, vinblastine, procarbazine and prednisolone) and ChlVPP (chlorambucil, vinblastine, procarbazine and prednisolone), are very similar to MOPP, involving the substitution of one vinca alkaloid for another (vinblastine for vincristine) and/or one alkylating agent for another (chlorambucil for mustine). Others, such as ABVD (doxorubicin, bleomycin, vinblastine and dacarbazine), contain different classes of drugs such as anthracyclines, and are also effective. There is good evidence that in some instances alternating courses of different types of chemotherapy such as MOPP/ABVD will produce better results. Various hybrid regimens have been evaluated and others are still the subject of clinical trials. Usually when chemotherapy is used, six to eight courses are sufficient.

Combined modality therapy refers to the elective use of chemotherapy and radiotherapy, usually in that order. It can be used to intensify treatment in patients with poor prognosis disease, or sometimes to allow a reduction in the total dose of radiotherapy and/or chemotherapy than if either modality was used alone, with the aim of diminishing treatment-related morbidity.

One of the greatest advances in recent years has been the introduction of high-dose chemotherapy with allogenetic bone marrow or peripheral blood stem cell support. This has been shown to improve outcome in patients with relapsed or poor prognosis disease.

The treatment of children with Hodgkin's disease differs from that of adults in that radiotherapy is less frequently used, largely because the adverse late effects on bone and soft tissue in the growing child can be circumvented by the use of chemotherapy. In addition, the prognosis for children is better than for adults with the same stage and type of disease, and treatment needs to be less intense.

Non-Hodgkin's lymphoma

Epidemiology

NHL is not one disease, but many. It embraces a spectrum from low-grade, indolent disease with an untreated natural history which may be measured in decades through to aggressive types which, if untreated may prove fatal within days of presentation.

NHL as a group is more common than Hodgkin's disease, but many of the subtypes are relatively rare. NHL seems to be becoming more common, but the reasons for this are not clear.

Usually, NHL is a disease of lymph nodes, but extranodal NHL is significantly more common than extranodal Hodgkin's disease. Children are more likely than adults to present with extranodal disease.

NHL can present at virtually any age, but different types are more common at different ages. For example, in children high grade lymphoblastic lymphoma predominates. Low grade NHL is exceptionally rare in childhood, and very uncommon in young adults, but is frequently encountered in the elderly. For most categories of NHL there is a small but distinct male predominance.

There is a geographical variation in the type of NHL encountered. For example, T-cell disease is more common in Japan (about 50% of NHL cases) than in Europe (about 15%), Burkitt's lymphoma is more common in parts of Africa, and human T-cell lymphotrophic virus type 1 (HTLV-1)-related T-cell lymphoma is more common in the Caribbean. For the most part, the aetiology of NHL is unknown, but some types are clearly related to viral infections such as human immunodeficiency virus (HIV), EBV and HTLV-1.

Pathology and classifications

Over the years, many different classifications of NHL have been used. For pathologists, the classification of NHL appears to be a source of perpetual joy. For clinicians, the regular arrival of new classifications often leads to confusion rather than enlightenment. Despite the profusion of classification systems with counterintuitive nomenclature, NHL can for practical clinical purposes largely be divided into just two groups: high-grade NHL and low-grade NHL.

The various classifications have come about partly as a result of increasing understanding about the biology of NHL and newer diagnostic techniques such as immunocytochemistry and cytogenetics, and partly because of a sensible desire to harmonize the nomenclature used by different groups in various countries. Problems have arisen because the same terminology is used in different classifications to describe separate clinicopathological entities, and what is regarded as one entity in one classification is split into several subtypes in another.

The first clinically relevant pathological classification in modern times was the Rappaport classification (1966). This pre-dated immunocytochemistry and the recognition of the T-cell and B-cell lineages. It was a morphological classification based on light microscopy, and divided cases of NHL by whether the individual cells were small or large and whether the architecture was follicular (or nodular) or diffuse. These simple categories correlated with prognosis. Small-cell and nodular subtypes had an indolent clinical course; they were low grade. Diffuse and large-cell NHL followed a much more aggressive course; in other words, it was high grade.

As newer histological techniques became available, a host of new classifications was proposed which led to much confusion. The Working Formulation for Clinical Use (1982) represented an American attempt at a practical classification and was widely adopted in the USA despite several flaws, perhaps the most important being that it ignored the T-cell and B-cell immunophenotypes.

In Britain and Europe the Kiel Classification (updated 1988) became more widely used. This classification, because it is still in current use, is outlined in Table 25.2. It too has its flaws in that it largely relates to nodal lymphoma and does not translate well to lymphomas arising in extranodal sites.

More recently, attempts have been made to draw together the American (Working Formulation) and European (Kiel Classification) systems of nomenclature. The Revised European–American Lymphoma Classification (the REAL Classification) was published in 1995 and it is hoped that this will become the new standard (Table 25.3). However the complexity of the REAL Classification, coupled with the liberal use of the designation 'provisional entity', means that we are unlikely to have come to the end of periodic revisions of lymphoma classification.

Whichever classification is used by each pathology department, the simplistic division of NHL into high-grade and low-grade subsets remains for the most part entirely valid.

Clinical presentation

Most patients seen by head and neck surgeons who are found eventually to have a lymphoma present with undiagnosed cervical lymphadenopathy. These patients should be investigated as any other patient who presents with a lump in the neck. The history may give useful clues and the examination should include not only the neck but the draining cutaneous sites and the upper

---

Table 25.2   The updated Kiel classification for non-Hodgkin's lymphoma

B-cell lymphomas	T-cell lymphomas

Low grade
Lymphocytic: chronic lymphocytic and
  prolymphocytic leukaemia; hairy cell leukaemia
Lymphoplasmacytic/cytoid (immunocytoma)
Plasmacytic
Centroblastic/centrocytic: follicular
  and/or diffuse diffuse
Centrocytic
	Low grade
	Lymphocytic: chronic lymphocytic and
	  prolymphocytic leukaemia
	Small, cerebriform cell: mycosis fungoides,
	  Sézary's syndrome
	Lymphoepithelioid (Lennert's lymphoma)
	Angioimmunoblastic (AILD)
	T-zone
	Pleomorphic, small cell (HTLV-1±)

High grade Centroblastic Immunoblastic Large-cell anaplastic (Ki-1 +) Burkitt's lymphoma Lymphoblastic	**High grade** Pleomorphic, medium and large cell (HTLV-1±) Immunoblastic (HTLV-1±) Large-cell anaplastic (Ki-1+) Lymphoblastic
Rare types	**Rare types**

Table 25.3 The Revised European–American Lymphoma (REAL) Classification

B-cell neoplasms

I. *Precursor B-cell neoplasm*
  1 Precursor B-lymphoblastic leukaemia/lymphoma

II. *Peripheral B-cell neoplasms*
  1 B-cell chronic lymphocytic leukaemia/prolymphocytic leukaemia/small lymphocytic lymphoma
  2 Lymphoplasmacytoid lymphoma (immunocytoma)
  3 Mantle cell lymphoma
  4 Follicle centre lymphoma, follicular (provisional cytological grades I, II, III) (provisional subtype: follicle centre lymphoma, diffuse, predominantly small cell)
  5 Marginal zone B-cell lymphoma
    (a) Extranodal (low-grade B-cell lymphoma of mucosa associated lymphoid tissue type)
    (b) Nodal (with or without monocytoid B-cells) (provisional entity)
  6 Splenic marginal B zone lymphoma (with or without circulating villous lymphocytes) (provisional entity)
  7 Hairy cell leukaemia
  8 Plasmacytoma/myeloma
  9 Diffuse large B cell lymphoma (subtype: primary mediastinal large B-cell lymphoma)
  10 Burkitt's lymphoma
  11 High-grade B-cell lymphoma, Burkitt like (provisional entity)

T-cell and postulated natural killer (NK) cell neoplasms

I. *Precursor T-cell neoplasm*
  1 Precursor T-lymphoblastic lymphoma leukaemia

II. *Peripheral T-cell and postulated NK cell neoplasms*
  1 T-cell chronic lymphocytic leukaemia/prolymphocytic leukaemia
  2 Large granular lymphocyte leukaemia
    (a) T-cell type
    (b) Natural killer cell type
  3 Mycosis fungoides/Sézary syndrome
  4 Peripheral T-cell lymphomas, unspecified (provisional cytological categories: medium sized cell; mixed medium and large cell; large cell) (subtypes: subcutaneous panniculitic T-cell lymphoma; hepatosplenic $\gamma\,\delta$ T-cell lymphoma)
  5 Angioimmunoblastic T-cell lymphoma
  6 Angiocentric lymphoma
  7 Intestinal T-cell lymphoma (with or without enteropathy)
  8 Adult T-cell leukaemia/lymphoma (HTLV 1+)
  9 Anaplastic large cell lymphoma (T- and null cell types)
  10 Anaplastic large cell lymphoma Hodgkin's like (provisional entity)

aerodigestive tract, and other superficial lymph node sites and the abdomen. Fine needle aspiration cytology may well point towards a lymphoma, but formal lymph-node biopsy will usually be required to yield a definitive diagnosis. Routine blood tests and a chest X-ray to evaluate the mediastinum should be performed prior to biopsy, but CT scans, bone marrow and any other staging investigations may usually be deferred until a definitive histopathological diagnosis has been made.

A substantial minority of patients with what turns out to be lymphoma presents to head and neck surgeons with symptoms other than neck-node enlargement. For example, otalgia and deafness in a child may be due to a nasopharyngeal tumour blocking the eustachian tube, a rapidly enlarging goitre in an old woman may be due to the development of a high-grade thyroid lymphoma, or nasal obstruction and discharge may prove to be due to a plasmacytoma. In such circumstances the differential diagnosis may be broad, and although lymphoma is not highest on the list, it should not be forgotten.

Staging

Nodal and extranodal NHL in adults is staged in the same way as Hodgkin's disease, using the Ann Arbor classification (Table 25.1). B symptoms are less common in advanced NHL than in Hodgkin's disease. In patients with certain high-grade NHL, especially if there is an extranodal head and neck primary tumour, central nervous system (CNS) spread is common and a lumbar puncture is often part of the staging process.

If a plasma cell tumour is diagnosed in the upper aerodigestive tract, it is important to ascertain whether it is a solitary plasmacytoma or whether there is any evidence of multiple myeloma. Blood should be sent for plasma protein electrophoresis and immunoglobulin measurements, and urine sent for Bence Jones protein estimations. Bone-marrow aspirates and trephines should be performed, and a radiological skeletal survey is better able to show bone involvement than a bone scan, as the lesions encountered in myeloma are not usually osteoblastic and do not provoke a periosteal reaction.

Table 25.4 The Murphy staging system for childhood non-Hodgkin's lymphoma

I	A single tumour (extranodal) or single anatomical area (nodal) with the exclusion of the mediastinum or abdomen
II	A single tumour (extranodal) with regional node involvement
	Two or more nodal areas on the same side of the diaphragm
	Two single (extranodal) tumours with or without regional node involvement on the same side of the diaphragm
	A primary gastrointestinal tract tumour, usually in the ileocaecal area, with or without involvement of associated mesenteric nodes only, grossly completely resected
III	Two single tumours (extranodal) on opposite sides of the diaphragm
	Two or more nodal areas above and below the diaphragm
	All the primary intrathoracic tumours (mediastinal, pleural, thymic)
	All extensive primary intra-abdominal disease, unresectable
	All paraspinal or epidural tumours, regardless of other tumour site(s)
IV	Any of the above with initial CNS and/or bone-marrow involvement

In children, extranodal disease is more common and an alternative staging classification, the Murphy staging system (Table 25.4), is used. This is a hybrid system which takes into account location, surgical treatment and spread into non-lymphoid structures.

Treatment

Once a patient with NHL has had their tumour characterized, classified and staged, it is possible to think about what treatment may be appropriate. As with any other patient with head and neck cancer, it is necessary also to take into account the patient's age, performance status, comorbidity, lifestyle factors, social support and personal wishes, before deciding on treatment.

The unusual case of localized, stage I, low-grade follicular NHL may possibly be cured by involved field radical radiotherapy. Many patients with low-grade NHL, however, have extensive disease, often with bone-marrow involvement, which although indolent must be considered to be incurable. The disease may not require specific treatment following diagnosis, unless or until symptoms require palliation. Simple chemotherapy with oral chlorambucil and prednisolone may be all that is required to make the patient symptom free and achieve a long remission. At relapse, if symptoms dictate, then the same treatment can be repeated. Alternatively, more intensive, but still relatively gentle chemotherapy with intravenous regimens such as cyclophosphamide and vincristine with oral prednisolone may be chosen. Low-

dose palliative radiotherapy is often effective at shrinking tumour masses and relieving symptoms. Eventually, the remission duration may shorten, the disease may become refractory to treatment or it may transform into a high-grade NHL. At this stage, treatment with alternative drugs such as fludarabine or anthracycline-containing regimens with their greater toxicity may be called for. The median survival of low-grade NHL is in the order of 10 years. As many patients are elderly, a substantial proportion will die of other causes before their lymphoma catches up with them. More aggressive initial treatment policies involving high-dose chemotherapy with autologous bone-marrow or peripheral blood stem cell support have been investigated in younger, fitter patients with low-grade NHL. Although some long-term remissions have been seen, this approach is associated with substantial treatment-related morbidity and even mortality, and it is not clearly superior to a more conservative treatment policy.

In contradistinction to low-grade NHL, where most patients will eventually die from their disease if they survive for long enough, high-grade NHL, despite a significant early mortality from progressive, refractory disease or from treatment toxity, is often curable. The initial treatment for fit patients with high-grade lymphoma nowadays is usually chemotherapy, and about half of adult patients may be cured. In children, the cure rate is closer to three-quarters. The standard chemotherapy regimen, CHOP, comprises cyclophosphamide, doxorubicin, vincristine and prednisolone. For patients with localized disease, especially in the head and neck, this is often followed by consolidation radiotherapy. Many other chemotherapy regimens have been evaluated. Some of these are associated with substantially greater toxicity but none has proved clearly superior. There is an increasing interest in high-dose chemotherapy with haemopoietic support for patients with refractory or relapsed disease, but the precise role of this approach remains to be determined. Many patients are elderly and relatively frail. Some more gentle regimens have been evaluated in this patient group. While overall the outcome may not be so good, some patients will still be cured. Radiotherapy can provide valuable palliation with minimal toxicity in patients who have relapsed or who are too frail for initial chemotherapy.

Patients with solitary plasmacytomas are usually treated with radiotherapy alone. A proportion will be cured, but many will eventually develop multiple myeloma. Patients with myeloma either at presentation or who develop it subsequently should receive chemotherapy. Myeloma is generally considered incurable and relatively gentle regimens of chemotherapy have traditionally been used. More recently, aggressive approaches using high-dose chemotherapy with total body irradiation and haemopoietic support have begun to yield promising results in selected patients. Prognostic factors include renal function, haemoglobin level, performance status and β_2-microglobulin level.

Sarcomas

Bone sarcomas

Osteosarcoma, which accounts for about one-third of primary bone tumours, usually arises in the limbs; only 10% occurs in the axial skeleton and so osteosarcoma in head and neck sites such as the mandible or maxilla is very rare. The peak incidence is in adolescence, earlier in females than males. Thereafter it is rare. Males are more commonly affected than females. There is sometimes a genetic basis. It may occur as part of the Li Fraumeni syndrome when there is familial clustering of breast cancer, brain tumours, leukaemia and bone and soft-tissue sarcomas, often occurring at younger ages in each succeeding generation. Osteosarcoma is the most common type of second malignant neoplasm in patients who have been treated for the familial type of retinoblastoma, usually presenting about 10 years after the original tumour. It is particularly likely to occur in the head and neck when there has been orbital irradiation, although it may also occur distantly. Other causes of osteosarcoma include irradiation and Paget's disease of bone. In these cases, the elderly are more often affected. Osteosarcoma is usually a high-grade tumour, but there are various subtypes of low-grade osteosarcoma. Metastases occur most commonly in the lungs and less frequently in the skeleton. Prior to the introduction of chemotherapy, surgery alone, which usually entailed amputation of the affected limb, cured about 20% of patients. The introduction of chemotherapy has now improved the survival rate to about 60%. A combination of doxorubicin and cisplatin seems to give results as good as those of more complex regimens. Advances in conservation surgery with growing endoprostheses have made amputation less common.

In the head and neck region, osteosarcoma usually presents in young adult males with pain and swelling of the maxilla or mandible. It is more commonly a well-differentiated, low-grade tumour such as a chondroblastic osteosarcoma. Distant metastases are unusual and the principal clinical challenge is complete excision, which gives better results than incomplete excision and radiotherapy. Preoperative chemotherapy can be beneficial.

Chondrosarcoma is the second most common primary bone tumour, comprising about one-fifth of cases. The peak incidence is in the middle aged and elderly, and again there is a male predominance. There is a spectrum of malignancy varying from well-differentiated tumours which have a tendency to recur locally but rarely metastasize, to highly malignant forms where metastasis is the rule. Mesenchymal chondrosarcoma is a high-grade metastasizing subtype, often presenting in the jaw with pain. Chemotherapy is probably indicated in fit patients with high-grade tumours and radiotherapy should be used for local control unless it has been possible to perform radical surgery.

Ewing's sarcoma is less common than osteosarcoma, comprising about 15% of primary bone tumours. It occurs between the ages of 5 and 30 years, with a peak incidence between 10 and 15 years, more frequently in males. Only 1–2% of cases occur in the head and neck. Histologically, Ewing's sarcoma is one of the small, round, blue cell tumours, like rhabdomyosarcoma, neuroblastoma and lymphoma. The cells usually contain glycogen, and there is a characteristic t(11;22) chromosomal translocation. The principal adverse prognostic factors are the presence of distant metastases and a large primary tumour volume. The advent of intensive multiagent chemotherapy has transformed the outlook for patients with Ewing's sarcoma, with survival rates rising from only about 10% in the era of local treatment alone to about 70% currently. Where possible without undue functional or cosmetic loss, surgery is recommended for local control, with postoperative radiotherapy if there is any doubt about the completeness of excision. Ewing's sarcoma is substantially more radiosensitive than osteosarcoma, and radical radiotherapy is a good local treatment if surgery is not thought to be appropriate, as for example may be the case in most head and neck sites.

Osteoclastoma or giant cell tumour of bone is a tumour of variable malignancy. Most commonly it is a low-grade lesion with a tendency to recur locally after inadequate surgery, but high-grade tumours which may metastasize to the lungs are encountered.

Chordoma is a tumour so called because it is assumed to arise from notochord remnants along the spine. Half occur on the sacrum, one-third in the clivus or base of skull, and the remainder in the cervical, thoracic or lumbar spine. It is usually a low-grade malignant tumour. Surgery is the recommended treatment wherever possible, but there is a tendency to local recurrence even after apparently satisfactory resection. Radiotherapy is used after incomplete resection, in inoperable cases and for palliation of recurrent disease. However, high doses are required and cure is seldom achieved. There is some suggestion that heavy particle (proton beam) therapy may be advantageous, but this is not available in the UK. Distant metastases may occur. Although chemotherapy has been used, it has no clearly defined role.

A variety of other primary bone sarcomas exist and all may occasionally present in the head and neck region. They include peripheral primitive neuroectodermal tumours, which are managed in a very similar way to Ewing's sarcoma, malignant fibrous histiocytoma of bone, which tends to be a high-grade spindle cell neoplasm and should be managed in a similar way to osteosarcoma.

Soft tissue sarcomas

'Soft-tissue sarcoma', like 'non-Hodgkin's lymphoma', is a simple term which belies the fact that it encompasses a broad range of entities, some clearly defined, others more obscure, occurring in many anatomical sites with a variety of natural histories. This diversity is explained by the fact that soft-tissue sarcomas are malignant mesenchymal tumours, and so can develop anywhere that mesenchyme is present and differentiate along the lines of any mesenchymal tissue. About 10% occur in the head and neck. As a group, soft-tissue sarcomas are rare and their heterogeneity means that any individual subtype is even rarer. They are therefore best managed in specialist multi-disciplinary sarcoma units which have the opportunity to gain experience and develop expertise.

In different published series, the proportion of different tumour types varies. Fibrosarcoma, liposarcoma and malignant fibrous histiocytoma are the more common types, each accounting for about 20% in most series. Leiomyosarcoma, neurosarcoma, synovial sarcoma and unclassified sarcomas each tend to account for about 10% in most series. Many other types such as alveolar soft part sarcoma, clear cell sarcoma and epitheliod sarcoma are rare. Kaposi's sarcoma is a distinct entity and is described later in the section on AIDS-related cancer. Rhab-domyosarcoma is the principal paediatric type, but is rare in adult life. The natural history and treatment of rhabdomyosarcoma are distinct from those of other soft-tissue sarcomas and this discussed separately.

Types of soft-tissue sarcoma

- Fibrosarcoma
- Liposarcoma
- Malignant fibrous histiocytoma
- Leiomyosarcoma
- Neurosarcoma
- Synovial sarcoma
- Unclassified sarcoma
- Alveolar soft part sarcoma
- Clear cell sarcoma
- Epithelioid sarcoma
- Kaposi's sarcoma
- Rhabdomyosarcoma

For practical clinical purposes it is not unreasonable to consider all of the non-rhabdomyosarcoma, non-Kaposi's sarcoma together as adult-type soft-tissue sarcoma, as the management policy for all of these will be broadly similar. The term adult-type soft-tissue sarcoma is an over-simplification as these non-rhabdomyosarcoma types do occur rarely in childhood and rhabdomyosarcoma can also occur in adults.

When a patient is suspected to have an adult-type soft-tissue sarcoma, the important features which determine management are the anatomical site, the tumour grade, size of the tumour, and the presence or absence of nodal or distant metastases. Several different staging systems are used. The TNM (tumour, node, metastasis) classification rather exceptionally takes histological grade into account as well as size and spread.

Most tumours are non-metastatic at presentation and local control is the principal issue. Radical surgery where possible offers the best prospects for local control. Postoperative radiotherapy will improve the likelihood of local control if there is any doubt about completeness of excision. If definitive surgery is not possible, then radical radiotherapy is indicated, although the results will not be so good as when surgery is undertaken. Tumour grade and size are predictors of the likelihood of metastatic disease developing. Adjuvant chemotherapy for high-risk patients has its proponents, but its true value is not entirely clear. When metastatic disease is present, treatment is essentially palliative and chemotherapy can sometimes be beneficial. Occasionally it is possible to resect a late-developing isolated pulmonary metastasis, and sometimes such patients become long-term survivors.

Rhabdomyosarcoma is a distinct clinicopathological entity and its management is substantially different from that of adult soft-tissue sarcoma. Cells are usually small, round and hyperchromatic, characterized by desmin positivity on immunocytochemistry. Several pathological classifications are in use by different international co-operative groups and a new proposed international classification is being formulated. The most common type is embryonal rhabdomyosarcoma, which carries a relatively favourable prognosis. Botryoid rhabdomyosarcoma is found as polypoidal outgrowths in hollow viscera such as the bladder, the vagina, the nasopharynx and the paranasal sinuses. It has a good prognosis and is characterized by a loose, myxoid and often oedematous stroma. There is a dense layer of tumour cells underneath the epithelium, referred to as the cambium layer. Alveolar rhabdomyosarcoma is a highly malignant subtype, with packeting of groups of cells by fibrous septa and a characteristic chromosomal translocation. It is more commonly found at extremity sites and distant metastases are common.

In addition to head and neck primary sites, rhabdomyosarcoma may occur in the genitourinary system, in limbs and rarely at other sites. In the head and neck, primary sites are divided into three main groups. If confined to the orbit without bone destruction, the prognosis is good. Tumours at parameningeal sites, such as the nasopharynx, nasal fossa, paranasal sinuses, pterygoid fossa, middle ear and mastoid, have a tendency to enter the cranial cavity through the neurovascular skull base foramina and are associated with a worse prognosis. Non-parameningeal head and neck sites include the face and cheek, the parotid, the oral cavity, the oropharynx and the larynx. If there is extension from a non-parameningeal site into a parameningeal one, such as from the parotid into the pterygoid region, the tumour is managed as a parameningeal one.

Patients usually present with symptoms related to the primary site as with any other cancer, or they may present with nodal or other metastases, and an occult primary tumour. For example, nasal obstruction, alteration in voice quality, lower cranial nerve palsies, otalgia and deafness may be caused by a nasopharyngeal tumour, whereas a middle ear tumour may present with unilateral deafness, otorrhoea, facial palsy and a fleshy polyp growing from the external auditory canal.

The initial rôle of the head and neck surgeon is limited to careful assessment of the primary tumour with clinical investigation including examination under anaesthesia (EUA) and biopsy. Radical resection is never part of the initial treatment of rhabdomyosarcoma at head and neck primary sites. Full evaluation of the extent of the primary with magnetic resonance imaging (MRI) and CT scanning is essential. Staging investigations are needed to evaluate sites such as the lungs and skeleton for metastatic disease.

The mainstay of treatment is with aggressive combination chemotherapy which should be carried out in a specialized paediatric oncology centre or adult sarcoma unit as appropriate. Radiotherapy is indicated in all cases of parameningeal tumours, or when there is residual disease after chemotherapy in the orbit or at other non-parameningeal sites. If complete remission is achieved, radiotherapy is withheld in the case of orbital and non-parameningeal tumours, but can be used if there is a subsequent relapse. Occasionally, radical surgery is indicated if there is residual disease after chemotherapy and radiotherapy.

Five year survival figures for orbital rhabdomyosarcoma are in the region of 90%, for non-parameningeal head and neck sites about 75% and for parameningeal sites about 60%.

Mucosal malignant melanoma

Cutaneous malignant melanoma is covered in Chapter 21, Tumours of the skin and ear. Mucosal malignant melanoma is much less commonly encountered as it represents only 1% of all cases, or 5% of those arising in the head and neck, and as it poses distinct management problems it is considered here separately.

Malignant melanoma of the head and neck mucosa is a disease of the middle aged and elderly, with a median age at presentation of about 70 years. The sex ratio varies in reported series. The primary site is more often in the nose or paranasal sinuses than in the oral cavity or pharynx. As tumours are often locally extensive at presentation it can be difficult to say exactly where the tumour originated. There is no TNM staging system for mucosal melanoma. Site-specific head and neck TNM staging classifications are limited to carcinoma. A simple system used in a few reports assigns tumours localized to the primary site as stage I, regardless of their local extent, those with nodal metastasis to stage II and those with haematogenous spread to stage III. According to this system, most patients present with stage I disease.

There are no controlled studies of treatment for mucosal melanoma. Because many patients are frail and elderly, and many have very extensive local disease at presentation, truly radical surgery is not often undertaken. Radical radiotherapy is often given if surgery is not deemed to be appropriate. Both radical surgery, if undertaken, and radical radiotherapy seem to result in local control rates of about 40%, but the groups receiving each treatment may not be comparable. There are anecdotal reports of successful chemotherapy for melanoma, but for the overwhelming majority of patients treated with chemotherapy no benefit is seen. The majority of

patients will be dead from disease by five years, with approximately equal proportions dying from metastatic disease with the primary controlled, uncontrolled local disease without distant spread, and both local and distant disease. Those who are alive and well at 5 years are likely to succumb to local relapse or metastasis after longer periods and very few are likely to be cured.

Neurogenic tumours

A variety of benign and malignant tumours of neural origin may present to the head and neck surgeon. They have in common an origin from neural crest cells. Here, three categories will be considered: paragangliomas, otherwise known as chemodectomas, nerve sheath tumours, and tumours of the sympathetic nervous system.

Paragangliomas

Paragangliomas are rare tumours which are thought to arise from chemoreceptor cells, hence the alternative name of chemodectoma. They are also called glomus tumours. They are usually benign, but approximately 5% are malignant and develop distant metastases in bone and lung.

Paragangliomas in the head and neck arise at four sites: the carotid body, the middle ear, the jugular bulb and on the vagus nerve. Carotid body tumours and glomus vagale present as lumps in the neck, while glomus tympanicum and glomus jugulare most commonly present with deafness, sometimes associated with tinnitus, vertigo, pain and cranial nerve palsies.

> *Name and location of head and neck paragangliomas*
>
> ■ Carotid body tumour: medial aspect of carotid bulb
> ■ Glomus vagale: nodose ganglion of the vagus nerve
> ■ Glomus tympanicum: middle ear
> ■ Glomus jugulare: the jugular bulb

Carotid body tumours occur with a high incidence in high-altitude places such as Peru, Colorado and Mexico City, where chronic hypoxia leads to carotid body hyperplasia. In the rest of the world it is a rare tumour. The average age of presentation is in the fifth decade and there is no sex predominance. One in 10 patients has a positive family history and some of this group have bilateral tumours or phaeochromocytoma.

The tumour arises from the chemoreceptor cells on the medial side of the carotid bulb and is firmly adherent to this area. Histology shows cells similar to normal carotid body cells: large, uniform epithelioid cells surrounded by a vascular stroma. The cells are not hormonally active.

Patients often present with a several years' history of a slowly enlarging painless lump in the region of the carotid bulb. About 30% present with a pharyngeal mass pushing the tonsil medially and anteriorly. Thus, biopsy of a pharyngeal swelling must never be taken from within the mouth. On palpation the mass is firm, rubbery (potato tumour) and pulsatile and refills in steps synchronous with the pulse after compression. A bruit may be present and the mass may decrease in size with carotid compression. It is said that it can be moved from side to side but not up and down: this is also true of most other lumps in the neck. Nerve involvement is rare.

The length of history differentiates this tumour from a metastatic gland. Such a history is, however, compatible with a branchial cyst or a tuberculous gland. Whenever a carotid body tumour is suspected a carotid angiogram should be performed to demonstrate a tumour circulation, to determine the extent of the tumour and to see whether there is a cerebral cross-circulation. This tumour must never be biopsied.

It is rare for a patient to die of an untreated carotid body tumour and metastases are exceptionally rare. Thus the mere presence of a carotid body tumour does not justify an attempt at removal. Indications for removal are patients in good health under the age of 50 years who have a small or medium-sized tumour, patients with tumours extending into the palate or pharynx that interfere with swallowing, speaking or breathing, or tumours with an aggressive growth pattern.

Although these tumours were originally thought to be radioresistant, cures have been reported in recent publications. Radiotherapy should be used in patients who refuse surgery, in poor-risk cases or in those with metastatic disease.

Removal of carotid body tumours should be undertaken in conjunction with a vascular surgeon. To remove a carotid body tumour, a long incision is made from the mastoid process to the clavicle down to the anterior border of the sternomastoid muscle: this is one of the few occasions when the incision is justified. The surgeon dissects down to the carotid sheath and finds the common carotid artery, the internal jugular vein and the vagus nerve. The common carotid artery is freed on all sides, with the vagus nerve being carefully preserved. A tape is placed loosely around the common carotid artery and tagged with an artery forceps. The tape is placed at this stage to allow easy and rapid occlusion of the carotid artery if the internal carotid artery is later damaged.

The common carotid artery is followed upwards, the surgeon dissecting along the adventitia and mobilizing the vagus nerve. On approaching the tumour large numbers of thin-walled veins, more brown than red in colour, will be encountered. These veins bleed very easily and are a source of difficulty in this procedure. This difficulty can be overcome by dissection with two dissecting forceps with fine points and no teeth. The tissue is grasped close to the adventitia of the artery with these forceps and pulled apart. Surprisingly, this produces much less bleeding than attempts at sharp dissection, which are slow, tedious and attended by steady bleeding. Continuing in this fashion, the surgeon frees the tumour from the internal carotid artery in particular with great care. It should always be possible to preserve the vagus nerve, but the hypoglossal nerve is often stretched and may be more difficult to preserve.

Glomus vagale or vagal paragangliomas arise from nests of paraganglionic tissue within the perineurium of the vagus nerve just below or at its ganglion nodosum. They are the rarest of the head and neck paragangliomas and are said to have the highest potential for metastasis. Characteristically, the tumours lie just below the base of the skull near the jugular foramen, are contiguous with the vagus nerve and replace the ganglion nodosum. Intravagal tumours, however, are not restricted to this site and may be found at various sites along the nerve and down to the level of the carotid artery bifurcation.

Vagal paragangliomas most commonly present as slowly growing and painless masses high in the anterolateral aspect of the neck. On examination the mass is often noted near the origin of the sternocleidomastoid muscle with a concomitant medial displacement of peritonsillar structures. Approximately one-half of the patients have had symptoms or signs for more than 3 years before diagnosis. Pharyngeal pain is usually a late sign and indicates irritation of the pharyngeal plexus, often preceding the onset of cranial nerve palsies. Pulsating tinnitus, deafness, syncope and vertigo may also be noted.

The diagnosis is confirmed by arteriography. Vagal paragangliomas are surrounded by a pharyngeal plexus of veins and consequently tend to appear larger upon arteriography than they really are. Vagal paragangliomas are more malignant than carotid body lesions, mainly because of their tendency to spread into the cranial cavity. Surgery is usually required. The approach used is that described below for parapharyngeal tumours. The numerous thin-walled veins should be dealt with in the same way as for carotid body tumours. The most dangerous part of the dissection is superiorly where the internal carotid artery loops over the tumour and then immediately enters the skull. Injury may occur at this site, so that the help of a vascular surgeon is often advisable. For disease which is inoperable because of either disease extent or the age, frailty or comorbidity of the patient, radical radiotherapy can be effective in halting tumour progression and alleviating symptoms in the long term.

Glomus tympanicum may present with deafness, pulsatile tinnitus, vertigo, headache and pain in the ear. Lower motor neurone facial nerve palsy may be present. Tumour may be visible on otoscopy as a bluish red discoloration of the tympanic membrane or as a pulsating mass.

Glomus jugulare presents with similar features, but palsies of the lower four cranial nerves may also be present because of tumour at the jugular foramen. With advanced disease there may be extension into the petrous temporal bone and intracranially, and it may not be possible to distinguish a glomus tympanicum from a glomus jugulare tumour.

Surgery is recommended for lesions confined to the middle ear and mastoid, when complete excision at one operation seems possible. Advances in operative technique mean that it is now possible to perform radical surgery safely for lesions extending into the petrous temporal bone or with intracranial disease. Such operations fall within the province of the neuro-otologist and skull-base surgeon rather than the head and neck surgeon, so details of the technique are not given here. For inoperable disease or when a patient refuses surgery, consideration should be given to treatment with radiotherapy.

Radiotherapy for paragangliomas does not require the 60–66 Gy level often used for cancers. Lower doses in the order of 35–50 Gy are associated with less morbidity and have been reported to be effective in achieving local control in the majority of patients. Regression of the tumour is usually slow but continues over a period of months to years. Some patients with widely metastatic paraganglioma have been successfully treated with targeted radionuclide therapy using iodine-131-labelled *meta*-iodobenzylguanidine ($[^{131}I]$-MIBG).

Nerve sheath tumours

The normal nerve fibre is ensheathed by Schwann cells and by loosely distributed endoneural fibroblasts. The Schwann cell is the parent cell of the common clinical tumours, the schwannoma and the neurofibroma. Schwannomas were previously called neuromas or neurilemmomas; both terms are incorrect. This tumour is solitary and encapsulated, being attached to or surrounded by the nerve. A paralysis of the associated nerve is thus unusual. Malignant change is also very unusual, if it occurs at all. The vagus nerve is the most common site of origin of this tumour. Usually the only symptom of these tumours is a mass which grows slowly, over a period of years, if at all. Diagnosis usually requires angiography to differentiate these tumours from paragangliomas, but the final diagnosis must usually wait until excision.

Neurofibromas may form part of either of the two syndromes collectively known as von Recklinghausen's disease or multiple neurofibromatosis, or rarely they may be single. There are two discrete diseases: neurofibromatosis type 1 (NF1) and neurofibromatosis type 2 (NF2). Both are inherited as autosomal dominant conditions, although there is no family history in about half of the cases of both NF1 and NF2. NF1 is by far the more common disease, with a prevalence of one in 5000. Café-au-lait spots, more than six in number, are present in all children by the age of 2 years, but some may disappear in adult life. Axillary or skinfold freckling is present in 70%, and 95% of adults will develop cutaneous neurofibromas. Lisch nodules may be detected on the iris of the eye in most patients. A small minority of patients will develop other nervous system tumours including optic pathway gliomas, other astrocytomas, plexiform neurofibromas, peripheral nerve neurofibromas, neurofibrosarcoma and spinal neurofibromas. Between one-third and one-half of patients with NF1 have neurodevelopmental problems. The responsible gene has been mapped to chromosome 17q 11.2. There is marked variation in expression of the disease within affected families.

NF2 has a prevalence of only one in 210 000. Multiple café-au-lait spots are very unusual and skinfold freckling is not seen. Cutaneous neurofibromas occur in only about one quarter of patients and tend to be fewer in number than is the case with NF1. The distinctive cutaneous feature of NF2 is the plaque. NF2 plaques are well circumscribed, raised cutaneous lesions usually less than 2 cm in diameter, with a rough surface, which may be slightly pigmented and are commonly hairy. Lisch nodules are not seen, but most patients will have cataracts which are usually asymptomatic. More than 90% of adults will develop bilateral acoustic neuromas. Almost half may have meningiomas or peripheral nerve schwannomas, and a quarter spinal schwannomas. Astrocytomas and ependymomas are unusual features and phaeochromocytomas may occur. The responsible gene is located on chromosome 22q 12.1. Members of the same family tend to have a similar severity of disease, but different families tend to fall into severe and mild forms.

The overall morbidity and mortality of NF2 far exceeds that of NF1 because of the intracranial and intraspinal lesions in NF2, and also because half the patients with NF1 have cutaneous stigmata only.

The nerve from which the tumour arises is only evident in one in three operations. It may be stretched over the capsule of the tumour, or the tumour can be in the central core of the nerve with the fibres spread around it. All simple tumours should be excised and an attempt made to rejoin or graft the nerve. Entry into the parapharyngeal space can be posterior to the submandibular gland, beneath the parotid – a cervical rather than a transparotid approach. Although some neurogenous tumours can be removed from the surface of the nerve it is inevitable that others are so closely integrated to the vagal trunk that a section of the cranial nerve has to be resected with secondary rehabilitation of the larynx.

Tumours of the sympathetic nervous system

Neuroblastoma is a disease of childhood, which is most common in the first year of life and is sometimes congenital. The tumours arise from the sympathetic chain, the majority are found in the abdomen, they are less common in the mediastinum and rarely present in the neck. If they arise in the neck they may be associated with Horner's syndrome, in which case there may be anisochromia of the ipsilateral iris due to failure of pigmentation as this is dependent upon sympathetic innervation. The staging system for neuroblastoma, as for many other cancers, ranges from stage 1 to stage 4 depending on whether the tumour is localized or there are distant metastases. In addition, however, there is the unique stage of stage 4S neuroblastoma, in which the S stands for special. This is found in infants (aged under 1 year by definition, but in practice nearly always before the age of 3 months) who have a small primary tumour which would be stage 1 or 2 but for the presence of distant metastases. These can affect the skin, the liver and the bone marrow, but not cortical bone. It is special because it can regress spontaneously. Increasing age and advancing stage are the strongest adverse prognostic factors, but there are also several biological features which influence prognosis. These include amplification of the N *myc* oncogene, chromosomal abnormalities including deletion of the short arm of chromosome 1, and elevated levels of lactate dehydrogenase, ferritin and neuron-specific enolase. Treatment is decided on the basis of age, stage and biology. At the most favourable end of the spectrum either observation or surgery alone is undertaken and the outlook is good. With advanced stage disease aggressive chemotherapy is used, often in conjunction with surgery and sometimes radiotherapy, followed perhaps by high-dose chemotherapy with autologous bone-marrow or peripheral blood stem cell support. Despite this intensive treatment, the prognosis in patients with stage IV disease over the age of 1 year is very poor and only a small minority is cured. Radionuclide therapy with $[^{131}I]$-MIBG is valuable in some cases, especially for the palliation of relapsed disease.

Ganglioneuroblastoma is a partly differentiated form of neuroblastoma and ganglioneuroma is the benign counterpart, which is usually treated with surgery alone.

Phaeochromocytoma is a tumour originating from the sympathetic nervous system. It is most commonly found in adults, located in the adrenal region, but rarely may be ectopic, for example in the neck. It usually presents with hypertension and symptoms of catecholamine excess. It is usually benign and surgery is usually curative. Rarely, however, it may metastasize, in which case $[^{131}I]$-MIBG therapy may be of value.

AIDS-related cancer

AIDS was first recognized in 1981 and is now known to be caused by HIV. During the 1980s both HIV infection and AIDS were associated with a grave short-term prognosis. Now, with the advent of triple therapy with anti-retroviral drugs and protease inhibitors, the outlook has improved substantially, although it is not yet possible to talk about curative treatment.

In western Europe and the USA, the three principal groups affected were originally homosexual men, intravenous drug abusers and recipients of blood products such as haemophiliacs. Now that all blood products are screened for HIV infection, just the first two groups remain at risk, but public-health campaigns have been effective in limiting the scale of the epidemic that was predicted in 1985. In sub-Saharan Africa the story is different and the epidemic progresses. The prevalence of HIV infection in the major cities in countries such as Uganda and Zimbabwe is very high. Transmission is principally heterosexual and maternofoetal. Public health measures have been less effective than in the West and there are inadequate resources for current drug treatments.

Clinically, AIDS is characterized by a constellation of opportunistic infections, such as *Pneumocystis carinii*

pneumonia, candidal oesophagitis and fungaemia and *Mycobacterium avium intracellulare* infection, and malignancies such as Kaposi's sarcoma, cerebral lymphoma and carcinoma of the cervix uteri.

The head and neck manifestations of AIDS include multifocal lymphoepithelial parotid cysts, benign lymphoid hyperplasia, cutaneous, oral and pharyngeal lesions of Kaposi's sarcoma, hairy leucoplakia of the tongue, and oral and pharyngeal candidiasis.

Kaposi's sarcoma was first described in 1872. The classical form is rare and indolent and usually affects the lower limbs of elderly people of Jewish or Mediterranean origin living in Europe and the USA. In 1950 an African variant was described. This endemic Kaposi's sarcoma is more aggressive and often multifocal. It is not associated with HIV infection. The epidemic form of Kaposi's sarcoma which led to the recognition of AIDS is HIV related, but the incidence in people with AIDS varies and it has become much less of a feature than it was in the early 1980s which is in keeping with the theory that it is caused by a coincidentally transmitted herpes virus. Pathologically, the different types of Kaposi's sarcoma appear similar, showing a proliferation of spindle cells with endothelial lined vascular clefts and a perivascular mononuclear cell infiltrate.

Because of its multifocal nature, surgery has little role in the treatment of Kaposi's sarcoma. Radiotherapy is valuable for localized superficial disease. Low doses such as 16 Gy in four fractions or a single dose of 8 Gy are often sufficient to bring about resolution. Mucosal surfaces in AIDS patients are very sensitive to radiation, and radiation mucositis can be severe and prolonged. For this reason it is best to avoid mucosal radiation or to limit the dose per fraction to 1 Gy per day. Chemotherapy can be effective and various regimens incorporating agents such as bleomycin, vinblastine and liposomal anthracyclines are often used.

NHL is much more common among patients with HIV infection than in those without. It is usually high grade and can be nodal or extranodal. It is commonly intracerebral, and this carries a poor prognosis regardless of treatment.

Patients with AIDS or HIV infection should be managed in dedicated multidisciplinary teams with a HIV physician and an oncologist experienced in the management of HIV-related malignancy.

Further reading

Chan J. K., Banks P. E., Cleary M. L., Delsol G., DeWolf-Peeters C., Fallini B. *et al.* (1995) A revised European–American classification of lymphoid neoplasms proposed by the International Lymphoma Study Group, *Am J Clin Pathol* **103**: 543–60.

Crist W., Gehan E. A., Ragab A. H., Dickman P. S., Donaldson S. S., Fryer C. *et al.* (1995) The Third Intergroup Rhabdomyosarcoma Study, *J Clin Oncol* **13**: 610–30.

Gaze M. N., Kerr G. R. and Smyth J. F. on behalf of the Scottish Melanoma Group (1990) Mucosal melanomas of the head and neck: the Scottish experience, *Clin Oncol* 2: 277–83.

Huson S. M. (1999) What level of care for the neuro-fibromatoses? *Lancet* 353: 1114–16.

Knowles D. M. (1996) Etiology and pathogenesis of AIDS related non-Hodgkin's lymphoma, *Haematol Oncol Clinics North Am* 10: 1081–10.

Lee F. -C. and Mitsuyasu R. T. (1996) Chemotherapy of AIDS related Kaposi's sarcoma, *Haematol Oncol Clinics N Am* 10: 1051–68.

Simpson J. K. and Gaze M. N. (1998) Current management of neuroblastoma, *Oncologist* 3, 253–62.

Souhami R. L., Craft A. W., Van Der Eijken J. W., Nooij M., Spooner D., Bramwell V. H. *et al.* (1997) Randomised trial of two regimens of chemotherapy in operable osteosarcoma: a study of the European Osteosarcoma Intergroup, *Lancet* 350: 911–17.

Swift P. S. (1996) The role of radiation therapy in the management of HIV related Kaposi's sarcoma, *Haematol Oncol Clinics N Am* 10: 1069–80.

Index